# MAGILL'S MEDICAL GUIDE

# HEALTH AND ILLNESS

## Volume II
### Factitious disorders — Numbness and tingling

## A Magill Book
*from the* Editors of Salem Press

SALEM PRESS, INC.
Pasadena, California     Englewood Cliffs, New Jersey

*Editor in Chief:* Dawn P. Dawson

*Project Editor:* Tracy C. Irons

*Editorial Consultant, Reference Matter:*
L. Fleming Fallon, Jr., M.D., M.P.H.

*Production Editor:* Joyce I. Buchea

*Proofreading Supervisor:* Yasmine A. Cordoba

*Layout:* James Hutson

*Illustrations:* Hans & Cassady, Inc., Westerville, Ohio

### Note to Readers

The material presented in *Magill's Medical Guide: Health and Illness* is intended for broad informational and educational purposes. Readers who suspect that they suffer from any of the physical or psychological disorders,
diseases, or conditions described in this publication should contact a physician
without delay; this work should not be used as a substitute for professional
medical diagnosis or treatment. This publication is not to be considered definitive on the covered topics, and readers should remember that the field of
health care is characterized by a diversity of medical opinions and constant
expansion in knowledge and understanding.

**Library of Congress Cataloging-in-Publication Data**
Magill's medical guide : health and illness / the editors of Salem Press
    p. cm.
   Includes bibliographical references and index.
   1. Medicine—Encyclopedias. I. Salem Press. II. Title: Medical guide.
RC41.M34  1995
610'.3—dc20                       94-44709
ISBN 0-89356-712-4 (set)          CIP
ISBN 0-89356-714-0 (vol 2)

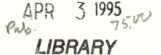
First Printing

PRINTED IN THE UNITED STATES OF AMERICA

# CONTENTS

MAGILL'S MEDICAL GUIDE

# HEALTH AND ILLNESS

## FACIAL PALSY. *See* BELL'S PALSY.

## FACTITIOUS DISORDERS

**SYSTEMS AFFECTED:** Psychic-emotional, most bodily systems

**SPECIALISTS:** Family physicians, internists, psychiatrists, psychologists

**DEFINITION:** Psychophysiological disorders in which individuals intentionally produce their symptoms in order to play the role of patient.

### CAUSES AND SYMPTOMS

Although factitious disorders cover a wide array of physical symptoms and are believed to be closely related to a subset of psychophysiological disorders (somatoform disorders), they are unique in all of medicine for two reasons. The first distinguishing factor is that whatever the physical disease for which treatment is sought and regardless of how serious, the patients who seek its treatment have deliberately and intentionally produced the condition. They may have done so in one of three ways, or in any combination of these three ways. First, patients fabricate, invent, lie about, and make up symptoms that they do not have; for example, they claim to have fever and night sweats or severe back pain that they actually do not have. Second, patients have the actual symptoms that they describe, but they intentionally caused them; for example, they might inject human saliva into their own skin to produce an abscess or ingest a known allergic food to cause the predictable reaction. Third, someone with a known condition such as pancreatitis has a pain episode but exaggerates its severity, or someone else with a history of migraines claims his or her headache to be yet another migraine when it is not.

The second element that makes these disorders unique (and at the same time both fascinating to study and frustrating to treat) is that the sole motivation for causing or claiming the symptoms is for these patients to become and remain patients, to assume the sick role wherein little can be expected from them. These patients are not malingerers, individuals who consciously use actual or feigned symptoms for some other gain (such as claiming a fever so one does not have to go to work or school, or insisting that one's post-traumatic stress is worse than it is to enhance the judgment in a lawsuit). In fact, it is the absence of any discernible external benefit that makes these disorders so intriguing.

Technically, psychiatrists and psychologists understand factitious disorders as having three subtypes. In the first, patients claim to have predominantly psychological symptoms such as memory loss, depression, contemplation of suicide, the hearing of voices, or false memory of childhood molestation. Characteristically, the symptoms worsen whenever the patients know themselves to be under observation. In the second, patients have predominantly physical symptoms that at least superficially suggest some general medical condition. In a more extreme form called Münchausen's syndrome, individuals will have spent much of their lives getting admitted to medical facilities and, once there, remaining as long as possible. While common complaints include vomiting, dizziness, blacking out, generalized rashes, and bleeding, the symptoms can involve any organ and seem limited only to the individuals' medical knowledge and experience with the medical system. The third subtype combines both psychological and physical complaints in such a way that neither predominates.

Regardless of subtype, factitious disorders are difficult to diagnose. Usually, the diagnosis is considered when the course of treating either a medical or a mental illness becomes atypical and protracted. Often, the person with a factitious disorder will present in a way which seems odd to the experienced clinician. The person may have an unusually extensive history of traveling, much familiarity with medical procedures and terminology, a complex medical and surgical history, few visitors during the hospitalization, behavioral disruptions and disturbances while hospitalized, exacerbation of symptoms while under observation, and/or fluctuating illness with new symptoms and complications arising as the workup proceeds. When present, these traits along with others make suspicion of factitious disorders reasonable.

No one knows how many people suffer with factitious disorders, but the condition is generally regarded as uncommon. It is certainly rarely reported, but this in part may be attributable to the difficulties in determining the diagnosis. While brief episodes of the condition occur, most people who claim a factitious disorder have it chronically, and they usually move on to another physician or facility when they are confronted with the true nature of their illness. It is therefore likely that some individuals are reported more than once by different hospitals and providers.

There is little certainty about what causes factitious disorders. This is true in large measure because those who know the most about the subject—patients with the disorder—are notoriously unreliable in providing information about their psychological state and often seem only dimly aware of what they are doing to themselves. It may be that they are generally incapable of putting their feelings into words. They are unaware of having inner feelings and may not know, for example, that they are sad or angry. It is possible that they experience emotions more physically, behaviorally, and concretely than do most others.

Another view suggests that people learn to distinguish their primitive emotional states through the responsivity of their primary caretaker. A normal, healthy, average mother responds appropriately to her infant's differing affective states, thereby helping the infant, as he or she develops, to distinguish, define, and eventually name what he or she is feeling. When a primary caretaker is, for any of several reasons, incapable of responding in consistently appropriate ways, the infant's emotional awareness remains undifferentiated and the child experiences confusion and emotional chaos.

It is possible, too, that factitious disorder patients are motivated to assume what sociology defines as a sick role wherein people are required to acknowledge that they are ill and are required to relinquish adult responsibilities as they place themselves in the hands of designated caretakers.

### TREATMENT AND THERAPY

Internists, family practitioners, and surgeons are the specialists most likely to encounter patients with factitious disorder, although psychiatrists and psychologists are often consulted in the management of these patients. These patients pose a special challenge because in a real sense they do not wish to become well even as they present themselves for treatment. They are not ill in the usual sense, and their indirect communication and manipulation often make them frustrating to treat using standard goals and expectations.

Sometimes mental and medical specialists' joint, supportive confrontation of these patients results in a disappearance of the troubling and troublesome behavior. During these confrontations, the health professionals are acknowledging that such extreme behavior evidences extreme distress in these patients, and as such is its own reason for psychotherapeutic intervention. These patients are not psychologically minded, however; they also have trouble forming relationships that foster genuine self-disclosure, and they rarely accept the recommendation for psychotherapeutic treatment. Because they believe that their problems are physical, not psychological, they often become irate at the suggestion that their problems are not what they believe them to be. —*Paul Moglia*

*See also* Hypochondriasis; Psychiatric disorders; Psychosomatic disorders.

### FOR FURTHER INFORMATION:

American Psychiatric Association. *Diagnostic and Statistical Manual of Mental Disorders*. Rev. 4th ed. Washington, D.C.: Author, 1994.

Ford, C. V. *The Somatizing Disorders: Illness as a Way of Life*. New York: Elsevier Biomedical, 1983.

Kenyon, F. E. "Hypochondriacal States." *The British Journal of Psychiatry* 129 (July, 1976): 1-14.

Viederman, M. "Somatoform and Factitious Disorders." In *The Personality Disorders and Neuroses*, edited by A. M. Cooper, A. J. Frances, and M. H. Sacks. New York: Basic Books, 1986.

## FAINTING. *See* DIZZINESS AND FAINTING.

## FATIGUE

**SYSTEMS AFFECTED:** All

**SPECIALISTS:** Family physicians, geriatric specialists, internists, psychiatrists

**DEFINITION:** A general symptom of tiredness, malaise, depression, and sometimes anxiety associated with many diseases and disorders; in some cases, no specific cause can be found.

**KEY TERMS:**

*physical deconditioning:* a condition that results when a person who has previously been exercising (has become conditioned) stops exercising

*psychogenic fatigue:* fatigue caused by mental factors, such as anxiety, and not attributable to any physical cause

*sleep apnea:* cessation of breathing during sleep, which may result from either an inhibition of the respiratory center (central apnea) or an obstruction to the flow of air (obstructive apnea)

*sleep disorders:* conditions resulting in sleep interruption, interfering with the restorative functions of sleep

*syndrome:* a collection of complaints (symptoms) and signs (abnormal findings on clinical examination) which do not match any specific disease

### CAUSES AND SYMPTOMS

Almost all people suffer form fatigue at some point in their lives. It is a nonspecific complaint including tiredness, lack of energy, listlessness, or malaise. Patients often confuse fatigue with weakness, breathlessness, or dizziness, which indicate the existence of other physical disorders. Rest or a change in the daily routine ordinarily alleviates fatigue in healthy individuals. Though normally short in duration, fatigue occasionally lasts for weeks, months, or even years in some individuals. In such cases, it limits the amount of physical and mental activity in which the person can participate.

Long-term fatigue can have serious consequences. Often, patients begin to withdraw from their normal activities. They may withdraw from society in general and may gradually become more apathetic and depressed. As a result of this progression, a patient's physical and mental capabilities may begin to deteriorate. Fatigue may be aggravated further by a reduced appetite and inadequate nutritional intake. Ultimately, these symptoms lead to malnutrition and multiple vitamin deficiencies, which intensify the fatigue state and trigger a vicious circle.

This fatigue cycle ends with a person who lacks interest and energy. Such patients may lose interest in daily events and social contacts. In later stages of fatigue, they may neglect themselves and lose track of their goals in life. The will to live and fight decreases, making them prime targets for accidents and repeated infections. They may also become potential candidates for suicide.

Physical and/or mental overactivity commonly cause recent-onset fatigue. Management of such fatigue is simple: Adequate physical and/or mental relaxation typically relieve it. Fortunately, many persistent fatigue states can be easily diagnosed and successfully treated. In some cases, however, fatigue does not respond to simple measures.

Fatigue can stem from depression. Depressed individuals often reflect boredom and a lack of interest, and frequently express uncertainty and/or anxiety about the future. These people usually appear "down." They may walk slowly with their head down, slump their shoulders, and sigh frequently. They often take unusually long to respond to questions or requests. They also show little motivation. Depressed individuals typically relate feelings of dejection, sadness, worthlessness, or helplessness. Often, they complain of feeling tired when they wake up in the morning, and no amount of sleep or rest improves their condition. In fact, they feel weary all day and frequently complain of feeling weak. They often have poor appetites and sometimes lose weight. Once these patients are questioned by a physician, however, it may become apparent that their state of fatigue actually fluctuates. At times they feel exhausted, while at other times (sometimes only minutes later) they feel refreshed and full of energy.

Other manifestations of depression include sleep disorders (particularly early morning waking), reduced appetite, altered bowel habits, and difficulty concentrating. Depressed individuals sometimes fail to recognize their condition. They may channel their depression into physical complaints such as abdominal pain, headaches, joint pain, or vaguely defined aches and pains. In older people, depression sometimes manifests itself as impaired memory.

Anxiety, another major cause of fatigue, interferes with the patient's ability to achieve adequate mental and physical rest. Anxious individuals often appear scared, worried, or fearful. They frequently report multiple physical complaints, including neck muscle tension, headaches, palpitations, difficulty in breathing, chest tightness, intestinal cramping, and trouble falling asleep. In some cases, both depression and anxiety may be present simultaneously.

Medications also constitute a major cause of fatigue. All drugs—prescription, over-the-counter, or recreational—can cause fatigue. Sleeping medications, antidepressants, antianxiety medications, muscle relaxants, allergy medications, cold medications, and certain blood pressure medications can lead to problems with fatigue.

An excessive intake of stimulants, paradoxically, sometimes leads to easy fatigability. Stimulants can interfere with proper sleeping habits and relaxation. Common culprits include caffeine and medications (such as some diet pills and nasal decongestants) that can be purchased without a prescription. So-called recreational drugs can also contribute to chronic fatigue. Depending on their tendencies, they function to cause fatigue in much the same way as the prescription and over-the-counter drugs already discussed. Cocaine and amphetamines, for example, act as stimulants. Narcotics such as heroin and barbiturates (downers) possess strong sedative qualities. Alcohol consumption in an attempt to escape loneliness, depression, or boredom may further exacerbate a sense of fatigue. Alcohol produces fatigue

in two ways. It has sedative qualities, and it also intensifies the sedative effects of other medications, if taken with them.

Other drugs that may induce fatigue include diuretics and those that lower blood pressure. These medications increase the excretions of many substances through the kidneys. If inappropriately given or regulated, these drugs may alter the blood concentration of other medications taken concurrently.

Painkillers can lead to fatigue in a different way. In some individuals, they irritate the lining of the stomach and cause it to bleed. Such bleeding usually occurs in small amounts and goes unnoticed by the patient. This slight blood loss can gradually lead to anemia and fatigue.

Medications are particularly likely to cause fatigue in elderly individuals. With many drugs, their elimination from the body through metabolism or excretion may decrease with age. This often leads to higher drug concentrations in the blood than intended, resulting in a state of constant sedation and lethargy. Also, elderly individuals' brains may be more sensitive to sedation than those of younger individuals. Finally, the elderly tend to take more medication for more illnesses than younger adults. The additive side effects of multiple medicines can add to fatigue problems.

Sleep deprivation or frequent sleep interruptions lead to fatigue. A change in environment can induce sleep disorders, especially if accompanied by unfamiliar noises, excessive lighting, uncomfortable temperatures, or an excessive degree of humidity or dryness. Total sleep time may be adequate under such conditions, but quality of sleep is usually poor. Nightmares can also interrupt sleep, and if numerous and recurring, they also cause fatigue.

Some sleep interruptions are not so readily apparent. In sleep apnea, a specific and increasingly diagnosed sleep disorder, the patient temporarily stops breathing while sleeping. This results in reduced oxygen levels and increased carbon dioxide levels in the blood. When a critical level is reached, the patient awakens briefly, takes a few deep breaths, and then falls asleep again. Many episodes of sleep apnea may occur during the night, making the sleep interrupted and less refreshing than it should be. The next day, the patient often feels tired and fatigued, but may not recognize the source of the problem. Obstructive sleep apnea normally develops in grossly overweight patients or in those with large tonsils or adenoids. Patients with obstructive sleep apnea usually snore while sleeping, and typically they are unaware of their snoring and/or sleep disturbance.

A number of diseases can lead to easy fatigability. In most illnesses, rest relieves fatigue and individuals awake refreshed after a nap or a good night's sleep. Unfortunately, they also tire quickly. Unlike psychogenic fatigue or fatigue induced by drugs, disease-related fatigue is not usually the patient's main symptom. Other symptoms and signs frequently reveal the underlying diagnosis. Individuals who suffer from severe malnutrition, anemia, endocrine system malfunction, chronic infections, tuberculosis, Lyme disease, bacterial endocarditis (a bacterial infection of the valves of the heart), chronic sinusitis, mononucleosis, hepatitis, parasitic infections, and fungal infections may all experience chronic fatigue.

In early stages of acquired immunodeficiency syndrome (AIDS), fatigue may be the only symptom. Persons at high risk for contracting the human immunodeficiency virus (HIV)—those with multiple sexual partners, homosexual men, those with a history of blood transfusion, or intravenous drug users—who complain of persistent fatigue should be tested for HIV infection.

Abnormalities of mineral or electrolyte concentrations—potassium, sodium, chloride, and calcium are the most important of these—may also cause fatigue. Such abnormalities may result from medications (diuretics are frequently responsible), diarrhea, vomiting, dietary fads, and endocrine or bone disorders.

Some less common medical causes of chronic fatigue include dysfunction of specific organs such as kidney failure or liver failure. Allergies can also produce chronic fatigue. Cancer can cause fatigue, but other symptoms usually surface and lead to a diagnosis before the patient begins to notice chronic weariness.

### TREATMENT AND THERAPY

When an individual's fatigue persists in spite of adequate rest, medical help becomes necessary in order to determine the cause. Common diseases known to be associated with fatigue should be considered. Initially, the physician makes detailed inquiries about the severity of the fatigue and how long ago it started. Other important questions include whether it is progressive, whether there are any factors that make it worse or relieve it, or whether it is worse during specific times of the day. An examination of the patient's psychological state may also be necessary.

The physician should ask about the presence of any symptoms that occur along with the general sense of fatigue. For example, breathlessness may indicate a cardiovascular or respiratory disease. Abdominal pain might arouse the suspicion of a gastrointestinal disease. Weakness may point to a neuromuscular collagen disease. Excessive thirst and increased urine output may suggest diabetes mellitus, and weight loss may accompany metabolic or endocrinal abnormalities, chronic infections, or cancer.

Whether they have been prescribed by a physician or purchased over-the-counter, the medications taken regularly by a patient should be reviewed. The doctor should also inquire about alcohol and tobacco use and dietary fads. A thorough physical examination may be required. During an examination, the doctor sometimes uncovers physical signs of fatigue-inducing diseases. Blood tests and other laboratory investigations may also be needed, especially because a physical examination does not always reveal the cause.

Often, however, despite an extensive workup, no specific cause for the persistent fatigue appears. At this stage, the diagnosis of chronic fatigue syndrome should be considered. In order to fit this diagnosis, patients must have several of the symptoms associated with this syndrome. They must have complained of fatigue for at least six months, and the fatigue should be of such an extent that it interferes with normal daily activities. Since many of the symptoms associated with chronic fatigue syndrome overlap with other disorders, these other fatigue-inducing conditions must be considered and ruled out.

In order to fit the diagnosis of chronic fatigue syndrome, patients must have at least six of the classic symptoms. These include a mild fever and/or sore throat, painful lymph nodes in the neck or axilla, unexplained generalized weakness, and muscle pain or discomfort. Patients may describe marked fatigue lasting for more than twenty-four hours that is induced by levels of exercise that would have been easily tolerated before the onset of fatigue. They may suffer from generalized headaches of a type, severity, or pattern that is different from headaches experienced before the onset of chronic fatigue. Patients may also have joint pain without swelling or redness and/or neuropsychologic complaints such as a bad memory and excessive irritability. Confusion, difficulty in thinking, inability to concentrate, depression, and sleep disturbances are also on the list of associated symptoms.

No one knows the exact cause of chronic fatigue syndrome. Researchers continue to study the disease and come up with hypotheses, though none have proven entirely satisfactory. One theory argues that since patients with chronic fatigue syndrome appear to have a reduced aerobic work capacity, defects in the muscles may cause the condition. This, however, constitutes only one of many theories concerning the syndrome and its origin.

Many patients with chronic fatigue syndrome relate that they suffered from an infectious illness immediately preceding the onset of fatigue. This pattern causes some scientists to suspect a viral origin. Typically, the illness that precedes the patient's problems with fatigue is not severe, and resembles other upper respiratory tract infections experienced previously. The implicated viruses include the Epsteirn-Barr virus, Coxsackie B virus, herpes simplex virus, cytomegalovirus, human herpesvirus 6, and the measles virus. It should be mentioned, however, that some patients with long-term fatigue do not have a history of a triggering infectious disease before the onset of fatigue.

Patients with chronic fatigue syndrome sometimes have a number of immune system abnormalities. Laboratory evidence exists of immune dysfunction in many patients with this syndrome, and there have been reports of improvement when immunoglobulin (antibody) therapy was given. The significance of immunological abnormalities in chronic fatigue syndrome, however, remains uncertain. Most of these abnormalities do not occur in all patients with this syndrome. Furthermore, the degree of immunologic abnormality does not always correspond with the severity of the symptoms.

Some researchers believe that the acute infectious disease that often precedes the onset of chronic fatigue syndrome forces the patient to become physically inactive. This inactivity leads to physical deconditioning, and the progression ends in chronic fatigue syndrome. Experiments in which patients with chronic fatigue syndrome were given exercise testing, however, do not support this theory completely. In the case of physical deconditioning, the heart rates of patients with chronic fatigue syndrome should have risen more rapidly with exercise than those without the syndrome. The exact opposite was found. The data were not determined consistent with the suggestion that physical deconditioning causes chronic fatigue syndrome.

A high prevalence of unrecognized psychiatric disorders exists in patients with chronic fatigue, especially depression. Depression affects about half of chronic fatigue syndrome patients and precedes other symptoms in about half of them as well. Yet a critical question remains unanswered concerning chronic fatigue syndrome: Are patients with this syndrome fatigued because they have a primary mood disorder, or has the mood disorder developed as a secondary component of the chronic fatigue syndrome?

No completely satisfactory treatment exists for chronic fatigue syndrome, since the cause remains a mystery. A group of researchers using intravenous immunoglobulin therapy met with varying degrees of success, but other investigators could not reproduce these results. Other therapeutic trials used high doses of medications such as acyclovir, liver extract, folic acid, and cyanocobalamine. A mixture of evening primrose oil and fish oil was also administered with some degree of success. Claims have also been made that patients administered magnesium sulfate improved to a larger extent than those receiving a placebo. Other therapeutic options include cognitive behavioral therapy, programs of gradually increasing physical activity, analgesics, nonsteroidal anti-inflammatory drugs (NSAIDs), and antidepressants. Finally, a number of self-help groups exist for chronic fatigue sufferers.

The prognosis and natural history of chronic fatigue syndrome are still poorly defined. Chronic fatigue syndrome does not kill patients, but it does significantly decrease the quality of life for sufferers. For the physician, management of this syndrome remains challenging. In addition to correcting any physical abnormalities present, the physician should attempt to find an activity that interests the patient and encourage him or her to become involved in it.

## PERSPECTIVE AND PROSPECTS

Fatigue is generally considered a normal bodily response, protecting the individual from excessive physical and/or mental activity. After all, the normal levels of performance for individuals who do not rest usually decline. In the case of overactivity, fatigue should be viewed as a positive warning sign. Using relaxation and rest (mental and/or physical), the individual can often alleviate weariness and optimize performance.

In some cases, however, fatigue does not derive from physical or mental overactivity, nor does it respond adequately to relaxation and rest. In these instances, it interferes with an individual's ability to cope with everyday life and enjoy usual activities. The patient begins referring to fatigue as the reason for not participating in normal physical, mental, and social activities.

Unfortunately, physicians, health care professionals, society, and even the patients themselves dismiss fatigue as a trivial complaint. As a result, sufferers seek medical help only after the condition becomes advanced. This dangerous, negative attitude can delay the correct diagnosis of the underlying pathology and threaten the patient's chances for a quick recovery.

The diagnosis and management of chronic fatigue syndrome prove challenging for both physician and patient. It is important to note that chronic fatigue syndrome often stems from nonmedical causes. While the possibility of a serious medical illness should be addressed, illness-related fatigue usually occurs along with other, more prominent symptoms. The causes of chronic fatigue syndrome are numerous and can take time to define. Patients need to answer all questions related to their complaints as thoroughly and accurately as possible, so that their physicians can reach accurate diagnoses using the minimum number of tests. Extensive testing for rare medical causes of fatigue can become extraordinarily expensive and uncomfortable, so doctors select the tests that they are ordering cautiously. They must balance the benefit, the cost, and the risk of each test to the patient. Such decisions should be based on their own experience and on the available data.

Open communication between the patient and doctor is of paramount importance. It ensures a correct diagnosis, followed by the most effective treatment. Follow-up visits and reassurance may be the best therapy in many cases. Professional counselors can offer assistance with fatigue-inducing psychological disorders. Examination of sleep and relaxation habits can reveal potential problems, and steps can be taken to ensure adequate rest.

Persistent fatigue should not be discarded lightly, and serious attempts should be made to determine its underlying causes. In this respect, it may be appropriate to recall one of Hippocrates' aphorisms, "Unprovoked fatigue means disease." —*Ronald C. Hamdy, Mark R. Doman, and Katherine Hoffman Doman*

***See also*** Apnea; Chronic fatigue syndrome; Depression; Dizziness and fainting; Narcolepsy; Sleep disorders; Sleeping sickness; Stress.

## FOR FURTHER INFORMATION:

Archer, James, Jr. *Managing Anxiety and Stress*. Muncie, Ind.: Excellerated Development, 1982. Anxiety is a common cause of persistent fatigue. This text examines the nature of anxiety. Contains several methods to combat anxiety and stress, ranging from management skills, personal relations, nutrition, and exercise to meditation and relaxation techniques. Arranged so that it can be used as a step-by-step guide to decreasing an individual's anxiety.

Feiden, Karyn. *Hope and Help for Chronic Fatigue Syndrome: The Official CFS-CFIDS Network*. New York: Prentice Hall, 1990. A complete review of chronic fatigue syndrome, presenting the many aspects of this disease. The history of this syndrome, symptomatology, theories of causation, and experimental therapies are addressed. Includes a section on surviving with this syndrome, recommending the use of support groups, social services, and self-help.

Goroll, Allan H., Lawrence A. May, and Albert G. Mulley. *Primary Care Medicine*. 2d ed. Philadelphia: J. B. Lippincott, 1987. The essential text for the medical office practice of adult medicine. It is problem-oriented and easily read even by individuals without medical training. The section on the causes of fatigue is the best available.

Pembrook, Linda. *How to Beat Fatigue*. Garden City, N.Y.: Doubleday, 1975. In this book, many aspects of fatigue are presented simply and thoroughly, including sleep, drugs and alcohol, nutrition, depression, and anxiety. Covers many of the causes of fatigue, with the exception of some of the physical causes.

Talley, Joseph. *Family Practitioner's Guide to Treating Depressive Illness*. Chicago: Precept Press, 1987. Depression is probably the most common cause of persistent fatigue. This well-written text examines the multiple facets of depression. It also reviews the various therapies available, different philosophies of depressive treatments, and the use of psychotherapy.

Trubo, Richard. *How to Get a Good Night's Sleep*. Boston: Little, Brown, 1978. An easy-to-read book that examines most facets of sleep, from the physiology of sleep to such sleep disorders as sleep apnea and nightmares. The text also includes an interesting section on dreams and dreaming.

## FEMALE GENITAL DISORDERS

**SYSTEM AFFECTED:** Reproductive (female)

**SPECIALISTS:** General surgeons, gynecologists, obstetricians, oncologists, surgeons

**DEFINITION:** All maladies affecting the reproductive organs of women.

**KEY TERMS:**

*cervix:* the narrow portion of the uterus situated at the upper end of the vagina

*cyst:* a closed sac having a distinct border which develops abnormally within a body space or structure

*estrogen:* the hormone responsible for female sexual characteristics, produced primarily by the ovaries

*Fallopian tubes:* tiny tubes that connect the ovaries to the uterus; after ovulation, the egg travels through these tubes, and its fertilization by sperm occurs here

*hormone:* a chemical compound produced at one site in the body which travels to other parts of the body to exert its effect

*hysterectomy:* the surgical removal of the uterus; in a total hysterectomy, the uterus, ovaries and Fallopian tubes are removed

*laparoscopy:* a surgical procedure in which an instrument is inserted into the abdominal cavity through tiny incisions in the abdomen; usually performed without hospitalization

### CAUSES AND SYMPTOMS

Diseases and disorders of the female genitals, both internal organs and outward anatomical structures, encompass a huge number of different types of conditions that can range in severity from merely physically annoying to life-threatening. These disorders affect the vulva, vagina, uterus, ovaries, and Fallopian tubes. Many develop from unknown causes, and others have clear-cut origins, such as sexually transmitted diseases. Some have immediately recognizable symptoms, while others are silent until the disease has progressed to a serious stage. Early recognition of symptoms or abnormalities and proper treatment can alleviate pain and save lives.

Endometriosis is a chronic, recurring disease in which the tissue that lines the uterus grows into the abdominal cavity. This tissue normally thickens with blood vessels in preparation for receiving a fertilized egg. In endometriosis, the tissue overgrows the uterus, invades the Fallopian tubes, and

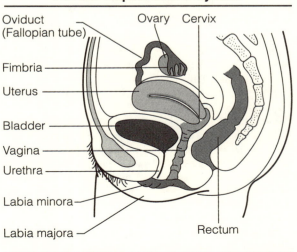

**Female Reproductive System**

Oviduct (Fallopian tube)

Ovary

Cervix

Fimbria

Uterus

Bladder

Vagina

Urethra

Labia minora

Labia majora

Rectum

## Sites of Common Nonmalignant Female Genital Disorders

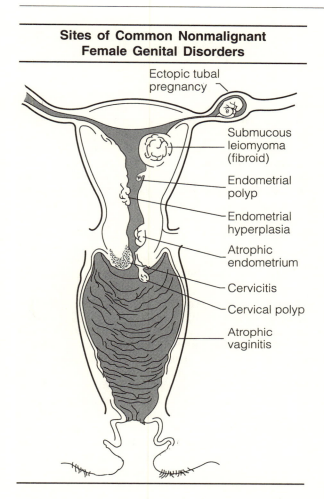

Ectopic tubal pregnancy

Submucous leiomyoma (fibroid)

Endometrial polyp

Endometrial hyperplasia

Atrophic endometrium

Cervicitis

Cervical polyp

Atrophic vaginitis

reaches the abdominal cavity, where it continues to grow. This abnormally growing tissue will attach to any nearby internal organs, such as the ovaries, bladder, Fallopian tubes, and rectum. The endometrial tissue responds to the same hormonal cues that signal the sloughing off of the uterine lining during menstruation; however, the blood from the endometrial tissue cannot leave the abdominal cavity, leading to inflammation. As the inflammation subsides, it is replaced with scar tissue. This process will repeat with each menstrual cycle, and the scarring can result in infertility, organ malfunction, or adhesions that bind organs together. Some women with endometriosis experience no symptoms, while many experience severe abdominal pain before, during, and after their menstrual periods. Endometrial tissue can be sometimes diagnosed with a pelvic exam, but a definitive diagnosis can only be reached with laparoscopy. The cause of endometriosis is unknown, but some evidence suggests an inherited tendency to develop endometriosis.

Vaginitis is a general term for infections of the vagina. The most common of these is commonly called a yeast infection, caused by the fungus *Candida albicans*. This fungus is usually a harmless organism which lives in nearly everyone's intestinal tract and in the vagina of 20 to 40 percent of American women. Symptoms are caused when the organism grows at an accelerated rate and include severe itching, vaginal discharge, and burning upon urination. Many situations may cause the enhanced growth of the fungus, including use of antibiotics which disturb the acid balance within the vagina, stress, use of oral contraceptives and corticosteroids, and the low estrogen levels that accompany the menopause.

Uterine fibroids are benign tumors made mainly of muscle tissue that can grow inside the uterus or along its outer surface. They grow slowly and are dependent on the hormone estrogen for continued growth. They are usually not problematic, but if they become very large they may cause extremely heavy bleeding during menstruation and can interfere with pregnancy and childbirth. Their cause is unknown, but they will shrink or disappear after the menopause.

Uterine prolapse occurs when the pelvic muscles are no longer able to support the pelvic organs, and the uterus "falls" into the vagina. A feeling of one's "insides falling out" is typical of this disorder, which is often precipitated by one or more difficult births.

Ovarian cysts form when an egg developing inside a follicle within the ovary does not ovulate but instead keeps growing. Small cysts will be painless, but larger ones (up to 7.5 centimeters in diameter) may cause abdominal pain. Most cysts will go away on their own, but some can rupture and cause severe pain.

The hallmark of cancer is uncontrolled cell growth. Cancer may prove fatal by causing destruction of a particular organ at the site of origin or by spreading throughout the body and damaging other organs and systems. All the organs of the female reproductive system can be affected by cancer. Cervical cancer begins in superficial layers of the cervix but may spread rapidly through the vagina and throughout the body. Cervical cancer can be detected in its early, most curable stages by a Pap smear. Endometrial cancer affects the glands which line the uterus. It can occur at any age, but the most common age of onset is sixty. Abnormal bleeding accompanies this disorder, which is diagnosed by examination of a biopsy of uterine tissue. Sarcomas of the uterus are malignant tumors of muscle tissue frequently confused with benign fibroids. This rare cancer is aggressive and difficult to treat. Ovarian cancer constitutes about 25 percent of female reproductive tract cancers, is difficult to detect and cure, and therefore has a high mortality rate. There are no early symptoms, and the cancer seems to occur frequently in those with a family history of the disease. Cancers of the Fallopian tubes and vagina are very rare, but vaginal cancer occurs with greater frequency in women whose mothers were treated with the synthetic estrogen diethylstilbestrol (DES) during the 1940's through the 1960's with the intent of preventing miscarriages. Cancer of the vulva, a form of skin cancer, is relatively easy to treat and has a high cure rate.

Sexually transmitted diseases (STDs) can involve any part of the female genital system. STDs of bacterial origin include gonorrhea and chlamydia, which are major precursors to pelvic inflammatory disease (PID) and syphilis. Untreated, these diseases can lead to serious complications. STDs with a viral cause include genital herpes, genital warts, and acquired immunodeficiency syndrome (AIDS). The causative agent of trichomoniasis is a protozoan. Each STD can be transmitted through direct sexual contact with an infected person, and each has its own set of symptoms and diagnostic criteria.

### TREATMENT AND THERAPY

A variety of treatments are available for endometriosis, depending on the severity of the disorder. Over-the-counter or prescription anti-inflammatory drugs may give immediate relief of pain, but the condition itself is frequently treated with hormone therapy. Birth control pills that are high in the hormone progestin and low in estrogen can help shrink endometriosis. Danazol, a synthetic male hormone, suppresses the production of estrogen by the ovaries, thereby helping to eliminate the condition, but it has undesirable side effects. In some cases, surgical removal of the tissue is necessary. In laparoscopy, an instrument is inserted through tiny abdominal incisions and used to remove the tissue. In the most severe cases, a complete hysterectomy (removal of the uterus and ovaries) is performed.

Yeast infections that result in vaginitis must be properly diagnosed by a physician. Two medications for yeast infections are available without a prescription: miconazole and clotrimazole, available under brand names in most pharmacies. If a severe infection does not respond to this treatment, cortisone may be prescribed. Yeast infections have a tendency to recur, and taking precautions to prevent additional episodes is advised. Some ways in which to reduce the chance of reinfection include eating a cup of yogurt daily, avoiding sweets, reducing stress, wearing cotton underwear, avoiding tight-fitting clothing, avoiding feminine-hygiene sprays, and using vinegar-and-water or povidone-iodine douches.

If no major discomfort is experienced by the woman when uterine fibroids are first detected, usually no treatment beyond regular observation is necessary. For those experiencing pain or difficulty in conception or pregnancy, the fibroids may be surgically removed in an operation called a myomectomy; in severe cases, a hysterectomy is performed. A laparoscope can be used to remove tumors on the outside of the uterus, or a hysteroscope can be inserted through the cervix, which uses a laser to burn away internal fibroids. Synthetic hormones called gonadotropin-releasing hormone agonists block the ovaries' production of estrogen, which leads to shrinking of the fibroids and the possible avoidance of surgery. Even with surgery, about 25 percent of fibroids grow back within five years.

A prolapsed uterus is frequently treated by hysterectomy, but other therapies are possible. Kegel exercises, designed to strengthen the muscles of the pelvic floor, are effective if done regularly for an extended period of time. A pessary, a ring-shaped device which fits around the cervix and props up the uterus, is another alternative, though an inconvenient one. Major surgery to resuspend the uterus is a surgical option to hysterectomy.

Ovarian cysts will usually be resorbed into the ovary within one to three menstrual cycles. Proper monitoring by a physician is needed to determine if the cysts have cleared. If the cyst does not disappear within three months or if it increases in size, ultrasound and/or laparoscopy will be used to determine if a different type of ovarian tumor is present, which would necessitate surgical removal.

Cancer treatment is highly specialized for the particular variety of the disease, its severity, and consideration of the affected individual. Typical treatments include surgical removal of the tumor and/or affected organ, radiation therapy, chemotherapy, and immunotherapy (the reinforcement of the immune system, generally administered after radiation or chemotherapy). When diagnosed in premalignant stages, cervical abnormalities may be treated by cryosurgery (freezing and killing the abnormal cells) or laser destruction of the abnormal cells. Advanced cervical cancer is treated by hysterectomy. Endometrial cancer is treated with total hysterectomy, including the uterus, ovaries, and Fallopian tubes, and if the cancer has spread, radiation and/or chemotherapy. The only known cure for uterine sarcoma is total hysterectomy, and removal of both the ovaries and the Fallopian tubes is performed for ovarian cancer. The tumors of vaginal cancer are eliminated surgically or with laser treatment.

Sexually transmitted diseases of bacterial origin are treated successfully with antibiotics. Drug therapy can also eliminate trichomoniasis. There are no cures for the virally transmitted STDs. Certain drugs can reduce the frequency of outbreaks of genital herpes, and genital warts may be removed by freezing, burning, or surgery. No cure exists for AIDS, and only experimental drugs are available to prolong life.

### PERSPECTIVE AND PROSPECTS

The diagnosis and treatment of female genital disorders and diseases have evolved from a state of some being considered psychosomatic to a field which spurs the continued development and improvement of diagnostic and treatment technologies. It is also a field which has been a major force in the mass screening of diseases and in public health issues. Many conditions such as endometriosis have historically been misdiagnosed and the associated pain dismissed as nonexistent—to the dismay of the suffering woman. This and other conditions such as prolapsed uterus and fibroids were typically treated with the drastic surgery of hysterectomy. Women have demanded that more research into the causes of these disorders, and options to hysterectomy, be developed. Laparoscopy has replaced hysterectomy in many cases, preserving the uterus and childbearing capacity.

The treatment of all female cancers has benefited from research into the cause and treatment of these disorders. For decades, the Pap smear has been routinely used with American women on an annual basis, and it has been responsible for saving thousands of lives through early detection of abnormal cervical cells that may progress to a cancerous state. Public education about the necessity of early cancer detection has helped to improve the survival chances of individuals with cancer, and sensitive blood tests can detect some cancers at their most treatable stages, long before any symptoms occur. Discovery of the hereditary nature of female genital cancers has established routine monitoring of those at risk for the disease, again resulting in early detection. New, better radiation and chemotherapy treatments, as well as improved immune system support, benefit all cancer patients. The connection between certain "cancer-fighting" foods and good health has led to a revision of Americans' eating habits.

While some sexually transmitted diseases are easily cured with antibiotics if caught early, those of viral origin are not and may have fatal consequences. Information through such diverse means as television and grade-school programs has educated people about this problem and the best ways to protect themselves from becoming victims of an incurable STD. Continuing research into diagnostic methods and treatment regimes in this area will lead to improved health for everyone. —*Karen E. Kalumuck*

*See also* Amenorrhea; Breast cancer; Breast disorders; Breast-feeding; Cervical, ovarian, and uterine cancers; Childbirth; Childbirth, complications of; Chlamydia; Conception; Cystitis; Dysmenorrhea; Ectopic pregnancy; Endometriosis; Gonorrhea; Herpes; Infertility in females; Infertility in males; Mastitis; Menopause; Menorrhagia; Menstruation; Miscarriage; Ovarian cysts; Pelvic inflammatory disease (PID); Postpartum depression; Pregnancy and gestation; Premature birth; Premenstrual syndrome (PMS); Sexually transmitted diseases; Stillbirth; Syphilis.

### FOR FURTHER INFORMATION:
Boston Women's Health Book Collective. *The New Our Bodies, Ourselves: A Book by and for Women.* New York: Simon & Schuster, 1992. Gives expanded and accessible information on a broad range of topics concerning women's health. An excellent reference book for all women. A listing of local, national, and international resources is included.

Curtis, L. R., G. B. Curtis, and M. K. Beard. *My Body, My Decision: What You Should Know About the Most-Common Female Surgeries.* Tucson, Ariz.: Body Press, 1986. A book written by female surgeons which gives practical and comprehensive information about the most common surgeries for women, elective and emergency. Designed to give women the ability to make informed decisions about their bodies.

Foley, Denise, and Eileen Nechas. *Women's Encyclopedia of Health and Emotional Healing: Top Women Doctors Share Their Unique Self-Help Advice on Your Body, Your Feelings, and Your Life.* Emmaus, Pa.: Rodale Press, 1993. A very readable and informative book filled with practical information and anecdotal examples covering all aspects of women's physical and emotional health.

Gray, Mary Jane, and Florence Haseltine. *The Woman's Guide to Good Health.* Yonkers, N.Y.: Consumer Reports Books, 1991. This practical and comprehensive guide is written by physicians and gives complete information about the myths, risks, and alternatives regarding female diseases, diagnosis, and treatment. A useful appendix includes a list of societies for support and further information.

Novotny, P. P. *What Women Should Know About Chronic Infections and Sexually Transmitted Diseases.* New York: Dell, 1991. This compact, easy-to-understand book gives complete and accurate information on the transmission, diagnosis, and prevention of all sexually transmitted diseases that affect women. A handy reference guide.

## FETAL ALCOHOL SYNDROME
**SYSTEMS AFFECTED:** Brain, muscular, nervous
**SPECIALISTS:** Neonatologists, obstetricians, perinatologists, public health specialists
**DEFINITION:** Growth retardation and mental or physical abnormalities in a child resulting from alcohol consumption by the mother during pregnancy.

Fetal alcohol syndrome was first identified in the early 1970's. Whether consumed as beer, wine, or hard liquor, alcohol is a teratogen, a toxic substance that can cause abnormalities in unborn children. The damage ranges from subtle to severe, depending on the quantity consumed and the stage of pregnancy when the exposure occurs. A critical period is in early pregnancy, when a woman may not know that she is pregnant. Even one or two drinks a day by the mother may have an effect on her child.

There are three diagnostic criteria for fetal alcohol syndrome: growth retardation, certain facial anomalies, and central nervous system impairment. Growth retardation begins in utero, causing low birth weight. Babies with low birth weight are at risk for delayed growth and development and even death. Growth impairment affects not only the skeleton but also the brain and face. The resulting head and facial abnormalities are characterized by thin lips; small, wide-set eyes; a short, upturned nose; a receding chin; and low-set ears. Fetal alcohol syndrome children have intelligence quotients (IQs) well below the mean of the population because of impaired brain growth that results in irreversible mental retardation. Fetal alcohol syndrome is a leading cause of mental retardation. Abnormalities often originate during the first trimester, when bones and organs are forming. Major organ systems such as the heart, kidney, liver, and skeleton can be impaired.

Less specific problems that result from alcohol damage are clumsiness, behavioral problems, a brief attention span, poor judgment, impaired memory, and a diminished capacity to learn from experience. These symptoms are often labeled "fetal alcohol effects."

Alcohol enters the fetal bloodstream as soon as the mother has a drink. It not only can damage the brain but also may impair the function of the placenta, which is the organ interface between maternal and fetal circulation. The exact mechanism for this damage is not completely understood. The most probable cause is that alcohol creates a glucose or oxygen deficit for the fetus. Because it is not known what dose of alcohol is safe, the best preventive measure is to abstain from alcohol during pregnancy and even when planning a pregnancy. —*Wendy L. Stuhldreher*

**See also** Alcoholism; Childbirth, complications of; Genetic diseases; Pregnancy and gestation.

# FEVER

**SYSTEMS AFFECTED:** All
**SPECIALISTS:** Family physicians, internists, pediatricians
**DEFINITION:** A symptom associated with a variety of diseases and disorders, characterized by body temperature above normal (98.6 degrees Fahrenheit, or 37 degrees centigrade or Celsius); considered very serious at 104 degrees Fahrenheit (40 degrees Celsius) and higher.

**KEY TERMS:**

*antipyretic drugs:* drugs that are employed to reduce fevers, such as sodium salicylate, indomethacin, acetophenetidin, and paracetamol

*ectotherms:* organisms that rely on external temperature conditions in order to maintain their internal temperature

*endotherms:* organisms that control the internal temperature of their bodies by the conversion of Calories to heat

*febrile response:* an upward adjustment of the thermoregulatory set point

*metabolic rate:* a measurement of the Calories that are converted into heat energy in order to maintain body temperature and/or for physical exertion

*pyrogens:* protein substances that appear at the outset of the process that leads to a fever reaction

*thermoregulatory set point:* the ultimate neural control that maintains the human internal body temperature at 37 degrees Celsius and can either raise or lower it

## CAUSES AND SYMPTOMS

Although the symptoms that often accompany a fever are familiar to everyone—shivering, sweating, thirst, hot skin, and a flushed face—what causes fever and its function during illness are not fully clear even among medical specialists. Considerable literature exists on the differences be-

tween warm-blooded organisms (endotherms) and cold-blooded organisms (ectotherms) in what is called the normal state, when no symptoms of disease are present. Cold-blooded organisms depend on temperature conditions in their external environment to maintain various levels of temperature within their bodies. These fluctuations correspond to the various levels of activity that they need to sustain at given moments. Thus, reptiles, for example, may "recharge" themselves internally by moving into the warmth of the sun. Warm-blooded organisms, on the other hand, including all mammals, utilize energy released from the digestion of food to maintain a constant level of heat within their bodies. This level—a "normal" temperature—is approximately 37 degrees Celsius (98.6 degrees Fahrenheit) in humans. An internal body temperature which rises above this level is called a febrile temperature, or a fever.

If the temperature in the surrounding environment is low, warm-blooded organisms must raise their metabolic rate (a measurement, in Calories, of converted energy) accordingly to maintain a normal internal body temperature. In humans, this rate of energy expenditure is about 1,800 Calories per day. If insufficient food is taken in to supply the necessary potential energy for this metabolic conversion into heat, the body will draw on its storage resource—fat—to fulfill this vital need. The potentially fatal condition called hypothermia, in which the body is too fatigued to maintain metabolic functions or has exhausted all of its stores of Calories, occurs when the internal temperature falls below normal. Although cold-blooded animals must also protect themselves against the danger that their body heat may fall too low to sustain life functions, they can support adjustments in their own internal temperature down to about 20 degrees Celsius. At the same time, metabolic expenditures, as measured in Calories, are very low in cold-blooded animals; for example, alligators must expend only 60 Calories per day to create the same amount of heat as 1,800 Calories per day in warm-blooded humans.

The question of internal temperature in warm-blooded animals is closely tied to management efficiency in the body. This function becomes critical when one considers abnormally high internal temperature, or fever. Generally speaking, all essential biochemical functions in the human body can be carried out at optimal levels of efficiency at the set point of 37 degrees Celsius. In the simplest of terms, any increase or decrease in temperature creates either more or less kinetic energy and has the potential to affect the chemistry of all body functions.

Endotherms are able to tolerate a certain range of involuntary change in their internal body temperature (brought about by disease or illness), but there is an upper limit of 45 degrees Celsius, which constitutes a high fever. If the self-regulating higher set point associated with fever goes beyond this point, destructive biochemical phenomena will occur in the body—in particular, a breaking down of protein molecules. If these phenomena are not checked, they can bring about death.

Modern scientific approaches to the internal body processes that lead to fever, like a medical discussion of the effects that occur once fever is operating in the body, are much more complicated. They revolve around the concept of a change in the set point monitored in the brain. When this change in the brain's normal (37 degree) thermostatic signal is called for, a process called phagocytosis begins, leading to a higher internal body heat level throughout the organism.

Phagocytosis, the ingestion of a solid substance (especially foreign material such as invading bacteria), involves the appearance in the host's system of large numbers of leukocyte cells. When these cells ingest the bacteria, small quantities of protein called leukocytic pyrogens are produced. According to most modern theories, these protein pyrogens trigger the biochemical reactions in the brain that alter the body's temperature set point. After this point, changes that occur throughout the system and raise the body's internal temperature depend on a component of the bacterial cell wall called endotoxin. By the end of the 1960's, researchers had drawn attention to at least twenty effects that activated endotoxins may have on the host organism. Key effects include enhancement of the production of new white blood cells (leukocytosis), enhancement of various forms of immunological resistance, reduction of serum iron levels, and lowering of blood pressure.

## Effects of Fever

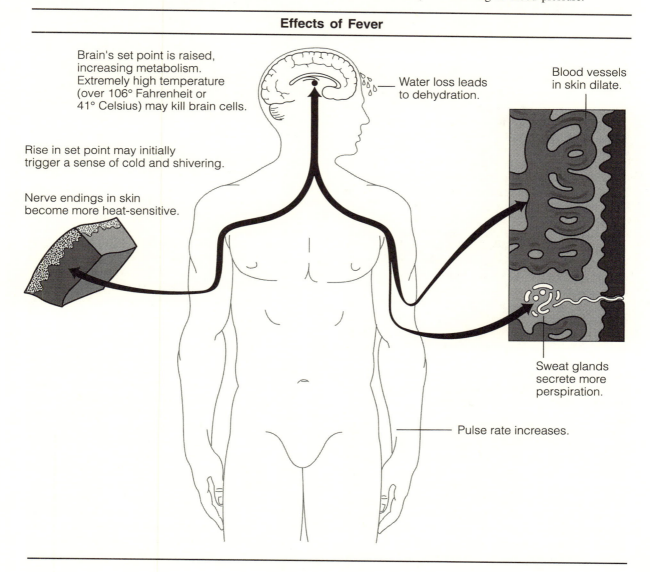

Brain's set point is raised, increasing metabolism. Extremely high temperature (over 106° Fahrenheit or 41° Celsius) may kill brain cells.

Rise in set point may initially trigger a sense of cold and shivering.

Nerve endings in skin become more heat-sensitive.

Water loss leads to dehydration.

Blood vessels in skin dilate.

Sweat glands secrete more perspiration.

Pulse rate increases.

Most, if not all, of these effects brought about by endotoxins are accompanied by higher levels of heat throughout the body, the definition of fever. Closer biochemical examination of the source of the added heat yielded the suggestion, made by P. B. Beeson in 1948, that the host's endotoxin-affected cells begin to produce a distinct form of protein, now called endogenous pyrogens. Pyrogens are thought to induce the first stage of fever by interacting with cells in tissues very close to the brain, specifically in the brain stem itself. Laboratory experiments in the first half of the twentieth century allowed researchers to produce almost immediate fever reactions when they injected pyrogen protein material into rabbits. Studies of the induced febrile state in laboratory animals, and therefore presumably also in humans, linked fever to immunological (virus-resistant and bacteria-resistant) reactions, not necessarily in the initially affected tissues around the brain but in various places throughout the organism.

Although scientific research has produced many hypotheses concerning the origins of fever in the body, experts admit that the process is not well understood. Matthew J. Kluger, in *Fever: Its Biology, Evolution, and Function* (1979), claims that "the precise mechanism behind endogenous pyrogens' effect on the thermoregulatory set-point is unknown."

### TREATMENT AND THERAPY

The febrile response has been noted in five of the seven extant classes of vertebrates on earth (Agnatha, such as lampreys, and Chondrichthyes, such as sharks, are excluded). Scientists have determined that its function as a reaction to bacterial infection can be traced back as far as 400 million years in primitive bony fishes. The question of whether the natural phenomenon of fever actually aids in combating disease in the body, however, has not been fully resolved.

In ancient and medieval times, it was believed that fever served to "cook" and separate out one of the four essential body "humors"—blood, phlegm, yellow bile, and black bile—that had become excessively dominant. Throughout the centuries, such beliefs even caused some physicians to try to induce higher internal body temperatures as a means of treating disease. Use of modern antipyretic drugs to reduce fever remained unthinkable until the nineteenth century.

It was the German physician Carl von Liebermeister who, by the end of the nineteenth century, set some of the guidelines that are still generally observed in deciding whether antipyretic drugs should or should not be used to reduce a naturally occurring fever during illness. Liebermeister insisted that the phenomenon of fever was not one of body temperature gone "out of control," but rather a sign that the organism was regulating its own temperature. He also demonstrated that part of the process leading to increased internal temperature could be seen in reactions that

actually reduce heat loss at the body's surface, notably decreases in skin blood flow and evaporative cooling through perspiration. Liebermeister determined that one of the positive effects of higher temperatures inside the body was to impede the growth of harmful microorganisms. At the same time, however, other side effects of fever during illness were deemed to be negative, such as loss of appetite and, in some cases, actual degeneration of key internal organs. Liebermeister's generation of physicians, therefore, tended to rely on antipyretic drugs only when high fevers persisted for long periods of time. Moderate fevers or even high fevers, if they did not continue too long, were deemed to contribute to the overall process of natural body resistance to disease.

In fact, a limited school of physicians followed the teaching of 1927 Nobel laureate Julius Wagner-Jauregg, who claimed that "fever therapy" methods should be adopted for the treatment of certain diseases. Wagner-Jauregg himself had pioneered this theory by inoculating victims of neurosyphilis with fever-producing malaria. Part of his argument in favor of this experimental therapy was that malaria, with its accompanying fever, was a treatable disease (through the use of quinine) and could be controlled at regular intervals during its "service" as a fighter against a disease that still had no known cure. Later use of fever therapy for treatment of other sexually transmitted diseases, specifically gonorrhea, proved to be moderately successful. When typhoid vaccine was used to induce fevers in some patients, however, side effects such as hypotension (low blood pressure) or cardiovascular shock introduced what some considered to be dangerous risk factors. Nevertheless, certain fields of medicine, especially those involved with eye diseases and related eye ailments, have proved that fever-inducing agents (specifically those contained in typhoid and typhoid-paratyphoid vaccines) also induce beneficial secretion of the anti-inflammatory hormone cortisol.

By the second half of the twentieth century, the medical use of antipyretic drugs, containing such components as salicylates and indomethacin, had become widespread. This phenomenon was not caused by any compelling reversal of earlier general assumptions that moderate levels of fever, being a natural body reaction, were not necessarily harmful to patients suffering from a wide variety of diseases. Rather, physicians may have opted to use such drugs as much for their pain-relieving qualities as for their fever-reducing characteristics. Although patients receiving such drug treatment notice a diminishing of severe pains or general aching, the cause of the disease has not been combated merely by the removal of such symptoms as fever and pain.

Modern medical science has tended to support further study of particular circumstances in which induced fevers can actually produce disease-combating reactions. A newly emerging field by the late 1970's, for example, involved studying the benefits of higher temperatures in newborn infants fighting viral infections. Although specific circumstances and the nature of disease prevent a generalized conclusion in terms of the use of induced fevers as a form of treatment, researchers have shown that an elevated body temperature serves to increase the speed at which white blood cells, the body's natural enemies against disease, move to infected areas.

## PERSPECTIVE AND PROSPECTS

Although doctors have been aware of the symptoms of fever since the beginnings of medical history, centuries passed before its importance as an indicator of disease was accepted. A certain degree of sophistication in the study of fevers became possible largely as a result of the development of the common thermometer, in a rudimentary form in the seventeenth century and then with greater technical accuracy in the eighteenth century. Systematic use of the thermometer in the eighteenth century enabled doctors to observe such phenomena as morning remission and evening peaking of fever intensity. Studies involving the recording of temperature in healthy individuals also yielded important discoveries. One such discovery was made in 1774, when use of the thermometer showed that, even in a room heated to the boiling point of water (100 degrees Celsius), healthy subjects maintained an internal body heat that was very close to the normal 37-degree level.

Medical reports as late as the end of the eighteenth century, however, indicate that even internationally recognized pioneers of science were still not close to understanding the causes of fever. The English doctor John Hunter, for example, declared himself opposed to the prevailing view that rising body heat came from the circulation of warmer blood throughout the body. Hunter suspected that the warmth was produced by an entirely different agent that was independent of the circulatory system. He never learned what that agent might be, however, and failed in defense of his theory that the source of added body heat was in the stomach. Even the famous French chemist Antoine-Laurent Lavoisier erred when he tried to explain fever in terms of some form of chemical "combustion" involving hydrogen and carbon. Lavoisier identified the lungs as the possible location for this spontaneous production of internal body heat.

Although these theories were identified as erroneous, the late eighteenth and early nineteenth centuries left one legacy that would develop into the twentieth century and is still practiced by physicians: systematic thermometry. In essence, thermometry involves the tracing of the upward or downward direction of fever during illness in order to judge the course of the disease and the effects brought about by different stages of treatment. In many diseases, for example, clinical records of the full course of previous cases can be studied by doctors responsible for treating an individual patient. With thermometry, the doctor is able to determine how far the body's struggle against a certain disease has progressed. If thermometry shows a marked departure from what clinical records have charted as the normal course of disease under certain forms of treatment, then the physician may look for signs of another disease. —*Byron D. Cannon*

**See also** Bacterial infections; Common cold; Heat exhaustion and heat stroke; Hyperthermia and hypothermia; Influenza; Rheumatic fever; Scarlet fever; Typhoid fever and typhus; Viral infections; Yellow fever; *specific diseases.*

## FOR FURTHER INFORMATION:

Brengelmann, George L. "Temperature Regulation." In *Physiology and Biophysics*, edited by T. C. Ruch and H. D. Patton. Philadelphia: W. B. Saunders, 1973. A general overview of the phenomenon of fever. Focuses more attention on the mechanism causing temperature change in the body than on the effects of this change on body functions.

Johnson, F. H., et al. *The Kinetic Basis of Molecular Biology*. New York: John Wiley & Sons, 1954. Although this basic text does not deal specifically with the phenomenon of fever, one needs to consult a general study of the effects of increased temperature on the essential functions that occur inside the body.

Kluger, Matthew J. *Fever: Its Biology, Evolution, and Function*. Princeton, N.J.: Princeton University Press, 1979. An accessible book-length study of the phenomenon of fever. Although some parts of the discussion are more technical in nature, the general level is comprehensible.

Myers, R. D., and T. L. Yaksh. "Thermoregulation Around a New 'Set-Point' Established in the Monkey by Altering the Ratio of Sodium to Calcium Ions Within the Hypothalamus." *Journal of Physiology* 218 (1971): 609-633. A somewhat specialized discussion of one of the key aspects of fever—the set point—covered in a general way.

Snell, E. S., and E. Atkins. "The Mechanisms of Fever." In *The Biological Basis of Medicine*, edited by E. Edward Bittar and Neville Bittar. New York: Academic Press, 1968. A concise review of the processes of fever. The level of technical detail and theory is comparable to that in Matthew Kluger's more recent and much longer monographic study (above).

## FIBROCYSTIC BREAST DISEASE. *See* BREAST DISORDERS.

## FOOD POISONING

**SYSTEM AFFECTED:** Gastrointestinal

**SPECIALISTS:** Epidemiologists, gastroenterologists, public health specialists, toxicologists

**DEFINITION:** Food-borne illness caused by bacteria, viruses, or parasites consumed in food and resulting in acute gastrointestinal disturbance that may include diarrhea, nausea, vomiting, and abdominal discomfort.

**KEY TERMS:**

*contamination:* infection of a food item by a pathogen

*foodborne infection:* disease caused by eating foods contaminated by infectious microorganisms, with onset occurring within twenty-four hours (for example, *Salmonella*)

*foodborne intoxication:* disease caused by eating foods containing microorganisms that produce toxins, with onset occurring within six hours (for example, botulism)

*microorganism:* an organism which is too small to be seen with the naked eye

*parasite:* an organism which lives on another organism (the host) and causes harm to the host while it benefits

*pathogen:* a disease-causing organism

*thermal death point:* the lowest temperature that can destroy a foodborne organism

## CAUSES AND SYMPTOMS

Often a person feeling the symptoms of nausea, vomiting, diarrhea, and abdominal discomfort assumes that he or she has contracted influenza. The presence of a true influenza virus, however, is uncommon. More likely, these symptoms are caused by eating food that contains undesirable bacteria, viruses, or parasites. This is called foodborne illness, or food poisoning. Most foodborne pathogens are colorless, odorless, and tasteless. Fortunately, there are recommendations based on scientific principles to help prevent foodborne illness.

Food poisoning is a worldwide problem. In developing countries, diarrhea is a factor in child malnutrition and is estimated to cause 3.5 million deaths per year. Despite advances in modern technology, foodborne illness is a major problem in developed countries as well. In the United States, an estimated 24 million cases of foodborne diarrheal disease occur each year, which means that about one out of ten people experience a food-associated illness in a given year.

Certain foods, particularly foods with a high protein and moisture content, provide an ideal environment for the multiplication of pathogens. The foods with high risk in the United States are raw shellfish (especially mollusks), underdone poultry, raw eggs, rare meats, raw milk, and cooked food that another person handled before it was packaged and chilled. In addition to those foods listed, some developing countries could add raw vegetables, raw fruits that cannot be peeled, foods from sidewalk vendors, and tap water or water from unknown sources. Most of the documented cases of foodborne illness are caused by only a few bacteria, viruses, and parasites.

Bacteria known as *Salmonella* are ingested by humans in contaminated foods such as beef, poultry, and eggs; they may also be transmitted by kitchen utensils and the hands of people who have handled infected food or utensils. Once the bacteria are inside the body, the incubation time is from eight to twenty-four hours. Since the bacteria multiply inside the body and attack the gastrointestinal tract, this disease is known as a true food infection. The main symptoms are diarrhea, abdominal cramps, and vomiting. The bacteria are killed by cooking foods to the well-done stage.

The major foodborne intoxication in the United States is caused by eating food contaminated with the toxin of *Staphylococcus* bacteria. Because the toxin or poison has already been produced in the food item that is ingested, the onset of symptoms is usually very rapid (between one-half hour and six hours). Improperly stored or cooked foods (particularly meats, tuna, and potato salad) are the main carriers of these bacteria. Since this toxin cannot be killed by reheating the food items to a high temperature, it is important that foods are properly stored.

Botulism is a rare food poisoning caused by the toxin of *Clostridium botulinim*. It is anaerobic, meaning that it multiplies in environments without oxygen, and is mainly found in improperly home-canned food items. Originally one of the sources of the disease was from eating sausages (the Latin word for which is *botulus*)—hence, the name "botulism." A very small amount of toxin, the size of a grain of salt, could kill hundreds of people within an hour. Danger signs include double vision and difficulty swallowing and breathing.

Though everyone is at risk for foodborne illness, certain groups of people develop more severe symptoms and are at a greater risk for serious illness and death. Higher-risk groups include pregnant women, very young children, the elderly, and immunocompromised individuals, such as patients with acquired immunodeficiency syndrome (AIDS) and cancer.

Bacteria known as *Listeria* were first documented in 1981 as being transmitted by food. Most people are at low risk of becoming ill after ingesting these bacteria; however, pregnant women are at high risk. *Listeria* infection is rare in the United States, but it does cause serious illness. It is associated with consumption of raw (unpasteurized) milk, nonreheated hot dogs, undercooked chicken, various soft cheeses (Mexican style, feta, Brie, Camembert, and blue-veined cheese), and food purchased from delicatessen counters. *Listeria* cause a short-term illness in pregnant women; however, this bacteria can cause stillbirths and spontaneous abortions. A parasite called *Toxoplasma gondii* is also of particular risk for pregnant women. For this reason, raw or very rare meat should not be eaten. (In addition, since cats may shed these parasites in their feces, it is recommended that pregnant women avoid cleaning cat litter boxes.)

As the protective antibodies from the mother are lost, infants become more susceptible to food poisoning. Botulism generally occurs by ingesting the toxin or poison; however, in infant botulism it is the spores that germinate and produce the toxin within the intestinal tract of the infant. Since honey and corn syrup have been found to contain spores, it is recommended that they not be fed to infants under one year of age, especially those under six months.

Determining whether a disease is caused by a foodborne organism is highly skilled work. The Centers for Disease Control (CDC) in Atlanta, Georgia, investigate diseases and their causes. It has been estimated that the true incidence of foodborne illness in the United States is ten to one hundred times greater than that reported to the CDC. The CDC report some of the more interesting cases and outbreaks in narrative form in the *Morbidity and Mortality Weekly Report*.

### TREATMENT AND THERAPY

In cases of severe food poisoning marked by vomiting, diarrhea, or collapse—especially in cases of botulism and ingestion of poisonous plant material such as suspicious mushrooms—emergency medical attention should be sought immediately, and, if possible, specimens of the suspected food should be submitted for analysis. Identifying the source of the food is especially important if that source is a public venue such as a restaurant, because stemming a widespread outbreak of food poisoning may thereby be possible. In less severe cases of food poisoning, the victim should rest, eat nothing, but drink fluids that contain some salt and sugar; the person should begin to recover after several hours or one or two days and should see a doctor if not well after two or three days.

The best "treatment" for food poisoning is prevention. While there is ample information regarding the prevention of food poisoning, many outbreaks still occur as a result of carelessness in the kitchen. Good food safety is basically good common sense, yet it can only make sense when one has acquired some knowledge of how foodborne pathogens spread and how to apply food safety steps to prevent foodborne illness. Based on the research literature, as well as on the suggestions made by the World Health Organization (WHO) and other groups, the recommendations are to cook foods well, to prevent cross-contamination, and to keep hot foods hot and cold foods cold.

Cooking foods well means cooking them to a high enough temperature in the slowest-to-heat part and for a long enough time to destroy pathogens that have already gained access to foods. Cooking foods well is only a concern when they have become previously contaminated from other sources or are naturally contaminated. There are a number of possible sources of contamination of food products.

Coastal water may contaminate seafood. Filter-feeding marine animals (such as clams, scallops, oysters, cockles, and mussels) and some fish (such as anchovies, sardines, and herring) live by pumping in sea water and sifting out organisms that they need for food. Therefore, they have the ability to concentrate suspended material by many orders of magnitude. Shellfish grown in contaminated coastal waters are the most frequent carriers of a virus called hepatitis A.

Contaminated eggs can be another vehicle of foodborne illness. Contamination of eggs can occur from external as well as internal sources. If moist conditions are present and there is a crack in the shell, the fecal material of hens carrying the microorganism can penetrate the shell and membrane of the egg and can multiply. In the early 1990's, *Salmonella enteritidis* began to appear in the intact egg, particularly in the northeastern part of the United States. It is hypothesized that contamination occurs in the oviduct of the hen before the egg is laid. Food vehicles in which *Salmonella enteritidis* has been reported include sandwiches dipped in eggs and cooked, hollandaise sauce, eggs Benedict, commercial frozen pasta with raw egg and cheese stuffing, Caesar salad dressing, and blended food in which cross-contamination had occurred. Foods such as cookie or cake dough or homemade ice cream made with raw eggs are other possible vehicles of foodborne illness.

Milk, especially raw milk, can be contaminated. Sources of milk contaminants could be an unhealthy cow (such as from mastitis, a major infection of the mammary gland of the dairy cow) or unclean methods of milking, such as not cleaning the teats well before attaching them to the milker or unclean utensils (milking tanks). If milk is not cooled fast enough, contaminants can multiply.

Modern mechanized milking procedures have reduced but not eliminated foodborne pathogens. Postpasteurization contamination may occur, especially if bulk tanks or equipment have not been properly cleaned and sanitized. In 1985 in Chicago, one of the largest salmonellosis outbreaks occurred, with the causal food being pasteurized milk. More than sixteen thousand people were infected, and ten died. A small connecting piece in the milk tank which allowed milk and microorganisms to collect was determined to be the source of the contamination. Bulk tanks should be properly maintained and piping should be inspected regularly for opportunities for raw milk to contaminate the pasteurized product.

Recommendations for cooking temperatures are not only based on the temperature required to kill foodborne pathogens but also on aesthetics and palatability. Generally, a margin of safety is built into the cooking temperature because of the possibility of nonuniform heating. Based on generally accepted temperature requirements, cooking red meat until 71 degrees Celsius (160 degrees Fahrenheit) will reach the thermal death point. Hamburger should be well cooked so that it is medium-brown inside. If pressed, it should feel firm and the juices that run out should be clear. Cooking poultry to the well-done stage is done for palatability. Tenderness is indicated when there is a flexible hip joint, and juices should run clear and not pink when the meat is pierced with a fork. Fish should be cooked until it loses its translucent appearance and flakes when pierced with a fork. Eggs should be thoroughly cooked until the yolk is thickened and the white is firm, not runny. Cooked or chilled foods that are served hot (that is, leftovers) should be reheated so that they come to a rolling boil.

Cross-contamination occurs when microorganisms are transmitted from humans, cutting boards, and utensils to food. Contamination between foods, especially from raw meat and poultry to fresh vegetables or other ready-to-eat foods, is a major problem.

One of the best ways to prevent cross-contamination is simply washing one's hands with soap and water. Twenty seconds is the minimum time span that should be spent washing one's hands. In order to prevent the spread of disease, it is also recommended that the hands be dried with a paper towel, which is then thrown away. Thoroughly washed hands can still be a source of bacteria, however, so one should use tongs and spoons when cooking to prevent contamination.

It is especially important to wash one's hands after certain activities, such as blowing the nose or sneezing, using the lavatory, diapering a baby, smoking, petting animals or pets, and before cooking or handling food.

Other sources of cross-contamination include utensils and cutting surfaces. If people use the same knife and cutting board to cut up raw chicken for a stir-fry and peaches for a fruit salad, they are putting themselves at great risk for foodborne illness. The bacteria on the cutting board and the knife could cross-contaminate the peaches. While the chicken will be cooked until it is well done, the peaches in the salad will not be. In this situation, one could cut the fruit first and then the chicken, and then wash and sanitize the knife and cutting board.

Cleaning and sanitizing is actually a two-step process. Cleaning involves using soap and water and a scrubber or dishcloth to remove the major debris from the surface. The second step, sanitizing, involves using a diluted chloride solution to kill bacteria and viruses.

Wooden cutting boards are the worst offenders in terms of causing cross-contamination. Since bacteria and viruses are small, they can adhere to and grow in the grooves of a wooden cutting board and spread to other foods when the cutting board is used again. Use of a plastic or acrylic cutting board prevents this problem.

The danger zone in which bacteria can multiply is a range of 4.4 degrees Celsius (40 degrees Fahrenheit) to 60 degrees Celsius (140 degrees Fahrenheit). Room temperature is generally right in the middle of this danger zone. The danger zone is critical because, even though they cannot be seen, bacteria are increasing in number. They can double and even quadruple in fifteen to thirty minutes. Consequently, perishable foods such as meats, poultry, fish, milk, cooked rice, leftover pizza, hard-cooked eggs, leftover refried beans, and potato salad should not be left in the danger zone for more than two hours. Keeping hot foods hot means keeping them at a temperature higher than 60 degrees Celsius. Keeping cold foods cold means keeping them at a temperature lower than 4.4 degrees Celsius.

Other rules are helpful for preventing contamination. When shopping, the grocery store should be the last stop so that foods are not stored in a hot car. When meal time is over, leftovers should be placed in the refrigerator or freezer as soon as possible. When packing for a picnic, food items should be kept in an ice chest to keep them cold or brought slightly frozen. Much serious illness and death could be prevented if such food safety rules were followed.

### Perspective and Prospects

When the lifestyle of people changed from a hunting-and-gathering society to a more agrarian one, the need to preserve food from spoilage was necessary for survival. As early as 3000 B.C., salt was used as a meat preservative and the production of cheese had begun in the Near East. The production of wine and the preservation of fish by smoking also was introduced at that time. Even though throughout history people had tried many methods to preserve foods and keep them from spoiling, the relationship between illness and pathogens or toxins in food was not recognized and documented until 1857. It was then that the French chemist Louis Pasteur demonstrated that the microorganisms in raw milk caused spoilage.

Stories from the American Civil War (1860-1865) demonstrate the problems of institutional feeding of many people for long periods of time. Gastrointestinal diseases were rampant during that time period. During the first year of the war, of the people who had diarrhea and dysentery, the morbidity rate was 640 per 1,000 and increased to 995 per 1,000 in 1862. More men died of disease and illness than were killed in battle.

Food can be contaminated by disease-causing organisms at any step of the food-handling chain, from the farm to the table. An important role of government and industry is to ensure a safe food supply. In the United States, setting and monitoring of food safety standards are the responsibility of the Food and Drug Administration (FDA) under the auspices of the U.S. Department of Health and Human Services and the Food Safety and Inspection Service (FSIS) under the auspices of the U.S. Department of Agriculture (USDA). The FDA is responsible for the wholesomeness of all food sold in interstate commerce, except meat and poultry, while the USDA is responsible for the inspection of meat and poultry sold in interstate commerce and internationally. Some major food safety laws and policies that have guided the provision of safe food are the Federal Food and Drugs Act in 1906; the Federal Meat Inspection Act in 1906-1907; the Food, Drug, and Cosmetic Act in 1938; and the Poultry Products Inspection Act in 1957. The food supply in the United States has been credited as being among the safest in the world.

Historically, the diseases of tuberculosis, scarlet fever, strep throat, typhoid fever, and diphtheria have been associated with raw or unpasteurized milk. The reporting of foodborne illness was initiated in the 1920's by the U.S.

Public Health Service (USPHS) when annual summaries of milkborne-disease outbreaks were recorded and reported. Later, reports of waterborne and foodborne diseases were added.

The public attitude about what is hazardous in the food supply and that of the FDA have often differed. The public generally believes that the safety of additives and chemical contaminants in food is of a higher priority than that of the microbiological and nutritional hazards—the exact opposite of the FDA's priorities. (For example, in the mid-1980's, the story about Alar, a chemical used to slow the ripening of apples, represented a very emotional topic. There was particular concern about the risks that this chemical might pose to children who ate large amounts of apple products.) As more reliable information is available about both areas of concern, the situation regarding priorities is likely to change. —*Martha M. Henze*

*See also* Alcoholism; Appendicitis; Diarrhea and dysentery; Gangrene; Gastrointestinal disorders; Indigestion; Intestinal disorders; Intoxication; Lead poisoning; Legionnaires' disease; Nausea and vomiting; Poisoning; Ulcers.

**FOR FURTHER INFORMATION:**

Cliver, Dean O., ed. *Foodborne Diseases*. San Diego: Academic Press, 1990. An exceptional college textbook providing chapters written by experts in the field. This important work provides not only background information but also in-depth reference information on the most common foodborne pathogens.

Jay, James Monroe. *Modern Food Microbiology*. 4th ed. New York: Van Nostrand Reinhold, 1992. This excellent textbook summarizes the current state of knowledge of the biology and epidemiology of the microorganisms that cause foodborne illness.

Jensen, Lloyd B. *Poisoning Misadventures*. Springfield, Ill.: Charles C Thomas, 1970. This book conveys, in a light narrative form, some of Jensen's personal observations of food poisonings in military camp and on the battlefield and of litigation in the courtroom. The anecdotes from the Civil War, as well as excerpts from medieval documents, provide interesting stories.

Lefferts, Lisa Y., and Stephen Schmidt. "The Safe Food Kitchen." *Nutrition Action Healthletter* 18 (September, 1991): 8-9. Published by the Center for Science in the Public Interest. This article, written for the general public, gives easy-to-follow food safety recommendations. Includes a section of precautions for microwave cooking.

Longree, Karla, and Gertrude Armbruster. *Quantity Food Sanitation*. 4th ed. New York: John Wiley & Sons, 1987. An excellent reference guide on food safety for quantity cooking in institutions such as hospitals and restaurants.

# FOOT DISORDERS

**SYSTEMS AFFECTED:** Muscular, skeletal
**SPECIALISTS:** Orthopedic surgeons, podiatrists

**DEFINITION:** Disorders involving the muscles, bones, nerves, or skin of the feet.

Because of the constant and heavy use of feet by humans as bipeds, they are prone to many problems. In spite of what is commonly believed, most cases of foot bone and joint abnormalities are developmental in origin instead of being caused by poorly fitting footwear.

*Developmental, muscle, and bone disorders of the feet.* Clubfoot, also called talipes, is one of the developmental, or congenital, disorders affecting the feet. It occurs in approximately 1 of every 1,000 live human births and is characterized by deformities such as the foot turning down and under, such that a child will walk on the top of his or her foot. Over time, tendon and ligament contraction reinforces the deformity; thus, either casting or surgery is needed for realignment.

Flat foot, or pes planus, is an abnormally flat arch in the foot, accompanied by a characteristic gait, both of which can occur in varying degrees. Muscle weakness, incorrect weight-bearing, a short Achilles tendon, and developmental defects may all contribute to this deformity. Flat foot may or may not produce a pathologic condition such as arthritis.

A bunion is the relocation of bone from the first metatarsal to the inner portion of the joint connecting it to the big toe. This prominence at the base of the big toe makes the soft tissue in the area subject to pressure from footwear, causing swelling and pain in the protective sac above the metatarsophalangeal joint in a condition called bursitis. Cortisone injections may relieve symptoms, but surgery is required in extreme cases to realign the first metatarsal. Flatfoot usually accompanies bunions and is a factor in their development.

Muscular imbalances inherent in the foot are the reason for the curvature of the individual bones of the toes. Abnormally curved bones produce hammertoe, or claw toe, which usually requires little treatment other than a padding of the shoes to avoid corn or callus development. Excessive muscle tension at the heel can produce bony growths called heel spurs or calcaneal exostoses. Inflammation may develop in a neighboring joint's bursa, causing a throbbing pain.

Apophysitis of the calcaneus or heel bone can occur in childhood while the heel is still in the process of fusing from two bones. Injury can result because the connecting, softer cartilage between the two bones has not yet been replaced with bone. This affliction usually disappears as a child grows.

*Nerve and skin disorders of the feet.* Factors including footwear, the structures of the foot itself, and harmful external forces acting on the foot may all contribute to the irritation and/or damage to the nerves of the foot. Morton's neuroma is the thickening of the nerve located between the metatarsals of the third and fourth toes, followed by the formation of a small benign tumor. Painful burning, numbness, or tingling sensations may be alleviated by wearing

## Common Foot Disorders

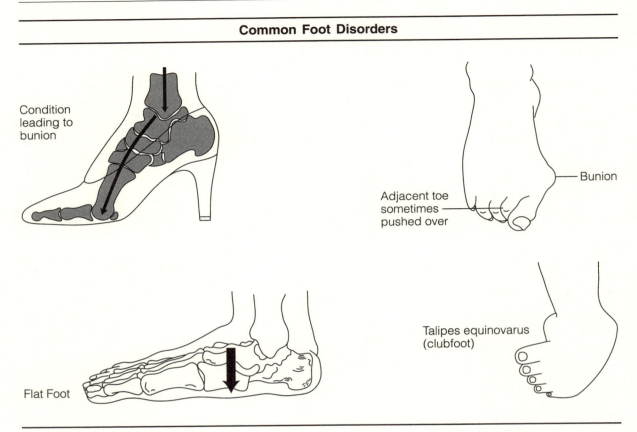

Condition leading to bunion

Bunion

Adjacent toe sometimes pushed over

Flat Foot

Talipes equinovarus (clubfoot)

more comfortable footwear or by the surgical removal of the tumor. Tarsal tunnel syndrome occurs when a nerve traveling along the bottom of the foot through a channel called the tarsal canal becomes compressed and damaged. Cortisone injections into this canal can relieve pressure on the nerve, and surgery can be used to treat severe cases.

The skin of the foot is subject to much pressure and rubbing; thus, it responds by producing changes, termed dermatologic disorders, which themselves cause pain. A corn, or heloma, is a small, sharply defined, raised area of thickened skin containing much of the fibrous protein called keratin. Calluses are also composed of keratin but are flatter and do not possess the defined borders of corns. Both types of thickened keratinized skin are usually attributed to incorrect positioning of the underlying bone.

Warts, or verrucae, are actually skin tumors caused by the human Papillomavirus. They occur most commonly on the sole of the foot, where they are named plantar warts. Warts can be transmitted from person to person, and the lymphatic communication between warts within an individual explains their ability to spread. Warts on the foot are invariably benign, however, and should not be treated with X-ray or radium therapy lest the surrounding areas undergo change themselves and eventually produce tumors.

Dermatitis venenata is often caused by chemicals used in the binding or dyeing of shoes. Angiokeratoma is a lesion on the bottom of the foot commonly mistaken for a wart. Fibroma is the name of the benign growth that may spread under the toenails as a result of insect bites in the vicinity or manifestations of other skin diseases.

Ingrown toenails, or onychocryptoses, occur when the free end of the toenail penetrates the surrounding soft tissue. Reasons for this painful disorder are commonly badly fitted footwear, nail disease, and foot or nail structural abnormalities.

*Systemic diseases affecting the feet.* Rheumatoid arthritis is a condition involving connective tissue, unknown in origin, in which the synovial membrane of joints proliferates while invading and even destroying cartilage and bone. Women acquire this disease three times more often than do men. Steroid hormones are sometimes applied to aid in the treatment of rheumatoid arthritis, but gold salt injection is the only therapy resulting in a permanent cure. The chances of a cure are greater when this disease occurs in children. The condition is then known as juvenile rheumatoid arthritis, or Still's disease.

Several normally fatal diseases may accompany rheumatoid arthritis. Systemic lupus erythematosus can be masked by the arthritic condition until inflammation spreads to small arteries of the body's organs. Polyarteritis nodosa also involves arteries throughout the body, and its true diagnosis may be prevented by the misleading arthritic condition. Scleroderma involves the thickening of the skin on the face, hands, and feet; depigmentation; loss of hair; and lesions. Sarcoidosis manifests itself in the hands and feet and causes microscopic lesions in the bone that eventually become visible by X-ray examination. Schoenlein-Henoch syndrome is an allergic reaction which can resemble the synovitis of rheumatic fever.

Rheumatic fever affects fibrous tissues in a widespread fashion involving the joints and later the heart. It is related to streptococcal infections and occurs as a migrating arthritis producing no lasting joint damage in the feet, but it can cause permanent damage to the cardiac valve. Osteoarthritis causes the degeneration of cartilage and the overgrowth of bone surfaces. The effects of this condition are limited to the joints, unlike rheumatoid arthritis, which can spread to nearby cartilage and bone. Staphylococci, streptococci, and coliform bacteria are the infective agents involved in pyogenic arthritis. In this condition, the organism is carried by the blood to the joint interior. Ulcers of the feet may be caused by a variety of conditions including diabetes mellitus, syphilis, anemia, and leprosy.

If there is sustained pain in the foot or ankle with no known cause such as injury, a continuously low leukocyte count, and negative laboratory tests for the presence of bacteria, then a viral infection is likely present. An elevated leukocyte count is often indicative of a bacterial infection.
—*Ryan C. Horst and Roman J. Miller*

*See also* Athlete's foot; Birth defects; Fracture and dislocation; Frostbite; Fungal infections; Warts.

## FRACTURE AND DISLOCATION

**SYSTEMS AFFECTED:** Joints, skeletal

**SPECIALISTS:** Emergency physicians, orthopedic surgeons

**DEFINITION:** A fracture is a break in a bone, which may be partial or complete; a dislocation is the forceful separation of bones in a joint.

**KEY TERMS:**

*anesthesia:* a state characterized by loss of sensation, caused by or resulting from the pharmacological depression of normal nerve function

*callus:* a hard, bonelike substance made by osteocytes which is found in and around the ends of a fractured bone; it temporarily maintains bony alignment and is resorbed after complete healing or union of a fracture occurs

*ecchymosis:* a purplish patch on the skin caused by bleeding; the spots are easily visible to the naked eye

*embolus:* an obstruction or occlusion of a vessel (most commonly, an artery or vein) caused by a transported blood clot, vegetation, mass of bacteria, or other foreign material

*epiphysis:* the part of a long bone from which growth or elongation occurs

*instability:* excessive mobility of two or more bones caused by damage to ligaments, the joint capsule, or fracture of one or more bones

*ischemia:* a local anemia or area of diminished or insufficient blood supply due to mechanical obstruction, commonly narrowing of an artery, of the blood supply

*osteoblast:* a bone-forming cell

*osteocyte:* a bone cell

*paralysis:* the loss of power of voluntary movement or other function of a muscle as a result of disease or injury to its nerve supply

*petechiae:* minute spots caused by hemorrhage or bleeding into the skin; the spots are the size of pinheads

*prone:* the position of the body when face downward, on one's stomach and abdomen

*pulse:* the rhythmical dilation of an artery, produced by the increased volume of blood forced into the vessel by the contraction of the heart

*transection:* a partial or complete severance of the spinal cord

### CAUSES AND SYMPTOMS

A fracture is a linear deformation or discontinuity of a bone produced by the application of a force that exceeds the modulus of elasticity (ability to bend) of a bone. Normal bones require excessive force to fracture. Bones may be weakened by disease or other pathology such as a tumor or tumor-related disease that reduces their ability to withstand an impact. Bones respond to stresses made upon them and can thus be strengthened through physical conditioning and made more resistant to fracture. This is a normal part of training in many athletic activities.

Fractures are classified according to the type of break or, more correctly, by the plane or surface that is fractured. A break that is at a right angle to the axis of the bone is called transverse. A fracture that is similar but at an angle, rather than perpendicular to the main axis of the bone, is called oblique. If a twisting force is applied, the break may be spiral, or twisted. A comminuted fracture is a break that results in two or more fragments of bone. If the pieces of bone remain in their original positions, the fracture is undisplaced. In a displaced fracture, the portions of bone are not properly aligned.

If bones do not penetrate the skin, the fracture is called closed, or simple. When bones protrude through the skin, the result is an open, or compound, fracture. Other types of fractures are associated with pathologic or disease processes. A stress fracture results from repeated stress or trauma to the same site of a bone. None of the individual stresses is sufficient to cause a break. If these stresses cause a callus to form, the bone will be strengthened and actual separation of fragments will not occur. A pathologic fracture occurs at the site of a tumor, infection, or other bone dis-

## Types of Fracture

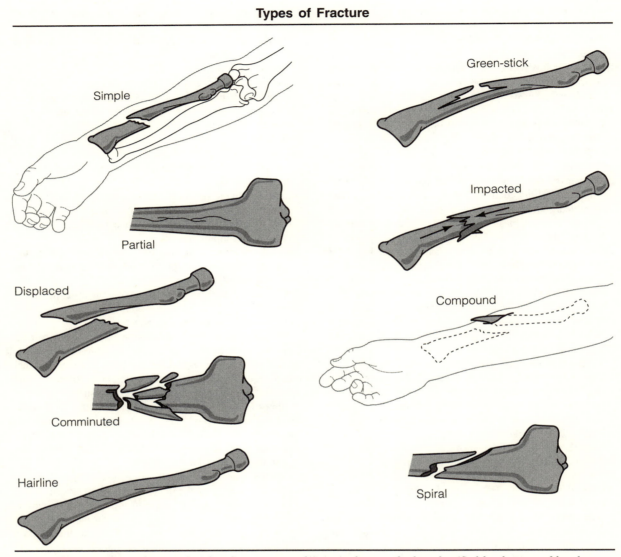

*All fractures are either simple (closed) or compound (open); they are further classified by the type of break.*

ease. A compression fracture results when bone is crushed; the force applied is greater than the ability of the bone to withstand it. A green-stick fracture is an incomplete separation of bone.

The diagnosis of a fracture is based on several criteria: instability, pain, swelling, deformity, and ecchymosis. The most reliable diagnostic criterion is instability. Pain is not universally present at a fracture site. Swelling may be delayed and occur at some time after a fracture is sustained. Deformity is obvious with open fractures but may not be apparent with other, undisplaced breaks.

Ecchymosis is a purplish patch caused by bleeding into skin; it will not be present if blood vessels are not broken.

A definitive diagnosis is made with two plane film X rays taken at the site of a fracture and at right angles to each other. If the fracture site is visually examined and palpated shortly after the injury occurs, an accurate tentative diagnosis may be made; this should be confirmed with X rays as soon as is convenient. Occasionally, an X ray will not show undisplaced or chip fractures. If a patient experiences symptoms of pain, swelling, or ecchymosis but has a negative X ray for fracture, the site should be immobilized and X-rayed again in two to three weeks.

Fractures occur most commonly in extremities: arms or legs. Such fractures must be evaluated to determine if injuries have occurred to other tissues such as nerves or blood vessels. The presence of bruising or ecchymosis indicates blood vessel damage. The existence of peripheral pulses indicates that arteries are not injured. Venous flow is more difficult to evaluate. For a relatively short period of time, however, venous bleeding may be of lesser importance and thereby tolerated.

Neurologic functioning may be assessed by the ability of the patient to contract muscles or sense skin touches or pinpricks. Temporary immobilization may be necessary before nerve status can be evaluated accurately.

An open fracture creates a direct pathway between the skin surface and underlying tissues. If the site becomes contaminated by bacteria, an opportunity for osteomyelitis (infection of the bone) is created. Inadequate treatment by the initial surgeon may result in skin loss, delayed union, loss of joint mobility, osteomyelitis, and even amputation.

Skin damage may or may not be related to a fracture. When skin integrity is broken over or near a fracture site, bone involvement must be assumed. The problem is infection of the fracture site; appropriate antibiotics are normally administered. If skin damage is extensive, final surgical reduction of the underlying fracture may have to be delayed until the skin is healed.

Delayed union refers to the inability of a fractured bone to heal. This is a potentially serious problem, as normal stability is not possible as long as a fracture exists. Joints may not function normally in the presence of a fracture. If a fracture heals improperly, bones may be misaligned and cause pain with movement, leading to limitations of motion. If the bones are affected by osteomyelitis, the infection may spread to the joint capsule and reduce the normal range of motion for the bones or the joint. Amputation may become necessary if infection becomes extensive in the area of a fracture. An infection which becomes firmly established in bones or spreads widely into adjacent muscle tissue may lead to cellulitis or gangrene and may compromise a portion of an extremity. Amputation may be performed if the pathologic process cannot be treated with antibiotics.

Adequate blood supply to tissues is critical for survival. In an extremity, the maximum time limit for complete ischemia (lack of blood flow) is six to eight hours; after that time, the likelihood of later amputation increases. Pain, pallor, pulselessness, and paralysis are indicators of impaired circulation associated with a fracture. When two of these signs are present, the possibility of vascular damage must be thoroughly explored.

Dislocations occur at joints and are caused by an applied force that is greater than the strength of the ligaments and muscles that keep a joint intact. The result is a stretching deformity or injury to a joint and abnormal movement of a bone out of the joint. Accidental trauma, commonly the result of an athletic injury or automobile accident, is the most common cause of a dislocation. Joints that are frequently dislocated include the shoulder and digits (fingers

and toes). Dislocations of the ankle and hip are infrequent but serious; they require immediate management. Dislocations may accompany fractures, but the two injuries need not occur together.

When dislocations are reduced, the bones of the joint are returned to normal position. Reduction is accomplished by relaxing adjacent muscles and applying traction or a pulling force to the bone until it returns to its normal position in the joint. For most dislocations of the shoulder, the victim lies in a prone position and the dislocated arm hangs down freely. Gradual traction is applied until reduction occurs. This can be accomplished by bandaging a pail to the arm and slowly filling it with water. Alternatively, a heavy book can be held by the victim and the muscles of the arm allowed to relax until the dislocation is reduced. Such treatments are usually reserved for situations in which medical assistance is unavailable. Digits are reduced in a similar manner, by gentle pulling of the end of the finger or toe. Ankle and hip dislocations are potentially more serious because these joints are more complex and have extensive blood supplies. Reduction of dislocated ankles and hips should be undertaken by qualified medical personnel in an expedited manner.

After reduction, all dislocations should be evaluated by competent medical personnel. With dislocated digits, later damage is relatively unlikely but can occur because of ligament damage sustained in the initial injury. Dislocations of the shoulder may be accompanied by a fracture of the clavicle or collar bone and may involve nerve damage in the shoulder joint. Dislocations of the ankle and hip may lead

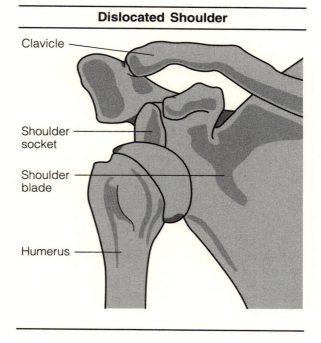

**Dislocated Shoulder**

Clavicle

Shoulder socket

Shoulder blade

Humerus

to avascular necrosis (damage to the bone as a result of inadequate blood supply) if not evaluated and reduced promptly.

## TREATMENT AND THERAPY

Fractures are usually treated by reduction and immobilization. Reduction, which refers to the process of returning the fractured bones to normal position, may be either closed or open. Closed reduction is accomplished without surgery by manipulating the broken bone through overlying skin and muscles. Open reduction requires surgical intervention in which the broken pieces are exposed and returned to normal position. Orthopedic appliances may be used to hold the bones in correct position. The most common of these appliances are pins and screws, but metal plates and wires may also be employed. Orthopedic appliances are usually made of stainless steel. These may be left in the body indefinitely or may be surgically removed after healing is complete. Local anesthesia is usually used with closed reductions; open reductions are performed in an operating room, under sterile conditions using general anesthesia.

Immobilization is generally accomplished by the use of a cast. Casts are often made of plaster, but they may be constructed of inflatable plastic. It is important to hold bones in a rigid, fixed position for a sufficient length of time for the broken ends to unite and heal. The cast must be loose enough, however, to allow blood to circulate. Padding is usually put in place before plaster is applied to form a cast. Whenever possible, the newly immobilized body part is elevated to reduce the chance of swelling in the cast, which would compromise the blood supply to the fracture site and body portion beyond the cast. Casts should be checked periodically to ensure that they do not impair circulation.

The broken bone and accompanying body part must be placed in an anatomically neutral position. This is done to minimize postfracture disability and improve the prospect for rehabilitation. The length of time that a fractured bone is immobilized is highly variable and dependent on a number of factors.

Traction may also be used to immobilize a fracture. Traction is the external application of force to overcome muscular resistance and hold bones in a desired position. Commonly, holes are drilled through bones and pins are inserted; the ends of these pins extend through the surface of the skin. Part of the body is fixed in position through the use of a strap or weights, and wires are attached to the pins in the body part to be stretched. Weights or tension is applied to the wires until the broken bone parts move into the desired position. Traction is maintained until healing has occurred.

Individual ends of a single fractured bone are sometimes held in position by external pins and screws. Holes are drilled through the bone, and pins are inserted. The pins on opposite sides of the fracture site are then attached to each other with threaded rods and locked in position by nuts. This process allows a fractured bone to be immobilized without using a cast.

Fractures of different bones require different amounts of time to heal. Further, age is a factor in fracture healing. Fractures in young children heal more quickly than do broken bones in adults. Older adults typically require even more time for healing. The availability of calcium and other nutrients also affects the speed with which a fracture heals.

Delayed union of fractures is a term applied to fractures that either do not heal or take longer than normal to heal; there is no precise time frame associated with delayed union. Nonunion refers to fractures in which healing is not observed and cannot be expected even with prolonged immobilization. X-ray analysis of a nonunion will show that the bone ends have hardened (sclerosed), that the ends of the marrow canal have become plugged, and that a gap persists between the ends of a fractured bone. Nonunion may be caused by inadequate blood supply to the fracture site, which leads to the formation of cartilage instead of new bone between the broken pieces of bone. Nonunion may also be caused by injury to the soft tissues that surround a fracture site. This damage impairs the formation of a callus and the reestablishment of an adequate blood supply to the fracture site; it is frequently seen in young children. Inadequate immobilization may also allow soft tissue to enter the fracture site, by slipping between the bone fragments, and may lead to nonunion. Respect for tissue and minimizing damage in the vicinity of a fracture, specially with open reduction, will minimize problems of nonunion. Subjecting the nonuniting fracture site to a low-level electromagnetic field will usually stimulate osteoblastic activity and lead to healing.

The epiphyseal plate is the portion of bone where growth occurs. Bony epiphyses are active in children until they attain their adult height, at which time the epiphyses become inactive and close. Once an epiphysis ceases to function, further growth does not occur. In children, a fracture involving the epiphyseal plate is potentially dangerous because bone growth may be interrupted or halted. This situation can lead to inequalities in the length of extremities or impaired range of movement in joints. Accurate reduction of injuries involving an epiphyseal plate is necessary to minimize subsequent deformity. A key factor is blood supply to the injured area: If adequate blood supply is maintained, epiphyseal plate damage is minimized.

Fractures of the spinal vertebrae are potentially very dangerous because they can cause injury to the nerves and tracts of the spinal cord. Fractures of the vertebrae are commonly sustained in automobile accidents, athletic injuries, falls from heights, and other situations involving rapid deceleration. When vertebrae are fractured, the spinal cord can be compromised. Spinal cord injury can be direct and cut all or a portion of the spinal nerves at the site of the fracture. The extent of the damage is dependent on the level of the injury. An accident that completely severs the spinal cord will lead to a complete loss of function for all structures below the level of injury. Since spinal nerves are arranged segmentally, cord damage at a lower level involves compromise of fewer structures. As the level of injury becomes higher in the spinal cord, more vital structures are involved. Transection of the spinal cord in the neck usually leads to complete paralysis of the entire body; it can cause death if high enough to cut the nerves controlling the lungs. Individuals in whom vertebral fractures and thus spinal cord injuries are suspected must have the spinal column immobilized before they are moved. Reduction of spinal cord fractures must be undertaken by a highly skilled person.

When bones having large marrow cavities such as the femur (thigh bone) are fractured, fat globules may escape from the marrow and enter the bloodstream. Such a fat globule is then called an embolus (plural is emboli). Fat emboli are potentially dangerous in that they can become lodged in the capillaries of the lungs. This causes pain and can lead to impaired oxygenation of blood, a condition called hypoxemia. About 10 to 20 percent of individuals sustaining a fractured femur also have central nervous system depression and skin petechiae (minute spots caused by hemorrhage or bleeding into the skin) in addition to hypoxemia in the two to three days after the injury. This triad of signs is called fat embolism syndrome. It is treated medically with oxygen, steroids, and anticoagulant drugs.

## PERSPECTIVE AND PROSPECTS

Fractures rarely threaten a patient's life directly, and injuries to the brain, heart, circulatory system, and abdominal cavity must receive priority of treatment. It is imperative, however, not to move a patient in whom a fracture is suspected without first immobilizing the potential fracture site. This is especially true with suspected fractures of the spine. Instability may not be apparent when a patient is lying down but can become catastrophic if the person is moved without proper preparation and immobilization.

Crush injuries of the spinal cord are relatively common among victims of osteoporosis. Osteoporosis is a pathological syndrome defined by a decrease in the density of a bone below the level required for mechanical support and is frequently associated with a deficiency of calcium, problems related to calcium in the body, or a rate of bone cell breakdown that is greater than the rate of bone cell remodeling. Crush fractures occur when the bones become so weak that the weight of the upper portion of the body is greater than the ability of the vertebrae to support it. These crush injuries may occur slowly over time and cause no serious injury to the underlying spinal cord. The resulting deformity of the spine, however, impairs movement. There is no treatment for osteoporotic crush fractures of the vertebrae.

Occupational exposures may lead to fractures and dislocations. Professional athletes are clearly at increased risk for skeletal injuries. These individuals are also usually well conditioned, however, and so can withstand increased impacts and blows to the body. Many are also trained in methods that minimize the force of impact; they know how to fall properly.

The vast proportion of workers are not conditioned and are given minimal training to avoid situations that lead to fractures. Accident analysis reveals that carelessness is the most common predisposing factor. Workers operating without safety equipment such as belaying lines or belts may become over-confident. In such a situation, slips or falls can occur, and fractures result. Unsafe equipment can lead to hazardous situations and cause fractures or dislocations. Machinery that is not properly maintained can fail; parts may become detached, hit nearby workers, and cause fractures.

Recreational activities also result in fractures. Individuals who once were well conditioned may engage in sports without proper equipment and sustain fractures or dislocations. Contact sports such as football, hockey, and basketball are primary examples of such activities. Riding bicycles and motorized recreational vehicles without proper safety equipment can lead to serious skeletal injuries. Activities such as rock climbing are inherently dangerous. With proper training and use of safety equipment, accidents can be reduced or their severity minimized. The keys to avoiding fractures and dislocations when participating in recreational activities are receiving proper instruction and training, employing adequate safety equipment, and using common sense by avoiding difficult or hazardous situations that are beyond one's physical abilities or skill level.

—*L. Fleming Fallon, Jr.*

**See also** Bone disorders; Head and neck disorders; Osteoporosis; Shock; Spinal disorders; Wounds.

## FOR FURTHER INFORMATION:

Rowe, C. R. "Acute and Recurrent Dislocations of the Shoulder." *Journal of Bone and Joint Surgery* 44A (July, 1962): 998-1008. This article is devoted solely to the treatment of shoulder dislocation, one of the most commonly dislocated joints. The language is fairly technical, as the text is intended primarily for orthopedic surgeons.

Sabiston, David C., Jr., ed. *Textbook of Surgery.* 14th ed. Philadelphia: W. B. Saunders, 1991. A standard textbook of surgery which contains an extensive discussion of different types of fractures and dislocations and how they are treated. Intended for practicing professionals, but can be generally understood by the layperson.

Schwartz, Seymour I., G. Tom Shires, Frank C. Spencer, and Wendy C. Husser. *Principles of Surgery.* 5th ed. New York: McGraw-Hill, 1989. A standard textbook of surgery containing sections on fractures and dislocations. Its intended audience is practicing surgeons, and thus the language is sometimes technical. Nevertheless, the serious reader can obtain much useful detail from this work.

Way, Lawrence W., ed. *Current Surgical Diagnosis and Treatment*. 10th ed. Norwalk, Conn.: Appleton and Lange, 1994. The diagnosis and treatment of fractures and dislocations is discussed in a brief and concise format emphasizing treatment modalities. The different section authors are recognized experts in their fields. The material is accessible to the general reader, but the sections are brief.

Wilmore, Douglas W., et al., eds. *Care of the Surgical Patient*. New York: Scientific American, 1992. This book should be understandable to lay readers even though it is written for professionals. Sections in part 1 discuss fractures and dislocations. The reputation of *Scientific American* for style and clarity is evident in this book. A good source for the general reader.

## FRIGIDITY. *See* SEXUAL DYSFUNCTION.

## FROSTBITE

**SYSTEMS AFFECTED:** Skin, other tissue adjacent to skin

**SPECIALISTS:** Emergency physicians, environmental medicine physicians, general surgeons

**DEFINITION:** Frostbite is localized freezing of tissue, usually of extremities exposed to low temperatures and resulting in ice crystals forming within cells, thereby killing them.

**KEY TERMS:**

*anticoagulant:* a drug that reduces the clotting of the blood

*basal metabolic rate:* the rate at which the body burns calories and produces heat energy while the body is at rest or not active

*gangrene:* the death of part of the body (such as an arm or leg) caused by the death of the cells in that structure

*hypothermia:* the process by which the body core temperature falls below that needed for the body to function normally

*hypoxia:* a lack of an adequate amount of oxygen to the tissues; results in a reduction of mental and physical capabilities

*maceration:* the process of breaking down tissue to a soft mass, either by soaking it or through infection or gangrene

*necrosis:* the death of body-tissue cells

*sludging:* an increase in red blood cell structures, known as platelets, which slows down the blood flow through vessels and promotes clotting of the blood

*sympathectomy:* the surgical process of removing or destroying nerves that may be afflicted by frostbite or other injury

*vascoconstriction:* a decrease in the diameter of vessels transporting blood throughout the body, reducing blood flow and oxygen transport

*windchill:* the effect of wind blowing across exposed flesh; increased heat is lost from the skin's surface, as if the air were much colder than the actual temperature indicates

### CAUSES AND SYMPTOMS

The effect of cold on the human body is to reduce the circulation of blood to surface areas, such as the feet, hands, and face. This reduction restricts the amount of heat lost by the body and helps to prevent the development of hypothermia. Blood constriction may become so severe in severely chilled areas of the body, however, that circulation almost totally ceases. People with poorer circulation, such as the elderly and the exhausted, are not as resistant to low temperatures as are fit or younger people.

If the skin's temperature falls below -0.53 degree Celsius, the tissue actually freezes and frostbite occurs. Rapid freezing causes ice crystals to form within a cell. These crystals rupture the cell wall and destroy structures within the cell, effectively killing it. If freezing is slow, ice crystals form between the cells; they grow by extracting water from the cells. The tissue may be injured physically by the ice crystals or by dehydration and the resulting disruption of osmotic and chemical balance within the cells; however, tissue death following frostbite is more likely to be attributable to interruption of the blood supply to the tissue than to the direct action of freezing. Cold also damages the capillaries in the affected areas, causing blood plasma to leak through their walls, thus adding to tissue injury and further impairing circulation by allowing the blood to sludge (to clot because of an increase in red blood cells) inside the vessels. All sensation of cold or pain is lost as circulation becomes seriously impaired. Unless the tissue is warmed quickly, the skin and superficial tissues actually begin to freeze. With continual chilling, the frozen area enlarges and extends to deeper areas. This condition is known as frostbite.

Frostbite was common among soldiers during Napoleon's campaign in Russia in the early 1800's, during World War II in Northern Europe, in the Korean War, and in fighting between Indian and Chinese troops in the Himalayas. Air crews, especially waist-gunners in the U.S. Air Force in World War II, were particularly prone to frostbite. In 1943, frostbite injuries among these bomber crews were greater than all other casualties combined.

Polar travelers before the 1920's suffered severely from frostbite. Mountain climbers are at risk from frostbite at higher elevations. Lower oxygen availability increases the danger of frostbite because the body cannot take in sufficient oxygen in this thinner air. The resulting condition, called hypoxia, reduces mental abilities, and precautions normally taken against the cold may be either inadequate or neglected altogether. High winds, often experienced in the mountains, speed heat loss from exposed skin surfaces. This windchill can be deadly to mountaineers and often produces hypothermia. Poor appetite at high elevations reduces the energy available for the production of body heat. The insulating layer of subcutaneous fat also decreases with longer periods of time spent at higher elevations; this in

## Frostbite

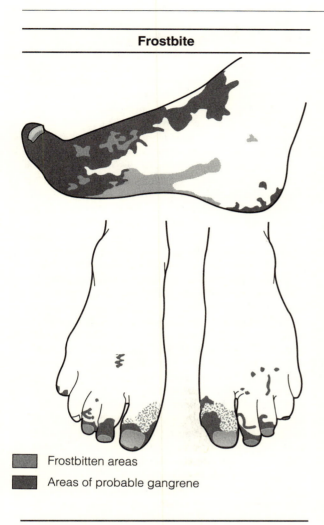

■ Frostbitten areas

■ Areas of probable gangrene

*Frostbite commonly affects the hands and feet.*

turn decreases the insulation of the surface areas of the body against freezing.

Inadequate food intake while mountain climbing increases the danger of frostbite, as the body does not have enough calories to keep its temperature constant. The occurrence of hypothermia also increases the risk of frostbite as heat is drawn away from extremities to protect the body's core temperature. At higher elevations, most humans function at only about 60 percent of the physiological efficiency that they have at sea level. Women have more resistance to cold and may be less likely to experience frostbite than are men.

Frostbite at high altitudes seems to be more common for the same temperature than at lower altitudes. More red blood cells are found in the blood of persons working at higher elevations, thickening the blood and reducing circulation to the extremities. This reduced circulation lowers the temperature of these extremities. The basal metabolic rate and cardiac output of the body also decrease as one goes higher; both of these actions reduce the body's ability to keep its feet, hands, and face warm.

Blood vessels move heat from the central body core to the skin; it radiates into the air from exposed surfaces. This heat loss is greatest in the hands, feet, and head, where the vessels are close to the skin's surface. Respiration loses body heat when cold air is inhaled into the lungs and body heat warms it; this heat is lost when the air is exhaled. Evaporation, moisture leaving the skin's surface, also draws heat from the body. In low temperatures, spilling gasoline on exposed skin will create frostbite because the evaporation of the fuel draws heat away from the body quickly. Convection carries body heat away by wind currents. This windchill factor, calculated for Fahrenheit temperatures by subtracting two times the windspeed from the air temperature, determines the amount of heat energy lost from the body's surface. Conduction transfers heat from one substance to another; for example, contact between the body and snow or metal will cause the skin to lose heat. Although many people work and live in subzero temperatures, frostbite is uncommon. Nevertheless, an accident that prevents one from moving, loss of the ability to shiver in order to generate heat, or inactivity may increase the chance of developing frostbite. Frostbite can occur in any cold environment. Warning symptoms of frostbite initially include tingling and pain in the afflicted tissues. The skin may be slightly flushed before freezing. It then turns white or a blotchy blue in color and is firm and insensitive to the touch. Tissue that is painful and then becomes numb and insensitive is frozen.

### TREATMENT AND THERAPY

Slight cases of frostbite, often termed frostnip or superficial frostbite, can be treated outdoors or in the field with little or no medical help. Such cases are usually reversible, with no permanent damage, as only skin and subcutaneous tissues are involved. The frozen part, although white and frozen on the surface, is soft and pliable when pressed gently before thawing. The area is often a cheek or the tip of the nose or the fingers. The frozen area, usually small, can be warmed manually. A hand is placed over the frostnipped area if it is a cheek or nose, and frozen fingers can be placed under the armpit or on a partner's bare stomach for warming. Tissue that has had only a minor amount of frostnip soon returns to normal color. A tingling sensation is felt when frostnipped tissue is thawed. After thawing, areas that have had more serious superficial frostbite become numb, mottled, or blue or purple in color and then will sting, burn, or swell for a period of time. Blisters, small ones called blebs, may occur within twenty-four to forty-eight hours. Blistering is more common where the skin is loose. Blister fluid is absorbed slowly; the skin may harden, become black (from gangrene), and be insensitive to touch. Throbbing or aching may persist for weeks. Gangrene occurring after frostnip is essentially superficial and extends only a few millimeters deep into the tissue. In two or three months, this type of frostbite will be mostly healed. With immediate treatment, frostnipped tissue will not progress to the much more serious injury of deep frostbite.

Tissues vary in their resistance to frostbite. Skin freezes at -0.53 Celsius, while muscles, blood vessels, and nerves are also highly subject to freezing. Connective tissue, tendons, and bones are relatively resistant to freezing, which explains why the blackened extremities of a frostbitten hand or foot can be moved: The tendons under the gangrenous skin remain intact and functional.

Deep frostbite includes not only skin and subcutaneous tissue but also deeper structures, including muscle, bone, and tendons. The affected area becomes cold, mottled, and blue or gray in color and may remain swollen for months. With deep frostbite, the tissues become quite hard to the touch. One to three days after thawing, the affected area becomes quite painful. Blisters, initially small blebs and then large, coalescing ones, may take weeks to develop. The patient should not be allowed to become alarmed about his or her condition; even mild cases of frostbite have a frightening appearance during blistering. Initially, the frozen part may be painless, but shooting and throbbing pains may occur for several months after thawing. Permanent loss of tissue is almost inevitable with deep frostbite. The affected extremity has a severely shriveled look. A limb may return to almost normal over some months, however, and amputation should never be carried out until a considerable period, probably at least six to nine months, has elapsed.

In cases of frostbite, surgical intervention must be minimal. Blackened frostbitten tissue will gradually separate itself from healthy, unfrozen tissue without interference; no efforts should be taken to hasten separation. Most cases of deep frostbite seem to heal in six to twelve months, and the gangrenous tissue, if it has not become infected with bacteria, is essentially superficial. Many unnecessary amputations have been carried out because of impatience at the slow recovery rate of tissue that has suffered deep frostbite; amputation is only necessary when infection has set in and it cannot be controlled with antibiotics.

If possible, deep frostbite should be treated under hospital care, not in the field or outdoors. The deep frozen tissue should remain frozen until hospital care is available. If frozen tissues are thawed, the patient will most likely be unable to move as the pain will be severe with any movement. Walking on feet that have been thawed after being frozen will cause permanent damage; however, walking on a frozen foot for twelve to eighteen hours or even longer produces less damage than inadequate warming. As frozen tissue thaws, cells exude fluid. If this tissue is refrozen, ice crystals form and cause more extensive, irreparable damage.

Rapid rewarming is the recommended treatment for deep frostbite and is a proven method of reducing tissue loss.

Rubbing the frostbitten area with the hand or snow—akin to rubbing the area with broken glass—should never be done. This treatment does not melt the intracellular ice crystals, nor does it increase circulation to the frozen area. It breaks the skin and allows infection to enter into the system. Vasodilator agents do not improve tissue survival. Local antibiotics in aerosol form can be used, but it is unwise to rely on this method alone for combating infection. Sympathectomy, the removal or destruction of affected nerves, does not improve cell survival. The use of the drug dextran early to prevent sludging has limited use and may have dangerous side effects. The use of hyperbaric oxygen or supplementary oxygen may increase the tissue tension of oxygen and save some cells partially damaged by cold injury.

Rewarming should be carried out in a water bath with water temperatures ranging from 37.7 to 42.2 degrees Celsius (100 to 108 degrees Fahrenheit). Higher temperatures will further damage already injured tissues. Rewarming in a large bathtub warms the frozen extremity more rapidly, resulting in less tissue loss in many cases, particularly where frostbite has been deep and extensive. A large container also permits more accurate control of the water temperature. If a bathtub is not available, a bucket, large wastebasket, dishpan, or other similar container can be used. During rewarming, hot water usually must be added to the bath occasionally to keep the temperature correct; in such cases the injured extremity should be removed from the bath and not returned to it until the water has been thoroughly mixed and its temperature measured. An open flame must not come into contact with the area to which heat is applied, since sensation is lost as a result of the frostbite and the tissue could be seriously burned.

For rewarming, the extremity should be stripped of all clothing, and any constricting bands, straps, or other objects that might stop circulation should be removed. The injured area should be suspended in the center of the water and not permitted to rest against the side or bottom. Warming should continue for thirty to forty minutes. The frostbitten tissues may become quite painful during this process, so it may be necessary to give painkillers to the patient in order to reduce discomfort during or after thawing of the frostbitten area. Aspirin (as well as codeine, morphine, or meperidine, if needed) may be given for pain. Aspirin or an anticoagulant increases blood circulation by reducing red blood cell platelet formation and thus reducing sludging. Phenoxybenzamine reduces vasoconstriction.

Following rewarming, the patient must be kept warm and the injured tissue elevated and protected from any kind of trauma. One should avoid rupturing blisters that have formed. Blankets or bedclothes should be supported by a framework to avoid pressure or rubbing of the injured area.

Subsequent care is directed primarily toward preventing infection. Cleanliness of the frostbitten area is extremely important. It should be soaked daily in a water bath at body temperature to which a germicidal soap has been added. If contamination of the water supply is a possibility, the bath water should be boiled and cooled before use. Dead tissue should not be cut or pulled away; the water baths remove such tissue more efficiently.

The afflicted area should be immobilized and kept sterile. Even contact with sheets can be damaging to a frostbitten limb. Sterile, dry cotton may be placed between the fingers or toes to avoid maceration. If infection appears present, as indicated by the area between the frostbitten tissue and healthy tissue becoming inflamed and feeling tender or throbbing, antibiotics such as ampicillin or cloxicillin should be given every six hours. Wet, antiseptic dressings should be applied if gangrene occurs in the damaged tissue. A tetanus toxoid booster shot, or human antitoxin if the patient has not been previously immunized against tetanus, should be given. Complete rest and a diet high in protein will help healing. Moderate movement of the afflicted area should be encouraged but should be limited to that done by a physical therapist, without assistance by the patient. Considerable reassurance and emotional support may be required by the patient, as the appearance of the frostbitten area can be alarming.

Amputation in response to infected, spreading gangrene may be needed eventually, but it should be delayed until the natural separation of dead from living tissue and bone has taken place. Radionucleotide scanning helps save frostbitten limbs. These scans accurately demonstrate blood flow in frostbitten extremities, thus predicting what tissue will survive.

### PERSPECTIVE AND PROSPECTS

Frostbite is an injury that can affect anyone who works or plays under cold conditions. Increased knowledge about what causes this injury, better equipment, and techniques that minimize its effect, however, have reduced its occurrence. Advances in medical knowledge regarding how the injury occurs within the afflicted tissues have produced treatment protocols that reduce the extent of permanent injury from frostbite.

Prevention is the most effective treatment for frostbite, which can occur only when the body lacks enough heat to keep the extremities above freezing. The overall body heat deficit results from inadequate clothing or equipment, reduced food consumption, exhaustion, injury or inactivity causing a lack of body movement, or some combination of these factors. Those playing or working in a cold environment should know the conditions under which frostbite may develop. For frostnip to occur, the windchill index must exceed 1,400 and the air temperature must be below the freezing point of exposed skin (-0.53 degree Celsius). An ambient temperature of -10 to -15 degrees Celsius is usually necessary for deep frostbite to develop.

Adequate clothing—especially boots that allow circulation to occur freely, mittens (not gloves) that cover the hands, and a head covering that protects the face, ears, and neck—must be worn. Boots should be well broken in and large enough to fit comfortably with several pairs of socks. The laces at the top of the boots should not be tight. Gaiters or overboots should be worn if deep or wet snow is anticipated. Windproof or insulated pants protect the legs from cold and help keep the feet warm. Dry socks and mitten liners should be carried. Moisture greatly reduces the insulative value of clothing, so it is necessary to stay dry; if clothing becomes wet or damp, one should change into dry items. Plastic bags, worn over bare feet, provide a vapor-barrier liner that is effective in helping keep one's feet dry and warm under cold conditions. Adequate ventilation avoids dampness from excessive perspiration. Dressing in layers—having several light shirts, jackets, or a windbreaker—is better than wearing only one heavy jacket.

Heat production, resulting from exercise or the protective mechanism of shivering, is just as important as clothing in maintaining body temperature. Injuries that cause the victim to go into shock or lie immobilized, even though adequate clothing may be worn, predispose the victim to frostbite.

Eating high-energy foods and taking in 6,000 or more kilocalories (Calories) a day may be necessary to keep body temperatures constant under very cold or physically demanding conditions. Adequate rest, including eight or more hours of sleep, helps to reduce fatigue, which in turn increases the body's ability to produce heat. Alcohol and tobacco should be strictly avoided. Alcohol dilates the blood vessels and, although this action temporarily warms the skin, results in increased loss of total body heat. Smoking constricts the blood vessels in the skin and so reduces heat flow to surface areas; this may be sufficient to initiate frostbite in exposed tissue. A person who has sustained frostbite in the past is usually more susceptible to more cold injury. Problems with arthritis may develop in extremities that have been frostbitten. —*David L. Chesemore*

*See also* Gangrene; Hyperthermia and hypothermia.

### FOR FURTHER INFORMATION:

Schuh, Dwight R. *Modern Survival: Outdoor Gear and Savvy to Bring You Back Alive*. New York: David McKay, 1979. This survival book contains a good discussion of frostbite and its prevention. It also discusses the other types of cold injuries that may occur.

Ward, Michael. "Frostbite." In *Mountain Medicine and Physiology*, edited by Charles Clarke, Michael Ward, and Edward Williams. London: Alpine Club, 1975. This chapter on frostbite was presented at a symposium for mountaineers, expedition doctors, and physiologists. It contains an excellent overview of frostbite and possible treatments; especially under expedition conditions. The other chapters are also interesting reading and provide valuable background for anyone who may be venturing into mountainous country.

_____. *Mountain Medicine: A Clinical Study of Cold and High Altitude.* New York: Van Nostrand Reinhold, 1976. Ward, a physician, has produced a comprehensive book on medical conditions, including frostbite, that one may encounter while mountaineering or trekking in the high country. It is extremely readable and is highly recommended as a book for novices to read before venturing into the cold outdoors.

Washburn, Brad. "Frostbite: What It Is, How to Prevent It—Emergency Treatment." *New England Journal of Medicine* 266 (1962): 974-989. One of the more readily available pioneer papers on frostbite. It is now a bit dated, but many of its suggestions for preventing frostbite are still used.

Wilkerson, James A., ed. *Medicine for Mountaineering.* 2d ed. Seattle: The Mountaineers, 1975. This book is a first-aid manual that goes beyond traditional treatment protocols. It was written for those who need information to care for serious injuries when organized medical help is not available. The information on frostbite and other problems is substantial. People in cold regions should keep this book (or a similar one) in their vehicles or backpacks.

# FUNGAL INFECTIONS

**SYSTEMS AFFECTED:** Skin, respiratory, immune

**SPECIALISTS:** Dermatologists, family physicians, immunologists, internists, pulmonologists

**DEFINITION:** Infections caused by fungi—simple, plantlike organisms—that range from minor skin diseases to serious, disseminated diseases of the lungs and other organs; patients whose immune systems are impaired are at greater risk of serious fungal infections.

**KEY TERMS:**

*asexual reproduction:* the production of new individuals without the mating of two parents of unlike genotype, such as by budding

*mycelium:* a collection of threadlike fungal strands (hyphae) making up the thallus, or nonreproductive portion, of a fungus

*mycosis:* a disease of humans, plants or animals caused by a fungus; the prefix *myco-* means fungus, hence mycology (the study of fungi)

*pleomorphic fungus:* a fungus whose morphology changes markedly from one phase of its life cycle to another, or according to changes in environmental conditions

*tinea:* a medical term for fungal skin diseases, such as ringworm and athlete's foot, caused by a variety of fungi

*yeast:* a unicellular fungus which reproduces by budding off smaller cells from the parent cell; yeasts belong to several different groups of fungi, and some fungi are capable of growing either as a yeast or as a filamentous fungus

## TYPES OF FUNGUS

The term "fungus" is a general one for plantlike organisms that do not produce their own food through photosynthesis but live as heterotrophs, absorbing complex carbon compounds from other living or dead organisms. Fungi were formerly classified in the plant kingdom (together with bacteria, all algae, mosses, and green plants); more recently, biologists have realized that there are fundamental differences in cell structure and organization separating the lower plants into a number of groups which merit recognition as kingdoms. Fungi differ from bacteria and actinomycetes in being eukaryotic, that is, in having an organized nucleus with chromosomes within the cell. One division of fungi, which is believed to be distantly related to certain aquatic algae, has spores that swim by means of flagella. These water molds include pathogens of fish and aquatic insect larvae and a few economically important plant pathogens, but none have yet been recorded as causing a defined, nonopportunistic human disease. The other division of fungi lacks flagellated spores at any stage in its life cycle. It encompasses most familiar fungi, including molds, mushrooms, yeasts, wood-rotting fungi, leaf spots, and all fungi reliably reported to cause disease in humans.

Fungi that lack flagellated stages in their life cycles are further divided into three classes and one form-class according to the manner in which the spores are produced. The first of these, the Zygomycetes (for example *Rhizopus*, the black bread mold), produce thick-walled, solitary sexual spores as a result of hyphal fusion; they are a diverse assemblage including many parasites of insects. Species in the genus *Mucor* cause a rare, fulminating, rapidly fatal systemic disease called mucormycosis, generally in acidotic diabetic patients. The Basidiomycetes, characterized by the production of sexual spores externally on a club-shaped structure called a basidium, is a large class that includes mushrooms, plant rusts (such as stem rust of wheat), and most wood-rotting fungi. There is one important basidiomycetous human pathogen (*Filobasidiella neoformans*), and a few confirmed opportunists. The Ascomycetes, including most yeasts and lichens, many plant pathogens (such as Dutch elm disease and chestnut blight), and a great diversity of saprophytes growing on wood and herbaceous material, produce sexual spores in a saclike structure called an ascus. One ascomycete, *Piedraia nigra*, regularly produces its characteristic fruiting bodies on its human host; others do so in culture. In addition, there is a form-class Deuteromycetes consisting of fungi that produce only asexual spores. Most are suspected of being stages in the life cycle of Ascomycetes, but some are Basidiomycetes or are of uncertain affinity. Human pathogens, at least as they occur on the host or in typical laboratory culture, are mostly Deuteromycetes.

Medical mycology would occupy only a single chapter in a book on the relationship of fungi to human affairs. Relatively few fungi have become adapted to living as parasites of human (or even mammalian) hosts, and of these, the most common ones cause superficial and cutaneous mycoses with annoying but scarcely life-threatening effects. Serious fungal diseases are mercifully rare among people with normally functioning immune systems.

The majority of fungi are directly dependent on green plants, as parasites, as symbionts living in a mutually beneficial association with a plant, or as saprophytes on dead plant material. One large, successful group of Ascomycetes lives in symbiotic association with algae, forming lichens. Fungi play a critical ecological role in maintaining stable plant communities. As plant pathogens, they cause serious economic loss, leading in extreme cases to famine. The ability of saprophytic fungi to transform chemically the substrate on which they are growing has been exploited by the brewing industry since antiquity and has been expanded to other industrial processes. Penicillin, other antibiotics, and some vitamins are extracted from fungi, which produce a vast array of complex organic compounds whose potential is only beginning to be explored and which constitutes a fertile field for those interested in genetic engineering.

This same chemical diversity and complexity also enable fungi to produce mycotoxins—chemicals that have an adverse effect on humans and animals. Saprophytic fungi growing on improperly stored food are a troublesome source of toxic compounds, some of which are carcinogenic. The old adage that "a little mold won't hurt you" is true in the sense that common molds do not cause acute illness when ingested, but it is poor advice in terms of long-term health.

A mycotoxicity problem of considerable medical and veterinary interest is posed by Ascomycetes of the order Clavicipitales, which are widespread on grasses. Some species of grasses routinely harbor systemic, asymptomatic infections by these fungi, which produce compounds toxic to animals that graze on them. From the point of view of the grass, the relationship is symbiotic, since it discourages grazing; from the point of view of range management, the relationship is deleterious to stock. *Claviceps purpurea*, a disease of rye, causes a condition known as ergotism in humans, with symptoms including miscarriage, vascular constriction leading to gangrene of the limbs, and hallucinations. Outbreaks of hallucinatory ergotism are thought by some authors to be responsible for some of the more spectacular perceptions of witchcraft in premodern times. Better control of plant disease and a decreased reliance on rye as a staple grain have virtually eliminated ergotism as a human disease in the twentieth century.

Fungi exhibit a bewildering variety of forms and life cycles; nevertheless, certain generalizations can be made. A fungus starts life as a spore, which may be a single cell or a cluster of cells and is usually microscopic. Under proper conditions, the spore germinates, producing a filament of fungal cells oriented end to end, called a hypha. Hyphae grow into the substrate, secreting enzymes that dissolve structures to provide food for the growing fungus and to

provide holes through which the fungus can grow. In an asexually reproducing fungus, some of the hyphae become differentiated, producing specialized cells (spores) which differ from the parent hypha in size and pigmentation and are adapted for dispersal, but which are genetically identical to the parent. In a sexually reproducing fungus, two hyphae (or a hypha and a spore from different individuals) fuse, their nuclei fuse, and meiosis takes place before spores are formed. Spores are often produced in a specialized fruiting body, such as a mushroom.

Fungus spores are ubiquitous. Common saprophytic fungi produce airborne spores in enormous quantities; thus it is difficult to avoid contact with them in all but the most hypersterile environments. In culture, fungi (including pathogenic species) produce large numbers of dry spores that can be transmitted in the air from host to host, making working with fungi in a medical laboratory potentially hazardous.

### FUNGAL DISEASES AND TREATMENTS

Human fungal diseases are generally placed in four broad categories according to the tissues they attack, and they are further subdivided according to specific pathologies and the organisms involved. The categories of disease are superficial mycoses, cutaneous mycoses, subcutaneous mycoses, and systemic mycoses.

*Superficial mycoses* affect hair and the outermost layer of the epidermis and do not evoke a cellular response. They include tinea versicolor and tinea nigra, deutermycete infections that cause discolored patches on skin, and black piedra, caused by an ascomycete growing on hair shafts. They can be treated with a topical fungicide, such as nystatin, or, in the case of piedra, by shaving off the affected hair.

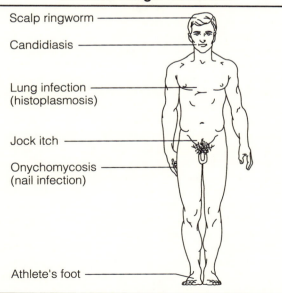

**Common Fungal Infections**

Scalp ringworm

Candidiasis

Lung infection (histoplasmosis)

Jock itch

Onychomycosis (nail infection)

Athlete's foot

*Cutaneous mycoses* involve living cells of the skin or mucous membrane and evoke a cellular response, generally localized inflammation. Dermatomycoses (dermatophytes), which affect skin and hair, include tinea capitis (ringworm of the scalp), tinea pedis (athlete's foot), and favus, a scaly infection of the scalp. Domestic animals serve as a reservoir for some cutaneous mycoses. The organisms responsible are generally fungi imperfecti in the genera *Microsporon* and *Trichophyton*. Cutaneous mycoses can be successfully treated with topical nystatin or oral griseofulvin.

*Candida albicans*, a ubiquitous pleomorphic fungus with both a yeast and a mycelial form, causes a variety of cutaneous mycoses as well as systemic infections collectively named candidiasis. Thrush is a *Candida* yeast infection of the mouth which is most common in infants, especially in infants born to mothers with vaginal candidiasis. Vaginal yeast infections periodically affect 18 to 20 percent of the adult female population and more than 30 percent of pregnant women. *Candida* also causes paronychia, a nailbed infection. Small populations of *Candida* are normally present in the alimentary tract and genital tract of healthy individuals; candidiasis of the mucous membranes tends to develop in response to antibiotic treatment, which disturbs the normal bacterial flora of the body, or in response to metabolic changes or decreasing immune function.

None of the organisms causing cutaneous mycoses elicits a lasting immune response, so recurring infections by these agents is the rule rather than the exception. Even in temperate climates, under modern standards of hygiene, cutaneous mycoses are extremely common.

*Subcutaneous mycoses*, affecting skin and muscle tissue, are predominantly tropical in distribution and not particularly common. Chromomycosis and maduromycosis are caused by soil fungi that enter the skin through wounds, causing chronic localized tumors, usually on the feet. Sporotrichosis enters through wounds and spreads through the lymphatic system, causing skin ulcers associated with lymph nodes. Amphotericin B, a highly toxic systemic antifungal agent, has been used to treat all three conditions; potassium iodide is used to treat sporotrichosis, and localized chromomycosis and maduromycosis lesions can be surgically removed.

*Systemic mycoses*, the most serious of fungal infections, have the ability to become generally disseminated in the body. The main nonopportunistic systemic mycoses known in North America are histoplasmosis, caused by *Histoplasma capsulatum;* coccidiomycosis, caused by *Coccidiodes immitis;* blastomycosis, caused by *Ajellomyces* (or *Blastomyces) dermatidis*; and cryptococcosis, caused by *Cryptococcus* (or *Filobasidiella) neoformans*. Similar infections, caused by related species, occur in other parts of the world.

Coccidiomycosis, also called San Joaquin Valley fever or valley fever, will serve as an example of the etiology of systemic mycoses. The causative organism lives in arid soils in the American southwest; its spores are wind-disseminated.

When inhaled, the fungus grows in the lungs, producing a mild respiratory infection which is self-limiting in perhaps 95 percent of the cases. The mild form of the disease is common in rural areas. In a minority of cases, a chronic lung disease whose symptoms resemble tuberculosis develops. There is also a disseminated form of the disease producing meningitis; chronic cutaneous disease, with the production of ulcers and granulomas; and attack of the bones, internal organs, and lymphatic system. A chronic pulmonary infection may become systemic in response to factors that undermine the body's immune system. Factors involved in individual susceptibility among individuals with intact immune systems are poorly understood.

Histoplasmosis (also known as summer fever, cave fever, or Mississippi Valley fever) is even more common; 90 percent of people tested in the southern Mississippi Valley show a positive reaction to this fungus, indicating prior, self-limiting lung infection. The fungus is associated with bird and bat droppings, and severe cases sometimes occur when previously unexposed individuals are exposed to high levels of innoculum in caves where bats roost. A related organism, *Histoplasma duboisii*, occurs in central Africa. Blastomycosis causes chronic pulmonary disease, chronic cutaneous disease, and systemic disease, all of which were usually fatal until the advent of chemotherapy with amphotericin B. The natural habitat of the fungus is unclear. *Cryptococcus neoformans* occurs in pigeon droppings and is worldwide in distribution. The subclinical pulmonary form of the disease is probably common; invasive disease occurs in patients with collagen diseases, such as lupus, and in patients with weakened immune systems. It is the leading cause of invasive fungal disease in patients with acquired immunodeficiency syndrome (AIDS).

Systemic fungal diseases are notoriously difficult to treat. Chemotherapy of systemic, organismally caused diseases depends on finding a chemical compound which will selectively kill or inhibit the invading organism without damaging the host. Therefore, the more closely the parasite species is related biologically to the host species, the more difficult it is to find a compound which will act in such a selective manner. Fungi are, from a biological standpoint, more like humans than they are like bacteria, and antibacterial antibiotics are ineffective against them. If a fungus has invaded the skin or the digestive tract, it can be attacked with toxic substances that are not readily absorbed into the bloodstream, but this approach is not appropriate for a systemic infection. Amphotericin, intraconazole, and fluconazole, the drugs of choice for systemic fungal infections, are highly toxic to humans. Thus, dosage is critical, close clinical supervision is necessary, and long-term therapy may not be feasible.

## PERSPECTIVE AND PROSPECTS

Medical mycology textbooks written before 1980 tended to focus on two categories of fungal infection: the common, ubiquitous, and comparatively benign superficial and cutaneous mycoses, frequently seen in clinical practice in the industrialized world, and the subcutaneous and deep mycoses, treated as a rare and/or predominantly tropical problem. Opportunistic systemic infections, if mentioned at all, were regarded as a rare curiosity.

The rising population of patients with compromised immune systems, including cancer patients undergoing chemotherapy, people being treated with steroids for various conditions, transplant patients, and people with AIDS, has dramatically changed this clinical picture. Between 1980 and 1986, more than a hundred fungi, a few previously unknown and the majority common inhabitants of crop plants, rotting vegetable debris, and soil, were identified as causing human disease. The number continues to increase steadily. Compared to organisms routinely isolated from soil and plants, these opportunistic fungi do not seem to have any special characteristics other than the ability to grow at human body temperature; however, the possibility that an opportunistic pathogen might mutate into a form capable of attacking healthy humans is worrisome.

Systemic opportunistic human infections have been attributed to *Alternaria alternata* and *Fusarium oxysporum*, common plant pathogens that cause diseases of tomatoes and strawberries, respectively. Several species of *Aspergillus*, saprophytic molds (many of them thermophilic) have long been implicated in human disease. Colonizing aspergillosis, involving localized growth in the lungs of people exposed to high levels of aspergillus spores (notably agricultural workers working with silage), is not particularly rare among people with normal immune systems, but the more severe invasive form of the disease, in which massive lung lesions form, and disseminated aspergillosis, in which other organs are attacked, almost always involve immunocompromised patients. *Ramichloridium schulzeri*, described originally from wheat roots, causes "golden tongue" in leukemia patients; fortunately this infection responds to amphotericin B. *Scelidosporium inflatum*, first isolated from a serious bone infection in an immunocompromised patient in 1984, is being isolated with increasing frequency in cases of disseminated mycosis; it resists standard drug treatment.

Oral colonization by strains of *Candida* is often the first sign of AIDS-related complex or full-blown AIDS in an individual harboring the human immunodeficiency virus (HIV). Drug therapy with fluconazole is effective against oral candidiasis, but relapse rates of up to 50 percent within a month of the cessation of drug therapy are reported. Reported rates of disseminated candidiasis in AIDS patients range from 1 to 10 percent. Invasive procedures such as intravenous catheters represent a significant risk of introducing *Candida* and other common fungi into the bloodstream of patients.

*Pneumocystis carinii*, the organism causing a form of pneumonia which is the single most important cause of death in patients with AIDS, was originally classified as a sporozoan—that is, as a parasitic protozoan—but detailed investigations of the life cycle, metabolism, and genetic material of *Pneumocystis* have convinced some biologists that it is actually an ascomycete, although an anomalous one that lacks a cell wall. Unfortunately, it does not respond to therapy with the antifungal drugs currently in use.

In general, antifungal drug therapy for mycoses in AIDS patients is not very successful. In the absence of significant patient immunity, it is difficult to eradicate a disseminated infection from the body entirely, making a resurgence likely once drug therapy is discontinued. Reinfection is also likely if the organism is a common component of the patient's environment.

Given the increasing number of lethal systemic fungal infections seen in clinical practice, there is substantial impetus for a search for more effective, less toxic antifungal drugs. A number of compounds, produced by bacteria and chemically dissimilar to both antibacterial antibiotics and the most widely used antifungal compounds, have been identified and are being tested. It is also possible that the plant kingdom, which has been under assault by fungi for all its long geologic history, may prove a source for medically useful antifungal compounds.

—*Martha Sherwood-Pike*

*See also* Athlete's foot; Candidiasis.

**FOR FURTHER INFORMATION:**
Ainsworth, C. G., and Alfred S. Sussman, eds. *The Fungi: An Advanced Treatise*. 4 vols. New York: Academic Press, 1965-1973. This multivolume review of mycological research, with individual chapters written by recognized specialists, is the best single reference book on general mycology. Volume 1 treats ultrastructure, growth, biochemistry, and the genetic control of physiology; volume 2 treats morphogenesis, reproduction, and inheritance; volume 3 covers ecology, parasitism, and evolution; volume 4 explores classification and identification. Chapter 8 in volume 3, "Fungal Parasites of Vertebrates," by Ainsworth, covers medical mycology.

British Society for Antimicrobial Chemotherapy Working Party. "Antifungal Chemotherapy in Patients with Acquired Immunodeficiency Syndrome." *Lancet* 340, no. 8820 (September 12, 1992): 648-650. Provides an overview of occurrence and therapies for the use of physicians in the British Isles. The article emphasizes candidiasis, cryptococcosis, histoplasmosis, and coccidiomycosis. The first two are common, life-threatening, and virtually impossible to cure in patients afflicted with AIDS. A technical preliminary overview of an area which is the subject of active, expanding research.

Campbell, Mary C., and Joyce L. Stewart. *The Medical Mycology Handbook*. New York: John Wiley & Sons, 1980. A practical, illustrated laboratory manual for medical technicians which contains considerable background information. It begins with a description of the types of fungal disease, then describes the specific diseases within each category. The second half includes keys and illustrations of pathogenic fungi in culture.

Christensen, Clyde. *The Molds and Man: An Introduction to the Fungi*. Minneapolis: University of Minnesota Press, 1951. An unspecialized book designed to acquaint the reader with "some of the arresting, unusual, little known and often wonderful aspects of the common fungi," although it is out of date with respect to mycotoxins and opportunistic infections. Chapter 9 treats fungal parasites of animals including humans, and chapter 10 discusses the industrial use of fungi.

Miller, Julie Ann. "Clinical Opportunities for Plant and Soil Fungi." *BioScience* 36, no. 10 (1986): 656-659. This article discusses the hundred-odd fungi that have been reported to cause opportunistic infections in immuno-compromised hosts, giving a few case histories and an overview of research underway to improve diagnostic procedures. The ubiquity of fungi and the relationship of the emerging epidemiological problem to the normal role of fungi in nature is emphasized. Aimed at a biologically literate audience of nonspecialists.

Rippon, John W. Medical Mycology: *The Pathogenic Fungi and Pathogenic Actinomycetes*. 3d ed. Philadelphia: W. B. Saunders, 1987. A standard medical mycology textbook for students of medicine and microbiology, with detailed descriptions of common mycoses and the organisms that cause them, as an aid to clinical diagnosis. There are also sections on general fungal biology and opportunistic infections.

# GALLBLADDER DISEASES

**SYSTEMS AFFECTED:** Gallbladder, gastrointestinal

**SPECIALISTS:** Gastroenterologists, general surgeons, internists

**DEFINITION:** A family of disorders affecting the gallbladder and causing abdominal pain or occasionally symptomless.

**KEY TERMS:**

*bile:* a complex solution formed by liver cells which is composed mainly of bile salts, fats, and cholesterol, which aids in fat digestion; it is secreted by the liver into a system of ducts connecting the liver, gallbladder, and intestinal tract

*biliary colic:* a distinct pain syndrome characterized by severe intermittent waves of right-sided, upper abdominal pain, often brought on by the ingestion of fatty foods; pain occurs when a gallstone obstructs the outflow of bile and usually resolves when the gallstone moves away from the outflow area

*cholecystectomy:* the surgical procedure that results in the removal of the gallbladder in its entirety; the two main techniques are the traditional open method and the laparoscopically aided method

*cholecystitis:* the disease that occurs when the gallbladder becomes inflamed or infected, which produces severe right-sided, upper abdominal pain, fever, and other signs of infection; a frequent indication for removal of the gallbladder

*cholelithiasis:* the presence of gallstones in the gallbladder

*gallbladder:* a muscular, walled sac located on the under surface of the liver which stores and concentrates bile; under stimulus from the intestine in response to a meal, the gallbladder contracts and expels bile into the digestive tract to aid in fat digestion

*gallstones:* particles that form in the gallbladder when the solubility of the components of bile is somehow altered, also resulting in the precipitation of cholesterol; the gallstones, which can grow very large, are made up mostly of cholesterol but can be pigmented or contain other substances

*laparoscopic cholecystectomy:* a procedure in which the gallbladder is removed with the help of a telescopic eyepiece which is attached to a tube inserted into the patient's body; the surgery is done using four small incisions and allows the patient to recover much faster than the traditional method of open surgery

## CAUSES AND SYMPTOMS

Gallbladder diseases affect a large number of patients and are among the most common causes of abdominal pain. Most gallbladder problems stem from the presence of gallstones, which may be present in as many as one of every ten adults. In the past, it was recommended that anyone with gallstones have their gallbladder taken out, but this is no longer the case. It is now known that many people with gallstones never experience difficulty because of them.

A very common gallbladder disease is biliary colic. This is usually manifested by severe right-sided, upper abdominal pain which is fairly repetitive in nature. The pain may literally take the patient's breath away, but an episode usually lasts less than thirty minutes. The patient may also complain of right-sided shoulder or back pain, often caused by irritation of the diaphragmatic nerves, which are located just above the liver on the right side. Many people may confuse the pain of biliary colic with indigestion, because in some patients it may be experienced in the middle of the upper abdomen. This pain is almost always brought on by eating, since the gallbladder contracts in response to food in the intestinal tract. The meal triggering such an episode often is described as rich and fatty, and many pa-

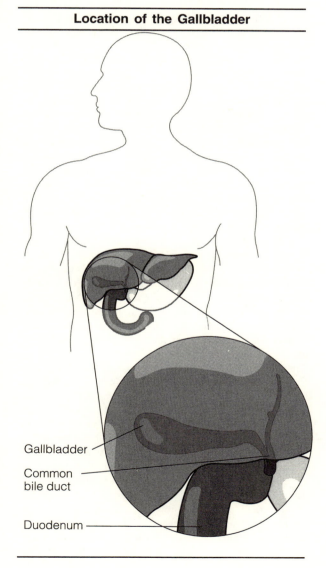

**Location of the Gallbladder**

Gallbladder

Common bile duct

Duodenum

tients soon learn what types of food to avoid. Biliary colic does not occur unless gallstones are present, as they tend to obstruct the outflow of bile from the gallbladder. The treatment for biliary colic usually consists of dietary manipulation, that is, the avoidance of fatty foods or other foods known to trigger the pain. Surgery is performed if the patient so desires, and removing the gallbladder should cure the problem.

When a diagnosis of gallstones is suspected, the physician will take down the patient's medical history and perform a physical examination. In most cases, however, such actions will yield no physical findings that are indicative of gallstone disease. Thus confirmation of this diagnosis is usually in the form of an imaging study of the gallbladder, in which the gallstones are either directly or indirectly visualized. The most commonly used imaging modality is the ultrasound test, which can be easily and rapidly performed with very reliable results. While the gallstones cannot actually be seen, they have a density which reflects, rather than transmits, sound waves. As a result, they create specific echoes and shadows that can be interpreted by the radiologists as gallstones. No patient should be treated for gallstone disease without such visualization being used to confirm the presence of gallstones.

A potentially serious type of gallbladder disease caused by gallstones is acute cholecystitis. In this condition, the outflow of bile is obstructed, usually by a gallstone that is stuck in the outflow tract, and severe inflammation and infection may develop. A patient with acute cholecystitis often complains of pain that does not go away promptly, may have chills or fever, and is usually found to have a very tender abdomen on the upper right side when examined by a physician. The treatment of this condition is not controversial, and most physicians would probably recommend removing the gallbladder surgically. The controversy that does exist is in regard to the timing of when the gallbladder should be removed—either immediately or electively, at a later date, if the patient recovers from acute cholecystitis with conservative management, including the use of antibiotics and the avoidance of eating until the inflammation subsides.

Inflammation and infection can also occur, although rarely, in gallbladders that do not produce gallstones. This happens in very select circumstances and is called acute acalculous cholecystitis. It usually afflicts very ill patients who have been in an intensive care unit for a long time, patients who have needed a heart-lung machine as a result of open heart surgery, or patients who are unable to eat for an extended period of time because of other problems. These patients are often fed only intravenously, which can lead to severe gallbladder problems. The exact mechanisms are not entirely known, but alterations in blood flow and an impaired ability to fight infection may play a role. Whatever the cause, the treatment often remains the same: re-

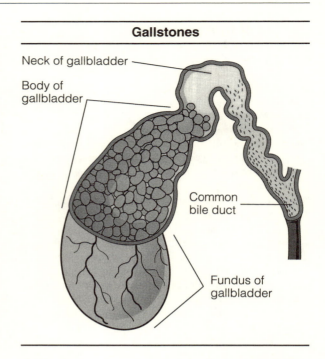

**Gallstones**

Neck of gallbladder

Body of gallbladder

Common bile duct

Fundus of gallbladder

moval of the gallbladder that does not respond to conservative therapy.

Gallstones can also move out of the gallbladder and cause serious problems. The main outflow tract of bile from the gallbladder and liver is the common bile duct, and this is a common place for gallstones to lodge. The end of this duct is surrounded by a small muscle called the sphincter of Oddi, which may not allow the passage of gallstones. If they become stuck there, they can completely obstruct the biliary system, and the patient will become jaundiced in appearance. Removal of the gallstones will cure the problem. The presence of these gallstones in the common bile duct is also associated with the development of pancreatitis, an inflammation of the pancreas which can be severe and life-threatening. Removal of the gallbladder at an appropriate time will prevent future bouts of pancreatitis.

The gallbladder can also be a source of cancer. Although cancer of the gallbladder is not common, it is estimated that one out of every one hundred gallbladders removed will have cancer in it. Therefore, all specimens removed must be examined by a qualified pathologist and all reports must be reviewed in their entirety by the surgeon. If the disease is limited to a minor thickness of the gallbladder, no further therapy is needed, but if the tumor is larger, further surgery—including removal of part of the liver—may be necessary. Gallbladder cancer grows silently in many patients, and it is often not detected until late in its course.

### TREATMENT AND THERAPY

Because there is no simple way to prevent gallbladder problems, surgery plays a large role in their management.

Removing the gallbladder, a relatively routine operation, results in a complete cure from the disease, with acceptably low complication rates and few long-term problems. While several exciting new ways of treating gallbladder and gallstone problems have been developed, the classic and standard method of therapy for gallbladder disease has been open cholecystectomy. This procedure entails making an incision across the upper right side of the abdomen a few inches below and parallel to the bottom of the rib cage. The muscles of the abdominal wall are cut, and the abdominal cavity is opened. The gallbladder, which is usually located right under this incision, is then removed and the incision closed in layers. This method of gallbladder removal has acceptable complication rates and is relatively safe and extremely effective. It allows the surgeon to inspect the entire abdomen and rule out other problems. One must consider, however, that this procedure constitutes major surgery. Most patients need to be in the hospital for a minimum of three to five days, and there is a considerable amount of pain with this incision. These problems have prompted surgeons to find a less invasive way of removing the gallbladder, thereby achieving better pain control and reducing the length of the hospital stay and the time lost from work and other activities.

A laparoscope is an optical instrument, composed of a tube connected to a telescopic eyepiece, that allows the surgeon to perform a procedure inside the patient's body. Although it has been employed in surgeries for many years, mainly in gynecological procedures, it was adapted only recently for removal of the gallbladder, as well as in other types of surgeries. Since then, laparoscopic cholecystectomy has become a procedure that all surgeons must know in order to stay current with the profession. The laparoscope and other surgical instruments are inserted directly into the abdomen through several small incisions, and the gallbladder is removed without a large incision having been made. The patients are often discharged the same day of the surgery, and they return to work much faster than with the open technique.

Despite its advantages, there are some pitfalls with laparoscopic cholecystectomy, and it cannot be used for all patients. There is an increased incidence of certain injuries to other organs and bile ducts at the time of the operation because less of the area can be seen than with an open operation. In addition, patients who have had previous upper abdominal surgery are also not candidates for this procedure, and for those with acute cholecystitis, severe inflammation may make this technique unsafe. For most patients, however, laparoscopic cholecystectomy can be performed easily and safely with minimal complications and excellent results. It is becoming the standard of care and will continue to change the way gallbladder surgery is performed. The laparoscope is also being used to perform appendectomies, ulcer surgeries, cancer surveillance, and all types of intra-abdominal surgery.

Radiologists and internists may play an important role in the management of patients with gallbladder disease. In certain circumstances, the techniques performed by these specialists may be indicated for extremely ill patients who might not be able to tolerate an operation, or for whom the anesthesia might be too hazardous. Invasive radiologists can actually place a tube into the gallbladder with help from their imaging techniques and remove infection from the gallbladder or troublesome gallstones. This procedure can alleviate symptoms in some patients, who may not even require any additional intervention. These practices are not common, however, and they are usually reserved for the very ill patient who might not survive an open operation or is at extremely high risk to develop a certain complication.

Gallstones can migrate out of the gallbladder and cause problems if they lodge in and obstruct the common bile duct. This places the patient at high risk for developing jaundice and infection in the biliary system. The standard method for dealing with this problem continues to be open surgery. In this procedure, the gallbladder is removed through an incision and the common bile duct is also opened. The gallstones are removed through a variety of techniques, and the duct is then closed. A tube is placed in the duct to keep it open, because otherwise it could scar and become narrowed. Many of these patients must be hospitalized for a number of days, making this surgery an expensive one.

Internists who specialize in the diseases of the abdomen have become proficient at performing endoscopic techniques. This development came about after the development of fiberoptics, which allow one to see through a tube, even if it is bent at a variety of angles. An endoscope, composed of surgical instruments, a light source, and fiberoptic cables, can be used to examine the lining of the stomach and intestines, allowing the diagnosis of many conditions.

Endoscopy is performed by inserting the endoscope through the mouth and into the patient's stomach and the first part of the intestines. From this location, the area where the common bile duct opens into the intestines can be seen, and this is often where gallstones become lodged. The gallstones can actually be removed with instruments attached to the scope, thus solving the patient's problem. Unfortunately, this technique does not remove the gallbladder, the source of the gallstones, and the patient is at some risk for a recurrence. This risk can be minimized by enlarging the opening where the duct enters the intestinal tract. This technique, too, is advantageous for patients who are elderly or ill and cannot withstand the trauma of surgery and anesthesia.

There are other options besides surgery or dietary changes for the treatment of patients with gallstones. Medicines are available that can dissolve the gallstones by changing the chemical nature and solubility of bile. Such drugs, however, are not ideal: They work only for certain types of gallstones, are expensive, and may produce side effects. In addition, there may be a recurrence of the gallstones when a patient stops taking these medicines. Such a result indicates that the bile-concentrating action of the gallbladder combines with a given patient's bile composition to create a gallstone-forming environment. Thus, gallstones will continue to form unless the gallbladder is removed or the bile is again altered when the taking of such medicines is resumed. Patients can also have the gallstones broken up into very small pieces, as is often done with kidney stones, by high-frequency sound waves aimed at the gallstones. This procedure, however, known as lithotripsy, has drawbacks: It works in only a small percentage of patients (those with a limited amount of small gallstones), and the results have not been uniformly consistent or satisfactory.

### PERSPECTIVE AND PROSPECTS

Diseases of the gallbladder and biliary system are common in modern industrialized societies. The exact etiologies are not entirely clear, but they may involve dietary mechanisms or other customs of the Western lifestyle. There is also evidence that genetic factors are important, as gallbladder disease often runs in families. Traditionally, the treatment of non-life-threatening gallbladder disease has been conservative, with dietary discretion being the most important factor. When that failed, or if the condition was more serious, the gallbladder was removed. Open cholecystectomy was long considered the best method for dealing with these problems. This operation has been recently challenged by endoscopic and laparoscopic techniques, which have become widely available and enjoyed great success. These new treatment options will become more important as increasing medical costs promote the refinement of less invasive and better techniques. Nevertheless, open cholecystectomy is sometimes the only option for a patient, and less invasive techniques can have limitations as well as complications.

Basic scientific research is also important in this field. Investigations into the mechanisms of gallstone formation are critical to the understanding of gallbladder diseases, as gallstones are the cause of many of these problems. As with many other diseases, prevention might be the key to eliminating many gallbladder diseases, making biliary colic, cholecystitis, and common bile duct diseases rare.

—*Mark Wengrovitz*

***See also*** Abdominal disorders; Gastrointestinal disorders; Intestinal disorders; Jaundice; Kidney stones; Liver cancer; Liver disorders; Obesity; Pain, types of; Pancreatitis; Stones.

### FOR FURTHER INFORMATION:

Blumgart, L. H., ed. *Surgery of the Liver and Biliary Tract.* 2 vols. Edinburgh, Scotland: Churchill Livingstone, 1988. This authoritative text offers a comprehensive, detailed description of the subject.

Cameron, John L., ed. *Current Surgical Therapy.* 4th ed. St. Louis: B. C. Decker, 1992. An excellent textbook that covers all surgical problems, including those related to gallbladder and gallstone removal.

Krames Communications. *The Gallbladder Surgery Book.* San Bruno, Calif.: Author, 1991. This helpful book provides the general reader with an understanding of the symptoms of gallbladder diseases, their most common causes, and treatment options.

————. *Laparoscopic Gallbladder Surgery.* San Bruno, Calif.: Author, 1991. This work offers information regarding laparoscopic cholecystectomy to patients who are facing gallbladder surgery.

Maingot, Rodney. *Maingot's Abdominal Operations.* Edited by Seymour I. Schwartz and Harold Ellis. 9th ed. 2 vols. Norwalk, Conn.: Appleton and Lange, 1989. This textbook, in its ninth edition, has long been considered the classic work on all surgical disciplines. Contains an excellent section on gallbladder diseases.

## GALLSTONES. *See* GALLBLADDER DISEASES.

## GANGLIONS. *See* CYSTS AND GANGLIONS.

## GANGRENE

**SYSTEMS AFFECTED:** All

**SPECIALISTS:** General surgeons, internists

**DEFINITION:** Necrosis (death of tissue) resulting from blood loss and bacterial invasion followed by putrefaction; may be initiated by a variety of diseases and conditions, and if left untreated may result in need for amputation or in death.

**KEY TERMS:**

*anaerobic:* referring to conditions that favor the growth of an organism in the absence of oxygen

*cellulitis:* an infection of the skin which, if left untreated, can abscess and kill the affected tissue

*collagenase:* an enzyme that breaks down the proteins of collagen tissue, a primary component of connective tissue (ligaments and tendons)

*debridement:* cleansing of a wound by removal of dirt, foreign objects, damaged tissue, and cellular debris, in order to promote healing

*exotoxin:* a toxic protein, such as an enzyme, excreted by microorganisms into the environment

*Gram's stain:* a stain used to classify bacteria as either gram-positive (they retain the primary stain of crystal violet when subjected to treatment with a decolorizer) or gram-negative (no coloration)

*hemolysis:* the premature breakdown of red blood cells

*hyaluronidase:* an enzyme that breaks down hyaluronic acid, the gel-like matrix of connective tissue

*lecithinase:* an enzyme that breaks down lecithin, a kind of phospholipid that is a component of human cells (such as red blood cells)

*necrosis:* localized tissue death that occurs in groups of cells in response to disease or injury

## CAUSES AND SYMPTOMS

The term "gangrene" is used when wounded or traumatized tissue has become so badly infected by bacteria that the tissue dies. The infection can be localized, but the threat of the gangrene spreading to other tissue is very serious: It can rapidly become fatal to the patient.

There are approximately thirty different clostridial bacteria species that can cause infection in the human body as they release toxins into the system. Five species of clostridia can cause gangrene. *Clostridium perfringens* is the most common culprit: This species is responsible for about 90 percent of invasive infections in damaged tissue. The other four species are *C. novyi, C. septicum, C. sordellii,* and *C. histolyticum.* Clostridia are bacilli (rod-shaped) bacteria. They are anaerobic and form spores that are heat-resistant. These spores are larger than the cells that produce them, but they are not motile.

*C. perfringens* is found in all types of soil, including desert sand and marine sediments. The spores produced by these bacteria can survive for years until conditions are right for germination. In addition to the soil, these bacteria are found in the mouth, vaginal tract, and intestinal tract. While these species can go undetected and be innocuous for a lifetime, they can cause gangrene in the intestinal tract and the adjoining peritoneum in persons with a bowel obstruction. They can also become dangerously active if freed into the abdominal cavity during invasive surgery or postoperatively if some of the intestine is isolated from the blood supply (ischemia). A type of gangrene, anaerobic puerperal sepsis, may result if the uterus is traumatized by surgical procedures such as septic instrumental abortions. This gangrene is especially dangerous, as mortality is high even with immediate treatment.

*C. perfringens* works anaerobically in tissue that has been deprived of oxygen. This deprivation can result from a decreased blood supply caused by damaged or crushed blood vessels or clots that block the flow of blood; the release of sulfhydryl groups or oxidases (oxygen-consuming enzymes) by traumatized tissue (from a wound, tourniquet, or foreign body); diseases that may damage the circulatory system, such as diabetes or arteriosclerosis; aerobic bacteria that use up the available oxygen in a given area; or chemicals introduced by soil or dirt that kill cells. Without living cells, there is no tissue to receive oxygen from the circulatory system. The anaerobes thrive in this oxygen-poor environment, since they also take advantage of and use the vitamins, amino acids, salts, and carbohydrates of damaged and dying cells. As the bacteria grow and reproduce in this environment, they infect neighboring tissue, including the lymphatic system. More cells are killed, which in turn provides a larger anaerobic environment in which the bacteria can increase in number. This spreading process can be very

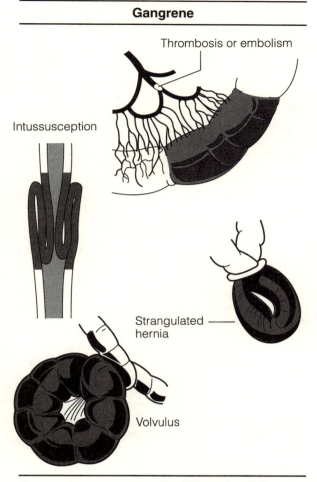

### Gangrene

Thrombosis or embolism

Intussusception

Strangulated hernia

Volvulus

*Gangrene may occur as a result of obstruction of the organs through a variety of means: strangulation, thrombosis, embolism, intussusception, volvulus, or other obstruction. The most dangerous form of gangrene, however (not pictured here), is gas gangrene, which results from infection by clostridial bacteria and usually occurs as a result of war wounds or other severe trauma.*

quick; a whole limb can become affected within a matter of hours. Bacteremia, toxemia, and hemolysis then develop, followed by circulatory failure, renal shutdown, and death.

Types of wounds that have a greater likelihood of developing anaerobic infections are jagged shrapnel wounds in soldiers on the battlefield, accidents (such as those caused by car wrecks) that result in crushed or torn limbs, wounds contaminated by dirty hands or instruments, and wounds resulting from human or animal bites. These wounds can be jeopardized by clostridial spores that are in the soil, or, as in the case of abdominal surgery, perforation of the large intestine may liberate clostridia into the area. The spores only germinate under anaerobic conditions; once they begin reproducing, however, they can maintain their own anaerobic environment.

Gangrenous infections can be divided into three categories: simple contamination, cellulitis, and gas gangrene. Simple contamination is infection with clostridia and/or streptococcal bacteria. Visible signs of simple contamination include a brown discharge of pus with a putrid odor. While this infection may increase in severity, it is possible that healing may result instead.

The second category of gangrenous infection is anaerobic cellulitis. Anaerobic cellulitis may be a worsened condition of simple contamination or may be the initial contamination of clostridia. It can develop within three or four days of exposure. Typically, the bacteria will multiply within connective tissue spaces and release gas. As gas is produced, the resulting pressure keeps the wound open and allows seepage of a foul-smelling discharge. This infection may remain localized or may spread, but little pain is associated with this form.

Gas gangrene, the most dangerous form of this type of infection, is also known as malignant edema. Its incubation period may be a mere four to six hours or may be as long as six weeks. Gas gangrene is not painless; the onset is sudden, with a feeling of increased weight in the affected area. The sufferer will feel critically ill, look pale, sweat, and be delirious, maniacal, or totally apathetic. The patient should be monitored for shock. The wound has not changed in appearance, but there may be an odorless discharge. Gas released is trapped between muscle fibers and can be found by palpitation. If treatment is not begun, toxemia, hemolytic anemia, and renal failure (caused by tubular necrosis) may occur; death then follows.

The seriousness of the invasion is determined by the location of the infection. The least worrisome is an infection of the subcutaneous skin layers that develops slowly, producing little pain with its inflammation. Even so, gas released from the bacteria may be trapped within the affected area and can be palpated (a sensation known as crepitance). This localized infection, referred to as clostridial anaerobic cellulitis, is not particularly dangerous.

Gas gangrene will more likely occur when the affected area is a deep infection of the muscle layers. The muscle cells are abundant in carbohydrates, a rich energy source for the pervasive bacteria. The bacteria release two byproducts as they consume cells: hydrogen gas and toxins. The gas collects and puts so much pressure on the sheets of muscles that the fibers begin to separate. In these gaps between fibers, the fluid accumulates and can further decrease the likelihood of the tissue's survival. The toxins emitted by the bacteria move quickly into more muscle cells, causing necrosis. This form of infection causes intense pain, and the rapid spread of the bacteria magnifies the symptoms. Affected muscle becomes pale, then fails to respond to stimuli. Following this stage, the muscle turns deep red and then black as the gangrene progresses. The skin covering the muscle also undergoes discoloration; a bronze tint colors the taut skin, and blisters filled with dark fluid appear. Eventually, even the skin blackens. The area is so inflamed that crepitance is hard to ascertain.

Though usually associated with skin and muscle, gangrene can also involve the lungs, pleural cavity, eye, brain, liver, or uterus.

## TREATMENT AND THERAPY

When gas gangrene occurs, it should be considered a medical emergency. Because gas gangrene spreads and infects so rapidly and endangers either a limb or the patient's life, the use of the laboratory in diagnosis is minimal before treatment: If the physician waits two or three days while the bacteria are cultivated and identified, the patient will likely lose a limb or may die.

The surest way to detect the presence of *C. perfringens* to diagnose gas gangrene is to aspirate some of the fluid that is seeping from the wound. Since these bacteria may normally inhabit the human environment, care must be taken not to contaminate the sample. Using needle and syringe aspiration rather than swabs will help keep the sample clean. If a section of tissue is removed to study, it must not be exposed to air; the bacteria would not survive the oxygen bath, and the readings would therefore be inaccurate. To ensure that no oxygen contamination has occurred, the syringe used to collect the fluid should be capped off and the sample should be injected into a transport container that is oxygen-free. This container would be a vial filled with nitrogen gas or carbon dioxide, filled with a reducing agent, or filled with a solution containing thioglycolate or cysteine.

Once the specimen has reached the laboratory, it should first be examined by microscope. In order for the bacteria to be seen in the microscope, a Gram's stain should be done. It is important to pinpoint the genus and species of bacteria so that proper treatment can begin as soon as possible. Since *C. perfringens* is gram-positive, the stain pattern and the bacterial size and shape immediately identify this bacteria as an anaerobe. Identifying characteristics would be a rod shape (either large and blunt-ended or long, skinny, and pointed), irregular staining, or the presence of cocci of different sizes. Not only can shape and size be detected, but an estimate of bacterial number can indicate the extent of the infection as well.

After a preliminary identification of the bacteria has been accomplished with staining and microscopy, cultivation and definitive identification follow. The specimen is inoculated onto several media (such as meat glucose, thioglycolate, and blood agar) and allowed to incubate anaerobically for forty-eight to seventy-two hours at 35 to 37 degrees Celsius. Then the samples are examined to detect colonization and the presence or absence of hemolysis. Final identification is made by compiling information about the results of the Gram's stain, the structure of the colony, biochemical reactions, and a determination of the end products released as glucose is fermented. This determination is made by infusing the colony with a glucose broth and monitoring the end products that are released using gas chromatography. Another test to detect *C. perfringens* measures lecithinase production. There is no value in examining the blood serum in a gangrene patient's blood.

Mortality rates for cases of gas gangrene that do not receive treatment range from 40 to 60 percent. Therefore, if signs indicate the presence of clostridia, immediate surgery is important to examine the affected tissue. The wound (and all tissue showing signs of bacterial invasion) should be thoroughly and aggressively debrided (cleansed) and the infected area removed. Depending on the extent of the infection, amputation of the area may be indicated to prevent further spread of the disease. Antibiotic therapy is also given in an attempt to stop bacterial growth; penicillin is the drug of choice.

If the infection has not progressed to the point that amputation is necessary, hyperbaric oxygen can sometimes be used for successful treatment. This treatment consists of putting the patient in a chamber of pure oxygen for a brief period several times a day. This environment is too rich for the bacteria to survive. The exposure to these conditions does not alter the oxygen-carrying capabilities or saturation of red blood cells. It does result in an important difference in the oxygen tension of the serum (and thereby the lymph in the interstitial tissue). The significance of this variation is that it may interrupt toxin synthesis and bacteria growth. This enhances the body's ability to combat the infection in that it allows normal phagocytic and host defense mechanisms to take control.

Although clostridial infections are not usually transmissible from one person to another, patients diagnosed with gas gangrene should be placed on drainage/secretion precautions. This simply means that those in contact with the patient should wear gowns and gloves and should wash their hands thoroughly after touching the patient or any contaminated articles. Those articles that are contaminated should be disposed of or cleaned thoroughly. Autoclaving of instruments and equipment should ensure adequate sterilization. Boiling and chemical disinfection is not enough to kill resistant spores contaminating other articles. To be rid of the infective organisms completely, dressings should be burned, bed linens autoclaved, and mattresses and pillows sterilized in an ethylene oxide chamber. The relatively small danger of transmission is to other patients with surgical or traumatic wounds.

Antitoxins have been developed for gas gangrene, but they are not reliable and have not come into practical use. Since there is no effective antitoxin against gangrene induced by *C. perfringens*, prevention lies in how the wound is treated. There must be a thorough debridement and an adequate dosage of antibiotics. In addition, final closure of the wound should be delayed for two or three days to allow complete drainage of the area. Any bandage or cast that must be applied should allow adequate circulation of air (an airless environment would encourage growth of *C. perfringens*).

## PERSPECTIVE AND PROSPECTS

The first anecdotes describing gangrene were in the seventeenth century. Since the Napoleonic Wars, gas gangrene has caused much death and disfigurement. In World War I, this was especially the case; as many as 10 percent of all wounded soldiers were infected. Many who would have survived their injuries succumbed to gas gangrene. In most of these cases, infection came through contaminated soil that had been fertilized with human and animal waste. The contamination most often was by several clostridial species.

Early surgical procedures carried the same risk; lack of sanitary conditions and poor (or absent) disinfection techniques led to far more deaths than injuries warranted. By the late 1800's, anaerobes were identified as the culprits causing putrefaction and infections associated with tissue necrosis, gas emissions in tissue, and a foul odor. The scientists credited with first isolating *C. perfringens* as the causative bacteria in gas gangrene were George Nuttall and William Welch in 1892. Though these bacteria were extensively studied, it was not until the 1960's that adequate diagnostic technology was available for clinical use. Because of this technology, there was a far smaller impact of gangrene on the battlefields of the Vietnam War. The threat of gangrene is still a reality, however, in the postoperative patient.

*C. perfringens* is also implicated in another common health hazard: food poisoning. This species is responsible for 3 percent of food poisoning outbreaks and 11 percent of single cases. Such food poisoning usually occurs with ingestion of meat, poultry, and gravies that are contaminated with *C. perfringens*. Most outbreaks are associated with restaurant, dormitory, or bulk food preparation and not with home cooking. Once the bacteria enter the intestinal tract, they make their presence obvious within eight to twenty-four hours. Typically, the disease is mild, producing discomfort in the form of abdominal pain and diarrhea. It usually runs its course in twenty-four hours. Medicinal treatment is unwarranted; the manifestations of this disease are often mild enough that the infection is undiagnosed.

*C. perfringens* may have the opportunity to multiply before the food is eaten. Contaminated dishes should be thoroughly reheated to prevent illness. Since *C. perfringens* produces endospores that are heat resistant, simply cooking or heating the food may be insufficient. Contamination is reinforced because heating also drives off oxygen, creating an environment in which the bacteria thrive. Therefore, those spores that survive the heating process are encouraged in this oxygen-poor medium to reproduce and grow quickly. Clostridial food poisoning can be avoided by refraining from eating foods that have been sitting out for prolonged periods. When there is a delay between preparation and eating, then food should be kept at very warm or very cool temperatures (above 60 degrees Celsius or below 5 degrees Celsius). *—Iona C. Baldridge*

*See also* Bacterial infections; Embolism; Food poisoning; Frostbite; Hernia; Infection; Poisoning; Thrombosis and thrombus; Wounds.

**FOR FURTHER INFORMATION:**

Jawetz, Ernest, Joseph L. Melnick, and Edward A. Adelberg. *Medical Microbiology*. 19th ed. Norwalk, Conn.: Appleton and Lange, 1991. A comprehensive microbiology text written primarily for medical students but also used by physicians and health science students. Some background is helpful in reading through the sections on microbiological principles, immunology, pathogenesis, and chemotherapy.

Morello, Josephine A., Helen Eckel Mizer, Marion E. Wilson, and Paul A. Granato. *Microbiology in Patient Care*. 5th ed. Dubuque, Iowa: Wm. C. Brown, 1994. This text is addressed to beginning students of health-related fields. It is divided into a section introducing the principles of microbiology and a section relating microbial diseases and their epidemiology. Well written and illustrated.

Pelczar, Michael J., Jr., E. C. S. Chan, and Noel R. Krieg. *Microbiology: Concepts and Applications*. New York: McGraw-Hill, 1993. A colorfully illustrated text for the undergraduate in microbiology with little background in chemistry and biology. After the history of microbiology is presented, fundamental concepts of microbiology are balanced with medical microbiology, environmental microbiology, and microbial genetics.

Schaechter, Moselio, Gerald Medoff, and David Schlessinger, eds. *Mechanisms of Microbial Disease*. Baltimore: Williams & Wilkins, 1989. A readable textbook designed for medical students, graduate students, and advanced undergraduate students. Combines microbiology with the study of infectious diseases, relating both subjects to the major human systems. This work is not intended to be an exhaustive reference volume.

Schuhardt, Vernon T. *Pathogenic Microbiology*. Philadelphia: J. B. Lippincott, 1978. A text for introductory pathology students. Bacterial infections are addressed, as are those caused by fungi, rickettsia, and viruses. The diseases are discussed relative to etiology, epidemiology, pathogenicity, symptoms, diagnosis, prevention, and treatment.

Slack, J. M., and I. S. Snyder. *Bacteria and Human Disease*. Chicago: Year Book Medical Publishers, 1978. This book was written for the beginning student who has very little background in bacteriology. The basic information given includes characteristics of pathogenic bacteria, how they cause disease, and which diseases they cause.

Youmans, Guy P., Philip Y. Paterson, and Herbert M. Sommers, eds. *The Biologic and Clinical Basis of Infectious Diseases*. 2d ed. Philadelphia: W. B. Saunders, 1980. Infectious disease is the primary focus of this text. Recognizes the direct relationship between disease and microbes and addresses their different modes of action. Also acknowledges the interactions between invading microorganisms and the host's defense mechanisms.

# GASTRITIS. *See* ABDOMINAL DISORDERS; GASTROINTESTINAL DISORDERS.

# GASTROENTERITIS. *See* ABDOMINAL DISORDERS; GASTROINTESTINAL DISORDERS.

# GASTROINTESTINAL DISORDERS

**SYSTEM AFFECTED:** Gastrointestinal

**SPECIALISTS:** Gastroenterologists, internists

**DEFINITION:** The many problems that can affect the gastrointestinal tract, such as infections, injuries, dysfunctions, tumors, congenital defects, and genetic abnormalities.

**KEY TERMS:**

*gastroenterologist:* a medical specialist in diseases of the gut

*endoscope:* any of several flexible fiber-optic scopes used to examine the inside of the gut; it is equipped with tools to cauterize wounds or remove tissue or gallstones

*intestines:* the section of the gut between the anus and the stomach, consisting of the rectum, colon, and small bowel (subdivided into the ileus, jejunum, and duodenum)

*motility:* the spontaneous movements of the gut during swallowing, digestion, and elimination

*mucosa:* the tissue lining the interior of the gastrointestinal tract, through which nutrients pass into the bloodstream

*stool:* the waste products excreted from the body upon defecation; feces

*tumor:* a mass of abnormal cells that can be cancerous

## CAUSES AND SYMPTOMS

What and how people eat, their digestion, and their toilet habits affect their health more than any other voluntary daily activity. Breathing, circulation, the brain's control of most bodily functions—these normally take place without conscious thought. The intake of nourishment and elimination of wastes, by contrast, afford a great variety of choices. Accordingly, poor or self-destructive eating and toilet habits lie behind many gastrointestinal (GI) disorders. Yet not all disorders result from an individual's habits. Many arise because of a person's cultural or physical environment, some are hereditary or congenital, and a fair amount have no known cause. All told, more than one hundred disorders may originate in the GI tract and its organs, including infections, cancer, dysfunctions, obstructions, autoimmune diseases, malabsorption of nutrients, and reactions to toxins taken in during eating, drinking, or breathing. Furthermore, diseases in other organs, systemic infections such as lupus, immune suppression such as that caused by acquired immunodeficiency syndrome (AIDS), reactions to altered body conditions as during pregnancy, and psychiatric problems can all reverberate to the gut.

The symptoms of GI disorders range from mildly annoying to life-threatening, although seldom does any single symptom except massive bleeding lead quickly to death. Indigestion, bloating, and gas send more people to gastroenterologists than any other set of symptoms, and they often reflect nothing more than overeating. Pain anywhere along the gut, aversion to food (anorexia), and nausea are general symptoms common to many disorders, although pain in the chest is likely to come from the esophagus while pain in the abdomen points to a stomach or intestinal problem. Red blood in the stool indicates bleeding in the intestines, black (digested) blood suggests bleeding in the upper small bowel or stomach, and vomited blood indicates injury to the stomach or esophagus—all dangerous signs indeed. Chronic diarrhea, fatty stool, constipation, difficulty in swallowing, hiccuping, vomiting, and cramps point to disturbances in the GI tract's orderly, wavelike contractions or absorption of nutrients and fluid. Pruritis (intense itching) can come from something as transient as a mild drug reaction or as serious as cancer. Dysentery (bloody diarrhea) usually comes from severe inflammation or lesions caused by viruses, bacteria, or other parasites. Malnourishment is a sign of badly disordered digestion, and ascites (fluid accumulation in body cavities) can result from serious disease in the liver or pancreas. Likewise, jaundice, the yellowing of the skin or eyes because of excess bile, signals problems in the liver, pancreas, or their ducts.

The large number and complexity of GI disorders do not allow a quick, comprehensive summary. Fortunately, many are uncommon, and the most frequent problems can be described through a tour of the GI tract. The GI tract is basically a tube that moves food from one end to the other, extracting energy and biochemical building blocks for the body along the way. So a disorder that interrupts the flow in one section of the intestines can have secondary effects on other parts of the gut. Disorders seldom affect one area alone.

*The esophagus.* The GI tract's first section, the esophagus, is simply a passageway from the mouth to the stomach. Although it rarely gets infected, the esophagus is the site of several common problems, usually relatively minor, if painful. Muscle dysfunctions, including slow, weak, or spasmodic muscular movement, can impair motility and make swallowing difficult, as can strictures, which usually occur at the sphincter to the stomach. The mucosal lining of the esophagus is not as hardy as in other parts of the gut. When acid backflushes from the stomach into the esophagus, it inflames tissue there and can cause burning and even bleeding, a condition popularly known as heartburn and technically called gastroesophageal reflux disease (GERD). Retching and vomiting, usually resulting from alcohol abuse or associated with a hiatal hernia, can tear the mucosa. Smokers and drinkers run the risk of esophageal cancer, which can spread down into the gut early in its development and then becomes deadly; however, it accounts for only about 1 percent of cancers. Most of these conditions can be cured or controlled if diagnosed early enough.

*The stomach.* In order to store food and prepare it for digestion lower in the gut, the stomach churns it into a homogenous mass and releases it in small portions into the small bowel; meanwhile, the stomach also secretes acid to kill bacteria. Bacteria that are acid-resistant, however, can multiply there. One type, *Helicobacter pylori*, is thought to be involved in the development of ulcers and perhaps cancer. Overuse of aspirins and other nonsteroidal anti-inflammatory drugs (NSAIDs) can also cause stomach ulcers. A variety of substances, including alcohol, can prompt inflammation and even hemorrhaging. Stomach cancer has been shown to strike those who have a diet high in salted, smoked, or pickled foods; the most common cancer in the world, although not in the United States, it has a low survival rate. When stomach muscle function fails, food accumulates until the stomach overstretches and rebounds, causing vomiting. Some foods can coalesce into an indigestible lump, and hair and food fibers can roll into a ball, called a bezoar; such masses can interfere with digestion.

*The small intestine.* The five to six meters of looped gut between the stomach and colon is called the small intestine. It secretes fluids, hormones, and enzymes into food passing through, breaking it down chemically and absorbing nutrients. Although cancers seldom develop in the small intestine itself, they frequently do so in the organs connected to it, the liver and pancreas. The major problem in the small bowel is the multitude of diseases causing diarrhea, dysentery, or ulceration: They include bacterial, viral, and parasitic disease; motility disorders; and the chronic, progressive inflammatory illness called Crohn's disease, which also ulcerates the bowel wall. Although most diarrhea is temporary, if its persists diarrhea severely weakens patients through dehydration and malnourishment. For this reason, diarrheal diseases caused by toxins in water or food are the leading cause of childhood death worldwide. Furthermore, the small bowel can become paralyzed, twisted, or kinked, thereby obstructing the passage of food. Sometimes its contents rush through too fast, a condition called dumping syndrome. All these disorders reduce digestion, and if they are chronic, then malnutrition, vitamin deficiency, and weight loss ensue.

*The large intestine.* The small intestine empties into the large intestine, or colon, the last meter of the GI tract; here the water content of digestive waste matter (about a liter a day) is reabsorbed, and the waste becomes increasingly solid along the way to the rectum, forming feces. Unlike the small bowel, which is nearly sterile under normal conditions, the colon hosts a large population of bacteria that ferments the indigestible fiber in waste matter, and some of the by-products are absorbed through the colon's mucosa. Bacteria or parasites gaining access from the outside world can cause diarrhea by interfering with this absorption (a condition called malabsorption) or by irritating the mucosa and speeding up muscle action. For unknown reasons, the colon can also become chronically inflamed, resulting in cramps and bloody diarrhea, an illness known as ulcerative colitis; Crohn's disease also can affect the colon. Probably because it is so often exposed to a variety of toxins, the colon is particularly susceptible to cancer in people over fifty years old: Colorectal cancer accounted for the second highest number of cancer deaths in 1993, with an equal proportion of men and women. As people age, the muscles controlling the colon deteriorate, sometimes forming small pouches in the bowel wall, called diverticula, that can become infected (diverticulitis). In ad-

## Gastrointestinal Tract

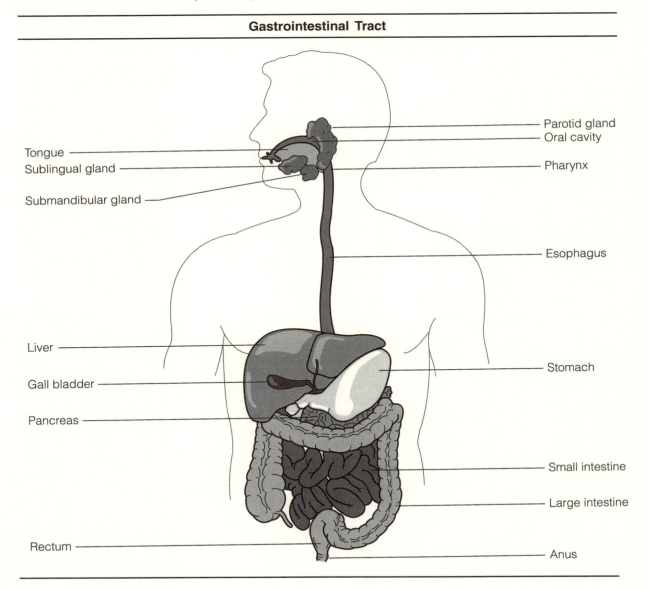

Tongue
Sublingual gland
Submandibular gland
Liver
Gall bladder
Pancreas
Rectum

Parotid gland
Oral cavity
Pharynx
Esophagus
Stomach
Small intestine
Large intestine
Anus

dition, small knobs called polyps can grow, and they may become cancerous. One of the most common lower GI disorders is constipation, which may derive from a poor diet, motility malfunction, or both.

*The rectum.* The last segment of the colon, the rectum collects and holds feces for defecation through the anus. The rectum is susceptible to many of the diseases affecting the colon, including cancer and chronic inflammation. The powerful anal sphincter muscle, which controls defecation, can be the site of brief but intensely painful spasms called proctalgia fugax, which strikes for unknown reasons. The tissue lining the anal canal contains a dense network of blood vessels called hemorrhoids; straining to eliminate stool because of constipation or diarrhea or simply sitting too long on a toilet can distend hemorrhoids, which may burn, itch, bleed, and become remarkably annoying. If infected, hemorrhoids or anal fissures may develop painful abscesses (sacs of pus). Extreme straining can cause the rectum to turn inside out through the anus, or prolapse.

*The liver.* The GI tract's organs figure prominently in many disorders. The liver is a large spongy organ that filters the blood, removing toxins and dumping them with bile into the duodenum. A number of viruses can invade the liver and inflame it, a malady called hepatitis. Acute forms of the disease have flulike symptoms and are self-limited. Some viruses, however, as well as alcohol or drug abuse and worms, cause extensive cirrhosis (the formation of abnormal, scarlike tissue) and chronic hepatitis. Although only recently common in the United States, viral hepatitis has long affected a large percentage of people in Southeast Asia; because hepatitis can trigger the mutation of normal cells, liver cancer is among the most common cancers worldwide. Hepatitis patients often have jaundice, as do those who, as a result of drug reactions, cancer, or stones, have blocked bile flow. Because of congenital or inherited errors of metabolism, excess fat, iron, and copper can build up in the liver, causing upper abdominal pain, skin discolorations, weakness, and behavioral changes; complications can include cirrhosis, diabetes mellitus, and heart disease.

*The gallbladder.* A small sac that concentrates and stores bile from the liver, the gallbladder is connected to the liver and duodenum by ducts. The concentrate often coalesces into stones, which seldom cause problems if they stay in one place. If they block the opening to the gallbladder or lodge in a duct, however, they can cause pain, fever, and jaundice. Although rare, tumors may also grow in the gallbladder or ducts, perhaps as a result of gallstone obstruction.

*The pancreas.* Lying just behind the stomach, the pancreas produces enzymes to break down fats and proteins for absorption and insulin to metabolize sugar; a duct joins it to the duodenum. The pancreas can become inflamed, either because of toxins (largely alcohol) or blockage of its duct, usually by gallstones. Either cause precipitates a painful condition, pancreatitis, that may last a few days, with full recovery, or turn into a life-threatening disease. If the source of inflammation is not eliminated, chronic pancreatitis may develop and with it the gradual loss of the pancreas' ability to make enzymes and insulin: Severe abdominal pain, malnutrition, diarrhea, and diabetes may develop. Pancreatic cancer, once rare in the United States, ranked fifth among cancers causing death during 1993. Scientists are unsure of the causes; pancreatitis, gallstones, diabetes, and alcohol have been implicated, but only smoking is well attested to increase the risk of contracting pancreatic cancer, which is very lethal and difficult to treat. Only about 1 percent of patients live more than a year after diagnosis.

*Functional diseases.* Finally, some disorders appear to upset several parts of the GI tract at the same time, often with no identifiable cause but with chronic or recurrent symptoms. Gastroenterologists call them functional diseases, and they afflict as much as 30 percent of the population in Western countries. People with irritable bowel syndrome (IBS) complain of abdominal pain, urgency in defecation, and bloating from intestinal gas; they often feel that they cannot empty their rectums completely, even after straining. Functional dyspepsia manifests itself as upper abdominal pain, bloating, early feelings of fullness during a meal, and nausea. Also included in this group are various motility disorders in the esophagus and stomach, whose typical symptom is vomiting, and pseudo-obstruction, a condition in which the small bowel acts as if it is blocked but no lesion can be found. Many gastroenterologists believe that emotional disturbance plays a part in some of these diseases.

## TREATMENT AND THERAPY

The majority of GI disorders are transient and pose no short-term or long-term threat to life. The body's natural defenses can combat most bacterial and viral infections in the gut without help. Even potentially dangerous noninfectious conditions, such as pancreatitis, resolve on their own if the irritating agent is eliminated. Many disorders require a gastroenterologist's help, however, and even despite help can make people semi-invalids. Regulation of diet and the use of drugs to combat infections or relieve pain are important treatments. If these fail, as is likely to happen in such serious conditions as chronic inflammatory disease and cancer, cures or palliation is yet possible because of gastroenterological technology, particularly endoscopy, and surgical techniques developed in the twentieth century.

While it is not true that GI disorders would necessarily disappear with improved diet, since genetic disorders would remain, gastroenterologists stress that proper nourishment is the first line of defense against trouble. For example, incidence of stomach cancer plummets in countries where people eat fresh foods and use refrigeration rather than salting and smoking to preserve food. Regions where fiber makes up a high percentage of the diet, such as Africa, have a far lower incidence of inflammatory bowel disease. Last, and certainly not least, groups that do not drink alcohol or smoke (such as Mormons) have far lower incidences of cancer and inflammatory disease throughout the GI tract. —*Roger Smith*

*See also* Abdominal disorders; Alcoholism; Appendicitis; Cholecystitis; Cirrhosis; Colitis; Colon cancer; Constipation; Crohn's disease; Diarrhea and dysentery; Diverticulitis and diverticulosis; Gallbladder diseases; Heartburn; Hemorrhoids; Hernia; Indigestion; Intestinal disorders; Jaundice; Liver cancer; Liver disorders; Nausea and vomiting; Obstruction; Pancreatitis; Peritonitis; Renal failure; Stomach, intestinal, and pancreatic cancers; Ulcers.

**FOR FURTHER INFORMATION:**

Janowitz, Henry D. *Indigestion: Living Better with Upper Intestinal Problems from Heartburn to Ulcers and Gallstones*. New York: Oxford University Press, 1992. Clear explanations of common ailments, especially those related to aging, to help people prevent or manage GI disorders. With charts and illustrations.

Sachar, David B., Jerome D. Waye, and Blair S. Lewis, eds. *Pocket Guide to Gastroenterology*. Rev. ed. Baltimore: Williams & Wilkins, 1991. In detailed outlines intended for physicians, this handbook contains a wealth of information from which general readers can profit despite the extensive use of medical terminology.

Thompson, W. Grant. *The Angry Gut: Coping with Colitis and Crohn's Disease*. New York: Plenum Press, 1993.

_____. *Gut Reactions: Understanding Symptoms of the Digestive Tract*. New York: Plenum Press, 1989. A gastroenterology professor, Thompson nevertheless writes for patients. Both books are excellent, reassuring sources on GI anatomy, general symptoms, and the treatment of common ailments. With illustrations and graphs.

# GENETIC DISEASES

**SYSTEMS AFFECTED:** All

**SPECIALISTS:** Geneticists, internists, obstetricians, pediatricians

**DEFINITION:** A variety of disorders transmitted from parent to child through chromosomal material; most people experience disease related to genetics in some form, and research into this area is yielding greater understanding of the relationship between disease and hereditary proclivities toward disease, as well as new strategies for early detection and prevention or therapy.

**KEY TERMS:**

*autosomal recessive disease:* a disease which is only expressed when two copies of a defective gene are inherited, one from each parent; present on non-sex-determining chromosomes

*chromosomes:* rod-shaped structures in each cell which contain genes, the chemical elements that determine traits

*deoxyribonucleic acid (DNA):* the chemical molecule that transmits hereditary information from generation to generation

*dominant gene:* a gene which can express its effect when an individual has only one copy of it

*gene:* the hereditary unit, composed of DNA, that resides on chromosomes

*inheritance:* the passing down of traits from generation to generation

*X-linked:* a term used to describe genes or traits that are located on the X chromosome; a male needs only one copy of an X-linked gene for it to be expressed

**CAUSES AND SYMPTOMS**

Hereditary units called genes determine the majority of the physical and biochemical characteristics of an organism. Genes are composed of a chemical compound called deoxyribonucleic acid (DNA) and are organized into rod-shaped structures called chromosomes that reside in each cell of the body. Each human cell carries forty-six chromosomes organized as twenty-three pairs, each composed of several thousand genes. Twenty-two of the chromosome pairs are homologous pairs; that is, similar genes are located at similar sites on each chromosome. The remaining chromosomes are the sex chromosomes. Human females bear two X chromosomes, and human males possess one X and one Y chromosome.

During the formation of the reproductive cells, the chromosome pairs separate and one copy of each pair is randomly included in the egg or sperm. Each egg will contain twenty-two autosomes (non-sex chromosomes) and one X chromosome. Each sperm will contain twenty-two autosomes and either one X or one Y chromosome. The egg and sperm fuse at fertilization, which restores the proper number of chromosomes, and the genes inherited from the baby's parents will determine its sex and much of its physical appearance and future health and well-being.

Genetic diseases are inherited as a result of the presence of abnormal genes in the reproductive cells of one or both parents of an affected individual. There are two broad classifications of genetic disease: those caused by defects in chromosome number or structure, and those resulting from a much smaller flaw within a gene. Within the latter category, there are four predominant mechanisms by which the disorders can be transmitted from generation to generation: autosomal dominant inheritance, in which the defective gene is inherited from one parent; autosomal recessive inheritance, in which one defective gene is inherited from each parent, who themselves show no signs of the disorder; X-linked chromosomal inheritance (often called sex-linked), in which the flawed gene has been determined to reside on the X chromosome; and multifactorial inheritance,

## Human Chromosomes

### Normal (pair)

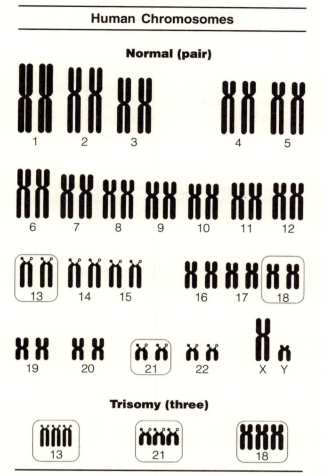

### Trisomy (three)

*Genetic diseases are caused by defects in the number of chromosomes, in their structure, or in the genes on the chromosome (mutation). Shown here is the human complement of chromosomes (23 pairs) and three errors of chromosome number (trisomies) that lead to the genetic disorders Patau's syndrome (trisomy no. 13), Edward's syndrome (no. 18), and the more common Down syndrome (trisomy no. 21).*

in which genes interact with each other and/or environmental factors.

Errors in chromosome number include extra and missing chromosomes. The most common chromosomal defect observed in humans is Down syndrome, which is caused by the presence of three copies of chromosome 21, instead of the usual two. Down syndrome occurs at a frequency of about one in eight hundred live births, this frequency increasing with increasing maternal age. The symptoms of this disorder include mental retardation, short stature, and numerous other medical problems. The most common form of Down syndrome results from the failure of the two cop-

ies of chromosome 21 to separate during reproductive cell formation, which upon fusion with a normal reproductive cell at fertilization produces an embryo containing three copies of chromosome 21.

Gross defects in chromosome structure include duplicated and deleted portions of chromosomes and broken and rearranged chromosome fragments. Prader-Willi syndrome results from a deletion of a small portion of chromosome 15. Children affected with this disorder are mentally retarded, obese, and diabetic. Cri du chat (literally, cat cry) syndrome is associated with a large deletion in chromosome 5. Affected infants exhibit facial abnormalities, are severely retarded, and produce a high-pitched, kittenlike wail.

Genetic diseases caused by defects in individual genes result when defective genes are propagated through many generations or a new genetic flaw develops in a reproductive cell. New genetic defects arise from a variety of causes, including environmental assaults such as radiation, toxins, or drugs. More than four thousand such gene disorders have been identified.

Manifestation of an autosomal dominant disorder requires the inheritance of only one defective gene from one parent who is afflicted with the disease. Inheritance of two dominant defective genes, one from each parent, is possible but generally creates such severe consequences that the child dies while still in the womb or shortly after birth. An individual who bears one copy of the gene has a 50 percent chance of transmitting that gene and the disease to his or her offspring.

Among the most common autosomal dominant diseases are hyperlipidemia and hypercholesterolemia. Elevated levels of lipids and cholesterol in the blood, which contribute to artery and heart disease, are the consequences of these disorders, respectively. Onset of the symptoms is usually in adulthood, frequently after the affected individual has had children and potentially transmitted the faulty gene to them.

Huntington's chorea causes untreatable neurological deterioration and death, and symptoms do not appear until affected individuals are at least in their forties. Children of parents afflicted with Huntington's chorea face the dilemma of making reproductive decisions without the knowledge of whether they themselves carry the defective gene; if so, they risk a 50 percent chance of transmitting the dread disease to their offspring.

Autosomal recessive genetic diseases require that an affected individual bear two copies of a defective gene, inheriting one from each parent. Usually the parents are simply carriers of the defective gene; their one normal copy masks the effect of the one flawed copy. If two carriers have offspring, 25 percent will receive two copies of the flawed gene and inherit the disease, and 50 percent will be asymptomatic carriers.

Cystic fibrosis is an autosomal recessive disease which occurs at a rate of about one in two thousand live births among Caucasians. The defective gene product causes improper chloride transport in cells and results in thick mucous secretions in lungs and other organs. Sickle-cell anemia, another autosomal recessive disorder, is the most common genetic disease among African Americans in the United States. Abnormality in the protein hemoglobin, the component of red blood cells that carries oxygen to all the body's tissues, leads to deformed blood cells that are fragile and easily destroyed.

X-linked genetic diseases are transmitted by faulty genes located on the X chromosome. Females need two copies of the defective gene to acquire such a disease, and in general women carry only one flawed copy, making them asymptomatic carriers of the disorder. Males, having only a single X chromosome, need only one copy of the defective gene to express an X-linked disease. Males with X-linked disorders inherit the defective gene from their mothers, since fathers must contribute a Y chromosome to male offspring. Half of the male offspring of a carrier female will inherit the defective gene and develop the disease. In the rare case of a female with two defective X-linked genes, 100 percent of her male offspring will inherit the disease gene, and, assuming that the father does not carry the defective gene, 50 percent of her female offspring will be carriers. There are more than 250 X-linked disorders, some of the more common being Duchenne's muscular dystrophy, which results in progressive muscle deterioration and early death; hemophilia; and red-green color blindness, which affects about 8 percent of Caucasian males.

Multifactorial inheritance, which accounts for a number of genetic diseases, is caused by the complex interaction of one or more genes with each other and with environmental factors. This group of diseases includes many disorders which, anecdotally, "run in families." Representative disorders include cleft palate, spina bifida, anencephaly, and some inherited heart abnormalities. Other diseases appear to have a genetic component predisposing an individual to be susceptible to environmental stimuli that trigger the disease. These include cancer, hypertension, diabetes, schizophrenia, alcoholism, depression, and obesity.

## Diagnosis and Detection

Most, but not all, genetic diseases manifest their symptoms immediately or soon after the birth of an affected child. Rapid recognition of such a medical condition and its accurate diagnosis are essential for the proper treatment and management of the disease by parents and medical personnel. Medical technology has developed swift and accurate diagnostic methods, in many cases allowing testing of the fetus prior to birth. In addition, tests are available that determine the carrier status of an individual for many autosomal recessive and X-linked diseases. These test results are used in conjunction with genetic counseling of individuals and couples who are at risk of transmitting a genetic disease to their offspring. Thus, such individuals can make informed decisions when planning their reproductive futures.

Errors in chromosome number and structure are detected in an individual by analyzing his or her chromosomes. A small piece of skin or a blood sample is taken the cells in the sample are grown to a sufficient number, and the chromosomes within each cell are stained with special dyes so that they may be viewed with a microscope. A picture of the chromosomes, called a karyotype, is taken, and the patient's chromosome array is compared with that of a normal individual. Extra or missing chromosomes or alterations in chromosome structure are determined, thus identifying the genetic disease. The analysis of karyotypes is the method used to determine the presence of Down, Prader-Willi, and cri du chat syndromes, among others.

Defects in chromosome number and structure can also be identified in the fetus, prior to birth, using two different sample collecting methods: amniocentesis and chorionic villus sampling. In amniocentesis, a needle is inserted through the pregnant woman's abdomen and uterus, into the fluid-filled sac surrounding the fetus. A sample of this fluid, the amniotic fluid, is withdrawn. The amniotic fluid contains fetal cells sloughed off by the fetus. The cells are grown for several weeks until there are enough to perform chromosome analysis. This procedure is performed only after sixteen weeks' gestation, in order to ensure adequate amniotic fluid for sampling.

Chorionic villus sampling relies on a biopsy of the fetal chorion, a membrane surrounding the fetus which is composed of cells that have the same genetic constitution as the fetus. A catheter is inserted through the pregnant woman's vagina and into the uterus until it is in contact with the chorion. The small sample of this tissue that is removed contains enough cells to perform karyotyping immediately, permitting diagnosis by the next day. Chorionic villus sampling can be performed between the eighth and ninth week of pregnancy. This earlier testing gives the procedure an advantage over amniocentesis, since the earlier determination of whether a fetus is carrying a genetic disease allows safer pregnancy termination if the parents choose this course.

Karyotype analysis is limited to the diagnosis of genetic diseases caused by very large chromosome abnormalities. The majority of hereditary disorders are caused by gene flaws that are too small to see microscopically. For many of these diseases, diagnosis is available through either biochemical testing or DNA analysis.

Many genetic disorders cause a lack of a specific biochemical which is necessary for normal metabolism. These types of disorders are frequently referred to as "inborn errors of metabolism." Many of these errors can be detected by the chemical analysis of fetal tissue. For example, galactosemia is a disease which results from the lack of galactose-1-phosphate uridyl transferase. Infants with this disorder cannot break down galactose, one of the major sugars in milk. If left untreated, galactosemia can lead to mental retardation, cataracts, kidney and liver failure, and death. By analyzing fetal cells obtained from amniocentesis or chorionic villus sampling, the level of this important chemical can be assessed, and if necessary, the infant can be placed on a galactose-free diet immediately after birth.

DNA analysis can be used to determine whether a genetic disease has been inherited when the chromosomal location of the gene is known, when the chemical sequence of the DNA is known, and/or when particular DNA sequences commonly associated with the gene in question, called markers, are known.

A sequence of four chemical elements of DNA—adenine (A), guanine (G), thymine (T), and cytosine (C)—make up genes. Sometimes the proper DNA sequence of a gene is known, as well as the changes in the sequence that cause disease. Direct analysis of the DNA of the individual suspected of carrying a certain genetic disorder is possible in these cases. For example, in sickle-cell anemia, it is known that a change in a single DNA chemical element leads to the disorder. To test for this disease, a tissue sample is obtained from prenatal sources (amniocentesis or chorionic villus sampling). The DNA is isolated from the cells and analyzed with highly specific probes that can detect the presence of the defective gene which will lead to sickle-cell anemia. Informed action may be taken regarding the future of the fetus or the care of an affected child.

Occasionally a disease gene itself has not been precisely isolated and its DNA sequence determined, but sequences very near the gene of interest have been analyzed. If specific variations within these neighboring sequences are always present when the gene of interest is flawed, these nearby sequences can then be used as a marker for the presence of the defective gene. When the variant sequences, called restriction fragment length polymorphisms, are present, so is the disease gene. Prenatal testing for cystic fibrosis has been done using restriction fragment length polymorphisms.

Individuals who come from families in which genetic diseases tend to occur can be tested as carriers. In this way, they will know the risk of passing a certain disease to offspring. For example, individuals whose families have a history of cystic fibrosis, but who themselves are not affected, may be asymptomatic carriers. If they have children with individuals who are also cystic fibrosis carriers, they have a 25 percent chance of passing two copies of the defective gene to their offspring. DNA samples from the potential parents can be analyzed for the presence of one defective gene. If both partners are carriers, their decision about whether to have children will be made with knowledge of the possible risk to their offspring. If only one or neither of them is a carrier, their offspring will not be at risk of inheriting cystic fibrosis, an autosomal recessive disease. Carrier testing is possible for many genetic diseases, as well as for disorders which appear late in life, such as Huntington's chorea.

Many of the gene flaws of multifactorial diseases, those that interact with environmental factors to produce disease, have been identified and are testable. Individuals armed with the knowledge of having a gene which puts them at risk for certain disorders can incorporate preventive measures into their lifestyle, thus minimizing the chances of developing the disease. For example, certain cancers, such as colon and breast cancer, have a genetic component. Individuals who test positive for the genes that predispose them to develop cancer can modify their diets to include cancer-fighting foods and receive frequent medical checkups to detect cancer development at its earliest, most treatable stage. Those with genes that contribute to arteriosclerosis and heart disease can modify their diets and increase exercise, and those with a genetic predisposition for alcoholism could avoid the consumption of alcohol.

## PERSPECTIVE AND PROSPECTS

The scientific study of human genetics and genetic disease is relatively new, having begun in the early twentieth century. There are many early historical records, however, which recognize that certain traits are hereditarily transmitted. Ancient Greek literature is peppered with references to heredity, and the Jewish book of religious and civil laws, the Talmud, describes in detail the inheritance pattern of hemophilia and its ramifications upon circumcision.

The Augustinian monk Gregor Mendel worked out many of the principles of heredity by manipulating the pollen and eggs of pea plants over many generations. His work was conducted from the 1860's to the 1870's but was unrecognized by the scientific community until 1900.

At about this time, many disorders were being recognized as genetic diseases. Pedigree analysis, a way to trace inheritance patterns through a family tree, was used since the mid-1800's to track the incidence of hemophilia in European royal families. This analysis indicated that the disease was transmitted through females (indeed, hemophilia is an X-linked disorder). In the early 1900's, Sir Archibald Garrod, a British physician, recognized certain biochemical disorders as genetic diseases and proposed accurate mechanisms for their transmission.

In 1953, Francis Crick and James D. Watson discovered the structure of DNA; thus began studies on the molecular biology of genes. This research resulted in the monumental discovery in 1973 that pieces of DNA from animals and bacteria could be cut and spliced together into a functional molecule. This recombinant DNA technology fostered a revolution in genetic analysis, in which pieces of human DNA could be removed and put into bacteria. The bacteria then replicate millions of copies of the human DNA, permitting detailed analysis. These recombinant molecules also produced the human gene product, thereby facilitating the analysis of normal and aberrant genes.

The recombinant DNA revolution spawned the development of the DNA tests for genetic diseases and carrier status. Knowledge of what a normal gene product is and does is exceptionally helpful in the treatment of genetic diseases. For example, Duchenne's muscular dystrophy is known to be caused by the lack of a protein called dystrophin. This suggests that a possible treatment of the disease is to provide functional dystrophin to the affected individual. Ultimately, medical science seeks to treat genetic diseases by providing a functional copy of the flawed gene to the affected individual. While such gene therapy would not affect the reproductive cells—the introduced gene copy would not be passed down to future generations—the normal gene product would alleviate the genetic disorder.
—*Karen E. Kalumuck*

*See also* Albinism; Birth defects; Cerebral palsy; Childbirth, complications of; Cleft palate; Color blindness; Congenital heart disease; Cystic fibrosis; Diabetes mellitus; Down syndrome; Dwarfism; Environmental diseases; Fetal alcohol syndrome; Gigantism; Hemophilia; Hydrocephalus; Mental retardation; Multiple sclerosis; Muscular dystrophy; Phenylketonuria; Porphyria; Reye's syndrome; Sickle-cell anemia; Spina bifida; Thalassemia.

**FOR FURTHER INFORMATION:**

Edlin, Gordon. *Human Genetics.* Boston: Jones and Bartlett, 1990. Presents excellent background on the principles of genetics and molecular biology for the nonscientist. This sound introduction is used to discuss human reproduction, heredity, and genetic disease in a clear, informative, and thorough style.

Gormley, Myra Vanderpool. *Family Diseases: Are You at Risk?* Baltimore: Genealogical Publishing, 1989. The author, a certified genealogist and syndicated columnist, explores the relationship between family trees and genetic diseases. Written in popular language, this book gives instruction on how to assess a family's genetic risk, information on the latest scientific breakthroughs, and direction for obtaining further information.

Maxon, Linda, and Charles Daugherty. *Genetics: A Human Perspective.* Dubuque, Iowa: Wm. C. Brown, 1992. This textbook, designed for persons with no science background, thoroughly covers the background information on cells and genetics needed for an informed understanding of human genetic disease. The discussion of scientific advances in the understanding, treatment, and diagnosis of genetic disease is a strong point of the text.

Millunsky, Aubrey. *Choices, Not Chances.* Boston: Little, Brown, 1989. The author is an outstanding medical geneticist and pediatrician who has written this informative, nontechnical guide for those interested in genetic disease.

Includes a broad discussion of particular diseases, genetic counseling, reproductive options, law, and ethics.

Pierce, Benjamin. *The Family Genetic Sourcebook.* New York: John Wiley & Sons, 1990. Pierce presents an excellent discussion of human inheritance patterns for the nonscientist and a catalog of more than one hundred genetic traits and diseases and their inheritance patterns. Includes a discussion of the history of genetics and instructions for constructing family trees.

Wingerson, Lois. *Mapping Our Genes.* New York: E. P. Dutton, 1990. Using an engaging narrative style and many anecdotal stories as illustrations, Wingerson provides an account of the history of scientific discoveries that have led to the human genome initiative, an effort to map the chromosomal location of all human genes. Good discussion of impact of scientific advances in genetics.

## GERMAN MEASLES. *See* CHILDHOOD INFECTIOUS DISEASES; RUBELLA.

## GESTATION. *See* PREGNANCY AND GESTATION.

## GIGANTISM

**SYSTEMS AFFECTED:** Endocrine, skeletal, brain
**SPECIALISTS:** Endocrinologists, neurosurgeons
**DEFINITION:** Gigantism is a rare endocrine disorder characterized by an overgrowth of all bones and body tissues. Along with acromegaly, in which the patient has excessively large hands, feet, and jaw, gigantism is a type of hyperpituitarism: The pituitary gland oversecretes growth hormone, usually because of the presence of a tumor. Gigantism begins during infancy or childhood and causes grotesque body changes to the skeleton and tissues, with heights that may be three times the normal figure. Removal of the pituitary tumor may prevent further growth, but the existing abnormalities are permanent and patients usually have a lowered life expectancy.

*See also* Congenital heart disease; Dwarfism; Endocrine disorders; Growth.

## GINGIVITIS

**SYSTEM AFFECTED:** Gums
**SPECIALISTS:** Dentists
**DEFINITION:** A superficial inflammation of the gums, gingivitis is associated with a destructive buildup of plaque on the gums and between the teeth. The plaque contains bacterial toxins and enzymes that cause irritation, resulting in red, swollen gums that bleed easily. The infection may progress slowly and almost unnoticeably until pockets form between the teeth and gums. If left untreated, the condition can result in periodontitis, in which the teeth detach from the gums. Good oral hygiene can help

## Development of Gingivitis

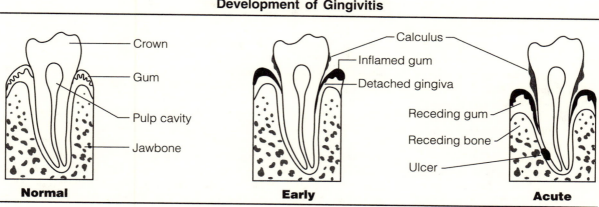

prevent plaque formation, but professional scaling of the teeth is necessary to remove the deposits that develop.

*See also* Caries, dental; Dental diseases; Endodontic disease; Periodontitis; Toothache.

## GLAUCOMA

**SYSTEM AFFECTED:** Visual

**SPECIALISTS:** Ophthalmologists

**DEFINITION:** A group of eye diseases characterized by an increase in the eye's intraocular pressure; early diagnosis through regular eye examinations can manage the effects of the disease, while late diagnosis may result in impaired vision or blindness.

**KEY TERMS:**

*aqueous humor:* the liquid filling the space between the lens and the cornea of the eye, which nourishes and lubricates them

*ciliary body:* a structure built of muscle and blood vessels which produces the aqueous humor

*cornea:* the curved, transparent membrane forming the front of the outer coat of the eyeball that serves primarily as protection and focuses light onto the lens

*intraocular pressure:* the degree of firmness of the eyeball, as controlled by the proper secretion and drainage of the aqueous humor

*lens:* a transparent, flexible structure, convex on both surfaces and lying directly behind the iris of the eye; it focuses light rays onto the retina

*ophthalmic laser:* a high-intensity beam of light which permits a surgeon to cut tissue precisely in the treatment of eye diseases

*optic disc:* the portion of the optic nerve at its point of entrance into the rear of the eye

*peripheral vision:* side vision, or the visual perception to all sides of the central object being viewed

*retina:* the thin, delicate, and transparent sheet of nerve tissue that receives visual stimuli and transmits them to the brain through the optic nerve

*tonometer:* an instrument used to measure the eye's intraocular pressure, thus checking for the presence of glaucoma

### CAUSES AND SYMPTOMS

Glaucoma is an eye disease caused by higher-than-normal pressure inside the eye. The intraocular pressure can increase slowly or suddenly for various reasons but always with detrimental results. Of all the possible causes of blindness, glaucoma is among the most common, but it is also the most preventable. If diagnosed early, it can be controlled and the loss of sight avoided. What complicates the problem is that the most common form of glaucoma shows no symptoms until extensive, irreversible damage has occurred.

To understand this disease, it is necessary to know what occurs within the eye when the intraocular pressure increases. The inner surface of the cornea is nourished by the aqueous humor, which is also called the aqueous fluid. This secretion from the ciliary body flows into the space behind the iris and then through the pupil into the space in front of the iris. Where the front of the iris joins the back of the cornea is a point called the venous sinus, at the anterior drainage angle. Here the aqueous humor is reabsorbed and transported to the bloodstream. In a normal eye, this drainage process works correctly and the balance between the amount secreted and the amount reabsorbed maintains a constant intraocular pressure. In glaucoma, the drainage part of the process works inefficiently. For a variety of reasons, some of which are not fully understood, the drainage mechanism is defective. The upset secretion-drainage balance causes the unwanted increase in intraocular pressure in one eye or, more commonly, in both. The iris is pushed forward, further inhibiting drainage of the aqueous fluid.

Even a very small elevation in intraocular pressure will affect the eye adversely, causing damage to its particularly delicate parts. Although the eye as a whole is quite tough, the optic nerve is vulnerable to increased pressure. This vital connection between the eye and the brain is damaged by the stress within the harder eyeball. The delicate nerve fibers and blood vessels of the optic disc, as the beginning of the optic nerve is called, then die. Once they die, they can never be regenerated or replaced, and blindness is the result. The destruction of the optic disc causes a condition called cupping. A normal optic disc is quite level with the retina. Glaucoma causes it to collapse, creating a genuine indentation. Thus, cupping is a definite sign of glaucoma.

The damage that glaucoma inflicts is progressive. The defect in drainage does not necessarily worsen, and the pressure, once elevated, does not necessarily continue to increase. Once begun, however, the killing of the optic nerve cells continues until the resulting loss of vision progresses to total blindness. The first nerve fibers to die are the ones near the outer edge of the optic disc, which originates near the periphery of the retina. The first decrease in vision, therefore, is in one's peripheral vision. Then, as each layer of nerve fibers dies, the visual field narrows and narrows.

This slow, progressive route to blindness is typical of the most common type of glaucoma, called chronic simple glaucoma. It is called "simple" because the rise in intraocular pressure does not result from any known underlying reason. Although individuals with a family history of glaucoma are more prone to the disease, it is not directly hereditary. Moreover, not everyone with a family history of glaucoma will develop the disease. For reasons that are not well understood, people of African ancestry have glaucoma in much greater numbers than those of European ancestry. In the United States, the incidence of glaucoma among African Americans is three times that of Caucasians.

In persons of all races, chronic simple glaucoma usually begins after the age of forty; however, the aging process does not seem to be a direct cause of glaucoma. Unlike the formation of senile cataracts, which result from inevitable eye changes as one grows older, glaucoma's development is not explained by the aging process. It can safely be said that glaucoma seems to occur in persons who have a tendency toward inadequate aqueous fluid drainage. As those persons grow older and their bodies lose their resiliency in general, the drainage problem reaches a point where it begins to raise the intraocular pressure beyond the normal range. Those with untreated chronic simple glaucoma are seldom aware of the disease before considerable damage has been done. The progressive death of nerve fibers is ordinarily very slow because the elevation of pressure is slight and causes no pain or blurriness of sight.

Chronic simple glaucoma makes up about 95 percent of all cases of the disease. Several other rare types together make up the other 5 percent. In chronic secondary glaucoma, the drainage defect is caused by some complication of a different eye problem. The causes of chronic secondary

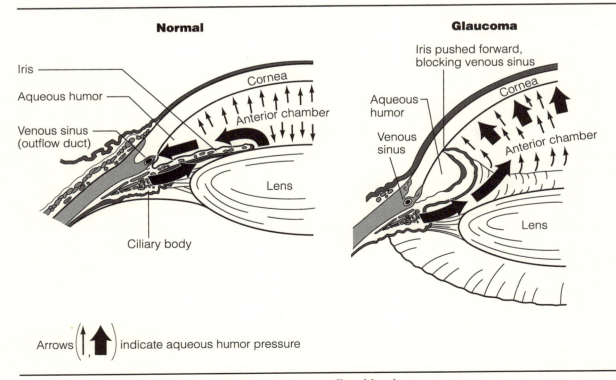

*A normal eye vs. an eye affected by glaucoma.*

glaucoma include inflammation from an eye infection, an allergic reaction, trauma to the eye, a tumor, or even the presence of a cataract. Medications such as corticosteroids can sometimes cause this type of glaucoma to develop. Whatever the cause, chronic secondary glaucoma exhibits the same increased pressure, slow nerve destruction, and ultimate loss of vision as chronic simple glaucoma.

A third variety, acute glaucoma, is both rare and dramatic in its onset. The increase in intraocular pressure is many times higher than that in chronic glaucoma. It also occurs very rapidly, sometimes within hours. The anterior drainage angle where drainage is accomplished is almost totally blocked. The eyeball becomes so hard that the elevated pressure can often be felt simply by touching the front of the eye. The great pressure causes terrible pain and immediate damage to the eye. When nausea, vomiting, and severe headaches accompany eye pressure, acute glaucoma should be suspected. Immediate treatment is required to prevent blindness. Acute glaucoma can be either simple or secondary. It is termed simple when a drainage area that has always been abnormally narrow suddenly becomes totally blocked. It is called secondary when it is precipitated by some other eye condition.

The rarest type of glaucoma, congenital glaucoma, is present at birth or develops during early infancy. It results from the incorrect formation of drainage canals while the eye is developing. Because a baby's eyeball is much smaller and softer than an adult's, this glaucoma is often recognized by the bulging of the eyes.

It is quite easy for an eye doctor to detect even the apparently symptomless chronic glaucoma, and the rate of successful treatment is high. It is unfortunate, then, that glaucoma is responsible for innumerable cases of permanent loss of vision. In the vast majority of these patients, the destruction of the eye could have been prevented. If everyone over the age of forty had an annual eye examination, blindness caused by glaucoma could be essentially eliminated.

### TREATMENT AND THERAPY

The treatments available for glaucoma include eyedrops, ointments, pills, and surgery, using both scalpels and lasers. In both acute and congenital glaucoma, there is no time for the use of medications. Patients need to be admitted to the hospital and operated on immediately if their eyesight is to be saved.

If diagnosed early, cases of both chronic simple and chronic secondary glaucoma can often be effectively treated by medications. The first drug given in the form of eyedrops was discovered in the nineteenth century. Called pilocarpine, it is obtained from the leaves or roots of a South American bush. The drug is classified as a miotic because it constricts the pupil of the eye. Constriction of the pupil draws it away from the drainage angle, automatically increasing the drainage of aqueous fluid and therefore decreasing the pressure. To be effective, it is generally used four times a day. Other glaucoma drugs act to decrease the secretion of the fluid, which also decreases the intraocular pressure. Timolol maleate, the most frequently prescribed drug for glaucoma, works in this fashion. It usually needs to be used twice a day. Some ophthalmologists prefer to use some of both types of drops for the same patient, decreasing pressure by both mechanisms. Others prescribe one medication that produces both effects. Dipivefrin is one such medication.

In either case, to avoid possible unpleasant side effects the most dilute concentration, to be used the fewest times each day, is prescribed first. If this does not control the pressure, more concentrated drops, to be used more times daily, must then be prescribed. The medications in these eyedrops can often be used more easily by elderly patients in the form of a gel, an ointment, or a tiny disc which is placed on the cornea. Although considerably more costly than frequent drops, these methods are less of a nuisance. The gels and ointments need only be used once a day, while the discs are time-released over an entire week.

If drops or gels do not produce the desired reduction in pressure, pills can be used, not to replace the drops but to supplement them. These tablets are essentially diuretics that decrease the production of aqueous humor. Taken once a day, or less frequently in a time-release capsule, acetazolamide is the drug most often prescribed.

There are also several fast-acting drugs that can be injected into a vein to lower pressure by rapidly pulling some aqueous fluid into blood vessels in the eye, bypassing the drainage angle. These are not used in the treatment of chronic glaucoma except as preparation for a planned surgery. They are, however, often used when patients are admitted to the hospital for acute glaucoma to prevent damage until emergency surgery can be performed.

In the great number of patients, chronic glaucoma can be controlled by one of these medications. In those rare cases when it cannot, surgery must be performed. Although initially successful, such surgeries must often be repeated in the future. As with the above medications, glaucoma surgery aims to decrease the intraocular pressure by decreasing secretion or increasing effective drainage.

Although surgery can never reverse the optic nerve damage that has already occurred, it is often effective in preventing further destruction. The first of these surgical procedures was developed in the mid-nineteenth century. Called an iridectomy or iridotomy, it attempts to provide a better access to the patient's drainage angle by removing part of the iris. A second type of surgical procedure, known as a trabeculectomy or filtering operation, attempts to control intraocular pressure by creating a new, wider drainage outlet for the aqueous humor. Until the use of lasers, both of these operations were done completely manually by a surgeon with steady hands using sharp blades on a tiny part of the eye.

To perform an iridectomy, the surgeon must cut a tiny hole into the edge of the iris with surgical scissors, allowing aqueous fluid to flow into the space between the iris and the cornea. Covered by the upper eyelid, this small hole is visible only by close examination and should not let in unwanted extra light or cause any discomfort to the patient.

The filtering operation, or trabeculectomy, can be performed in several different ways, but each involves the eye surgeon's use of a knife called a scalpel to create an artificial canal through the outer wall of the patient's eye. The passageway created, known as a fistula or filtering bleb, permits the aqueous humor to drain properly from the inner eye. By removing a part of the abnormal tissue from the drainage angle, the surgeon unclogs the drainage mechanism.

A different approach to glaucoma control does not involve cutting. It attempts to help the patient by destroying part of the source of the excess fluid, the oversecreting ciliary body. When a cold probe is applied to the ciliary body, the procedure is termed cryotherapy; when a hot probe is used, the method is called cyclodiathermy. No incision is required in either case because the probes are applied externally. A very common side effect of these two procedures, however, is fairly severe inflammation. Even when inflammation does not occur, the desired result may be only partially achieved. Both cryotherapy and cyclodiathermy are less commonly done than either iridectomy or trabeculectomy, and the procedures are usually only performed on older patients.

Many of these manual procedures are being replaced by several types of laser therapy. A laser is a precisely directed beam of high-intensity light that can function as a surgical knife. Laser surgery is generally safer than the older methods because it is less invasive to the body, as no incision is made in the eye. It can be done on an outpatient basis with only a local anesthetic. Recovery time, the likelihood of complications, and postoperative discomfort are all lessened. Patients with acute glaucoma, chronic simple glaucoma, and certain types of secondary glaucoma (depending on the cause) can be successfully treated with lasers.

Both iridotomy and trabeculectomy can be performed by the use of an instrument called the argon laser. This particular laser is relatively low-powered, but it is efficient and very popular with ophthalmologists. After a drop of anesthetic is placed in the eye, the surgeon aims the highly focused argon beam at a precise location within the affected eye. The beam need only be directed into the eye for one-tenth of a second to achieve its effect. In an iridotomy, the laser simply drills a tiny hole in the iris for the fluid to circulate freely, while in a trabeculectomy several laser cuts are made on the clogged drainage angle to open it. A more sophisticated ophthalmic laser is the YAG laser. After a drop of anesthetic is placed on the eye, a weak "aiming beam" of helium-neon laser light is shone directly into the afflicted eye to pinpoint the area to be treated. This is fol-lowed by two to five bursts of the YAG laser, which drills a hole for better drainage.

All the above treatments for glaucoma, whether medical or surgical, have the potential for serious side effects and complications. Consequently, research continues to seek therapies with better rates of success and fewer complications.

## PERSPECTIVE AND PROSPECTS

The development of ways to diagnose glaucoma has paralleled the general development of the ophthalmologist's tools. These devices in turn reflect the links between the science of those branches of physics that study pressure, lenses, mirrors, and light and the science that studies the normal and abnormal functioning of the eye.

In 1851, the German doctor Hermann von Helmholtz invented the ophthalmoscope, which enables one to study the interior of the eye. His instrument focuses a beam of light into the patient's eye and then magnifies its reflection. If this test reveals early signs of cupping of the optic disc, glaucoma can be diagnosed long before other symptoms have appeared.

Intraocular pressure can be measured with an instrument called a tonometer. The two basic varieties are called Schiötz tonometry and applanation tonometry. Both only became possible after biochemists developed anesthetic drops to put in the eye so that the patient would not feel the device touching the very sensitive cornea. The earlier of the two devices, developed in 1905 by the Norwegian physician Hjalmar Schiötz, is a very simple device that is still the most widely used tonometer in the world. With the patient lying down and looking upward, the physician places the hand-sized instrument directly on the cornea. A simple lever is moved by the pressure within the eye to indicate whether that pressure is within the normal range or dangerously high. The Goldman applanation tonometer is considered even more accurate and is often used to confirm the results of the simpler Schiötz device. An orange dye called fluorescein is added to the anesthetic. The patient, in a sitting position, rests the head against a bar to steady it. The doctor uses a tonometer to touch the cornea while simultaneously peering into it with a well-illuminated microscope.

More specialized glaucoma examination may require gonioscopy, visual field tests, or tonography. The gonioscope has mirrors and facets to provide an illuminated view of the drainage angle, a normally dark corner at a 90 degree angle from the examiner. Excessive narrowing of the angle is a dangerous indication of glaucoma. There are many kinds of visual field tests, but all give a map of the central area where vision is sharp and more acute, versus the peripheral area where it is weaker. Since damage to the optic nerve always causes a narrowing of the visual field, this mapping is very important. The ability to measure the field has grown from oculokinetic perimetry—using an inexpensive test chart, pencil, record sheet, and human examiner—

to the expensive and sophisticated automated perimetry, which generates a computer analysis for the physician. Tonography does not measure the visual field but again attacks the problem by measuring the intraocular pressure. Unlike the ordinary use of tonometry, which involves momentary contact with the cornea, tonography uses the tonometer for four minutes to massage the eye. In a normal eye, pressure will drop; in a glaucoma patient, it will not.

All these tests, developed through years of ophthalmic research, have given medical science invaluable tools to diagnose glaucoma and prevent blindness.

—*Grace D. Matzen*

**See also** Astigmatism; Cataracts; Visual disorders.

**FOR FURTHER INFORMATION:**

Eden, John. *The Physician's Guide to Cataracts, Glaucoma, and Other Eye Problems.* Yonkers, N.Y.: Consumer Reports Books, 1992. This excellent book provides the reader with nontechnical yet truly accurate explanations of the functioning of the normal eye and of the disease conditions glaucoma and cataracts. Also contains a very useful chapter on commonsense eye care, as well as a very extensive glossary.

Galloway, N. R. *Common Eye Diseases and Their Management.* New York: Springer-Verlag, 1985. While this text may be difficult material for the general reader, it is useful for obtaining more precise medical information. Intended for medical students but accessible to nonscientists because of the author's writing style.

Glasspool, Michael. *Eyes: Their Problems and Treatments.* New York: Arco, 1984. Written in outline form, so that specific information is easy to locate. Includes clear discussions of the various side effects of glaucoma medications. This is a well-illustrated volume, but it contains no glossary.

Neal, Helen. *Low Vision.* New York: Simon & Schuster, 1987. Interesting approach to ophthalmology, providing technical material in a light, readable style. Aims to give the reader a solid understanding of how to avoid eye problems. Includes in its lengthy appendix several lists of further resources, organizations, and products for the visually impaired.

Rubman, Robert H., and Howard Rothman. *Future Vision.* New York: Dodd, Mead, 1987. Rubman, a doctor, brings to this volume his extensive knowledge of and skill in practicing ophthalmology. Rothman, an accomplished freelance writer of science materials, makes Rubman's knowledge genuinely accessible to the nonscientist. Includes a useful list of national organizations and a lengthy glossary.

Samz, Jane. *The Encyclopedia of Health: Vision.* New York: Chelsea House, 1990. Contains a rather brief treatment of the topic of glaucoma. This volume is more useful for understanding the normal eye, eye tests in general, and a diversity of other eye diseases. Includes lists of helpful organizations and further readings, as well as a brief glossary.

## GLOMERULONEPHRITIS

**SYSTEM AFFECTED:** Kidneys

**SPECIALISTS:** Internists, nephrologists

**DEFINITION:** The filtering units of the kidneys are known as glomeruli, and inflammation of these structures is called glomerulonephritis. There are two main types: acute and chronic. Acute glomerulonephritis follows an infection, usually by streptococcal bacteria but also by the viruses that cause chickenpox, mumps, syphilis, measles, and malaria. After the underlying infection is cured, the kidney disorder generally disappears without treatment. Chronic glomerulonephritis, however, has no cure and develops slowly and without symptoms. Renal failure often results, and dialysis or kidney transplantation may be required. The chronic form may be caused by other renal disorders or systemic disorders such as lupus erythematosus.

**See also** Kidney disorders; Lupus erythematosus; Renal failure; Stones; Streptococcal infections.

## GOITER

**SYSTEM AFFECTED:** Endocrine

**SPECIALISTS:** Endocrinologists, internists

**DEFINITION:** A goiter is an enlargement of the thyroid, the butterfly-shaped gland found over the trachea and below the larynx in the neck. It may be attributable to inflammation (as from an autoimmune disorder) or to a benign

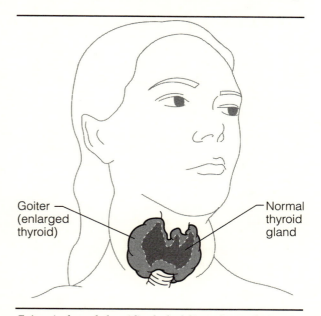

Goiter — (enlarged thyroid)

Normal thyroid gland

*Goiter (enlarged thyroid); dashed lines show relative size of normal thyroid.*

or malignant tumor, or the condition may be classified as simple goiter. Simple goiter is either endemic, related to such nutritional factors as the iodine deficiency characteristic of malnutrition, or sporadic, following the ingestion of certain foods or drugs. Goiters can also occur as a result of benign nodules that usually strike middle-aged women. Regardless of the cause, the enlarged thyroid gland can reach enormous proportions, resulting in respiratory and circulatory problems. Treatment depends on the cause and may include hormone replacement or surgery.

*See also* Endocrine disorders; Hyperparathyroidism and Hypoparathyroidism; Thyroid disorders.

## GONORRHEA

**SYSTEMS AFFECTED:** Reproductive, visual

**SPECIALISTS:** Gynecologists, obstetricians, public health specialists, urologists

**DEFINITION:** One of the most common and treatable sexually transmitted diseases, gonorrhea is an infection of the urogenital tract. In men, the symptoms may be painful urination and a yellow discharge from the penis; in women, the symptoms may be painful urination, a cloudy discharge and blood from the vagina, and abdominal discomfort. Some people have no symptoms, however, and become lifetime carriers of the disease. Gonorrhea can also be transmitted from mother to baby during childbirth, affecting the eyes and possibly causing blindness. Adults may also contract conjunctivitis associated with gonorrhea. If left untreated, the disease can become serious, resulting in blindness, systemic infection, and pelvic inflammatory disease in women.

*See also* Acquired immunodeficiency syndrome (AIDS); Blindness; Chlamydia; Conjunctivitis; Female genital disorders; Herpes; Male genital disorders; Pelvic inflammatory disease (PID); Sexually transmitted diseases; Syphilis.

## GOUT

**SYSTEM AFFECTED:** Joints

**SPECIALISTS:** Internists, rheumatologists

**DEFINITION:** A form of arthritis of the peripheral joints, often characterized by painful, recurrent acute attacks and resulting from deposits of uric acid in joint spaces.

**KEY TERMS:**

*acute gout:* a very painful gout attack, most common in the left big toe; usually the first indicator of occurrence of the disease

*arthritis:* any of more than a hundred related diseases, including gout, that are characterized by joint inflammation

*cartilage:* a tough, white, fibrous connective tissue attached to the bone surfaces that is involved in movement

*corticosteroid:* a fatlike steroid hormone made by the adrenal glands, or similar synthetic chemicals manufactured by pharmaceutical companies

*gene:* a piece of the hereditary material deoxyribonucleic acid (DNA) that carries the information needed to produce an inheritable characteristic

*genetic engineering:* also called recombinant DNA research; a group of scientific techniques that allow scientists to alter genes

*hyperuricemia:* the presence of abnormally high uric acid levels, which usually leads to gout symptoms

*rheumatologist:* a physician who studies rheumatoid arthritis and related diseases

*secondary gout:* gout symptoms caused by other diseases and by therapeutic drugs

*synovial fluid:* the thick, clear, lubricating fluid that bathes joints and helps them to move smoothly

*tophaceous gout:* chronic gout that may be characterized by tophi, severe joint degeneration, and/or serious kidney problems

*tophi:* lumps in the cartilage and joints of chronic gout sufferers, caused by crystals of uric acid

### CAUSES AND SYMPTOMS

Gout, once called the affliction of kings, is a hereditary disease that causes inflammation of the peripheral joints. It is also called gouty arthritis because arthritis means joint inflammation and describes more than a hundred related diseases. Gout has afflicted humans since antiquity, and it was first described by Hippocrates in the fifth century B.C. It usually first presents itself as an extremely painful swelling of the big toe of the left foot in men over the age of forty. Gout attacks, termed acute gout, are quite rare in premenopausal women. In fact, more than 90 percent of all gout sufferers are men. The prevalence of gout is extremely high in Pacific Islanders, with 10 percent of adult males afflicted. One characteristic portrayal of gout sufferers, which may come from the "affliction of kings" concept, is of obese and obviously affluent individuals. This is partly a misconception because gout is a very democratic disease, found in the poor as often as in the wealthy. Nevertheless, acute gout attacks are often brought on by very rich meals or by drinking sprees, so obesity is accurately portrayed as a contributing factor.

An acute gout attack may occur in almost any joint, with the most common sites after the big toe being the ankles, fingers, feet, wrists, elbows, and knees. Such attacks are not often seen in the shoulders, hips, or spine and, if they do occur, appear only after a gout sufferer has had many previous attacks in other joints. Acute gout of the big toe occurs so often that it has been given its own name, podagra. Common explanations for the very frequent occurrence of podagra are that considerable pressure is placed on the big toe in the process of walking and that most people are right-handed and are therefore "left-footed," putting more pressure on the left foot than on the right one in walking or in sports.

An acute gout attack is preceded by feelings of weakness, nausea, chills, and excessive urination. Then, the area that

## Gout

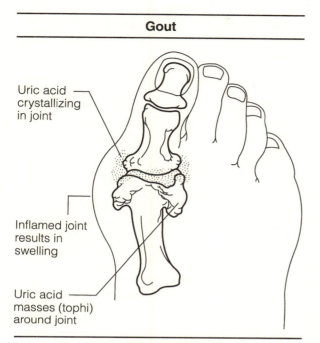

Uric acid crystallizing in joint

Inflamed joint results in swelling

Uric acid masses (tophi) around joint

*The big toe is a common site for gout.*

is affected becomes red to purple, swollen, and so tender that the slightest touch is very painful. This pain is so severe that many sufferers describe it as being crushing, or even excruciating. Acute gout attacks come on suddenly, and many victims report suddenly being jolted awake by pain in the night. Fortunately, such attacks are few and far between and usually last only from a few days to a week. In addition, more than half of those who have one attack of podagra will never have another gout attack.

The problems associated with acute gout are attributable to a chemical called uric acid. Uric acid does not dissolve well in the blood and other biological fluids, such as the synovial fluid in joints. When overproduced by the body or excreted too slowly in urine, undissolved uric acid forms sharp crystals. These crystals and their interactions with other joint components cause the pain felt by gout sufferers. It is interesting to note that gout is caused by the overproduction of uric acid in some individuals and by uric acid underexcretion in others. Many of the foods that seem to cause gout are rich in chemicals called purines, which are converted to uric acid in the course of preparation for excretion by the kidneys.

Much more dangerous to gout victims than the acute attacks is leaving the disease untreated. When this happens, crystals of uric acid produce lumps or masses in the joints throughout the body and in the kidneys. In the joints, the masses, called tophi, lead to inflammation, scarring, and deformity that can produce an irreversible degenerative process. Tophi are most common in the fingers and the carti-

lage of various parts of the body, and external tophi are found in the cartilage of the ears of gout sufferers. The visible tophi, however, are only representative, and undetected uric acid masses may be widely spread throughout the body. Such untreated gout is called chronic or tophaceous gout.

Tophaceous gout is another disease with a long history. It was first described by the Greek physician Galen in the second century A.D. Another extremely dangerous aspect of tophaceous gout is unseen kidney stones, which will cause great pain on urination, produce high blood pressure, and even cause fatalities in 3 to 5 percent of afflicted persons.

The prime indicator of gout is high blood levels of uric acid, called hyperuricemia; however, this condition, without other symptoms, does not always signal existent, symptomatic gout. Therefore, the best indicator of the presence of the disease is a combination of hyperuricemia, acute attacks, and observed uric acid in the synovial fluid of all troublesome, gouty joints.

Some investigators propose that gout sufferers are highly intelligent because such famous individuals as Michelangelo, Leonardo da Vinci, Martin Luther, Charles Darwin, and Benjamin Franklin were afflicted with the disease. This trend, however, may indicate that famous people are usually able to afford a lifestyle that causes the predilection to high uric acid levels (for example, the eating of purine-rich foods and high alcohol consumption). Rheumatologists who have studied gout would argue that alcoholism is a better predictor for the disease because it is very common in heavy drinkers. In fact, studies in which gout patients were given purine-rich diets or purine-rich diets plus alcoholic beverages showed that alcohol increased the number and severity of gout attacks.

Gout is also associated with a number of other diseases, including Down syndrome, lead poisoning, some types of diabetes, psoriasis, and kidney disease. Furthermore, a number of therapeutic drugs used in chemotherapy for cancer, diuretics, and some antibiotics can cause acute gout symptoms. These types of gout are differentiated from the hereditary disease already described—so-called primary gout—by the term "secondary gout." Drug-induced secondary gout goes away quickly when administration of the offending drug is stopped.

Another group of diseases that have symptoms somewhat similar to gout are called pseudogout. They have an entirely different cause (mineral crystals in the joints), occur in men and women with equal frequency, usually begin in extreme old age, and are treated quite differently.

It is also interesting that while premenopausal women are nearly gout-free, the disease becomes fairly common after the menopause. This fact supports a role for female hormones in preventing the disease. Primary gout in women is usually much more severe and destructive than gout in men. In those families in which maternal gout is observed, it is likely that occurrence of the disease in male offspring will occur earlier than is usual, such as near the age of thirty.

## TREATMENT AND THERAPY

Once primary gout has been diagnosed, three methods are available for treating it: therapeutic drugs, surgery, and special diets. Most often, gout treatment uses therapeutic drugs, with the drug of choice being colchicine. Colchicine treatment can be traced back for thousands of years, to Egypt in 1500 B.C. Originally, it was given as an extract of the meadow saffron plant, *Colchicum autumnale*. In modern times, the pure chemical has been isolated for medicinal use.

Colchicine is reportedly a specific remedy for gout and has no effect on any other type of arthritis. In fact, the reversal of severe joint pain with colchicine is often used as a diagnostic tool that tells physicians that the joint disease being treated is indeed gout. Colchicine can be utilized to treat acute gout attacks or can be taken routinely for long periods of time. Its actions in the handling of acute attacks are quick and profound. In some cases, however, colchicine will have side effects, including severe stomach cramps, nausea, and diarrhea. When these effects occur, colchicine use is discontinued until they disappear and then its reuse is instituted.

Most of the basis for colchicine action is its decrease of the inflammation that causes the pain of gout attacks. This action is believed to be attributable to colchicine interaction with white blood cells that destroy uric acid crystals and subsequent prevention of the cells from releasing inflammatory factors. Other drugs that work in this way are nonsteroidal anti-inflammatory drugs (NSAIDs) such as aspirin, ibuprofen, indomethacin, naproxin, and phenylbutazone. Colchicine and NSAIDs are usually given by mouth. In some cases, anti-inflammatory steroid hormones called corticosteroids, such as prednisone and prednisolone, are used to treat acute gout. The corticosteroids are given by injection into the gouty joint. Despite the rapid, almost miraculous effects of these steroids, they are best avoided unless absolutely necessary because they can lead to serious medical problems.

Another group of antigout medications consists of the uricosuric drugs. Two favored examples of such drugs are probenecid (Benemid) and sulfinpyrazone (Anturane). The uricosuric drugs prevent the occurrence of hyperuricemia and eventual tophaceous gout by increasing uric acid excretion in the urine, therefore lowering the uric acid levels in the blood. This lowering has two effects: the prevention of the attainment of uric acid levels in the blood and joints that lead to crystal or tophus formation and the eventual dissolution of crystals and tophi as blood levels of uric acid drop.

Uricosuric drugs have no effect, however, on an acute gout attack and can sometimes make such attacks even more painful. For this reason, uricosuric drug therapy is always started after all acute gout attack symptoms have subsided. Aspirin blocks the effects of the uricosuric drugs

and should be replaced with acetaminophen (for example, Tylenol) whenever they are utilized for chemotherapeutic purposes. Side effects of excessive doses of uricosuric drugs can include headache, nausea and vomiting, itching, and dizziness. Their use should be discontinued immediately when such symptoms occur. Later reuse of the uricosuric drugs is usually possible.

The third category of antigout drugs is a single chemical, allopurinol (usually, Lopurin or Zyloprim). This drug lowers the body's ability to produce uric acid. It is highly recommended for all gout-afflicted people who have kidney disease that is severe enough for kidney stones to form. It has undesired side effects, however, that include skin rashes, drowsiness, a diminished blood count, and severe allergic reactions. As a result, the use of allopurinol is disqualified for many patients. One advantage of allopurinol chemotherapy over the use of uricosuric agents is the fact that it can be taken along with aspirin.

The end result of a chemotherapeutic regimen with uricosuric drugs and/or allopurinol is the lowering of the blood and urinary uric acid levels so that crystals and tophi do not form or, where formed, redissolve. Often, their combination with colchicine is useful for preventing the occurrence of gout attacks during the initial chemotherapy period.

While surgery is not a common treatment for gout, people who have large tophi that have opened up, become infected, or interfere with joint mobility may elect to have them removed in this fashion. In some cases, severe disability or joint pain caused by the degenerative effects of long-term tophaceous gout is also corrected surgically. Care should be taken, however, to evaluate the consequences of such surgery carefully because the postoperative healing process is often quite slow and many other problems can be encountered.

Media sources often praise special diets in treating gout, without firm proof of their effectiveness. The finding that gout is usually a hereditary disease resulting from metabolic defects that either prevent uric acid excretion or cause its accumulation has pointed out that most dietary factors have a relatively small effect on the disease. Consequently, chemotherapy is much more effective than dietary intervention for diminishing gout symptoms. Nevertheless, there are several incontestable dietary aspects essential to the well-being of persons afflicted with gout.

First, dieting is quite useful, and overweight gout sufferers should lose weight. Such action is best taken slowly and under medical supervision. In fact, excessively fast weight loss can temporarily worsen gout symptoms by elevating blood uric acid levels. In addition, excesses of a number of foods should be avoided by gout sufferers because they are overly rich in the purines that give rise to uric acid when the body processes them. Some examples are the organ meats (liver, kidneys, and sweetbreads), mushrooms, anchovies, sardines, caviar, gravy and meat extracts, shellfish, wine, and beer. Modest intake of these foods is allowable. For example, the daily intake of one can of beer, a glass of wine, or an ounce or two of hard liquor is permissible. The gout sufferer should remember that excessive alcohol intake often brings on acute gout attacks and, even worse, will contribute to worsening tophus and kidney stone formation.

Another adjunct to the prevention or diminution of gout symptoms is the daily intake of at least a half gallon of water or other nonalcoholic beverages. This will help to flush uric acid out of the body, in the urine, and may help to dissipate both tophi and kidney stones. Plain water is best, as it contains no calories that will increase body weight, potentially aggravating gout and leading to other health problems.

### PERSPECTIVE AND PROSPECTS

Many sources agree that primary gout is under control in most afflicted people, who can look forward to a normal life without permanent adverse effects of the disease. Those individuals who seek medical treatment at the first appearance of gout symptoms may combine chemotherapy, an appropriate diet regimen, and alcohol avoidance to prevent all but a few acute attacks of the disease. In addition, they will not develop tophi or kidney problems.

Even those afflicted persons who put off treatment until kidney stones or tophi appear can be helped easily. Again, an appropriate diet and the wise choice of chemotherapy agents will prevail. Only the patients who neglect all gout treatment until excessive joint damage and severe kidney disease occur are at serious risk, yet even with these individuals, remission of most severe symptoms is usually possible. The long-term neglect of gout symptoms is unwise, however, because severe tophaceous gout can be both deforming and fatal.

Currently, the eradication of most primary gout, not gout treatment, is seen as the desired goal of research. It is believed that a prime methodology for the eradication of gout will be the use of genetic engineering for gene replacement therapy. Primary gout sufferers are victims of gene lesion diseases: Their bodies lack the ability, because of defective genes, to control either the production or the excretion of uric acid. It is hoped that gene replacement technology will enable medical science to add the missing genes back into their bodies. Other research aspects viewed worthy of exploration in the attempts to vanquish primary gout are the understanding of how to cause white blood cells to destroy uric acid crystals in the joints more effectively and safely and to decode the basis for the gout-preventing effects of female hormones related to their presence in premenopausal women. —*Sanford S. Singer*

*See also* Alcoholism; Arthritis; Down syndrome; Lead poisoning; Obesity; Urinary disorders.

### FOR FURTHER INFORMATION:

Barnhart, Edward R., ed. *The Physician's Desk Reference.*
45th ed. Oradell, N.J.: Medical Economics, 1991. This atlas of prescription drugs includes those used against gout—their manufacturers, useful dose ranges, metabolism and toxicology, and contraindications. This text, found in most public libraries, is useful for both physicians and patients.

Berkow, Robert, and Andrew J. Fletcher. *The Merck Manual of Diagnosis and Therapy.* 15th ed. Rahway, N.J.: Merck Sharp & Dohm Research Labs, 1987. Contains a brief but useful exposition of the characteristics, etiology, diagnosis, and treatment of gout and its relationship to other forms of arthritis. Designed for physicians, the material is also useful for less specialized readers. Information on related topics is also included.

Devlin, Thomas E. *Textbook of Biochemistry: With Clinical Correlations.* New York: Wiley-Liss, 1992. This college textbook presents considerable information on gout, hormones, genetic engineering, and related topics. Includes chemical structures, diagrams, and references useful to the reader. All descriptions are simple but scholarly.

Fries, James F. *Arthritis: A Comprehensive Guide to Understanding Your Arthritis.* Reading, Mass.: Addison-Wesley, 1986. Covers gout and pseudogout in a chapter on crystal arthritis, discussing the features, prognosis, and treatments of both problems. Crystal arthritis types are very well differentiated and integrated into the consideration of arthritis. Recommended for teachers.

Keough, Carol. *Natural Relief for Arthritis.* Emmaus, Penn.: Rodale Press, 1983. This well-written book on arthritis contains a useful chapter on gout covering its causes, symptoms, and treatment. Also explains the difference between gout and pseudogout and why gout is a type of arthritis.

Kushner, Irving. *Understanding Arthritis: What It Is, How It's Treated, How to Cope with It.* New York: Charles Scribner's Sons, 1984. This book is published under the auspices of the Arthritis Foundation. Its chapters on gout and pseudogout differentiate the diseases. Offers valuable information on gout symptoms, possible causes, and treatment.

Scriver, Charles R., et al., eds. *The Metabolic Basis of Inherited Disease.* 6th ed. 2 vols. New York: McGraw-Hill, 1989. This classic medical text contains an excellent chapter on gout describing the symptoms, diagnosis, biochemistry, and genetics of the disease in great detail. Aimed at health science professionals, the book contains much important information for the diligent general reader as well. Important pictures, diagrams, and large number of handy references are included.

# GRIEF AND GUILT

**SYSTEM AFFECTED:** Psychic-emotional

**SPECIALISTS:** Family physicians, psychiatrists, psychologists

**DEFINITION:** Grief and accompanying guilt are common reactions to the fact or eventuality of serious losses of various kinds, especially death; every person eventually experiences grief, and while grief is normal, its effects can be incapacitating.

**KEY TERMS:**

*abnormal grief:* an unhealthy response to a loss, which may include anger, an inability to feel loss, withdrawal, and deterioration in health

*grief:* a multifaceted physical, emotional, psychological, spiritual, and social reaction to loss

*guilt:* a cognitive and emotional response often associated with the grief experience in which a person feels a sense of remorse, responsibility, and/or shame regarding the loss

*loss:* the sudden lack of a previously held possession, physical state, or social position or the death of a loved one

## CAUSES AND SYMPTOMS

During life, people unavoidably experience a variety of losses. These may include the loss of loved ones, important possessions or status, health and vitality, and ultimately the loss of self through death. "Grief" is the word commonly used to refer to an individual's or group's shared experience following a loss. The experience of grief is not a momentary or singular phenomenon. Instead, it is a variable, and somewhat predictable, process of life. Also, as with many phenomena within the range of human experience, it is a multidimensional process including biological, psychological, spiritual, and social components.

The biological level of the grief experience includes the neurological and physiological processes that take place in the various organ systems of the body in response to the recognition of loss. These processes, in turn, form the basis for emotional and psychological reactions. Various organs and organ systems interact with one another in response to the cognitive stimulation resulting from this recognition. Human beings are self-reflective creatures with the capacity for experiencing, reflecting upon, and giving meaning to sensations, both physical and emotional. Consequently, the physiological reactions of grief that take place in the body are given meaning by those experiencing them.

The cognitive and emotional meanings attributed to the experience of grief are shaped by and influence interactions within the social dimensions of life. In other words, how someone feels or thinks about grief influences and is influenced by interactions with family, friends, and helping professionals. In addition, the individual's religious or spiritual frame of reference may have a significant influence on the subjective experience and cognitive-emotional meaning attributed to grief.

The grief reactions associated with a loss such as death vary widely. While it is very difficult and perhaps unfair to generalize about such an intensely personal experience, several predictors of the intensity of grief have become evi-

dent. The amount of grief experienced seems to depend on the significance of the loss, or the degree to which the individual subjectively experiences a sense of loss. This subjective experience is partially dependent on the meaning attributed to the loss by the survivors and others in the surrounding social context. This meaning is in turn shaped by underlying belief systems, such as religious faith. Clear cognitive, emotional, and/or spiritual frameworks are helpful in guiding people constructively through the grief process.

People in every culture around the world and throughout history have developed expectations about life, and these beliefs influence the grief process. Common questions in many cultures include "Why do people die?" "Is death a part of life, or a sign of weakness or failure?" "Is death always a tragedy, or is it sometimes a welcome relief from suffering?" and "Is there life after death, and if so, what is necessary to attain this afterlife?" The answers to these and other questions help shape people's experience of the grief process. As Elisabeth Kübler-Ross states in *Death: The Final Stage of Growth* (1975), the way in which a society or subculture explains death will have a significant impact on the way in which its members view and experience life.

Another factor that influences the experience of grief is whether a loss was anticipated. Sudden and/or unanticipated losses are more traumatic and more difficult to explain because they tend to violate the meaning systems mentioned above. The cognitive and emotional shock of this violation exacerbates the grief process. For example, it is usually assumed that youngsters will not die before the older members of the family. Therefore, the shock of a child dying in an automobile crash may be more traumatic than the impact of the death of an older person following a long illness.

Death and grief are often distasteful to human beings, at least in Western Judeo-Christian cultures. These negative, fearful reactions are, in part, the result of an individual's difficulty accepting the inevitability of his or her own death. Nevertheless, in cultures which have less difficulty accepting death and loss as normal, people generally experience more complicated grief experiences. The Micronesian society of Truk is a death-affirming society. The members of the Truk society believe that a person is not really grown up until the age of forty. At that point, the individual begins to prepare for death. Similarly, some native Alaskan groups teach their members to approach death intentionally. The person about to die plans for death and makes provisions for the grief process of those left behind.

In every culture, however, the grief-stricken strive to make sense out of their experience of loss. Some attribute death to a malicious intervention from the outside by someone or something else; death becomes frightening. For others, death is in response to divine intervention or is simply the completion of "the circle of life" for that person. Yet for most people in Western societies, even those who come to believe that death is a part of life, grief may be an emotional mixture of loss, shock, shame, sadness, rage, numbness, relief, anger, and/or guilt.

Kübler-Ross points out in her timeless discourse "On the Fear of Dying" (*On Death and Dying*, 1969) that guilt is perhaps the most painful companion of death and grief. The grief process is often complicated by the individual's perception that he or she should have prevented the loss. This feeling of being responsible for the death or other loss is common among those connected to the deceased. For example, parents or health care providers may believe that they should have done something differently in order to detect the eventual cause of death sooner or to prevent it once the disease process was detected.

Guilt associated with grief is often partly or completely irrational. For example, there may be no way that a physician could have detected an aneurysm in her patient's brain prior to a sudden and fatal stroke. Similarly, a parent cannot monitor the minute-by-minute activities of his adolescent children to prevent lethal accidents. Kübler-Ross explains a related phenomenon among children who have lost a parent by pointing out the difficulty in separating wishes from deeds. A child whose wishes are not gratified by a parent may become angry. If the parent subsequently dies, the child may feel guilty, even if the death is some distance in time away from the event in question.

The guilt may also involve remorse over surviving someone else's loss. People who survive an ordeal in which others die often experience "survivor's guilt." Survivors may wonder why they survived and how the deceased person's family members feel about their survival, whether they blame the survivors or wish that they had died instead. As a result, survivors have difficulty integrating the experience with the rest of their lives in order to move on. The feelings of grief and guilt may be exacerbated further if survivors believe that they somehow benefited from someone else's death. A widow who is suddenly the beneficiary of a large sum of money attached to her husband's life insurance policy may feel guilty about doing some of the things that they had always planned but were unable to do precisely because of a lack of money.

Lastly, guilt may result when people believe that they did not pay enough attention to, care well enough for, or deserve the love of the person who died. These feelings and thoughts are prompted by loss—loss of an ongoing relationship with the one who died, as well as part of the empathetic response to what it might be like to die oneself.

Feelings of guilt are not always present, even if the reaction is extreme. If individuals experience guilt, however, they may "bargain" with themselves or a higher power, review their actions to find what they did wrong, take a moral inventory to see where they could have been more loving or understanding, or even begin to act self-destructively. Attempting to resolve guilt while grieving loss is doubly

complicated and may contribute to the development of what is considered an abnormal grief reaction.

The distinctions between normal and abnormal grief processes are not clear-cut and are largely context-dependent; that is, what is normal depends on standards that vary among different social groups and historical periods. In addition, at any particular time the variety of manifestations of grief depend on the individual's personality and temperament; family, social, and cultural contexts; resources for coping with and resolving problems; and experiences with the successful resolution of grief.

Despite this diversity, the symptoms that are manifested by individuals experiencing grief are generally grouped into two different but related diagnostic categories: depression and anxiety. It is normal for the grieving individual to manifest symptoms related to anxiety and/or depression to some degree. For example, a surviving relative or close friend may temporarily have difficulty sleeping, or feel sad or that life has lost its meaning. Relative extremes of these symptoms, however, in either duration or intensity, signal the possibility of an abnormal grief reaction.

In *Families and Health* (1988), family therapist William Doherty and family physician Thomas Campbell identify the signs of abnormal grief reactions as including periods of compulsive overactivity without a sense of loss; identification with the deceased; acquisition of symptoms belonging to the last illness of the deceased; deterioration of health in the survivors; social isolation, withdrawal, or alienation; and severe depression. These signs may also include severe anxiety, abuse of substances, work or school problems, extreme or persistent anger, or an inability to feel loss.

### TREATMENT AND THERAPY

There is no set time schedule for the grief process. While various ethnic, cultural, religious, and political groups define the limits of the period of mourning, they cannot prescribe the experience of grief. Yet established norms do influence the grief experience inasmuch as the grieving individuals have internalized these expectations and standards. For example, the typical benefit package of a professional working in the United States offers up to one week of paid "funeral" leave in the event of the death of a significant family member. On the surface, this policy begins to prescribe or define the limits of the grief process.

Such a policy suggests, for example, that a mother or father stricken with grief at the untimely death of a child ought to be able to return to work and function reasonably well once a week has passed. Most individuals will attempt to do so, even if they are harboring unresolved feelings about the child's death. Coworkers, uncomfortable with responding to such a situation and conditioned to believe that people need to "get on with life," may support the lack of expression of grief.

Helpful responses to grief are as multifaceted as is grief itself. Ultimately, several factors ease the grief process.

These include validating responses from significant others, socially sanctioned expression of the experience, self-care, social or religious rituals, and possibly professional assistance. Each person responds to grief differently and requires or is able to use different forms of assistance.

Most reactions to loss run a natural, although varied, course. Since grief involves coming to grips with the reality of death, acceptance must eventually be both intellectual and emotional. Therefore, it is important to allow for the complete expression of both thoughts and feelings. Those attempting to assist grief-stricken individuals are more effective if they have come to terms with their own feelings, beliefs, and conflicts about death, and any losses they personally have experienced.

Much of what is helpful in working through grief involves accepting grief as a normal phenomenon. Grief-related feelings should not be judged or overly scrutinized. Supportive conversations include time for ventilation, empathic responses, and sharing of sympathetic experiences. Helpful responses may take the form of "To feel pain and sadness at this time is a normal, healthy response" or "I don't know what it is like to have a child die, but it looks like it really hurts" or "It is understandable if you find yourself thinking that life has lost its purpose." In short, people must be given permission to grieve. When it becomes clear that the person is struggling with an inordinate amount of feelings based on irrational beliefs, these underlying beliefs—not the feelings—may need to be challenged.

People tend to have difficulty concentrating and focusing in the aftermath of a significant loss. The symptoms of anxiety and depression associated with grief may be experienced, and many of the basic functions of life may be interrupted. Consequently, paying attention to healthy eating and sleeping schedules, establishing small goals, and being realistic about how long it may take before "life returns to normal" are important.

While the prescription of medication for the grief-stricken is fairly common, its use is recommended only in extreme situations. Antianxiety agents or antidepressants can interfere with the normal experiences of grief that involve feeling and coming to terms with loss. Sedatives can help bereaved family members and other loved ones feel better over the short term, with less overt distress and crying. Many experts believe, however, that they inhibit the normal grieving process and lead to unresolved grief reactions. In addition, studies suggest that those who start on psychotropic medication during periods of grief stay on them for at least two years.

The grief process is also eased by ritual practices that serve as milestones to mark progress along the way. Some cultures have very clearly defined and well-established rituals associated with grief. In the United States, the rituals practiced continue to be somewhat influenced by family, ethnic, and regional cultures. Very often, however, the ritu-

als are confined to the procedures surrounding the preparation and burial of the body (for example, viewing the body at the mortuary, a memorial service, and interment). As limited as these experiences might be, they are designed to ease people's grief. Yet the grief process is often just beginning with the death and burial of the loved one. Consequently, survivors are often left without useful guidelines to help them on their way.

Another common, although unhelpful, phenomenon associated with the process is for the grief-stricken person initially to receive a considerable amount of empathy and support from family, friends, and possibly professionals (such as a minister or physician) only to have this attention drop off sharply after about a month. The resources available through family and other social support systems diminish with the increasing expectation that the bereaved should stop grieving and "get on with living." If this is the case, or if an individual never did experience a significantly supportive response from members of his or her social system, the role of psychotherapy and/or support groups should be explored. Many public and private agencies offer individual and family therapy. In addition, in many communities there are a variety of self-help support groups devoted to growth and healing in the aftermath of loss.

## PERSPECTIVE AND PROSPECTS

The grief process, however it is shaped by particular religious, ethnic, or cultural contexts, is reflective of the human need to form attachments. Grief thus reflects the importance of relationships in one's life, and therefore it is likely that people will always experience grief (including occasional feelings of guilt). Processes such as the grief experience, with its cognitive, emotional, social, and spiritual dimensions, may affect an individual's psychological and physical well-being. Consequently, medical and other health care and human service professionals will probably always be called upon to investigate, interpret, diagnose, counsel, and otherwise respond to grief-stricken individuals and families.

In the effort to be helpful, however, medical science has frequently intervened too often and too invasively into death, dying, and the grief process—to the point of attempting to disallow them. For example, hospitals and other institutions such as nursing homes have become the primary place that people die. It is important to remember that it has not always been this way. Even now in some cultures around the world, people die more often in their own homes than in a "foreign" institution.

In the early phases of the development of the field of medicine, hospitals as institutions were primarily devoted to the care of the dying and the indigent. Managing the dying process was a primary focus. More recently, however, technological advances and specialty development have shifted the mission of the hospital to being an institution devoted to healing and curing. The focus on the recovery process has left dying in the shadows. Death has become equated with failure and associated with professional guilt.

It is more difficult for health care professionals to involve themselves or at least constructively support the grief process of individuals and families if it is happening as a result of the health care team's "failure." In a parallel fashion, society has become unduly fixated on avoiding death, or at least prolonging its inevitability to the greatest possible extent. The focus of the larger culture is on being young, staying young, and recoiling from the effects of age. As a result, healthy grief over the loss of youthful looks, stamina, health, and eventually life is not supported.

Medical science can make an important contribution in this area by continuing to define the appropriate limits of technology and intervention. The struggle to balance quantity of life with quality of life (and death) must continue. In addition, medical science professionals need to redouble their efforts toward embracing the patient, not simply the disease; the person, not simply the patient; and the complexities of grief in death and dying, not simply the joy in healing and living.  —*Layne A. Prest*

***See also*** Death and dying; Depression; Manic-depressive disorder; Midlife crisis; Neurosis; Postpartum depression; Psychiatric disorders; Stress; Suicide.

### FOR FURTHER INFORMATION:

Doherty, William J., and Thomas L. Campbell. *Families and Health*. Beverly Hills, Calif.: Sage Publications, 1988. Doherty and Campbell write from the valuable perspective of two health care providers—a family therapist and a family physician. They place the grief experience within the context of health care delivery and, more important, within the context of the biological, psychological, and social aspects of people's lives.

Kübler-Ross, Elisabeth, ed. *Death: The Final Stage of Growth*. Englewood Cliffs, N.J.: Prentice-Hall, 1975. A valuable companion to Kübler-Ross' earlier work, this book contains insightful perspectives on variations in culture, the impact of institutions, and the importance of ritual in the dying and grieving processes.

_____. *On Death and Dying*. New York: Macmillan, 1969. This book is, and will remain, a classic in the field. Kübler-Ross shares the experience of many years working with dying patients and their families. In addition to discussing the typical stages through which people progress in the death and dying process, she details the many specifics and variations of people's grief and guilt reactions to death and dying.

Staudacher, Carol. *Beyond Grief: A Guide for Recovering from the Death of a Loved One*. Oakland, Calif.: New Harbinger, 1987. A clear and readable guide to the grief process. The author provides specific examples relevant for some of the most painful grief experiences: those following the death of a spouse, child, or parent at an early age.

# GROWTH

**SYSTEMS AFFECTED:** All

**SPECIALISTS:** Endocrinologists, obstetricians, pediatricians

**DEFINITION:** The development of the human body from conception to adulthood; growth occurs at different rates for different systems over this period, and varies by sex and individual as well.

**KEY TERMS:**

*accretion:* a type of growth in which new, nongrowing material is simply added to the surface

*allometric growth:* unequal rates of growth of different body parts, or in different directions

*developmental biology:* broadly, the study of ontogeny; narrowly, the study of how gene action is controlled

*embryonic stage:* that part of ontogeny during which organs are formed

*fetal stage:* that part of ontogeny after the organs are formed but before birth takes place

*interstitial growth:* growth throughout a structure, usually in all directions

*isometric growth:* equal rates of growth of all parts, or in all directions

*ontogeny:* the entire developmental sequence, from conception through the various embryonic stages, birth, childhood, maturity, senescence, and death; also, the study of this sequence

*ossification:* the formation of bone tissue

### PROCESS AND EFFECTS

The human body grows from conception until adult size is reached. Adult size is reached in females around the age of eighteen and in males around twenty or twenty-one, but there is considerable variation in either direction. (Nearly all numerical measurements of growth and development are subject to much variation.) On the average, males end up with a somewhat larger body size than females because of these two or three extra years of growth.

Growth begins after conception. The first phase of growth, including approximately the first month after conception, is called embryonic growth, and the growing organism is called an embryo. During embryonic growth, the most important developmental process is differentiation, the formation of the various organs and tissues. After the organs and tissues are formed, the rest of prenatal growth is called fetal growth and the developing organism is called a fetus. Respiratory movements begin around the eighteenth week of gestation, during the fetal stage; limb movements (such as kicking) begin to be felt by the mother around the twenty-fourth week, with a considerable range of variation. At birth, the average infant weighs about 3.4 kilograms (7.5 pounds) and measures about 50 centimeters (20 inches) in length.

Growth continues after birth and throughout childhood and adolescence. From the perspective of developmental biology, childhood is defined as the period from birth to

## Median Heights and Weights from Childhood to Adulthood

| | Boys | | Girls | |
|---|---|---|---|---|
| Age | Height (cm) | Weight (kg) | Height (cm) | Weight (kg) |
| 2 | 87 | 12 | 87 | 12 |
| 3 | 95 | 15 | 94 | 14 |
| 4 | 103 | 17 | 102 | 16 |
| 5 | 110 | 19 | 108 | 18 |
| 6 | 117 | 21 | 115 | 20 |
| 7 | 122 | 23 | 121 | 22 |
| 8 | 127 | 25 | 127 | 25 |
| 9 | 132 | 28 | 132 | 28 |
| 10 | 138 | 31 | 138 | 33 |
| 11 | 143 | 35 | 145 | 37 |
| 12 | 150 | 40 | 152 | 42 |
| 13 | 157 | 45 | 157 | 46 |
| 14 | 163 | 51 | 160 | 50 |
| 15 | 169 | 57 | 162 | 54 |
| 16 | 174 | 62 | 162 | 56 |
| 17 | 176 | 66 | 163 | 57 |
| 18 | 177 | 69 | 164 | 57 |

puberty, which generally begins at twelve years of age, and adolescence continues from that point to the cessation of skeletal growth at around the age of eighteen in females and twenty or twenty-one in males. The long period of adulthood that follows is marked by a stable body size, with little or no growth except for the repair and maintenance of the body, including the healing of wounds. After about age sixty, there may be a slight decline in body height and in a few other dimensions.

By one year of age, the average baby is 75 centimeters (30 inches) long and weighs 10 kilograms (22 pounds). (There is actually a slight decline in weight in the first month of postnatal life, but this is usually regained by age three months.) For ages one to six, the average weight (in kilograms) can be approximated by the equation "weight = age x 2 + 8." For ages seven to twelve, growth takes place more rapidly: Average weight (in kilograms) can be approximated by "weight = age x 3.5 - 2.5," while average height (in centimeters) can be approximated for ages two to twelve by the equation "height = age x 6 + 77." Head circumference has a median value of about 34.5 centimeters at birth, 46.3 centimeters at an age of one year, 48.6 centimeters at age two, and 49.9 centimeters at age three. All these figures are about 1 centimeter larger in boys than in girls, with considerable individual variation. Median heights and weights, when differentiated by sex, reveal that boys and girls are generally similar until age fourteen, after which boys continue to gain in both dimensions (see table).

Growth of the teeth takes place episodically. In most children, the first teeth erupt between five and nine months of age, beginning with the central incisors, the lower pair generally preceding the upper pair. The lateral incisors (with the upper pair first), the first premolars, the canines, and the second premolars follow, in that order. All these teeth are deciduous teeth ("baby teeth") that will eventually be shed, to be replaced during late childhood by the permanent teeth. At one year of age, most children have between six and eight teeth.

## Growth from Infancy to Adulthood

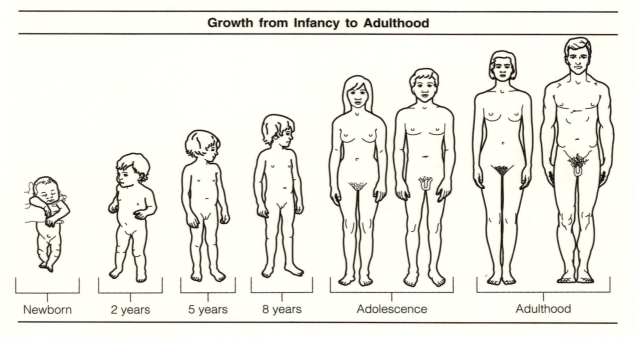

Newborn    2 years    5 years    8 years    Adolescence    Adulthood

Growth takes place in several directions. Growth at the same rate in all directions is called isometric growth, which maintains similar proportions throughout the growth process. Isometric growth occurs in nautilus shells and a variety of other invertebrates. Most of human growth, however, is allometric growth, which takes place at different rates in different directions. Allometric growth results in changes in shape as growth proceeds. Moreover, different parts of the body grow at different rates and in different directions. During fetal development, for example, the head develops in advance of the fore and hind limbs, and the fetus at about six months of age has a head which is about half its length. The head of a newborn baby is about one-third of its body length, compared to about one-seventh for an adult. In contrast, the legs make up only a small part of the body length in either the six-month-old fetus or the newborn baby, and their absolute length and proportionate length both increase throughout childhood and adolescence.

Growth of the skeleton sets the pace for growth of the majority of the body, except for the nervous system and reproductive organs. Most parts of the skeleton begin as fast-growing cartilage. The process in which cartilage tissue turns into bone tissue is called ossification, which begins at various centers in the bone. The first center of ossification within each bone is called the diaphysis; in long bones, this ossification usually takes place in the center of the bone, forming the shaft. Secondary centers of ossification form at the ends of long bones and at certain other specified places; each secondary center of ossification is called an epiphysis. In a typical long bone, two epiphyses form, one at either end. Capping the end of the bone, beyond the epiphysis, lies an articular cartilage. Between the epiphysis and the diaphysis, the cartilage that persists is called the epiphyseal cartilage; this becomes the most rapidly growing region of the bone. During most of the growth of a long bone, the increase in width occurs by accretion, a gradual process in which material is added at a slow rate only along a surface. In the case of a bone shaft, increase in width takes place only at the surface, beneath the surrounding membrane known as the periosteum. By contrast, the epiphyseal cartilage grows much more rapidly, and it also grows by interstitial growth, meaning that growth takes place throughout the growing tissue in all directions at once. As the epiphyseal cartilage grows, parts of it slowly become bony, and those bony portions grow more slowly.

During the first seven or eight years of postnatal life, the growth of the epiphyseal cartilage takes place faster than its replacement by bone tissue, causing the size of the epiphyseal cartilage to increase. Starting around age seven, the interstitial growth of the epiphyseal cartilage slows down, while the replacement of cartilage by bone speeds up, so that the epiphyseal cartilage is not growing as fast as it turns into bone tissue; the size of the epiphyseal cartilage therefore starts to decrease. At the time of puberty, the hor-

monal influences create an adolescent growth spurt during which the individual's bone growth increases for about a one-year period. In girls, the adolescent growth spurt takes place about two years earlier than it does in boys—the average age is around twelve in girls, versus about fifteen in boys—but there are tremendous individual variations both in the extent of the growth spurt and in its timing. At age fourteen, most girls have already experienced most of their adolescent growth spurt, while most boys are barely beginning theirs. Consequently, the average fourteen-year-old girl is a bit taller than the average fourteen-year-old boy.

At around eighteen years of age in females and twenty or twenty-one years of age in males, the replacement of the epiphyseal cartilage by bone is finally complete, and bone growth ceases. The age at which this occurs, and the resulting adult size, both vary considerably from one individual to another. For the rest of adult life, the skeleton remains more or less constant in size, diminishing only slightly in old age.

Most of the other organs of the body grow in harmonious proportion with the growth of the skeleton, reaching a maximum growth rate during the growth spurt of early adolescence and reaching a stable adult size at around age eighteen in women and age twenty or twenty-one in men. The nervous system and reproductive system, however, constitute major exceptions to this rule. The nervous system and brain grow faster at an earlier age, reaching about 90 to 95 percent of their adult size by one year of age. The shape of the head, including the shape of the skull, keeps pace with the development of the brain and nervous system. For this reason, babies and young children have heads that constitute a larger proportion of their body size than do the heads of adults.

The growth of the reproductive system also follows its own pattern. Most reproductive development is delayed until puberty. The reproductive organs of the embryo form slowly and remain small. The reproductive organs of children, though present, do not reach their mature size until adolescence. These organs, both the internal ones and the external ones, remain small throughout childhood. Their period of most rapid growth marks the time of puberty, which spans ages eleven through thirteen, with a wide range of variation. At this time, the pituitary gland begins secreting increased amounts of the follicle-stimulating hormone (FSH), which stimulates the growth and maturation of the gonads (the ovaries of females and the testes of males). The ovaries or testes then respond by producing increased amounts of the sex hormones testosterone (in males) or estrogen (in females), which stimulate the further development of both primary and secondary sexual characteristics. Primary sexual characteristics are those which are functionally necessary for reproduction, such as the presence of a uterus and ovaries in females or the presence of testes and sperm ducts in males. Secondary sexual characteristics are those which distinguish one sex from another, but which are not functionally necessary for reproduction. Examples of secondary sexual characteristics include the growth of breasts or the widening of the hips in females, the growth of the beard and deepening of the voice in males, and the growth of hair in the armpits and pubic regions of both sexes.

Growth takes place psychologically and socially as well as physically. Newborn babies, though able to respond to changes in their environment, seem to pay attention to such stimuli only on occasion. At a few weeks of age, the baby will respond to social stimuli (such as the sound of the mother's voice) by smiling. Babies usually can grasp objects by five months of age, depending on the size and shape of the object. By six months, most babies will show definite signs of pleasure in response to social stimulation; this may include an open-mouth giggle or laugh. At seven months of age, most babies will respond to adult facial expressions and will show different responses to familiar adults as opposed to strangers. The age at which babies learn to crawl varies greatly, but most infants learn the technique by nine or ten months of age. Social imitation begins late in the first year of life. Also, by this time, children learn object permanence, meaning that they will search for a missing object if they have watched it being hidden. Walking generally develops around eighteen months of age, but the time of development varies greatly.

Jean Piaget (1896-1980) was a pioneer in the study of the social and cognitive development of children. Piaget identified four stages of cognitive and social growth, which he called sensorimotor, preoperational, concrete operational, and formal operational. In the sensorimotor stage, from birth to about two years of age, infants begin with reflexes such as sucking or finger curling (in response to touching their palms). Starting with these reflexes, they gradually learn to understand their senses and apply the resulting information in order to acquire important adaptive motor skills that can be used to manipulate the world (as in picking up things) or to navigate about and explore the world (as in walking). Socially, infants develop ways to make desirable stimuli last by such acts as smiling. In the preoperational stage, which lasts from about two to six years of age, children acquire a functional use of their native language. Their imagination flourishes, and pretending becomes an important and frequent activity. Most of the thinking at the preoperational stage is egocentric, however, which means that the child perceives the world only from his or her own point of view and has difficulty seeing other points of view.

The concrete operational stage spans the years from about seven to eleven years of age. This is the stage at which children learn to apply logic to concrete objects. For example, they realize that liquid does not change volume when poured into a taller glass, and they develop the ability to arrange objects in order (for example, by size) or to classify them into groups (for example, by color or shape). The final stage is called the formal operational stage, beginning around age twelve. This is the stage of adolescence and adulthood, when the person learns to manipulate abstract concepts in such areas as ethical, legal, or mathematical reasoning. This is also the stage at which people develop the ability to construct hypothetical situations and to use them in arguments.

## COMPLICATIONS AND DISORDERS

Disorders of growth include dwarfism, gigantism, and several other disorders such as achondroplasia (chondrodystrophy). Dwarfism often results from an insufficiency of the pituitary growth hormone, also called somatostatin or somatotrophic hormone. Some short-statured individuals are normally proportioned, while others have proportions differing from those of most other people. An overabundance of growth hormone causes gigantism, a condition marked by unusually rapid growth, especially during adolescence. In some individuals, the amount of growth hormone remains normal during childhood but increases to excessive amounts during the teenage years; these individuals are marked by acromegaly, a greater than normal growth which affects primarily the hands, feet, and face.

Achondroplasia, also called chondrodystrophy, is a genetically controlled condition caused by a dominant gene. In people having this condition, the epiphyseal cartilages of the body's long bones turn bony too soon, so that growth ceases before it should. Those exhibiting chondrodystrophy therefore have short stature and childlike proportions but rugged faces that look older than they really are.

Inadequate growth can often result from childhood malnutrition, particularly from insufficient amounts of protein. If a child is considerably shorter or skinnier than those of the same age, that child's diet should be examined for the presence of malnutrition. Intentional malnutrition is one of the characteristic features of anorexia nervosa. The opposite problem, overeating, can lead to obesity, although obesity can also result from many other causes, including diabetes and other metabolic problems.

## PERSPECTIVE AND PROSPECTS

As a phenomenon, growth of both wild and domestic animals was well known to ancient peoples. Hippocrates (460-377 B.C.), considered the father of medicine, wrote a treatise on embryological growth, and Aristotle (384-322 B.C.) wrote a longer and more complete work on the subject. During the Renaissance, Galileo Galilei (1564-1642) studied growth mathematically and distinguished between isometric and allometric forms of growth, arguing that the bones of giants would be too weak to support their weight.

The most important era in the study of human embryonic development was ushered in by the Estonian naturalist Karl Ernst von Baer (1792-1876), who discovered the human ovum. From this point on, detailed studies of human embryonic and postnatal development proceeded at a rapid pace, especially in Germany. Much of the modern understanding of growth in more general or mathematical terms derives from the classic studies of the British anatomist D'Arcy Wentworth Thomson (1860-1948). In the twentieth century, Piaget became a leader in the study of childhood social and cognitive growth phases. —*Eli C. Minkoff*

*See also* Aging; Childbirth; Conception; Hypertrophy; Malnutrition; Menopause; Menstruation; Pregnancy and gestation; Puberty and adolescence; Sexuality; Vitamin and mineral deficiencies; Weight loss and gain.

## FOR FURTHER INFORMATION:

Anson, B. J. *An Atlas of Human Anatomy*. 2d ed. Philadelphia: W. B. Saunders, 1963. This atlas contains excellent color-coded illustrations, including several on various stages of growth.

Behrman, R. E., ed. *Nelson Textbook of Pediatrics*. 14th ed. Philadelphia: W. B. Saunders, 1992. Contains a considerable amount of useful information, including graphs and growth charts. Offers advice for the monitoring of growth development in children and adolescents.

Gasser, R. F. *Atlas of Human Embryos*. Hagerstown, Md.: Harper & Row, 1975. This text includes superior black-and-white illustrations, most of which are photomicrographs. All of the illustrations are thoroughly labeled and explained.

Gray, Henry. *Gray's Anatomy*. Edited by Peter L. Williams et al. 37th ed. New York: C. Livingstone, 1989. The classic work on anatomy, containing the most thorough descriptions. The excellent color illustrations provide much realistic detail in most cases and well-selected highlights in a few. Developmental stages are covered in detail.

Hollinshead, W. H. *Textbook of Anatomy*. 4th ed. Philadelphia: Harper & Row, 1985. A very thorough, up-to-date, detailed reference work. Provides helpful descriptions and illustrations, including descriptions of the immature stages of growth.

King, B. G., and M. J. Showers. *Human Anatomy and Physiology*. 6th ed. Philadelphia: W. B. Saunders, 1969. A good general work on the subject. This text includes a section on growth and development.

Moore, K. L. *The Developing Human*. 4th ed. Philadelphia: W. B. Saunders, 1988. Excellent descriptions and illustrations of all developmental stages of human growth are provided in this useful work.

Oski, F. A., ed. *Principles and Practice of Pediatrics*. Philadelphia: J. B. Lippincott, 1990. Contains many good descriptions and illustrations of different stages of development, various disorders common in children, and several treatments for these disorders.

Thompson, D. W. *On Growth and Form*. Edited by John Tyler Bonner. Abridged ed. Cambridge, England: Cambridge University Press, 1966. A classic treatment on the numerical relationships involved in relative growth rates and growth patterns in both animals and humans.

# GUILLAIN-BARRÉ SYNDROME (GBS)

**SYSTEMS AFFECTED:** Brain, nervous, muscular

**SPECIALISTS:** Internists, neurologists

**DEFINITION:** An acute degeneration of peripheral motor and sensory nerves, known to physicians as acute inflammatory demyelinating polyneuropathy, a common cause of acute generalized paralysis.

**KEY TERMS:**

*antibody:* a substance produced by plasma cells which usually binds to a foreign particle; in GBS, antibodies bind to myelin protein

*antigen:* any substance that stimulates white blood cells to mount an immune response

*areflexia:* loss of reflex

*autoimmune disorder:* a condition in which the immune system attacks the body's own tissue instead of foreign tissue

*B cell:* a type of white blood cell that produces antibodies

*CSF protein:* a protein in the cerebrospinal fluid which is usually very low

*demyelination:* a loss of the myelin coating of nerves

*electromyogram:* the external recording of electrical impulses from muscles

*macrophage:* a white blood cell that engulfs foreign protein; in GBS, it also attacks myelin

*motor weakness:* muscle weakness resulting from the failure of motor nerves

*nerve conduction velocity:* the speed at which a nerve impulse travels along a nerve

*neurogenic atrophy:* shrinkage of muscle caused by a loss of nervous stimulation

*neuropathy:* a condition in which nerves are diseased, are inflamed, or show abnormal degeneration

*phagocytosis:* the process of engulfing particles

*polyneuropathy:* neuropathy found in many areas

## CAUSES AND SYMPTOMS

Guillain-Barré syndrome (GBS) is an acute disease of the peripheral nerves, especially those that connect to muscles. It causes weakness, areflexia (loss of reflex), ataxia (difficulty in maintaining balance), and sometimes ophthalmoplegia (eye muscle paralysis). GBS demonstrates a variable, multifocal pattern of inflammation and demyelination of the spinal roots and the cranial nerves, although the brain itself is not obviously affected. By the 1990's, it was the most common cause of generalized paralysis in the United States, averaging two cases per 100,000 people per year. The disease was first described in the early 1900's by Georges Guillain and Jean-Alexander Barré, two French neurologists. Little was known of the cause of GBS or the mechanism for its symptoms, however, until the 1970's. Since then, symposia sponsored by the National Institute of Neurological and Communicative Disorders and Stroke have shed more light on this condition.

Most individuals with GBS have a rapidly progressing muscular weakness in more than one limb and also experience paresthesia (tingling) and numbness in the hands and feet. These sensations have the effect of reducing fine muscle control, balance, and one's awareness of limb location. The prevailing scientific opinion regarding GBS is that it is an autoimmune disorder involving white blood cells, which for some unknown reason attack nerves and/or produce antibodies against myelin, the insulating covering of nerves. The weakness is usually ascending in nature, beginning with numbness in the toes and fingers and progressing to total limb weakness. The demyelination is more prominent in the nerves of the trunk and occurs to a lesser extent in the more distal nerves. The brain and spinal cord are protected from GBS by the blood-brain barrier, although antibodies to myelin have been found in the cerebrospinal fluid of some patients.

With GBS, there is often a precipitating event such as surgery, pregnancy, upper respiratory infection, viral infection (such as cytomegalovirus), or vaccination. Preexisting debilitating illnesses such as systemic lupus erythematosus (SLE) or Hodgkin's disease also seem to predispose a person to GBS. GBS has been diagnosed in patients having heart transplants in spite of the fact that they are receiving immunosuppressive drugs. The increased risk with such surgery may be attributable to the stress associated with the procedure. Most patients who come down with GBS have had some prior condition that placed stress on the immune system prior to the appearance of GBS.

The patient with GBS is frequently incapable of communicating as a result of paralysis of the vocal cords. Typically, motor paralysis will worsen rapidly and then plateau after four weeks, with the patient bedridden and often in need of respiratory support. Autonomic nerves can also be affected, causing gastrointestinal disturbances, adynamic ileus (loss of function in the ileum of the small intestine), and indigestion. Other, less common symptoms include pupillary disturbances, pooling of blood in limbs, heart rhythm disturbances, and a decrease in the heart muscle's strength. These patients are usually hypermetabolic because considerable caloric energy goes into an immune response that is self-destructive and into mechanisms that are attempting to repair the damage.

In addition to the loss of myelin, cell body damage to nerves may result and may be associated with permanent deficits. If the nerve cell itself is not severely damaged, regrowth and remyelination can occur. Antibodies to myelin proteins and to acidic glycolipids are seen in a majority of patients. Blood serum taken from patients with GBS has been shown to block calcium channels in muscle, and experiments in Germany have found that cerebrospinal fluid from GBS patients blocks sodium channels.

Like most autoimmune conditions, GBS is cyclic in nature; the patient will have "good" days and "bad" days because the immune system is sensitive to the levels of steroid hormones in the body, which are known to fluctuate. In addition to paralysis, there is significant pain with GBS. Many of the nerve fibers that register the pain response (nociceptors) are nonmyelinated and therefore are not interrupted in GBS. Pain management can be difficult, requiring the use of such drugs as fentanyl, codeine, morphine, and other narcotics. The course of the disease is variable and is a function of the level of reactivity of the patient's immune system. The autoimmune attack is augmented in those patients experiencing activation of serum complement protein induced by antibodies. Recovery usually takes months, and frequently the patient requires home health care. Complications can lead to death, but most patients recover fully, though some have residual weakness.

The physician must be careful to distinguish GBS from lead poisoning, chemical or toxin exposure, polio, botulism, and hysterical paralysis. Diagnosis can be confirmed using cerebrospinal fluid (CSF) analysis. GBS patients have protein levels greater than 0.55 gram per deciliter of CSF. Macrophages are frequently found in the CSF, as well as some B cells. Nerve conduction velocity will be decreased in these patients to a value that is 50 percent of normal in those nerves that are still functioning. These changes can take several weeks to develop. With GBS, macrophages and T cells have been shown to be in contact with nerves, as evidenced in electron micrographs. T-cell and macrophage activation in these individuals point to an immune response gone awry, possibly precipitated by a virus or exposure to an antigen that is foreign but similar in appearance to one of the proteins in myelin. T cells, upon encountering an unrecognizable antigen, will produce interleukin 2, initiate attack, and recruit macrophages to participate. The use of an anti-T-cell drug theoretically should improve nerve function, but researchers at the University of Western Ontario failed to find any benefit from the infusion of an anti-T-cell monoclonal antibody. Unexpectedly, GBS has been found in patients testing positive for the human immunodeficiency virus (HIV) who are asymptomatic, in spite of the fact that their T cells are under attack from the HIV virus and are diminished in number. Although myelin proteins are thought to be the immunogens, other candidates include gangliosides in the myelin. Antiganglioside antibodies have been seen in a majority of the GBS patients. This trait may distinguish GBS from amyotrophic lateral sclerosis (Lou Gehrig's disease) and multiple sclerosis, which seem to involve different myelin proteins as antigens.

In GBS, the white blood cells attack peripheral motor nerves more often than other types of nerves, implying a biochemical difference between motor and sensory nerves that has yet to be discovered. One possible cause of this disease is a similarity between a protein or glycolipid that is present normally in myelin and coincidentally on an infectious agent, such as a virus. The immune system responds to the agent, resulting in a sensitization of the macrophages and T cells to that component of myelin. B cells are then stimulated to produce antibodies against this antigen, and they unfortunately cross-react with components of the myelin protein. The severity of the disease will depend on the number of macrophages and lymphocytes activated and whether serum complement-binding antibodies are being produced. Serum complement proteins are activated by a particular class of antibodies, resulting in the activation of enzymes in the blood that potentiate tissue destruction and neurogenic atrophy. Serum complement levels can be determined by a serum complement fixation test.

In severe cases of GBS, intercostal muscles are more severely compromised and respiratory function needs to be monitored closely. The immune response will subside when T-suppressor cells have reached their peak levels. Halting the autoimmune response will not reverse the symptoms immediately, since it takes time for antibody levels to decrease and for the nerves to regrow and remyelinate, which occurs at the rate of 1 to 2 millimeters per day. Some nerves will undergo retrograde degeneration and be lost from the neuronal pool. Other nerves will have more closely spaced nodes and conduct impulses at a lower velocity. Nerve sprouting will also occur, which will result in one nerve's being responsible for more muscle fibers or serving a larger sensory area and in decreased fine motor control.

### TREATMENT AND THERAPY

In Guillain-Barré syndrome, the amount of muscle and nerve involvement can be assessed by performing an electromyogram, which can reveal the amount of motor nerve interruption and the conduction velocity of the nerves that continue to function. Based upon the assumption that an autoimmune response is in progress, corticosteroids such as prednisolone and methylprednisolone are sometimes administered in high doses. The benefits of such drugs have been shown to be marginal, while the side effects are considerable.

More recently, a procedure known as plasmapheresis has been tried with better results, especially when performed in the first two weeks. This procedure involves removing 250 milliliters (a little more than a pint) of plasma from the blood every other day and replacing this volume with a solution containing albumin, glucose, and appropriate salts. Six treatments are typical and usually result in a faster recovery of muscle control than for those not receiving plasmapheresis. Because relapses may occur if the patient produces new antibodies to myelin, immunosuppressants are given to the patient after plasmapheresis. Another procedure, intravenous immunoglobulin therapy, is in the clinical trial stage and is based on the strategy of blocking the binding of antibodies to nerves.

Cyclosporine, a T-cell inhibitor, is also being tried, with some promising results. Some researchers note, however, that transplant patients, who routinely take cyclosporine, have a higher-than-normal risk of developing GBS. Others emphasize that no one knows what their risk for GBS would be without the administration of cyclosporine. Because of the variability of the body's immune response, the benefits of this drug will depend on whether, in a given individual, it is an antibody response or T-cell response. Cyclosporine will benefit those who have a strong T-cell response. T-cell reactivity can be tested with the mixed lymphocyte assay, and T-cell counts can be done.

Cerebrospinal fluid filtration is also being tried in order to remove reactive white blood cells and antibodies. Serum so filtered loses its nerve-inhibiting effect, as evidenced by its application to in vitro nerve and muscle cells. GBS has been mimicked in animal models, which show antibody and T-cell reactivity to myelin protein. Guillain-Barré syndrome has many of the characteristics of an autoimmune disease and could serve as a model for an acquired autoimmune condition.

### PERSPECTIVE AND PROSPECTS

Guillain-Barré syndrome is an example of a delicate physiological balance gone awry. The immune system has the difficult task of distinguishing between self and enemy, and if it detects the latter it must either inactivate or eliminate the intruder. Mistakes in recognition or communication between immune cells can cause either an unintended attack or the failure to attack when appropriate. GBS probably represents an unnecessary attack on self tissue, in this case myelin, and may be considered a form of hyperimmunity. Many diseases fall into this category. They include rheumatoid arthritis, juvenile diabetes, Crohn's disease, ulcerative colitis, Graves' disease, multiple sclerosis, amyotrophic lateral sclerosis, ankylosing spondylitis (inflammation of the joints between the vertebrae), and systemic lupus erythematosus. The other type of response, hypoimmune, is seen in cancer and immunodeficiency diseases such as acquired immunodeficiency syndrome (AIDS).

Questions that arise with GBS are the same ones that arise in many other diseases. It must be determined why the immune system chose this time to initiate an attack against a self-antigen. The answer could be a mistake in recognition, an error in translating the deoxyribonucleic acid (DNA) code in the bone marrow cells, an alteration of the antigen by some environmental factor, or an alteration of an antigen-detector protein on a white blood cell. Researchers also try to discover if there is a genetic predisposition for GBS. Seeking answers about GBS may shed light on other conditions as well, and treatments beneficial to GBS patients have a high probability of benefiting patients with other immune disorders. GBS is a reminder that physiological stress can translate to immunological stress, and under stress the immune system can make mistakes. Failure to react can result in diseases such as cancer, and unnecessary action can lead to diseases such as GBS.

—*William D. Niemi*

*See also* Ataxia; Autoimmune disorders; Motor neuron diseases; Neuralgia, neuritis, and neuropathy; Numbness and tingling; Paralysis; Stress.

354 • GUILLAIN-BARRÉ SYNDROME (GBS)

## FOR FURTHER INFORMATION:

Barr, Murray L., and John A. Kierman. *The Human Nervous System*. 6th ed. Philadelphia: J. P. Lippincott, 1993. A softbound text designed for a medical school introductory course in the basic sciences. Provides a good foundation for understanding the nervous system, with some discussion of demyelination. Contains good diagrams, photographs, and references.

Daubel, Jasper R., Thomas J. Reagan, Burton A. Sandok, and Barbara F. Westmoreland. *Medical Neurosciences*. 2d ed. Boston: Little, Brown, 1986. This textbook emphasizes anatomy and pathways in the body. Provides clinical descriptions of the more common neurological diseases and could serve as a reference book.

Kuffler, Stephen W., John G. Nicholls, and A. Robert Martin. *From Neuron to Brain*. 2d ed. Sunderland, Mass.: Sinauer Associates, 1984. An excellent and detailed neurobiology text that can help the reader understand the basis and consequences of demyelinating conditions such as Guillain-Barré syndrome.

Lechtenberg, Richard. *Synopsis of Neurology*. Philadelphia: Lea & Febiger, 1991. A pocket-sized book with summary descriptions of the most common neurological syndromes. Covers diagnostic techniques and symptoms associated with neurological problems, including Guillain-Barré syndrome.

Merrill, Jean E., Michael C. Graves, and Donald G. Mulder. "Autoimmune Disease and the Nervous System: Biochemical, Molecular, and Clinical Update." *Western Journal of Medicine* 156, no. 6 (1992): 639-646. This review summarizes information published on the immunological aspects of many of the classic autoimmune conditions up to 1992.

Noback, Charles R., Norman L. Strominger, and Robert J. Demarest. *The Human Nervous System*. 4th ed. Philadelphia: Lea & Febiger, 1991. A concise, easy-to-read paperback that offers a good balance of physiology and anatomy. Well illustrated.

Pearlman, Alan L., and Robert C. Collins. *Neurobiology of Disease*. New York: Oxford University Press, 1990. An advanced text that provides detailed descriptions of most neurological abnormalities. Contains a good description of Guillain-Barré syndrome and a chapter devoted to demyelinating disease.

# HAIR LOSS AND BALDNESS

**SYSTEMS AFFECTED:** Endocrine, skin

**SPECIALISTS:** Dermatologists, endocrinologists, plastic and reconstructive surgeons

**DEFINITION:** Symptoms of genetic factors, endocrine disorders, and aging which occur in both men and women, although more frequently in men, affecting more than one-half of the male population.

**KEY TERMS:**

*alopecia:* a condition in which all hair falls out, not only that on the scalp but also eyebrows, eyelashes, and even body hair

*follicle:* a small, saclike cavity for secretion or excretion

*hair shaft:* the hair itself, consisting of the central part (medulla), the middle part (cortex), and the outer part (cuticle)

*psoriasis:* a chronic skin disease characterized by scaly, reddish patches

*seborrhea:* a dermatologic condition characterized by an excessively dry (seborrhea oleosa) or oily skin (seborrhea sicca)

### CAUSES AND SYMPTOMS

The major reason that hair on the scalp thrives more lavishly than on other parts of the body is that scalp hairs are produced by the largest follicles found in human skin. Throughout the early years of infancy, these follicles increase in size, shedding their hairs about every two to six years to clear a path for a new hair that grows thicker and longer than the one that it replaced. In the mid-teens, nearly every follicle in an individual's scalp is generating an actively growing hair, and by the late teens scalp hair reaches its adult size, populating the scalp in numbers that will never again be equaled.

For most adults entering their twenties, this situation reverses, and hair loss begins to occur—either permanently or temporarily. At this stage in their development, nearly every man and more than 80 percent of women find their hairlines receding. As the years progress, the shedding continues, and the density of scalp hair continues to diminish. Nearly all the permanent hair loss that affects the human scalp is produced by the natural aging process and/or common baldness.

Common, or male pattern, baldness (baldness is classified into various groups depending on its pattern on the scalp) affects at least 20 million Americans. The term "baldness" is often used when a definite hairline recession, a bald spot on the crown, thinning over the top of the scalp, or a combination of the three is detected. The sides and rear scalp fringe areas are usually spared, except for the inevitable thinning that accompanies age. These regions appear to be capable of generating enough two-to-six-year hair cycles to keep them well covered for most, if not all, of a male's average life span.

The less frequent causes of permanent hair loss can be categorized into three groups. The first involves injury to follicles created by constant tension or pulling of scalp hair. Tight ponytails or chignons, worn over a number of years, often result in permanent bald patches on the sides of the head. In addition, tight rollers and the process of hair weaving kill follicles. The second infrequent cause of permanent hair loss is physical injury, such as a laceration or burn. If hair is ironed as a method of straightening over a period of years, hair follicles will become damaged. The third cause involves various inflammatory skin disorders and growths that occasionally affect the scalp. For example, a scalp wen, or cyst, tends to occur in families and requires no treatment unless it appears to be growing. Removal involves a simple office procedure and eliminates the bald spot that results from pressure of the enlarging cyst upon adjacent scalp follicles.

Nearly all humans lose some scalp hair every day. The number of falling hairs, however, often varies considerably from day to day. This daily variation in hair loss is not an indication of abnormality. An average of thirty to sixty hairs may be shed from the scalp each day. While days, weeks, and months may pass with little to no hair loss, large numbers of hairs may be lost over similar time periods. The yearly average, however, remains fairly constant.

## Patterns of Hair Loss

Male pattern

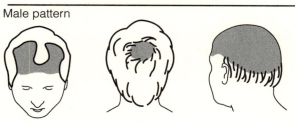

Women (rare, after pregnancy)

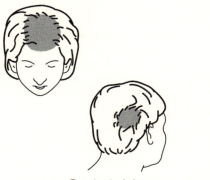

Patchy hair loss
(from infection, disease or stress)

This daily variation in hair loss merely reflects the fact that hair follicles act independently of one another. Their three-year growth and three-month rest cycles occur randomly. Aside from the tendency to lose more hair in the autumn, chance dictates the periods when the scalp will contain more resting hairs (hairs having small whitish roots).

Dandruff and its two related conditions of seborrhea and psoriasis, both scaly-scalp conditions, may create a significant diffuse hair loss. Because these conditions are so common, they account for most of the shedding that requires medical treatment. In most cases, these problems can be controlled without medical assistance.

Temporary hair loss can result from alopecia areata, pregnancy, severe illness, surgery, certain medications, hormonal disorders, or dieting. Alopecia areata is a condition that usually produces temporary shedding of scalp—and occasionally body—hair. In most cases, the hair regrows spontaneously or after medical therapy has ended. Occasionally, if this problem begins during childhood, all the scalp and body hair may be lost permanently. Extensive shedding may follow pregnancy or the discontinuation of birth control pills. After several months, however, the hair usually begins to regrow. Hair loss may also result from a severe illness associated with high fever (usually influenza) or an extensive surgical procedure. In the case of surgery, the cause is related to changes in body chemistry. Various medications can also create hair loss. The main offenders are the amphetamines, blood thinners, antithyroid drugs, anticancer drugs (as well as radiation treatments), and birth control pills. Hormonal disorders, particularly thyroid dysfunction, can create a thinning problem, but this condition is rarely an isolated symptom. In rare instances, improper nutrition can result in hair loss, such as in the case of dieters who eliminate protein from their daily food intake.

The conditions responsible for temporary shedding usually create a thinning problem quite rapidly. Aside from hair breakage or forcible extraction (hair pulling), the problem is usually one of increased numbers of resting hairs, resulting in massive hair loss. (The two conditions primarily responsible for creating permanent hair loss—aging and common baldness—usually develop slowly, over many years. Thinning occurs simply because the scalp follicles are no longer capable of producing new hairs.)

If something occurs to double the number of resting hairs from their normal 15 to 30 percent, then hundreds of hairs may fall each day. If this lasts for several months, about one-third of the scalp's hair may be lost. A loss of about 30 to 40 percent is required before thinning becomes obvious. After the shedding abates, it may take years for the scalp hair to return to its original density, since the new hairs can grow only about an inch every two months.

### TREATMENT AND THERAPY

Scientific research in the area of hair loss has produced a drug that has been relatively effective in some individuals.

The drug minoxidil was originally used as an antihypertensive medication; however, 70 percent of patients taking it reported unexpected hair growth, occasionally in such undesirable places as the forehead. A 0.2 percent minoxidil solution for external use was devised by a major drug company in the United States and marketed under the name Rogaine. The Food and Drug Administration approved Rogaine as the only prescription drug that effectively combats baldness.

Although it is uncertain how the drug works, it is believed that minoxidil enables shrunken follicles to grow back to a size capable of producing sturdy, visible hairs. Minoxidil has been shown to have promising, though limited, results. It is best at filling in those patchy gaps that herald the beginnings of baldness. Between one-third and one-half of men in some studies exhibited "significant" or "cosmetically acceptable" hair growth. Minoxidil is not a cure, however, and it requires a lifetime commitment. When the drug is stopped, hair thins out within months.

Another nonsurgical method for achieving permanent hair is hair weaving, a process that originated in the African American culture in the nineteenth century. Weaving hair involves braiding it tightly so that a toupee or smaller weft (section of hair) can be attached permanently. All that is required is a sufficient amount of hair remaining on the scalp to serve as an anchor for a hairpiece.

The braids are usually formed from the thicker hair found on the sides and back of the scalp. A semicircular ridge is created that holds a hairpiece firmly in place. If enough hair is still growing on top of the scalp, it can be twisted into smaller braids to anchor individual wefts. This type of weave permits better aeration and easier cleansing of the scalp.

A hair "fusion," "bonding," or "linking" is exactly like a weave except that the hairpiece or wefts are glued, instead of tied, onto the braided hair. This so-called chemical bond is insoluble in water and quite caustic. Frequent hair breakage has limited the usefulness of this method.

While weaved or fused hair does not grow, it still requires regular care and maintenance to keep it looking acceptable. The scalp hair used to anchor the weave naturally continues to grow. As it grows, the attached hair starts to ride above the scalp. Thus the weave or fusion must be reanchored frequently (as often as every three weeks). In addition, the tension placed on the anchoring scalp hair creates accelerated shedding, and this hair loss is often irreversible.

Hair implants, also known as medical or suture implants, have become the principal method for fixing a hairpiece securely to the scalp. Implants are usually not permanent, are only quasi-medical, and are to be distinguished from transplants, with which they share a resemblance in name only. Implants are stitches made from either stainless steel or nylon-type materials that are sewn into the scalp and tied into rings. Like the weave hair braids, the knotted stitches act as anchors, holding a hairpiece or several wefts against the barren scalp. If the implants secure a hairpiece, only two or perhaps six stitches are needed. If the implants anchor many smaller wefts of hair, however, more than a dozen stitches must be sewn into the scalp. A physician must perform this procedure, since only someone with a medical license can inject a local anesthetic and sew stitches into the scalp. The problems generated by sewing and leaving stitches in the scalp, however, are pain, infection, and scarring.

In the 1970's, a surgical procedure known as tunnel grafting was developed. This procedure is not available in implant clinics. A 2.5-by-7.5 centimeter rectangle of skin is removed from behind each ear. The two pieces are immediately grafted to the front and back of the scalp to form two loops that serve as anchors for a hairpiece. While the operation is relatively simple to perform, extreme care must be taken to ensure proper graft acceptance and healing. Although this method avoids the pitfalls of implanted stitches, it still retains two of the problems common to any kind of artificial anchoring device. Since only two loops are available to fix a hairpiece, the hairpiece can still lift off the scalp. In addition, the skin loops are as vulnerable to injury as suture loops. Scalp lacerations resulting from forcible removal of the hairpiece have occurred.

From the discovery of hair transplants in the 1960's to 1978, it has been estimated that approximately one million people—both men and women—underwent such transplants. As with implants, a medical license is mandatory in order to inject a local anesthetic into the scalp and make the surgical incisions required for a hair transplant. Doctors who specialize in hair transplants are usually dermatologists, some are plastic surgeons, and a few acquire the training that enables them to perform this procedure.

Even the baldest scalp contains thousands of transplantable hair follicles. To move them where they are most needed, three surgical methods have been developed, employing scalp grafts known variously as "flaps," "strips," and "plugs." While all three methods are used, most hair transplants are performed with plug grafts because they are simpler and safer to work with and yield the most satisfying results. The transplant candidate need only be bald enough to justify undergoing the procedure and be endowed with enough side and rear fringe scalp hair to make the procedure worthwhile.

To create a flap or "full thickness" graft, a surgeon cuts out three sides of a rectangular patch of scalp from above the ears and swings it over to the bald area to create a new hairline. Thus is a major hospital procedure requiring considerable surgical expertise. Although a fairly large portion of bald scalp can be provided with instant hair-density, this method is fraught with problems. To ensure a proper take, or graft survival, the blood vessels feeding the transplant must remain intact while they are moved along with it. Because the vessels are quite fragile, they are frequently damaged, resulting in poor graft survival and catastrophic hair loss.

To alleviate this problem, a variation of this type of transplant, known as a free flap procedure, was developed by a team of Japanese surgeons. The free flap is cut out on all four sides, completely severing the blood supply. After setting the graft into its new location, the surgeons meticulously reestablish its blood supply to the recipient blood vessels using a delicate microsurgical technique.

Even if this technical obstacle is surmounted, however, other aesthetic problems remain. The first problem involves the surgical scar that delineates the border between the forehead and the transplanted hairline. Little can be done to minimize this scar. The other problem concerns the unnatural direction in which the newly transplanted hair grows. A flap graft cannot provide hair that will grow in the direction of the hair that has been lost. Hairs growing from the sides of the scalp exit much closer to the surface than in other areas. When transplanted to the frontal area, these hairs lie much too flat against the scalp. Thus, while a flap may provide a faster way to achieve a high-density transplant, the problems of graft survival and poor aesthetic results have limited its usefulness.

A surgical strip graft is a narrow rectangular patch of scalp, cut out on all four sides, that is usually transplanted to create a hairline. Unlike the larger flap, its blood supply need not be moved along with it or be laboriously reestablished. After the strip is placed into its new location, the adjacent bald scalp sends new blood vessels directly into it. Like a flap graft, however, it must be sewn into place. If it is used to create a hairline, an unsightly scar will mark its border with the forehead as well. While this procedure can be performed in an office rather than at a hospital, extreme care must be taken to avoid damaging this delicate graft. Despite the most painstaking precautions, poor takes result quite often. Areas of nongrowth are common, and not infrequently the entire graft becomes almost completely devoid of hair.

A "hair transplant" usually refers to a procedure in which a small cylinder of hair-bearing scalp, or plug, is taken from the rear or side fringe areas and transferred to either the bald crown or the scalp's frontal region. While this transplant method requires several sessions to approach the density of hair acquired with a flap graft, the ease with which it can be performed, coupled with its superior aesthetic results, make it the logical choice for surgically replacing hair.

The surgeon uses a trephine, or "punch," to remove the cylindrical section of scalp, properly called a donor graft rather than a plug. The graft is quite small, measuring about 0.8 centimeter deep by 0.5 centimeter in diameter. The hair follicle is intimately related to all three skin layers. The bulb—or hair-producing portion of the follicle—lies within and is cushioned by the fat, or adipose, layer. The entire follicle is supported by and receives its nourishment from the fibrous portion of skin, or dermis, which is about 0.6 centimeter thick in the scalp. The skin mantle, or epidermis, provides the opening, or "pore," through which the hair exits to the surface of the scalp.

When a donor graft is removed, all three skin layers must be included. The hair is actually superfluous to the procedure: The hair follicle is all that is essential. After removing the hair-bearing donor grafts, the physician next punches out identical sections of bald scalp. The term "plug" actually refers to the hairless cylinder of scalp that is taken from the bald area. The donor graft is placed into the void left by the removal of the bald plug. Light pressure is applied for several seconds to allow the blood to clot and hold the graft in place. Because these grafts are so small and clotting occurs so rapidly, stitches are not required to fix them in place.

Within hours, new blood vessels move into the graft from the surrounding skin to feed the new section. Within several days, as healing continues, the graft and its adjacent host skin become one. Keeping the grafts small facilitates easy penetration by these vital blood vessels. When larger grafts, or strips, are used, the blood supply may not reach all the hair follicles, and they die.

Because of their small size, the rounded edges of the grafts blend into the host skin quite evenly, creating an acceptable hairline. While they might appear obvious on close inspection, they are always less noticeable than the borders left by flaps and strips. Because the grafts are small and are taken from the rear half of the scalp, where the hairs grow out in the same manner as the front and crown hairs, they can be directed to duplicate exactly the original pattern of growth in the bald host areas. This method is a minor office procedure that, in the hands of an experienced physician, is considered safe, with little discomfort experienced by the patient.

## PERSPECTIVE AND PROSPECTS

The observation that eunuchs are not subject to gout or baldness was made by Hippocrates in the year 400 B.C. and is contained in the *Hippocratic Corpus* as a short medical truth or aphorism. Aristotle, himself balding, was interested in the fact that eunuchs did not become bald and were unable to grow hair on their chests. These observations were either forgotten or overlooked for the next twenty-five centuries, and medical science remained baffled by male pattern baldness until James B. Hamilton, an anatomist, in 1949 again made the observation that eunuchs did not become bald. His suggestion that androgens are a prerequisite and incitant in male pattern baldness and his later classification of the patterns and grades of baldness are landmarks in the study of male pattern baldness. Subsequent investigations of hair loss confirmed the significance of androgens

in male pattern baldness, and Hamilton's classification remains in use.

Hamilton demonstrated conclusively that the extent and development of male pattern baldness were dependent on the interaction of three factors: androgens, genetic predisposition, and age. In summary, he found that genetic, endocrine, and aging factors are interdependent. No matter how strong the inherited predisposition, male pattern alopecia will not result if androgens are missing. Neither are the androgens able to induce baldness in individuals not genetically predisposed to baldness. The action of aging is demonstrated by the immediate loss of hair upon exposure to androgens in the sixth decade of life, whereas hair in young men exposed to androgens tends to remain much longer.

Over the centuries, men have tried every imaginable approach to retain hair. They have shampooed their scalps with tar, petroleum, goose dung, and cow urine. They have stuck their heads into rubber caps connected to vacuum pumps to suck recalcitrant hairs to the surface. In the 1960's, hair transplants became the most efficient and aesthetically pleasing method of retaining scalp hair. Research in the area of drug treatment continues.

—*Genevieve Slomski*

**See also** Aging; Pregnancy and gestation; Psoriasis; Skin disorders.

### FOR FURTHER INFORMATION:

Baccaredda-Boy, Aldo, et al., eds. *Biopathology of Pattern Alopecia*. New York: S. Karger, 1968. In this collection of essays, scientists who initiated the modern era of male pattern baldness research investigate the various etiologies and treatment of the condition. Somewhat technical but accessible to the general reader. Contains a bibliography.

Feinberg, Herbert S. *All About Hair*. Alpine, N.J.: Wallingford Press, 1978. Written by a practicing dermatologist, this book is intended for the general reader. Explains in clear, nontechnical language the composition of hair, as well as the causes and treatment of hair thinning or loss. Contains illustrations.

Montagna, William, and Richard A. Ellis. *The Biology of Hair Growth*. New York: Academic Press, 1958. A somewhat dated but useful overview of biological factors that affect hair growth. Etiologies of hairfall is also discussed.

Norwood, O'Tar T., and Richard C. Shiell. *Hair Transplant Surgery*. 2d ed. Springfield, Ill.: Charles C Thomas, 1984. The authors discuss the surgical techniques for transplanting hair. Accessible to the general reader. Includes bibliographical references.

Setterberg, Fred. "The Naked Truth About Baldness." In *Health* 3 (September/October, 1989): 112-118. This article summarizes for the general reader the main causes of permanent hair loss and discusses treatment options such as transplants and the drug minoxidil.

# HALITOSIS

**SYSTEMS AFFECTED:** Gastrointestinal, respiratory
**SPECIALISTS:** Dentists, family physicians, otolaryngologists
**DEFINITION:** Halitosis, commonly known as bad breath, is usually the result of such habits as drinking alcohol, smoking, and eating pungent foods, including onions and garlic; over time, the offensive odor may no longer be noticeable to the patient. The odor is eliminated if these habits are stopped. Halitosis may also be attributable to chronic infections of the mouth, throat, and lungs. Poor oral or dental hygiene, sinusitis, tonsillitis, and bronchiectasis (distortion and consequent damage of the bronchi in the lungs) may be responsible for the foul breath; treatment consists of addressing the underlying condition.

*See also* Abdominal disorders; Alcoholism; Caries, dental; Dental diseases; Gastrointestinal disorders; Indigestion; Nasopharyngeal disorders; Pharyngitis; Sinusitis; Sore throat; Tonsillitis.

# HALLUCINATIONS

**SYSTEMS AFFECTED:** Brain, nervous, psychic-emotional
**SPECIALISTS:** Neurologists, psychiatrists, psychologists
**DEFINITION:** The perception of sensations without relevant external stimuli.

Society often associates hallucinations with psychotic behavior, because schizophrenia and other forms of mental illness frequently involve hallucinations. Another widely publicized example of these symptoms is the use of hallucinogenic drugs, for example, LSD (lysergic acid diethylamide) or marijuana. One must also consider the role of hallucinations in religious experiences and megalomania; such perceptions occur when ordinary people are subjected to extraordinary stimuli.

Medical science has resisted the study of hallucinations and treated them as symptoms of mental illness. Increasing evidence shows, however, that they arise from specific brain and nervous system structures involving specific biological experiences and common reactions to stimuli. Consequently, people suffering from drug abuse, alcoholism, and disorders similar to Alzheimer's disease, in which severe loss of memory can provoke illusions, are subject to hallucinations.

Since a hallucination can be the result of physical causes as well as the traditional mental unbalance of schizophrenia or manic depression, it is difficult to categorize its symptoms. An individual experiencing hallucinations at times other than waking or falling asleep should see his or her doctor. If the incidents are attributable to a serious illness, early detection is possible. If they are an effect of a particular medication, the prescription should be changed immediately. —*K. Thomas Finley*

*See also* Addiction; Alcoholism; Alzheimer's disease; Brain disorders; Dementia; Intoxication; Manic-depressive disorder; Narcolepsy; Paranoia; Poisonous plants; Psychiatric disorders; Psychosis; Schizophrenia; Sleep disorders; Stress.

**FOR FURTHER INFORMATION:**

Johnson, Fred H. *The Anatomy of Hallucinations.* Chicago: Nelson-Hall, 1978.

Siegel, Ronald K. *Fire in the Brain: Clinical Tales of Hallucination.* New York: E. P. Dutton, 1992.

Slade, P. D., and R. P. Bentall. *Sensory Deception: A Scientific Analysis of Hallucinations.* Baltimore: The Johns Hopkins University Press, 1988.

# HARE LIP. *See* CLEFT PALATE.

# HAY FEVER. *See* ALLERGIES; RHINITIS.

# HEAD AND NECK DISORDERS

**SYSTEMS AFFECTED:** Brain, nervous, muscular, skeletal
**SPECIALISTS:** Dentists, emergency physicians, maxillofacial surgeons, neurologists, neurosurgeons, otolaryngologists, sports medicine physicians
**DEFINITION:** Physical trauma or neurological problems affecting the head and neck, including the spinal cord.

The head and neck region of the human body houses a sophisticated collection of structures including the special sense organs (structures for breathing, speaking, and eating) and the brain, brain stem, and cervical (neck) portion of the spinal cord. A multitude of disorders or injuries can occur in this complex region.

*Trauma to the head and neck.* Head or neck trauma can result from a harsh blow on the head, as can occur in a fall or with a strike from an object. These injuries are commonly seen in young, basically healthy persons who come to emergency rooms during evenings or weekends as a result of sports accidents, automobile accidents, or domestic or street violence. In the older age group, strokes and aneurysms are more common problems. Some of these accidents or events can cause permanent nerve and brain damage to the injured person.

Concussions and contusions of the head are common results of head trauma, which induces an internal neurological response. A concussion is a loss of consciousness or awareness of one's surroundings that may last a few minutes or days. Sometimes a concussion appears only as a moderately decreased level of awareness and not a total loss of consciousness. There is no evidence of a change in the brain's structure but, oddly, there is a change in the way in which the brain operates so that alertness is altered. Concussion is presumably a temporary change in brain chemistry, and the damage is reversible unless repeated head blows, such as a professional boxer may experience, are endured. Concussions may occur from other trauma, such as loss of blood flow to the brain, but such trauma is more closely associated with the more urgent threat of permanent brain damage. A contusion is popularly referred to as a bruise.

The color associated with a fresh bruise is attributable to an aggregation of blood in an area that was damaged, causing many small blood vessels to rupture and release blood into the surrounding tissue. A bruise around the eye, temple, or forehead causes a black eye.

Automobile accidents rank as one of the common causes of head and neck injury. One of the more familiar complaints after a car accident is the condition called whiplash. Whiplash is the lay person's term for hyperextension of the neck, whereby the head is thrust backward (posteriorly) abruptly and beyond the normal range of neck motion. Hyperflexion occurs when the head is abruptly thrust in the forward (anterior) direction—sometimes as a recoil from hyperextension. The pain of whiplash originates from the damage to the anterior longitudinal ligament along the neck region of the spinal cord. This ligament can be overly stretched or even torn as a result of a sudden snap or jerk of the neck. Furthermore, the bony vertebrae may also grind against one another after the trauma, causing additional irritation, swelling, and pain in the neck area.

One of the common troubles of a gun or knife wound to the head and neck region is superficial and deep lacerations (cuts). If left unsutured, a deep scalp wound can cause death by hemorrhage. Superficial lacerations to the face may also cause considerable bleeding; such wounds generally are not life-threatening, but they often require stitches in order to heal.

Trauma to the head and neck area can arise from spontaneous internal events such as a stroke, an embolus, or an aneurysm. Each of these conditions is serious and potentially life-threatening because of the risk of losing blood flow to the brain and other vital tissues of the head and neck region.

*Neurological problems of the head and neck.* Although the bony cranium offers some protection to the head, the neck is, in some regards, more vulnerable to intrusion. Breathing can be interrupted by severing the left or right phrenic nerve, each of which innervates its corresponding half of the most important muscle of breathing, the diaphragm.

The left or right vagus nerve may also be severed. The vagus nerves supply the sympathetic system of the thorax and abdomen, and they also innervate the vocal cords. Severance of one of the vagus nerves causes a hoarseness of the voice as a result of the loss of function of one-half of the vocal cords. If both vagus nerves are damaged—a rare event—then the ability to speak is forever lost.

The sympathetic trunk is another nerve at risk in the neck. Severance of this nerve leads to Horner's syndrome, which consists of a group of signs including ptosis (drooping eyelids), constricted pupils, a flushed face as a result of vasodilation, and dry skin on the face and neck because of the inability to sweat.

Transection (the complete severance) of the lower cervical spinal cord causes upper and lower limb paralysis and

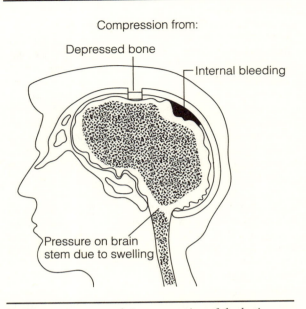

Compression from:

Depressed bone

Internal bleeding

Pressure on brain stem due to swelling

*Head trauma may result in compression of the brain, consequent distortions, and severe neurological reactions.*

trouble with urination, and damage to the upper cervical cord can cause death because of loss of innervation to the muscles of respiration. Hemisection (partial severance) of the cervical spinal cord can also cause Horner's syndrome. Damage to the spinal cord can occur from a knife or gun wound or from crushing or snapping the cord by sudden impact, as with an injury from an earthquake or an automobile accident.   *—Mary C. Fields*

***See also*** Alzheimer's disease; Amnesia and memory loss; Ataxia; Brain disorders; Cluster headaches; Coma; Concussion; Dementia; Encephalitis; Epilepsy; Guillain-Barré syndrome (GBS); Hallucinations; Headaches; Hemiplegia; Laryngitis; Meningitis; Migraine headaches; Motor neuron diseases; Multiple sclerosis; Nasopharyngeal disorders; Neuralgia, neuritis, and neuropathy; Numbness and tingling; Palsy; Paralysis; Paraplegia; Parkinsonism; Pharyngitis; Quadriplegia; Seizures; Sinusitis; Spinal disorders; Tics; Unconsciousness; Voice and vocal cord disorders.

**FOR FURTHER INFORMATION:**

Kunz, Jeffrey R. M., and Asher J. Finkel, eds. *The American Medical Association Family Medical Guide*. New York: Random House, 1987. The perfect beginner's guide, not only to head and neck medicine but to any common medical topic as well.

Moore, Keith L. *Clinically Oriented Anatomy*. 3d ed. Baltimore: Williams & Wilkins, 1992. Moore addresses the normal human anatomy and offers clinical commentary for the sake of relevance. Enhanced by multicolored, detailed sketches. Expertly written.

# HEADACHES

**SYSTEM AFFECTED:** Brain

**SPECIALISTS:** Family physicians, internists, neurologists

**DEFINITION:** A general term referring to pain localized in the head and/or neck, which may signal mere tension or serious disorders.

**KEY TERMS:**

*cluster headache:* a severe type of headache, characterized by excruciating pain; attacks occur in groups, or clusters

*migraine headache:* a type of headache characterized by pain on one side of the head, often accompanied by disordered vision and gastrointestinal disturbances

*prophylactic treatment:* a treatment focusing on preventing disease, illness, or their symptoms from occurring

*symptomatic treatment:* a treatment focusing on aborting disease, illness, or their symptoms once they have occurred

*tension-type headache:* a type of headache characterized by bandlike or caplike pain over the head

## CAUSES AND SYMPTOMS

In 1988, an ad hoc committee of the International Headache Society developed the current classification system for headaches. This system includes fourteen exhaustive categories of headache with the purpose of developing comparability in the management and study of headaches. Headaches most commonly seen by health care providers can be classified into four main types: migraine, tension-type, cluster, and "other" acute headaches.

Migraine headaches have been estimated to affect approximately 12 percent of the population. The headaches are more common in women, and they tend to run in families; they are usually first noticed in the teen years or young adulthood. For the diagnosis of migraine without aura ("aura" refers to visual disturbances or hallucinations, numbness and tingling on one side of the face, dizziness, or impairment of speech or hearing—symptoms that occur twenty to thirty minutes prior to the onset of the headache), the person must experience at least ten headache attacks, each lasting between four and seventy-two hours with at least two of the following characteristics: The headache is unilateral (occurs on one side), has a pulsating quality, is moderate to severe in intensity, or is aggravated by routine physical activity. Additionally, one of the following symptoms must accompany the headache: nausea and/or vomiting, or sensitivity to light or sounds. The person's medical history, a physical examination, and (where appropriate) diagnostic tests must exclude other organic causes of the headache, such as brain tumor or infection. Migraine with aura is far less common.

Migraines may be triggered or aggravated by physical activity, by menstruation, by relaxation after emotional stress, by ingestion of alcohol (red wine in particular) or certain foods or food additives (chocolate, hard cheeses, nuts, fatty foods, monosodium glutamate, or nitrates used in processed meats), by prescription medications (including birth control pills and hypertension medications), and by changes in the weather. Yet the precise pathophysiology of migraines is unknown. It had been posited that spasms in the blood vessels of the brain, followed by the dilation of these same blood vessels, cause the aura and head pain; however, studies using sophisticated brain and cerebral blood-flow scanning techniques indicate that this is likely not the case and that some type of inflammatory process may be involved related to the permeability of cerebral blood vessels and the resultant release of certain neurochemicals.

Tension-type headaches are the most common type of headache; its prevalence is approximately 79 percent. Tension-type headaches are not hereditary, are found more frequently in females, and are first noticed in the teen years of young adulthood, although they can appear at any time of life. For the diagnosis of tension-type headaches, the person must experience at least ten headache attacks lasting from thirty minutes to seven days each, with at least two of the following characteristics: The headache has a pressing or tightening (nonpulsating) quality, is mild or moderate in intensity (may inhibit but does not prohibit activities), is bilateral or variable in location, and is not aggravated by physical activity. Additionally, nausea, vomiting, and light or sound sensitivity are absent or mild. Furthermore, the patient's medical history and physical or neurological examination exclude other organic causes for the headache apart from the following: oral or jaw dysfunction, muscular stress, or drug overuse. Tension-type headache sufferers describe these headaches as a bandlike or caplike tightness around the head, and/or muscle tension in the back of the head, neck, or shoulders. The pain is described as slow in onset with a dull or steady aching.

Tension-type headaches are believed to be precipitated primarily by emotional factors but can also be stimulated by muscular and spinal disorders, jaw dysfunction, paranasal sinus disease, and traumatic head injuries. The pathophysiology of tension-type headaches is controversial. Historically, tension-type headaches were attributed to sustained muscle contractions of the pericranial muscles. Studies indicate, however, that most patients do not manifest increased pericranial muscle activity and that pericranial muscle blood flow and/or central pain mechanisms might be involved in the pathophysiology of tension-type headaches. It is also believed that muscle contraction and scalp muscle ischemia play some role in tension-type headache pain.

Cluster headaches are the least frequent of the headache types and are thought to be the most severe and painful. Cluster headaches are more common in males, with estimates of 0.4 to 1.0 percent of males being affected. Traditionally, these headaches first appear at about thirty years of age, although they can start later in life. There is no genetic predisposition to these headaches. For the diagnosis of cluster headaches, the person must experience at least ten severely painful headache attacks, typically on one side of the face and lasting from fifteen minutes to three hours. One of the following symptoms must accompany the headache on the painful side of the face: a bloodshot eye, tearing, nasal congestion, nasal discharge, forehead and facial sweating, contraction of the pupils, or drooping eyelids. Physical and neurological examination and imaging must exclude organic causes for the headaches, such as tumor or infection. Cluster headaches often occur once or twice daily, or every other day, but can be as frequent as ten attacks in one day, recurring on the same side of the head during the cluster period. The temporal "clusters" of these headaches give them their descriptive name.

A cluster headache is described as a severe, excruciating, boring, sharp, and burning pain through the eye. The pain is occasionally throbbing but always unilateral. Radiation of the pain to the teeth has been reported. Duration of a headache can range from ten minutes to three hours, with the next headache in the cluster occurring sometime the same day. Cluster headache sufferers are often unable to sit or lie still and are in such pain that they have been known, in desperation, to hit their heads with their fists or to smash their heads against walls or floors.

Cluster headaches can be triggered in susceptible patients by alcohol consumption, subcutaneous injections of histamine, and sublingual use of nitroglycerine. Because these agents all cause the dilation of blood vessels, these attacks are believed to be associated with dilation of the temporal and ophthalmic arteries and other extracranial vessels. There is no evidence that intracranial blood flow is involved. Cluster headaches have been shown to occur more frequently during the weeks before and after the longest and shortest days of the year, lending support for the hypothesis of a link to seasonal changes. Additionally, cluster headaches often occur at about the same time of day in a given sufferer, suggesting a relationship to the circadian rhythms of the body. Vascular changes, hormonal changes, neurochemical excesses or deficits, histamine levels, and autonomic nervous system changes are all being studied for their possible role in the pathophysiology of cluster headaches.

Acute headaches, using the International Headache Society's classification scheme, constitute many of the headaches not mentioned above. Distinct from the other headache types, which are often considered to be chronic in nature, acute headaches often signify underlying disease or a life-threatening medical condition. These headaches can display pain distribution and quality similar to those seen in chronic headaches. The temporal nature of acute headaches, however, often points to their seriousness. Acute headaches of concern are usually the first or worst headache the patient has had or are headaches with recent onset that are persistent or recurrent. Other signs that cause a high

index of suspicion include an unremitting headache that steadily increases without relief, accompanying weakness or numbness in the hands or feet, an atypical change in the quality or intensity of the headache, headache upon exertion, recent head trauma, or a family history of cardiovascular problems. Such headaches can point to hemorrhage, meningitis, stroke, tumor, brain abscess, hematoma, and infection, which are all potentially life-threatening conditions. A thorough evaluation is necessary for all patients exhibiting the danger signs of acute headache.

## TREATMENT AND THERAPY

Because there are several hundred causes of headaches, the evaluation of headache complaints is crucial. Medical science offers myriad evaluation techniques for headaches. The initial evaluation includes a complete history and physical examination to determine the factors involved in the headache complaint, such as the general physical condition of the patient, neurological functioning, cardiovascular condition, metabolic status, and psychiatric condition. Based on this initial evaluation, the health care professional may elect to perform a number of diagnostic tests to confirm or reject a diagnosis. These tests might include blood studies, X rays, computed tomography (CT) scans, psychological evaluation, electroencephalograms (EEGs), magnetic resonance imaging (MRI), or studies of spinal fluid.

Once a headache diagnosis is made, a treatment plan is developed. In the case of acute headaches, treatment may take varying forms, from surgery to the use of prescription medications. For migraine, tension-type, and cluster headaches, there are several common treatment options. Headache treatment can be categorized into two types: abortive (symptomatic) treatment or prophylactic (preventive) treatment. Treatment is tailored to the type of headache and the type of patient.

A headache is often a highly distressing occurrence for patients, sometimes causing a high level of anxiety, relief-seeking behavior, and a dependency on the health care system. The health care provider must consider not only biological elements of the illness but also possible resultant psychological and sociological elements as well. An open, communicative relationship with the patient is paramount, and treatment routinely begins with soliciting patient collaboration and providing patient education. Patient education takes the form of normalizing (or "decatastrophizing") the headache experience for patients, thereby reducing their fears concerning the etiology of the headache or about being unable to cope with the pain. Supportiveness, understanding, and collaboration are all necessary components of any headache treatment.

There are a number of abortive pharmacological treatments for migraine headaches. Ergotamine tartrate (an alkaloid or salt) is effective in terminating migraine symptoms by either reducing the dilation of extracranial arteries or in some way stimulating certain parts of the brain.

Isomethaptine, another effective treatment for migraine, is a combination of chemicals that stimulates the sympathetic nervous system, provides analgesia, and is mildly tranquilizing. Another class of medications for migraines are nonsteroidal anti-inflammatory drugs (NSAIDs); these drugs, as the name implies, work on the principle that inflammation is involved in migraine. Both narcotic and nonnarcotic pain medications are often used for migraines, primarily for their analgesic properties; the concern in prescribing potent narcotic pain medications is the potential for their overuse. Antiemetic medications prevent or arrest vomiting and have been used in the treatment of migraines. Sumatriptan, a vasoactive agent that increases the amount of the neurochemical serotonin in the brain, shows promise in treating migraines that do not respond to other treatments.

Prophylactic treatments for migraines include beta-blockers, methysergide, and calcium channel blockers, which are believed to interfere with the dilation or contraction of extracranial arteries by acting on the sympathetic nervous system or on the central nervous system itself. Antidepressants, medications used typically for the treatment of depression, have also been found to prevent migraine attacks; there appears to be an analgesic effect from certain antidepressants that is effective for chronic migraines. Antiseizure medications have been found to be useful for some migraine patients, although the mechanism of action is unknown. NSAIDs have also been used as a preventive measure for migraines.

There are several nonpharmacological treatment options for migraine headaches. These include stress management, relaxation training, biofeedback (a variant of relaxation training), psychotherapy (both individual and family), and the modification of headache-precipitating factors (such as avoiding certain dietary precipitants). Each of these treatments has been found to be effective for certain patients, particularly those with chronic migraine complaints. For some patients, they can be as effective as pharmacological treatments. The exact mechanism of action for their effect on migraines has not been established. Other self-management techniques include lying quietly in a dark room, applying pressure to the side of the head or face on which the pain is experienced, and applying cold compresses to the head.

The abortive treatment options for tension-type headaches include narcotic and nonnarcotic analgesics, because of their pain-reducing properties. More often with tension-type headaches, the milder over-the-counter pain medications (such as aspirin or acetaminophen) are used. NSAIDs, simple muscle relaxants, or antianxiety drugs can also be used. Muscle relaxants and antianxiety drugs are believed to relax smooth muscles, reducing scalp muscle ischemia and therefore head pain.

Prophylactic treatments for tension-type headaches include antidepressants, narcotic and nonnarcotic analgesics, muscle relaxants, and antianxiety drugs. Occasionally, "trigger-point injections" are used to relieve tension-type headaches. Trigger points are areas within muscles, primarily in the upper back and neck, that are hypersensitive; when stimulated, they can cause headaches. These trigger points can be injected with a local anesthetic or steroid to decrease their sensitivity or to eliminate possible inflammation in the area.

Nonpharmacological treatment of tension-type headaches is similar to that for migraines and includes stress management, relaxation training, biofeedback, and psychotherapy. Psychotherapy has been found to be a very important adjunct to any treatment of tension-type headaches because the illness, particularly when chronic, can lead to a pain syndrome characterized by family dysfunction, medication overuse, and vocational disruptions. Other self-management techniques include taking a hot shower or bath, placing a hot water bottle or ice pack on the head or back of the neck, exercising, and sleeping.

For cluster headaches, one of the most excruciating types of headache, the most common abortive treatment is administering pure oxygen to the patient for ten minutes. The exact mechanism of action is unknown, but it might be related to the constriction of dilated cerebral arteries. Ergotamine tartrate or similar alkaloids given orally, intramuscularly, or intravenously can also abort the attack in some patients. Nasal drops of a local anesthetic (lidocaine hydrochloride) or cocaine have been used to interrupt the activity of the trigeminal nerve that is believed to be involved in cluster attacks. The efficacy of these treatments is inconclusive.

Prophylactic treatment of this headache type is crucial. Ergotamine, methysergide, calcium channel blockers, antiseizure medications, and steroidal anti-inflammatory medications have been used with some success in the prevention of cluster attacks. The mechanism of action for these medications is unknown. Lithium carbonate, a drug commonly prescribed for manic-depressive disorder, has been found to be effective for some cluster patients. This medication is believed to affect certain regions of the brain, possibly the hypothalamus.

While no nonpharmacological treatment strategies are routinely offered to cluster headache patients, surgery is an option in severe cases, particularly if the headaches are resistant to all other available treatments. Percutaneous radio frequency thermocoagulation of the trigeminal ganglion is a surgical procedure that destroys the trigeminal nerve pathway, the chief nerve pathway to the face. Modest successes have been found with this extreme treatment option.

## PERSPECTIVE AND PROSPECTS

Headaches are among the most common complaints to physicians and quite likely have been a problem since the beginning of humankind. Accounts of headaches can be found in the clinical notes of Arateus of Cappadocia, a first century physician. Descriptions of specific headache subtypes can be traced to the second century in the writings of the Greek physician Galen. Headaches are a prevalent health problem that affects all ages and sexes and those from various cultural, social, and educational backgrounds.

The lifetime prevalence estimates of headaches is 93 percent for males and 99 percent of females. Studies in the United States estimate that 65 to 85 percent of the population will experience a headache within a year. Data from cross-cultural studies echo the significance of this public health problem: Frequent, severe headaches are reported by 10.4 percent of men and 35.3 percent of women in Thailand; 17.6 percent of men and 20.2 percent of women in urban Africa report a history of recurrent headaches; 57 percent of men and 73 percent of women in Finland report at least one headache in the previous year; and 39 percent of men and 60 percent of women in New Zealand also report an annual headache frequency.

As these data indicate, the prevalence of headaches is greater in women, although the reason is unknown. Age seems to be a mediating factor as well, with significantly fewer people sixty-five years of age or older reporting headache problems. There are no socioeconomic differences in prevalence rates, with persons in high-income and low-income brackets having similar rates. There are data to suggest that people with college educations or higher report headaches more often than those with only some high school education. The only vocational area that has been tied to increased rates of headaches are people who work at computer terminals.

The total economic costs of headaches are staggering. Headaches constitute approximately 1.7 percent of all visits to physician offices. Of visits to hospital emergency rooms, 2.5 percent are for headaches. The expenses associated with advances in assessment techniques and routine health care have risen rapidly. The cost in lost workdays adds to this economic picture. Thirty-six percent of headache sufferers in one study reported missing one or more days of work in the previous year because of headaches. The scientific study of headaches is necessary to understand this prevalent illness. Efforts, such as those by the International Headache Society, to develop accepted definitions of headaches will greatly assist efforts to identify and treat headaches.

—*Oliver Oyama*

*See also* Anxiety; Cluster headaches; Head and neck disorders; Migraine headaches; Neuralgia, neuritis, and neuropathy; Sinusitis; Stress.

**FOR FURTHER INFORMATION:**

Bakal, Donald A. *The Psychobiology of Chronic Headache*. New York: Springer, 1982. This text synthesizes the psychological and biological theories of headaches into a conceptual model encompassing the different variables that interact to produce headaches.

Blanchard, Edward B., and Frank Andrasik. *Management of Chronic Headaches: A Psychological Approach*. New York: Pergamon Press, 1985. The authors review the evaluation and treatment of headaches from a psychological perspective. Alternative, nonpharmacological treatments for headaches are described in detail. The chapters are practical and offer a guide for managing headaches derived from the authors' experiences at a headache clinic.

Diamond, Seymour. "Migraine Headaches." *The Medical Clinics of North America* 75, no. 3 (May 1, 1991): 545-566. Diamond is one of the world's authorities on headaches. His article is well organized and comprehensively addresses the subject of migraines in a readable and interesting format. A practical guide to treating the headache patient.

Headache Classification Committee of the International Headache Society. "Classification and Diagnostic Criteria for Headache Disorders, Cranial Neuralgias, and Facial Pain." *Cephalalgia* 8, supp. 7 (1988): 1-96. This article in a medical journal presents the International Headache Society's classification system for headaches. Clinicians and researchers alike rely on a universal diagnostic system to direct their work in the study of headaches.

Rapoport, Alan M., and Fred D. Sheftell. *Headache Relief*. New York: Simon & Schuster, 1991. The book takes the often-complicated theory, evaluation, and treatment of headaches and explains each area in very understandable terms for the lay reader. The authors describe a "how-to" approach to treating headaches.

Raskin, Neil H. *Headache*. 2d ed. New York: Churchill Livingstone, 1988. A review of headaches from a technical perspective. The reader looking for a thorough resource study of headaches will find this text useful. The review of common headache types is comprehensive and reflects the research on headaches in the mid-1980's.

Saper, Joel R., ed. *Headache Disorders: Current Concepts and Treatment Strategies*. Boston: John Wright/PSG, 1983. This text covers a number of areas within the topic of headaches, including the assessment and treatment of the various types. An excellent review of the work on headaches conducted prior to 1983.

# HEARING LOSS

**SYSTEMS AFFECTED:** Auditory, nervous

**SPECIALISTS:** Audiologists, geriatric specialists, neurologists, occupational medicine physicians, otolaryngologists

**DEFINITION:** Loss of sensitivity to sound pressure changes as a result of congenital factors, disease, traumatic injury, noise exposure, or aging.

**KEY TERMS:**

*aging process:* the process in which physiological, neurological, and biological changes affect behavior and function

*auditory:* referring to the ear and to the sense of hearing

*auditory cortex:* that portion of the temporal lobe in the human brain where the ascending auditory pathway terminates *auditory nerve:* the cochlear branch of the eighth cranial nerve

*neural hearing loss:* hearing impairment caused by a loss of the neural tissue that constitutes the ascending pathway of the auditory system

*ossicles:* three small bones located in the middle ear that convey sound pressure changes from the tympanic membrane (eardrum) to the oval window of the cochlea; the bones are commonly referred to as the hammer (malleus), anvil (incus), and stirrup (stapes)

*phonology:* the study of the sounds that make up any verbal language system

*sensory hearing loss:* hearing impairment caused by a loss of sensory cells (nerve cells) in the cochlea

*Physiology of the Ear.* The normal, young ear is capable of detecting frequencies (tones) from as low as 20 hertz to as high as 20,000 hertz. (Hertz is the current notation for cycles per second.) Actually, in terms of frequency, humans can hear as low as 2 hertz, but about 20 hertz is required for a perception of "tonality." This is an amazing range. At the very low end of the frequency scale, one is not certain whether a tone is being "heard" or whether the sensation is a "tactile" one. (There is some neuroanatomical speculation that the organ of hearing is a very specialized tactile sensor.) At the very high end of the frequency scale, one can detect the highest strings of the violin, the rustle of leaves as they are disturbed by the wind, and the distinctive cry of birds and animals. A host of other sounds in between the lowest and highest frequencies can also be perceived. The subjective, psychological correlate of frequency is pitch. In general, the higher the frequency of a sound, the higher is the perceived pitch.

The ear performs an amazing feat in dealing with the broad range of intensities. Intensity is directly proportional to the magnitude of sound pressure change. The ear is so sensitive to small changes in sound pressure that the normal ear is capable of detecting pressure changes no greater than the diameter of a hydrogen molecule. At the other end of this continuum, the human ear can withstand great amplitude changes in sound pressure without damage. In terms of sound pressure units, the range from the weakest sound detected to the loudest sound tolerated represents a ratio of 10,000,000:1. In other words, the most intense sound pressure that is bearable is on the order of 10,000,000 times as great as the softest one that is perceptible under optimum listening conditions.

Intensity is expressed in decibels. Essentially, the higher the decibel value, the more intense or louder the sound. The ear is sensitive to a range of intensities from about 0 decibels to about 135 decibels. At the very extreme of this range, pain is experienced and permanent damage can occur if the sound intensity is prolonged. The psychological cor-

## Anatomy of the Inner Ear

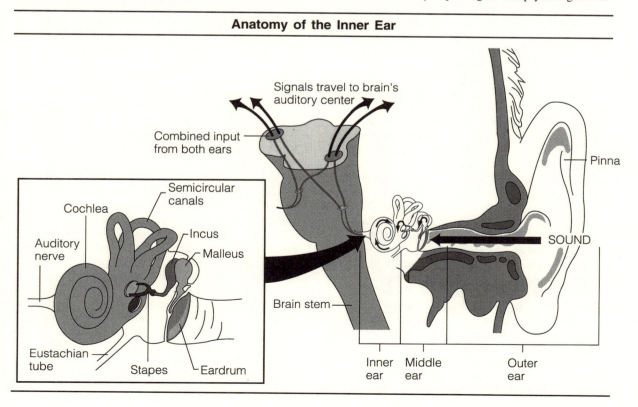

relate of intensity is loudness. Under ideal conditions, if the intensity is increased by 9 decibels, the signal is perceived as being twice as loud.

The ability to process acoustic information correctly depends on the critical relationship between frequency and intensity. The critical frequency range needed to understand the English phonological system extends from about 300 hertz to 4,000 hertz. Theoretically, if one heard no other sounds above 4,000 hertz and below 300 hertz, one would experience no difficulty in understanding the intended message. Relative to intensity, a listener would have no difficulty in information processing if speech were presented at 65 decibels at a distance of one meter. In addition to the listener's distance from the speech source, speech understanding is also influenced by ambient background noise. For adequate processing to occur, speech must be louder than the ambient noise.

Sound is produced by a generating source such as a musical instrument, sounds of nature, or the vibrations of the human vocal cords that create a voice. The resulting series of sound pressure changes represent all the frequency and intensity characteristics generated at the source. These sound pressure changes travel through the atmosphere at a constant speed (approximately 335 meters per second at sea level). They are channeled through the external ear canal and strike the eardrum (tympanic membrane). The eardrum is sensitive to negative and positive changes in sound pressure and moves in concert with these changes. The greater the sound pressure, the greater is the magnitude of movement. Similarly, the higher the frequency, the more rapid are the movements of the eardrum. In the middle ear of the hearing system are three small bones, called ossicles. The first of these, the hammer (malleus), is attached to the eardrum. The second, the anvil (incus), is attached by ligaments to the malleus and to the third ossicle, the stirrup (stapes), which in turn attaches to the oval window membrane of the cochlea. As the eardrum is displaced in a negative or positive direction by sound pressure changes in the external ear canal, there is an absolute and corresponding movement of the ossicles.

In the cochlea, there are three anatomical divisions: the scala vestibuli, the scala tympani, and the scala media. Each of these spaces is filled with a fluid. The fluid of the scala media is chemically different from the fluid in the other two spaces. Housed in the scala media are all the specialized nervous tissues that respond to the movement of the fluid. These specialized nerve cells are situated on top of an anatomical structure called the basilar membrane. The wave forms generated within the fluid are caused by the movement of the stapes bones, as the oval window membrane communicates directly with the fluid of the cochlear space. The rate at which the stapes moves will cause the basilar membrane to be displaced at a site-specific location along its length. High-frequency sounds generate amplitude

changes of the membrane at the apical portion. The movement of the membrane causes the small nerve cells (hair cells) to "fire," creating a neural discharge that travels from the cochlea to the temporal cortex of the brain. The neural events generated by sound pressure changes are interpreted by the brain.

## CAUSES, SYMPTOMS, AND TREATMENTS

In the truest sense, hearing loss is any reduction in threshold sensitivity for any frequency, including those below or above the range for the normal hearing of speech. The real issue, however, is whether minor changes in sensitivity create significant problems in understanding speech and other information-bearing acoustic signals. For example, it is known that loss of threshold sensitivity below 300 hertz and above 4,000 hertz has a minimal affect on understanding speech information. It is when hearing loss exists within this critical frequency range that an individual may experience appreciable difficulty in understanding intended messages. The question becomes, then, "What conditions may cause a permanent or temporary loss of hearing, and how is such a loss managed by medical, surgical, or rehabilitative intervention?"

*Conductive Hearing Loss.* Any barrier or impedance that keeps sound from reaching the cochlea of the human auditory system at its intended loudness is termed "conductive hearing loss." A very common cause of conduction loss is a buildup of earwax (cerumen) in the external ear canal. The production of earwax in the ear canal is essential. It prevents the skin of the ear canal from drying and sloughing off, and it may serve to trap minute foreign particles and keep them from causing damage to the external canal. Normally, earwax will migrate out of the ear and create no conduction problem. It is when the earwax accumulates to an amount sufficient to block sound from entering the ear that something needs to be done. In most cases, earwax can be removed by irrigation. A physician washes out the earwax using a special liquid solution that does not damage the tissue of the ear canal or the eardrum itself.

Another cause of conductive hearing loss is a hole (perforation) in the eardrum, which can be created by a number of conditions, including injury. Depending on the size and location of the hole, surgery (tympanoplasty) is often successful in restoring normal hearing function. For some persons, otosclerosis (a disease causing hardening and fixing of the three small bones in the middle-ear space) results in significant conductive hearing impairment. Otosclerosis prevents these tiny bones from moving efficiently as the eardrum moves, and hearing sensitivity is reduced. Fortunately, advances in surgical procedures have allowed the surgeon to replace the stapes bone with a suitable prosthesis, reinstating relatively normal activity of the ossicles and greatly improving hearing ability.

Congenital malformation of the pinna or the ear canal, known as atresia, is an infrequent cause of conductive hear-

## Causes of Hearing Loss

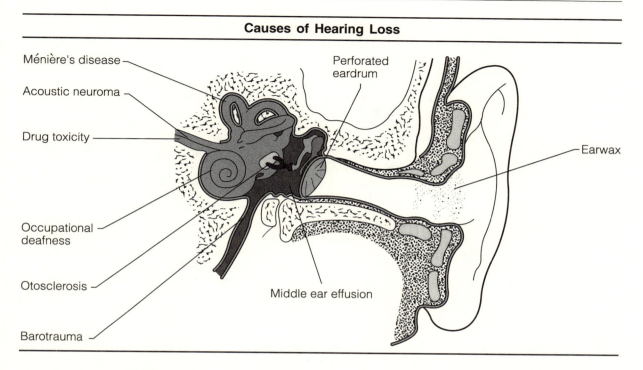

Ménière's disease
Acoustic neuroma
Drug toxicity
Occupational deafness
Otosclerosis
Barotrauma
Perforated eardrum
Earwax
Middle ear effusion

ing loss. Often, when the pinna is malformed, there is no opening into the ear canal. In some cases, the ear canal has failed to develop. Depending on the severity of the malformation, of either the pinna or the ear canal, surgery may be successful in restoring function. Other causes of conductive hearing loss include Eustachian tube malfunction, disruption of the ossicular chain (the three tiny bones in the middle ear), and swelling (edema) of the external ear canal.

A frequently occurring cause of conductive pathology is otitis media. Otitis media may refer to inflammation involving the middle-ear space or to a disorder in which the middle ear is filled with a watery fluid. In some cases, the fluid may harbor bacteria, creating significant medical problems if this condition is not treated early. Such middle-ear effusions are more common in children than in adults. If fluid is present in the middle ear, its mass will restrict the movement of the ossicles and create hearing impairment. Generally, patients with otitis media can be successfully treated through medical or surgical intervention.

It must be noted that conductive pathology does not affect the behavior of inner-ear structures; that is, the inner ear is capable of normal auditory performance. If the conductive pathology is eliminated by appropriate treatment, normal hearing will be restored. Severity of the condition may prevent the restoration of hearing, however, even if an aggressive treatment program is followed.

*Sensorineural Hearing Loss.* As a major classification of hearing loss, this term is somewhat misleading. Actually, there are two types of hearing loss within this classification.

One is a sensory loss which involves the destruction of nerve cells (hair cells) in the cochlea. The other is a neural loss which involves neural cells in the ascending auditory pathway from the cochlea to the brain. It is possible to experience one type of loss without the other. Some examples of sensory loss include the following: loss of nerve cells resulting from traumatic injury to the cochlea, such as from whiplash, sharp blows to the head, or sudden, brief, and intense noises; loss of sensory cells from viral infections such as measles; loss of sensory cells caused by ototoxic drugs such as those in the mycin group (such as streptomycin or kanamycin); congenital problems associated with a lack of embryonic development; and exposure to loud and continuous (long-term) noise, a very common cause of hearing loss in adults. This last type of impairment is different from traumatic injury resulting from sudden, intense noise because it may take months or years for hearing loss caused by long-term noise to manifest itself. Research has also established a clear correlation between the normal aging process and sensory hearing impairment.

When sensory hearing impairment occurs, it is permanent. At the moment, there is no way of regenerating sensory tissue after the cell body has died. The only exception to this rule is found in those patients suffering from Ménière's disease. This disorder is often characterized by vertigo, dizziness, vomiting, and hearing loss. In the initial stages, however, the loss of sensitivity to sound is the result of changes in cellular physiology rather than of necrosis (death) of the nerve cells.

Examples of neural hearing loss are found among those hearing-impaired individuals with tumors, acoustic neuromas (benign tumors), cysts, and other anomalous conditions affecting the transmission of nerve impulses from the cochlea to the brain. Depending on the magnitude of the disorder, neural hearing loss has a much more devastating effect on speech understanding and signal processing than does sensory loss. As with sensory hearing impairment, neural hearing loss is a rather frequent occurrence associated with the aging process. For a sizable portion of those who experience hearing impairment, components of both sensory and neural loss are present. If the cause of the hearing deficit is entirely neural in nature, then the impairment is referred to as a retrocochlear loss.

For some types of neural pathology, medical or surgical intervention can be undertaken successfully. Acoustic neuromas are often removed after they have been confirmed by audiologic, otologic, radiologic, and other diagnostic modalities. The size and location of the neuroma or tumorous growth will often dictate whether hearing can be preserved following surgery.

For those millions suffering from hearing impairment, it is the loss of speech discrimination ability that is of greatest concern. Thousands of studies have been undertaken to investigate the correlation between the magnitude, type, and length of hearing loss and the degree of speech recognition difficulty. One of the essential findings of these studies indicates that, in general, hearing loss is more pronounced for the high frequencies (above 1,000 hertz), whether the loss is caused by disease, drugs, noise, or the aging process. Another major finding is that one's ability to identify vowel and consonant information is frequency-dependent. Vowel identification is dependent on frequencies from about 200 hertz to 1,000 hertz, while consonant identification is dependent on frequencies above 1,000 hertz. A listener understands about 68 percent of speech sounds if nothing above 1,500 hertz is heard and about 68 percent of speech if nothing below 1,500 hertz is heard.

## Perspective and Prospects

Hearing loss is quite common and affects some twenty million Americans, ranging from infants to the elderly. The primary reason for preserving hearing is to maintain social adequacy in communication skills. Hearing conservation programs have been instituted by public and private schools, industry, military installations, construction organizations, and more recently, by the U.S. government. In 1970, the Occupational Safety and Health Act (OSHA) was passed, making it mandatory for employers to provide safe work areas for workers exposed to noise levels exceeding government standards.

For the hearing impaired, understanding of speech is related to the degree of loss and the type of impairment. Because medical or surgical care cannot always ameliorate the loss, rehabilitation programs may take the form of speech or lipreading to improve communication skills. These rehabilitative programs constituted the treatment of choice until the introduction of wearable electric hearing aids.

Before the advent of electric hearing aids, however, the early ear trumpets were very effective for some in restoring speech recognition ability. Through ingenious design, some of the ear trumpets were "acoustically tuned" to provide more amplification in the higher frequencies than in the lower, but the volume of sound was determined by the person talking—often a major problem for the hearing impaired.

With the development of the vacuum tube in the early part of the twentieth century, electric hearing aids became the treatment of choice when medical or surgical intervention was not indicated in resolving the hearing loss. It was possible not only to control the loudness of the hearing aid sound (volume) but also to shape the frequency response of the instrument to match the acoustic needs of the patient. In the second half of the twentieth century, there were significant advances in hearing aid technology. Transistor technology makes it possible to reduce the size of the hearing aid device without sacrificing performance. Computer science has also been used in the design of hearing aids. With digital technology, it is now possible to program electroacoustic characteristics into the hearing aid, which extends its utility.

Recently, major emphasis has been given to hearing conservation. Such continuing efforts have been instrumental in conserving the hearing of tens of thousands who might otherwise suffer from hearing losses sufficient to create problems in speech understanding. Although such programs are too late for millions of hearing-impaired individuals, advances in rehabilitative practices and the scientific application and use of hearing aids have provided them with a quality of life that was not possible only a generation ago.
—*Robert Sandlin*

***See also*** Aging; Ear infections and disorders; Ménière's disease; Nasopharyngeal disorders; Neuralgia, neuritis, and neuropathy.

## For Further Information:

Gerber, Sanford. *Introductory Hearing Science.* Philadelphia: W. B. Saunders, 1974. Somewhat more than a basic text, but one that clearly outlines the various aspects of hearing science, from the measurement of sound and hearing to the use and description of hearing aid devices for the acoustically impaired. Suitable for those readers who have some basic knowledge of how the ear works and the fundamentals of sound, but can be understood by those having little or no previous knowledge of acoustics or the auditory system.

Green, David M. *An Introduction to Hearing.* New York: John Wiley & Sons, 1971. An excellent reference for the serious student seeking a deeper understanding of hearing and auditory mechanisms. Contains an abundance of graphs and charts to aid the interested reader in understanding the concepts presented.

Myklebust, Helmer. *Auditory Disorders in Children*. New York: Grune & Stratton, 1954. A classic work which continues to serve as a standard text for analyzing hearing disorders in children. The incidence of hearing loss is reviewed, as are the probable causes of hearing disorders. Although the book is dated, the content serves as an excellent introduction to the problems found among hearing-impaired children.

Pascoe, David. *Hearing Aids: Who Needs Them?* St. Louis: Big Bend Books, 1991. This easy-to-read text presents an abundance of data relative to hearing, hearing aid devices, and their use. Answers many questions that may arise concerning hearing aid use in direct and simple terms. One of the most significant aspects of this book is that it explains, in reasonable detail, how to use and evaluate hearing aids.

Sanders, Derek. *Aural Rehabilitation*. New York: Prentice-Hall, 1971. An invaluable text by Sanders, who was a recognized authority on aural rehabilitation. Recommended for those wanting useful information on rehabilitation practices for the hearing-impaired child or adult.

Yost, William, and Donald Nielsen. *Fundamentals of Hearing*. New York: Holt, Rinehart & Winston, 1977. This relatively modest text describes, in easy-to-understand terms, the organ of hearing and its contribution to an individual's behavior. Simple auditory theory is examined, as is the nature of the ear's response to acoustic energy.

# HEART ATTACK

**SYSTEM AFFECTED:** Heart

**SPECIALISTS:** Cardiologists, emergency physicians, internists

**DEFINITION:** Myocardial infarction; the sudden death of heart muscle characterized by intense chest pain, sweating, shortness of breath, or sometimes none of these symptoms.

**KEY TERMS:**

*atherosclerosis:* narrowing of the internal passageways of essential arteries caused by the buildup of fatty deposits

*atria:* the chambers in the right and left top portions of the heart that receive blood from the veins and pump it to the ventricles

*fibrillation:* wild beating of the heart, which may occur when the regular rate of the heartbeat is interrupted

*myocardium:* the muscle tissue that forms the walls of the heart, varying in thickness in the upper and lower regions

*sinoatrial node:* the section of the right atrium that determines the appropriate rate of the heartbeat

*ventricles:* the chambers in the right and left bottom portions of the heart that receive blood from the atria and pump it to the arteries

## CAUSES AND SYMPTOMS

Although varied in origin and effect on the body, heart attacks (or myocardial infarctions) occur when there are interruptions in the delicately synchronized system either supplying blood to the heart or pumping blood from the heart to other vital organs. The heart is a highly specialized muscle whose function is to pump life-sustaining blood to all parts of the body. The heart's action involves the development of pressure to propel blood through arriving and departing channels—veins and arteries—that must maintain that pressure within their walls at critical levels throughout the system.

The highest level of pressure in the total cardiovascular system is to be found closest to the two "pumping" chambers on the right and left lower sections of the heart, called ventricles. Dark, bluish-colored blood, emptied of its oxygen content and laden with carbon dioxide waste instead of the oxygen in fresh blood, flows into the upper portion of the heart via the superior and inferior venae cavae. It then passes from the right atrium chamber into the right ventricle. Once in the ventricle, this blood cannot flow back because of one-way valves separating the "receiving" from the "pumping" sections of the total heart organ.

After this valve closes following a vitally synchronized timing system, constriction of the right ventricle by the myocardium muscle in the surrounding walls of the heart forces the blood from the heart, propelling it toward the oxygen-filled tissue of the lungs. Following reoxygenation, bright red blood that is still under pressure from the thrust of the right ventricle flows into the left atrium. Once channeled into the left ventricle, the pumping process that began in the right ventricle is then repeated on the left by muscular constriction, and oxygenated blood flows out of the aortic valve under pressure throughout the cardiovascular system to nourish the body's cells. Because the force needed to supply blood under pressure from the left ventricle for the entire body is greater than the first-phase pumping force needed to move blood into the lungs, the myocardium surrounding the left ventricle constitutes the thickest muscular layer in the heart's wall.

The efficiency of this process, as well as the origins of problems of fatigue in the heart that can lead to heart attacks and eventual heart failure, is tied to the maintenance of a reasonably constant level of blood pressure. If pulmonary problems (blockage caused by the effects of smoking or environmental pollution, for example) make it harder for the right ventricle to push blood through the lungs, the heart must expend more energy in the first stage of the cardiovascular process. Similarly, and often in addition to the added work for the heart because of pulmonary complications, the efficiency of the left ventricle in handling blood flow may be reduced by the presence of excessive fat in the body, causing this ventricle to expend more energy to propel oxygenated blood into vital tissues.

Although factors such as these may be responsible for overworking the heart and thus contributing to eventual heart failure, other causes of heart attacks are to be found much closer to the working apparatus of the heart, particularly in the coronary arteries. The coronary arteries begin at the top of the heart and fan out along its sides. They are responsible for providing large quantities of blood to the myocardium muscle, which needs continual nourishment to carry out the pumping that forces blood forward from the ventricles. The passageways inside these and other key arteries are vulnerable to the process known as atherosclerosis, which can affect the blood supply to other organs as well as to the heart. In the heart, atherosclerosis involves the accumulation, inside the coronary arteries, of fatty deposits called atheromas. If these deposits continue to collect, less blood can flow through the arteries. A narrowed artery also increases the possibility of a variant form of heart attack, in which a sudden and total blockage of blood flow follows the lodging of a blood clot in one of these vital passageways.

A symptomatic condition called angina pectoris, characterized by intermittent chest pains, may develop if atherosclerosis reduces blood (and therefore oxygen) supply to the heart. These danger signs can continue over a number of years. If diagnosis reveals a problem that might be resolved by preventive medication, exercise, or recommendations for heart surgery, then this condition, known as myocardial ischemia, may not necessarily end in a full heart attack.

A full heart attack occurs when, for one of several possible reasons including a vascular spasm suddenly constricting an already clogged artery or a blockage caused by a clot, the heart suddenly ceases to receive the necessary supply of blood. This brings almost immediate deterioration in some of the heart's tissue and causes the organ's consequent inability to perform its vital functions effectively.

Another form of attack and disruption of the heart's ability to deliver blood can come either independently of or in conjunction with an arterially induced heart attack. This form of attack involves a sustained interruption in the rate of heartbeats. The necessary pace or rate of myocardial contractions, which can vary depending on the organism's rate of physical exertion or age, is regulated in the sinoatrial node in the right atrium, which generates its own electrical impulses. The ultimate sources for the command to the sinoatrial node are to be found in the network of nerves coming directly from the brain. There are, however, other so-called local pacemakers located in the atria and ventricles. If these sources of electrical charges begin giving commands to the myocardium that are not in rhythm with those coming from the sinoatrial node, then dysrhythmic or premature beats may confuse the heart muscle, causing it to beat wildly. In fact, the concentrated pattern of muscle contractions will not be coordinated and instead will be dispersed in different areas of the heart. The result is fibrilla-

## Pain Associated with Heart Attack

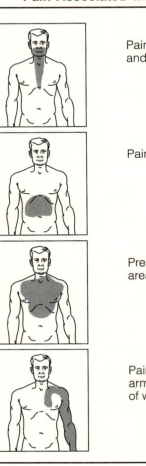

Pain radiating up into jaw and through to back.

Pain felt in upper abdomen.

Pressure in the central chest area from mild to severe.

Pain radiating down left arm; may cause sensation of weakness in the arm.

tion, a series of uncoordinated contractions that cannot combine to propel blood out of the ventricles. This condition may occur either as the aftershock of an arterially induced heart attack or suddenly and on its own, caused by the deterioration of the electrical impulse system commanding the heart rate. In patients whose potential vulnerability to this form of heart attack has been diagnosed in advance, a heart physician may decide to surgically implant a mechanical pacemaker to ensure coordination of the necessary electrical commands to the myocardium.

### TREATMENT AND THERAPY

Extraordinary medical advances have helped reduce the high death rates formerly associated with heart attacks. Many of these advances have been in the field of preventive medicine. The most widely recognized medical findings are related to diet, smoking, and exercise. Although controversy remains, there is general agreement that cholesterol absorbed by the body from the ingestion of animal fats plays a key role in the dangerous buildup of platelets inside arterial passageways. It has been accepted that regular, although not necessarily strenuous, exercise is an essential long-term preventive strategy that can reduce the risk of heart attacks. Exercise also plays a role in therapy after a heart attack. In both preventive and post-attack contexts, it has been medically proven that the entire cardiovascular system profits from the natural muscle-strengthening process (in the heart's case) and general cleansing effects (in the case of oxygen intake and stimulated blood flow) that result from controlled regular exercise.

The actual application of medical scientific knowledge to assist in the campaign against the deadly effects of heart disease involves multiple fields of specialization. These may range from the sophisticated use of electrocardiograms (ECGs) to monitor the regularity of heartbeats, to specialized drug therapies aimed at preventing heart attacks in people who have been diagnosed as high-risk cases, to coronary bypass surgery or even heart transplants. In the 1980's, highly specialized surgeons at several university and private hospitals began performing operations to implant artificial hearts in human patients.

In the case of ECGs, it has become possible, thanks to the use of portable units that record the heartbeat patterns of persons over an extended period of time, to gain a much more accurate impression of the actual functioning of the heart. Previous dependence on electrocardiographic data gathered during an appointed and limited examination provided only minimal information to doctors.

The domains of preventive surgery and specialized drug treatment to prevent dangerous blood clotting are vast. Statistically, the most important and widely practiced operations that were developed in the later decades of the twentieth century were replacement of the aortic valve, the coronary bypass operation, and with greater or lesser degrees of success, the actual transplantation of voluntary donors' hearts in the place of those belonging to heart disease patients. Coronary bypass operations involve the attachment to the myocardium of healthy arteries to carry the blood that can no longer pass through the patient's clogged arterial passageways; these healthy arteries are taken by the heart surgeon from other areas of the patient's own body.

Another sphere of medical technology, that of balloon angioplasty, held out a major nonsurgical promise of preventing deterioration of the arteries leading to the heart. This sophisticated form of treatment involves the careful, temporary introduction of inflatable devices inside clogged arteries, which are then stretched to increase the space within the arterial passageway for blood to flow. By the 1990's, however, doctors recognized one disadvantage of balloon angioplasty. By stretching the essential blood vessels being treated, this procedure either stretches the plaque with the artery or breaks loose debris that remains behind, creating a danger of renewed clogging. Thus another tech-

nique, called atherectomy, was developed to clear certain coronary arteries, as well as arteries elsewhere in the body.

Atherectomy involves a motorized catheter device resembling a miniature drill that is inserted into clogged arteries. As the drill turns, material that is literally shaved off the interior walls of arteries is retrieved through a tiny collection receptacle. Early experimentation, especially to treat the large anterior descending coronary artery on the left side of the heart, showed that atherectomy was 87 percent effective, whereas, on the average, angioplasty removed only 63 percent of the blockage. In addition, similar efforts to provide internal, nonsurgical treatment of clogged arteries using laser beams were being made by the early 1990's.

## PERSPECTIVE AND PROSPECTS

The modern conception of cardiology dates from William Harvey's seventeenth century discovery of the relationship between the heart's function as a pump and the circulatory "restoration" of blood. Harvey's much more scientific views replaced centuries-old conceptions of the heart as a blood-warming device only.

Although substantial anatomical advances were made over the next two centuries that helped explain most of the vital functions of the heart, it was not until the early decades of the twentieth century that science developed therapeutic methods to deal with problems that frequently cause heart attacks. Drugs that affect the liver's production of substances necessary for normal coagulation of blood, for example, were discovered in the 1930's. A large variety of such anticoagulants have since been developed to help thin the blood of patients vulnerable to blood clotting. Other drugs, including certain antibiotics, are used to treat persons whose susceptiblitity to infection is known to be high. In these cases, the simple action of dislodging bacteria from the teeth when brushing can cause an invasion of the vital parts of the heart by an infection. This bacterial endocarditis, the result of the actual destruction of heart tissue or the sudden release of clots of infectious residue, could lead to a heart attack in such individuals although they have no other symptoms of identifiable heart disease.

The most spectacular advance in the scientific treatment of potential heart attack victims, however, has been in the field of cardiac surgery. Many advances in open heart surgery date from the late 1950's, when the development of heart and lung replacement machines made it safe enough to substitute electronic monitors for some of the organism's normal body functions. Before the 1950's, operations had been limited to surgical treatment of the major blood vessels surrounding the heart.

Various technical methods have also been developed that help identify problems early enough for drug therapy to be attempted before the decision to perform surgery is made. The use of catheters, which are threaded into the coronary organ using the same vessels that transport blood, became the most effective way of locating problematic areas. The process known as angiography, which uses X rays to trace the course of radio-opaque dyes injected through a catheter into local heart areas under study, can actually tell doctors if drug therapy is having the desired effects. In cases where such tests show that preventive drug therapy is not effective, an early decision to perform surgery can be made, preventing the source of coronary trouble from multiplying the patient's chances of suffering a heart attack.

—*Byron D. Cannon*

*See also* Angina; Arrhythmias; Atherosclerotic disease; Cholesterol; Embolism; Heart disease; Heart failure; Hyperlipidemia; Hypertension; Ischemia; Mitral insufficiency; Palpitations; Phlebitis; Strokes and TIAs; Thrombosis and thrombus.

### FOR FURTHER INFORMATION:

Amundsen, Louis R., ed. *Cardiac Rehabilitation*. New York: Churchill Livingston, 1981. This text examines the types and levels of exercise that should be performed following a heart attack.

Burch, George E., and Travis Winsor. *A Primer of Electrocardiography*. 5th ed. Philadelphia: Lea & Febiger, 1966. Especially valuable for its discussion regarding technical methods of diagnosing disorders of the heartbeat.

Keen, Harry, John Jarrett, and Arthur M. Levy, eds. *Triumphs of Medicine*. London: Paul Elek, 1976. Several of the chapters in this historical view of medical discoveries are relevant to understanding how modern cardiology developed.

Lynch, James J. *The Broken Heart*. New York: Basic Books, 1977. This book deals mainly with the patient's state of mind after a heart attack. Explores the lives of individuals who know they are living under the shadow of heart disease.

Wallwork, John, and Rob Stepney. *Heart Disease*. Oxford, England: Basil Blackwell, 1987. After a comprehensive survey of what constitutes a healthy heart, the authors offer a discussion of specific cardiac problems, as well as both preventive and post-heart attack treatments.

# HEART DISEASE

**SYSTEMS AFFECTED:** Heart, circulatory

**SPECIALISTS:** Cardiologists, family physicians, internists

**DEFINITION:** One of the leading causes of death in many industrialized nations; heart diseases include atherosclerotic disease, coronary artery disease, cardiac arrhythmias, and stenosis, among others.

### KEY TERMS:

*cardiac arrhythmia:* a disturbance in the heartbeat

*coronary arteries:* blood vessels surrounding the heart that provide nourishment and oxygen to heart tissue

*nodes:* areas of electrochemical transmission within the heart that regulate the heartbeat

*plaque:* an accumulation of matter within artery walls that can impede blood flow

### CAUSES AND SYMPTOMS

The heart is a fist-sized organ located in the upper left quarter of the chest. It consists of four chambers: the right and left atria on top and the right and left ventricles at the bottom. The chambers are enclosed in three layers of tissue: the outer layer (epicardium), the middle layer (myocardium), and the inner layer (endocardium). Surrounding the entire organ is the pericardium, a thin layer of tissue that forms a protective covering for the heart. The heart also contains various nodes that transmit electrochemical signals, causing heart muscle tissue to contract and relax in the pumping action that carries blood to organs and cells throughout the body.

Signals from the brain cause the heart to contract rhythmically in a sequence of motions that move the blood from the right atrium down through the tricuspid valve into the right ventricle. From here, blood is pushed through the pulmonary valve into the lungs, where it fulfills one of its major functions: to pick up oxygen in exchange for carbon dioxide. From the lungs, the blood is pumped back into the heart, entering the left atrium from which it is pumped down through the mitral valve into the left ventricle. Blood is then pushed through the aortic valve into the main artery of the body, the aorta, from which it starts its journey to the organs and cells. As it passes through the arteries of the gastrointestinal system, the blood picks up nutrients which, along with the oxygen that it has taken from the lungs, are brought to the cells and exchanged for waste products and carbon dioxide. The blood then enters the veins, through which it is eventually returned to the heart. The heart nourishes and supplies itself with oxygen through the coronary arteries, so called because they sit on top of the heart like a crown and extend down the sides.

The heart diseases collectively include all the disorders that can befall every part of the heart muscle: the pericardium, epicardium, myocardium, endocardium, atria, ventricles, valves, coronary arteries, and nodes. The most significant sites of heart diseases are the coronary arteries and the nodes; their malfunction can cause coronary artery disease and cardiac arrhythmias, respectively. These two disorders are responsible for the majority of heart disease cases.

Coronary artery disease occurs when matter such as cholesterol and fibrous material collects and stiffens on the inner walls of the coronary arteries. This plaque that forms may narrow the passage through which blood flows, reducing the amount of blood delivered to the heart, or may build up and clog the artery entirely, shutting off the flow of blood to the heart. In the former case, when the coronary artery is narrowed, the condition is called ischemic heart disease. Because the most common cause of ischemia is narrowing of the coronary arteries to the myocardium, another designation of the condition is myocardial ischemia, referring to the fact that blood flow to the myocardium is

## Anatomy of the Heart

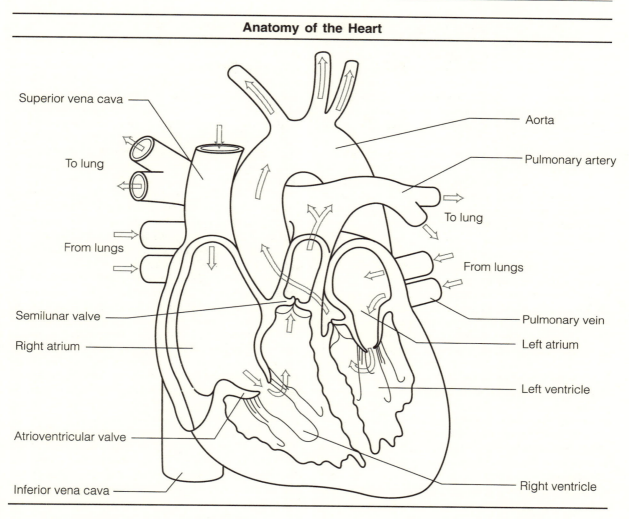

Superior vena cava

To lung

From lungs

Semilunar valve

Right atrium

Atrioventricular valve

Inferior vena cava

Aorta

Pulmonary artery

To lung

From lungs

Pulmonary vein

Left atrium

Left ventricle

Right ventricle

impeded. Accumulation of plaque within the coronary arteries is referred to as coronary atherosclerosis.

As the coronary arteries become clogged and then narrow, they can fail to deliver the required oxygen to the heart muscle, particularly during stress or physical effort. The heart's need for oxygen exceeds the arteries' ability to supply it. The patient usually feels a sharp, choking pain, called angina pectoris. Not all people who have coronary ischemia, however, experience anginal pain; these people are said to have silent ischemia.

The danger in coronary artery disease is that the accumulation of plaque will progress to the point where the coronary artery is clogged completely and no blood is delivered to the part of the heart serviced by that artery. The result is a myocardial infarction (commonly called a heart attack), in which some myocardial cells die when they fail to receive blood. The rough, uneven texture of the plaque instead may cause the formation of a blood clot, or throm-

bus, which closes the artery in a condition called coronary thrombosis.

Although coronary ischemia is usually thought of as a disease of middle and old age, in fact it starts much earlier. Autopsies of accident victims in their teens and twenties, as well as young soldiers killed in battle, show that coronary atherosclerosis is often well advanced in young persons. Some reasons for these findings and for why the rates of coronary artery disease and death began to rise in the twentieth century have been proposed. While antibiotics and vaccines reduced the mortality of some bacterial and some viral infections, Western societies underwent significant changes in lifestyle and eating habits that contributed to the rise of coronary heart disease: high-fat diets, obesity, and the stressful pace of life in a modern industrial society. Further, cigarette smoking, once almost a universal habit, has been shown to be highly pathogenic (disease-causing), contributing significantly to the development of heart disease, as well as lung cancer, emphysema, bronchitis, and other disorders. In the early and middle decades of the twentieth century, coronary heart disease was considered primarily an ailment of middle-aged and older men. As women began smoking, however, the incidence shifted so that coronary artery disease became almost equally prevalent, and equally lethal, among men and women.

Other conditions such as hypertension or diabetes mellitus are considered precursors of coronary artery disease. Hypertension, or high blood pressure, is an extremely common condition that, if unchecked, can contribute to both the development and the progression of coronary artery disease. Over the years, high blood pressure subjects arterial walls to constant stress. In response, the walls thicken and stiffen. This "hardening" of the arteries encourages the accumulation of fatty and fibrous plaque on inner artery walls. In patients with diabetes mellitus, blood-sugar (glucose) levels rise either because the patient is deficient in insulin or because the insulin that the patient produces is inefficient at removing glucose from the blood. High glucose levels favor high fat levels in the blood, which can cause atherosclerosis.

Cardiac arrhythmias are the next major cause of morbidity and mortality among the heart diseases. Inside the heart, an electrochemical network regulates the contractions and relaxations that form the heartbeat. In the excitation or contraction phase, a chain of electrochemical impulses starts in the upper part of the right atrium in the heart's pacemaker, the sinoatrial or sinus node. The impulses travel through internodal tracts (pathways from one node to another) to an area between the atrium and the right ventricle called the atrioventricular node. The impulses then enter the bundle of His, which carries them to the left atrium and left ventricle. After the series of contractions is complete, the heart relaxes for a brief moment before another cycle is begun. On the average, the process is repeated sixty to eighty times a minute.

This is normal rhythm, the regular, healthy heartbeat. Dysfunction at any point along the electrochemical pathway, however, can cause an arrhythmia. Arrhythmias range greatly in their effects and their potential for bodily damage. They can be completely unnoticeable, merely annoying, debilitating, or frightening. They can cause blood clots to form in the heart, and they can cause sudden death.

The arrhythmic heart can beat too fast (tachycardia) or too slowly (bradycardia). The contractions of the various chambers can become unsynchronized, or out of step with one another. For example, in atrial flutter or atrial fibrillation, the upper chambers of the heart beat faster, out of synchronization with the ventricles. In ventricular tachycardia, ventricular contractions increase, out of synchronization with the ventricles. In ventricular tachycardia, ventricular contractions increase, out of synchronization with the upper chambers. In ventricular fibrillation, ventricular contractions lose all rhythmicity and become uncoordinated

to the point at which the heart is no longer able to pump blood. Cardiac death can then occur unless the patient receives immediate treatment.

An arrhythmic disorder called heart block occurs when the impulse from the pacemaker is "blocked." Its progress through the atrioventricular node and the bundle of His may be slow or irregular, or the impulse may fail to reach its target tissues. The disorder is rated in three degrees. First-degree heart block is detectable only on an electrocardiogram (ECG), in which the movement of the impulse from the atria to the ventricles is seen to be slowed. In second-degree heart block, only some of the impulses generated reach from the atria to the ventricles; the pulse becomes irregular. Third-degree heart block is the most serious manifestation of this disorder: No impulses from the atria reach the ventricles. The heart rate may slow dramatically, and the blood flow to the brain can be reduced, causing dizziness or loss of consciousness.

Disorders that affect the heart valves usually involve stenosis (narrowing), which reduces the size of the valve opening; physical malfunction of the valve; or both. These disorders can be attributable to infection (such as rheumatic fever) or to tissue damage, or they can be congenital. If a valve has narrowed, the passage of blood from one heart chamber to another is impeded. In the case of mitral stenosis, the mitral valve between the left atrium and the left ventricle is narrowed. Blood flow to the left ventricle is reduced, and blood is retained in the left atrium, causing the atrium to enlarge as pressure builds in the chamber. This pressure forces blood back into the lungs, creating a condition called pulmonary edema in which fluid collects in the air sacs of the lungs. Similarly, malfunctions of the heart valves that cause them to open and close inefficiently can interfere with the flow of blood into the heart, through it, and out of it. This impairment may cause structural changes in the heart that can be life-threatening.

Heart failure may be a consequence of many disease conditions. It occurs primarily in the elderly. In this condition, the heart becomes inefficient at pumping blood. If the failure is on the right side of the heart, blood is forced back into the body, causing edema in the lower legs. If the failure is on the left side of the heart, blood is forced back into the lungs, causing pulmonary edema. There are many manifestations of heart failure, including shortness of breath, fatigue, and weakness.

Numerous diseases afflict the tissues of the heart wall—the epicardium, myocardium, and endocardium, as well as the pericardium. They are often caused by bacterial or viral infection, but they may also result from tissue trauma or a variety of toxic agents.

### TREATMENT AND THERAPY

The main tools for diagnosing heart disease are the stethoscope, the electrocardiograph (ECG), and the X ray. With the stethoscope the doctor listens to heart sounds, which provides information about many heart functions such as rhythm and the status of the valves. The doctor can determine whether the heart is functioning normally in pumping blood from one chamber into the other, into the lungs, and into the aorta. The ECG gives the doctor a graph representation of heart function. Twelve to fifteen electrodes are placed on various parts of the body, including the head, chest, legs, and arms. The activities of the heart are printed on a strip of paper as waves or tracings. The doctor analyzes the printout for evidence of heart abnormalities, changes in heart function, signs of a heart attack, or other problems. Generally, the electrocardiographic examination is conducted with the patient at rest. In some situations, however, the doctor wishes to view heart action during physical stress. In this case, the electrodes are attached to the patient and the patient is required to exercise on a treadmill or stationary bicycle. The physician can see what changes in heart function occur when the cardiac workload is increased. The X ray gives the doctor a visual picture of the heart. Any enlargements or abnormalities can be seen, as well as the status of the aorta, pulmonary arteries, and other structures.

Another standard diagnostic tool is the echocardiograph. High-frequency sound waves are pointed at the heart from outside the body. The sound waves bounce against heart tissue and are shown on a monitor. The general configuration of the heart can be seen, as well as the shape and thickness of the chamber walls, the valves, and the large blood vessels leading to and from the heart. Velocity and direction of blood flow through the valves can be determined.

Various procedures can help the doctor assess the degree of ischemia within the heart. In one test, a radioactive isotope is injected into a vein and its dispersion in the heart is read by a scanner. This procedure can show which parts of the heart are being deprived of oxygen. In another test using a radioactive isotope, the reading is made while the patient exercises, in order to detect any changes in expansion and contraction of the heart wall that would indicate impaired circulation. The coronary angiogram gives a picture of the blockage within the coronary arteries. A thin tube called a catheter is threaded into a coronary artery and a dye that is opaque to X rays is released. The X-ray picture will reveal narrowings in the artery resulting from plaque buildup.

The main goals of therapy in treating heart diseases are to cure the condition, if possible, and otherwise help the patient live a normal life and prevent the condition from becoming worse. In coronary artery disease, the physician seeks to maintain blood flow to the heart and to prevent heart attack. Hundreds of medications are available for this purpose, including vasodilators (agents that relax blood vessel walls and increase their capacity to carry blood). Chief among the coronary vasodilators are nitroglycerin and other drugs in the nitrate family. Also, calcium channel blockers are often used to dilate blood vessels. Beta-blocking agents are used because they reduce the heart's need for oxygen and alleviate the symptoms of angina. In addition, various support measures are recommended by physicians to stop plaque buildup and halt the progress of the disease. These include losing weight, reducing fats in the diet, and stopping smoking. The physician also treats concomitant illnesses that can contribute to the progress of coronary artery disease, such as hypertension and diabetes.

Sometimes medications and diet are not fully successful, and the ischemia continues. In a relatively new procedure, the cardiologist can unblock a clogged artery by a procedure called angioplasty. The physician threads a catheter containing a tiny balloon to the point of the blockage. The balloon is inflated to widen the inner diameter of the artery, and blood flow is increased. This procedure is often successful, although it may have to be repeated. When it is not successful, coronary bypass surgery may be indicated. In this procedure, clogged coronary arteries are replaced with healthy blood vessels from other parts of the body.

When coronary artery disease progresses to a heart attack, the patient should be treated in the hospital or similar facility. The possibility of sudden death is high during the attack and remains high until the patient is stabilized. Emergency measures are undertaken to minimize the extent of heart damage, reduce heart work, keep oxygen flowing to all parts of the body, and regulate blood pressure and heartbeat.

Cardiac arrhythmias can be managed by a variety of medications and procedures. Digitalis, guanidine, procainamide, tocanamide, and atropine are widely used to restore normal heart rhythm. In acute situations, the patient's heart rhythm can be restored by electrical cardioversion, in which an electrical stimulus is applied from outside the body to regulate the heartbeat. When a slowed heartbeat cannot be controlled by medication, a pacemaker may be implanted to regulate heart rhythm.

Treatment of heart valve disorders and disorders of the heart wall is directed at alleviating the individual condition. Antibiotics and/or valve replacement surgery may be required. In many cases, valve disorders can be completely corrected. Cardiac transplantation remains a possible treatment for some heart patients. This is an option for comparatively few patients because there are ten times as many candidates for heart transplants as there are available donor hearts.

### PERSPECTIVE AND PROSPECTS

Heart disease became a major killer in the United States in the twentieth century. In the early decades, the best that the medical community could do was to treat symptoms. Since then, the emphasis has shifted to prevention. Hundreds of investigative studies have been undertaken to determine the causes of the most prevalent heart dysfunction, coronary artery disease. Many of these studies have involved tens of thousands of subjects, and they point to a general consensus that coronary artery disease is a multifactorial disorder, the primary elements of which are cholesterol and other fatty substances circulating in the bloodstream, smoking, diabetes, high blood pressure, stress, and obesity.

The reasons that mortality from heart disease is declining include improved medications and treatment modalities, and much credit has to be given to the success of preventive measures. Millions of Americans have stopped smoking and have begun watching their diets. Entire industries are devoted to helping Americans eat more intelligently. While fast-food outlets continued to offer high-fat standards, such as hotdogs and hamburgers, they have also added salads and leaner selections.

Perhaps most important, medical and sociological authorities have turned their attention to children. Because advanced atherosclerosis has been detected in young men and women, cholesterol-watching has become a major preoccupation with parents and school dieticians. In addition, national programs have been instituted to discourage smoking among the young. Whether the rates of coronary heart disease will be lower in these individuals than in their parents remains to be seen, but the success of these measures in the older populations indicates that the prognosis is good.

The prognosis is also good for other heart diseases. New drugs continue to be licensed for the treatment of arrhythmias, and more versatile and reliable pacemakers increase the prospects of a normal life for many patients. Improvements in heart surgery have been particularly impressive, especially those for managing congenital heart defects in neonates and infants. Heart transplants have been successfully performed on these patients, and numerous other procedures promise significant improvement in the prospects of young people with heart disease.

Rheumatic fever, however, one of the major causes of heart disease in children, remains a threat. No vaccine is available for immunization against the streptococcus strains that cause rheumatic fever, but fortunately there are effective antibiotics to control infection in these patients. Rheumatic fever usually develops subsequent to a throat infection. Careful monitoring of the child with a sore throat can avoid progression of the infection to rheumatic fever.

—*C. Richard Falcon*

**See also** Aneurysms; Angina; Arrhythmias; Atherosclerotic disease; Cholesterol; Claudication; Congenital heart disease; Diabetes mellitus; Eclampsia; Embolism; Endocarditis; Heart attack; Heart failure; Hyperlipidemia; Hypertension; Ischemia; Mitral insufficiency; Obesity; Palpitations; Phlebitis; Strokes and TIAs; Thrombosis and thrombus; Varicosis; Venous insufficiency.

**FOR FURTHER INFORMATION:**

Cohen, Lawrence S., Marvin Moser, and Barry L. Zaret, eds. *Yale University School of Medicine Heart Book*. New York: Hearst Books, 1992. This text will give the reader a clear understanding of the various heart diseases, as well as current methods of treating and preventing them.

Dranov, Paula. *Heart Disease*. New York: Random House, 1990. Devoted to helping the reader become knowledgeable about heart disease and how it is being treated.

Editors of the University of California, Berkeley, Wellness Letter. *The Wellness Encyclopedia*. Boston: Houghton Mifflin, 1991. A good general medical text with exemplary coverage of the heart diseases, preventive measures, and current therapeutic modalities.

Kowalski, Robert E. *Eight Steps to a Healthy Heart*. New York: Warner Books, 1992. In addition to outlining how to avoid heart disease, this book advises patients with heart disease about how to get the most benefit from their therapy.

Larson, David G., ed. *Mayo Clinic Family Health Book*. New York: William Morrow, 1990. This large reference work was written for the lay reader. The sections on the heart diseases are exemplary for clarity and thoroughness.

# HEART FAILURE

**SYSTEM AFFECTED:** Heart

**SPECIALISTS:** Cardiologists, internists, vascular surgeons

**DEFINITION:** A condition in which the heart cannot pump enough blood to meet the needs of the body because its ability to contract is impaired.

**KEY TERMS:**

*congestive heart failure:* the stage of heart failure that occurs when a backup of pressure results in accumulation of fluid in the veins and tissues

*coronary arteries:* the arteries that supply blood to the heart muscle

*diuretic:* a drug that stimulates the kidneys to eliminate more salt and water from the body

*edema:* the accumulation of fluid around the cells in tissue

*ejection fraction:* the ratio of the stroke volume to the residual volume, expressed as a percentage

*hormone:* a chemical messenger released by a gland which is carried by the blood to its target

*inotropic agent:* a drug that improves the ability of the heart muscle to contract

*optimal length:* the length of a heart muscle cell at which stimulation can elicit the maximum possible force development

*residual volume:* the blood volume left in the heart chamber at the end of a heartbeat

*stroke volume:* the blood volume leaving either the right or the left side of the heart with each beat; each side usually ejects the same volume per beat

*vasodilator:* a drug that relaxes blood vessels

## CAUSES AND SYMPTOMS

The circulation of the blood has many functions. It is essential for the delivery of oxygen, nutrients, and elements of the immune system to tissues. It also contributes to regulation and communication between different parts of the body by moving chemical messengers from where they are produced to where they have a biological effect. The delivery of warm blood to the surface of the skin is one essential element in temperature control. The blood pressure determines how much water can move across the exchange surfaces in the kidneys, thus effecting water balance in the body. The movement of blood through the kidneys, the lungs, and all tissues is important for waste removal.

All these functions depend on the ability of the heart to contract and eject blood. Blood is pumped, in two serial circuits, from the right heart through the lungs into the left heart and from the left heart around the body back to the right heart. In each circuit, the blood travels through large arteries, then to smaller arterioles, to capillaries (where exchange takes place), and back via small venules and veins to the heart. Heart failure describes the situation in which heart function is reduced. While still able to beat, the heart is unable to meet the circulatory needs of the body. That is, the heart muscle is unable to contract enough to pump the blood adequately.

The severity of the heart failure can be gauged by the ejection fraction, a measure of the pumping capacity of the heart. It is the percentage calculated from the stroke volume (the volume of blood leaving a heart chamber with each beat) divided by the residual volume (the volume left in the heart chamber at the end of a heartbeat). Thus the ejection fraction measures how much blood in the heart chamber can actually leave when the heartbeat occurs. In normal, healthy hearts, this value is 100 percent: The amount that stays in the heart is approximately equal to the amount that leaves it. In mild or moderate heart failure, it ranges approximately between 15 and 40 percent: Less blood leaves the heart with each beat, and more blood remains behind.

The pressure inside the heart at the end of a heartbeat is another index of heart performance. If the heart is failing and more blood is left behind in the heart at the end of a beat, the pressure inside the heart at the end of the beat will be increased. In cases of severe failure, the pressure in the arteries outside the heart will fall.

In failure, the heart cannot supply enough blood for all the functions of the circulation. This fact accounts for the variety of symptoms that accompany heart failure: labored breathing; light-headedness; generalized weakness; cold, pale, or even bluish skin tone; and accumulation of fluid in the extremities and/or lungs. Possible other symptoms include distended neck veins, accumulation of fluid in the abdomen, abnormal heart rate and rhythm, and chest pain.

The specific symptoms of the condition depend on the type of failure, its severity, its underlying causes, and the ways in which the body attempts to compensate. There are several ways to categorize types of heart failure: acute or chronic, forward or backward, and right-sided or left-sided.

Acute heart failure refers to a sudden decrease in heart function. It can be caused by toxic quantities of drugs, anesthetics, or metals or by certain disease states, such as infections. Most often, however, it is caused by a sudden blockage of the coronary arteries supplying the heart muscle. A sudden blockage caused by a blood clot can induce a heart attack and subsequent heart failure, causing chest pain and often abnormal heart rate or rhythm. These effects are sometimes so rapid that there is little time for the body to attempt compensation.

Chronic heart failure is a progressive reduction in heart function that develops over time. It can be caused by inherited or acquired diseases, allergic reactions, connective tissue or metabolic abnormalities, high blood pressure, and anatomical defects. The most common cause, however, is coronary artery disease. This disease narrows blood vessels and leads to a reduction in the amount of blood reaching the heart muscle. It causes reduced oxygen availability and, eventually, a reduction in the ability of the heart muscle to contract.

In the early stages of chronic failure, the hormone and nervous systems promote compensation in the heart, blood vessels, and kidneys to help the heart continue to pump enough blood. These systems stimulate the heart muscle directly to make it beat harder. They also take advantage of the fact that modest stretching of the heart muscle increases its ability to contract. By stimulating the blood vessels to contract, more blood moves back toward the heart, causing a cold, pale, or even bluish skin tone. Stimulation of the kidney to retain water and sodium results in an increase in blood volume, which also moves more blood back to the heart. In each case, the heart muscle is stretched by these increases and, therefore, can contract harder.

Yet these reactions do not constitute a long-term solution. The heart muscle can become fatigued from overwork and can become overstretched. A resulting accumulation of fluid in the heart reduces its ability to contract. Compensation fails, and the additional fluid in the blood starts to back up in the circulation. This condition is called backward heart failure. At the same time, the heart is unable to pump hard enough to move the blood forward against the higher resistance caused by the contraction of the blood vessels. This condition is termed forward heart failure. Congestive heart failure is the stage that occurs when the backup of pressure is worsened by fluid retention and blood vessel contraction. The congestion, or accumulation of fluid, occurs in the veins and tissues.

Left-sided or right-sided heart failure can occur alone or together. The right side of the heart pumps blood to the lungs to be oxygenated, and the left side of the heart pumps oxygenated blood to the organs of the body. Normally, these two sides are well matched so that the same volume moves through each side. When the right heart cannot contract properly, however, blood accumulates upstream in the veins and somewhat less blood reaches the lungs to pick up oxygen, resulting in distended veins and shortness of breath. It is primarily a backward heart failure. Fluid can back up in the veins and increase pressure in the capillaries so that it starts to leak out of the circulation into the surrounding tissues. This leads to an accumulation of fluid (called edema), especially in the liver and lower extremities. In isolated right-sided heart failure, this pressure rarely backs up to such an extent that it causes problems through the rest of the circulation to the left side of the heart.

In contrast, when the left side of the heart cannot contract properly, it can back up pressure so badly that it creates a pressure overload against which the right side of the heart must pump. This increase in the workload on the right side of the heart frequently leads to two-sided heart failure. This outcome is especially common since the disease conditions that exist in the left side are likely to exist on the right as well. In left-sided heart failure, blood accumulates upstream in the lungs, increasing pressure enough to cause a leakage of fluid into the lungs (pulmonary edema). This leakage interferes with oxygen uptake and therefore causes shortness of breath. It also results in inadequate blood flow to the body's tissues, including the muscles and brain, resulting in generalized weakness and light-headedness. Left-sided heart failure is thus both a backward and a forward failure.

### TREATMENT AND THERAPY

Treatments for cardiac failure, like its symptoms, depend on a variety of factors. The first goal of treatment is to avoid any obvious precipitating causes of the failure, such as alcohol, drugs, the cessation of necessary essential medications, acute stress, a salt-loaded diet, overexercise, infection, illness, or surgery. The next approach is to take the simplest measures to reduce distension of the heart by controlling salt and water retention and to decrease the workload of the heart by altering the circulatory needs of the tissues. The former can be achieved by dietary salt restriction, restriction of fluid consumption, or mechanical removal of fluid accumulating around the lungs or abdomen. The latter can be accomplished with bed rest and weight loss.

Typically, drug therapy is also required in order to treat heart failure. No single agent meets all the requirements for optimal treatment, which includes rapid relief of labored breathing and edema, enhanced heart performance, reduced mortality, reduced progression of the underlying disease, safety, and minimal side effects. Therefore, drugs are used in combination to achieve control over sodium and water retention, improve heart contraction, reduce heart work, and protect against blood clots.

The purpose of therapy with diuretic drugs (drugs that increase salt and water loss through the kidneys) is three-fold: to reduce the pooling of fluid that can take place in the lungs, abdomen, and lower extremities; to minimize the buildup of back pressure from the accumulation of blood in the veins; and to reduce the circulating blood volume. All these things will lessen the overstretch of the heart mus-

cle and bring it to a level of stretch that is closer to its optimum. Care must be taken, however, not to reduce severely the water content of the blood, which could reduce the stretch on the heart muscle to below the optimum and consequently impair heart contraction. One way to monitor how much water is lost or retained is for patients to empty their bladders and then weigh themselves each day before breakfast. If weight changes steadily or suddenly, then sodium and water loss may be too great or too little. In either case, an adjustment is in order. Some generic diuretic drugs used to treat heart failure include furosemide, ethacrynic acid, the thiazides, and spironolactone.

The purpose of therapy with inotropic drugs (drugs that increase the contractile ability of heart muscle) is to improve the pumping action of the heart. This effect causes an increase in stroke volume (more blood moves out of the heart per beat) and helps compensate for forward failure. The increased output also reduces the backup of blood returning to the heart and thus also compensates for backward failure.

Digitalis, a derivative of the foxglove plant which originated as a Welsh folk remedy, is still the most frequently used inotropic drug for the treatment of chronic heart failure. Because it improves heart muscle contraction, it reverses to some extent all the symptoms of heart failure. Digitalis exerts its effects by increasing the accumulation of calcium inside the heart muscle cells. Calcium interacts with the structure of the shortening apparatus inside the cell to make more contractile interactions within the cell possible. Its disadvantages are that it becomes toxic in high doses and that it can severely damage performance of an already healthy heart.

Other inotropic agents also act to improve contraction by increasing calcium levels within the heart muscle cells. Some of them mimic the naturally produced hormones and neurotransmitters that are released and depleted in early stages of heart failure. These are called the sympathomimetic drugs. They include drugs such as dopamine, terbutaline, and levodopa. While these drugs improve heart performance, they can have serious side effects: increased heart rate, palpitations, and nervousness. One group of inotropic agents improves cardiac contraction while relaxing blood vessels. These drugs, called phosphodiesterase inhibitors, stop the breakdown of an essential cellular messenger molecule which helps to manage calcium levels and other events inside both heart cells and blood vessel cells. Examples of these drugs include amrinone and milrinone. Their use is not common because they can cause stomach upset and fatigue and because they are not clearly superior to other treatments.

The purpose of therapy with vasodilator drugs (drugs that relax the blood vessels) is to decrease the work of the heart. The resulting expansion of the blood vessels makes it easier for blood to be pumped through them. It also leaves room for pooling some of the blood in the veins, decreasing the amount of blood returning to the heart and so reducing overstretching as well. Some of the vasodilators, such as hydralazine, pinacidil, dipyridamole, and the nitrates, act directly on the blood vessels. Other vasodilators, such as angiotensin-converting enzyme (ACE) inhibitors and adrenergic inhibitors, inhibit the release of naturally produced substances that would make the blood vessels contract. Sometimes it is hard to predict the effects of vasodilators because they may act differently in different blood vessels and the body may attempt to offset the effects of the drug by releasing substances that contract blood vessels. Vasodilator drug therapy is usually added to other treatments when the symptoms of heart failure persist after digitalis and diuretic therapy are used.

The purpose of therapy with antithrombotics (blood clot inhibitors) is to prevent any further obstruction of the circulation with blood clots. Because heart failure changes the mechanics of blood flow and is the result of damaged heart muscle, it can increase the formation of blood clots. When blood clots form an obstruction in the large blood vessels of the lungs, it is often fatal. Clots can also lodge in the heart to cause further damage to heart muscle or in the brain, where they could cause a stroke. Both the short-acting clot inhibitor heparin and oral agents such as aspirin are used to prevent these effects.

The combination of all these drug therapies, while unable to reverse the permanent damage of heart failure, makes it possible to treat the condition. Individuals treated for heart failure can lead comfortable, productive lives.

If the heart failure progresses to acutely life-threatening proportions and the patient is in all other ways healthy, the next alternative is surgical replacement of the heart. Artificial hearts are sometimes used as a transition to heart transplant while a donor is sought. Yet transplantation is not a perfect solution. Transplanted hearts do not have the nervous system input of a normal heart and so their control from moment to moment is different. They are also subject to rejection. Nevertheless, they provide an enormous improvement in quality of life for severe heart failure patients.

## PERSPECTIVE AND PROSPECTS

The vital significance of the pulse and heartbeat have been part of human knowledge since long before recorded history. Pulse taking and herbal treatments for poor heartbeat have been recorded in ancient Chinese, Egyptian, and Greek histories. Digitalis has been used in treatment for at least two hundred years. It was first formally introduced to the medical community in 1785 by the English botanist and physician William Withering. He learned of it from a woman folk healer named Hutton who used it with other extracts to treat more than one kind of swelling. Withering identified the foxglove plant as the source of its active ingredient and characterized it as having effects on the pulse as well as on fluid retention. The plant is indigenous to both the United Kingdom and Europe and may well have been employed as a folk remedy for far longer. It is still the most widely used agent for the treatment of heart failure.

The developments in physiology and medicine during the nineteenth century set the stage for greater understanding and further treatments of heart failure. It was then that the stethoscope and blood pressure cuff were created for diagnostic purposes. In basic science, cell theory, hormone theory, and kidney physiology led to a better understanding of how heart muscle contraction and fluid balance might be coordinated in the body. The concepts and techniques required to keep organs and tissues alive outside the body with an artificial circulation system were conceived and introduced. Anesthesia and sterile techniques essential for cardiac surgery were developed.

These ideas and accomplishments contributed to important discoveries in the early twentieth century that greatly enhanced the understanding of the early compensatory responses to heart failure. For example, it was found that when heart muscle is stretched, it will contract with greater force on the next beat and that heart muscle usually operates at a muscle length that is less than optimal. Thus, when the amount of blood returning to the heart increases and stretches the muscle in the walls of the heart, the heart will contract with greater force, ejecting a greater volume of blood. This phenomenon, called the Frank-Starling mechanism, was first demonstrated in isolated heart muscle by the German physiologist Otto Frank and in functional hearts by the British physiologist Ernest Henry Starling in 1914.

Subsequent developments in the second half of the twentieth century, such as more specific vasodilator and diuretic drugs as well as the heart-lung machine, have led to the options of more complete drug therapy, artificial hearts (first introduced to replace a human heart by William DeVries in 1982), and heart transplant (first performed by Christiaan Barnard in 1967) as options for the treatment of heart failure. —*Laura Gray Malloy*

*See also* Arrhythmias; Atherosclerotic disease; Cholesterol; Congenital heart disease; Edema; Endocarditis; Heart attack; Heart disease; Hyperlipidemia; Hypertension; Ischemia; Mitral insufficiency; Obesity; Palpitations; Strokes and TIAs.

## FOR FURTHER INFORMATION:

Campbell, Neil A. *Biology.* 2d ed. Redwood City, Calif.: Benjamin/Cummings, 1990. An accessible general textbook with an excellent treatment of cardiovascular function and disease in chapter 38. Contains outstanding illustrations and a glossary. A college-level text that is suitable for the high school student as well.

Cohn, Peter F., and Joan K. Cohn. *Heart Talk: Preventing and Coping with Silent and Painful Heart Disease.* Boston: Harcourt Brace Jovanovich, 1987. This review of heart disease emphasizes one cause of heart failure, coronary artery disease. Does an excellent job of reviewing in lay person's terms what is known about both symptomatic (painful) and nonsymptomatic (silent) heart disease. Includes descriptions of individual experiences and chapters about treatment of and living with heart failure. Provides a glossary and guidelines about exercise and diet. A readable general account that is an excellent resource for high school students.

Davis, Goode P., Jr., Edwards Park, and the editors of U.S. News Books. *The Heart: The Living Pump*. Washington, D.C.: U.S. News Books, 1981. A beautifully illustrated and photographed volume for the general public, this book provides the best summary of all aspects of cardiac function. Historical, experimental, and clinical aspects of the heart's function are presented simply and accurately. The treatment and prevention of cardiovascular disease are given ample consideration, as are experimental and clinical techniques. Includes a glossary. Excellent for high school or college students.

Dox, Ida G., B. John Melloni, and Gilbert M. Eisner. *The HarperCollins Illustrated Medical Dictionary*. New York: HarperCollins, 1993. A home medical dictionary with more than 26,000 medical terms and 2,500 illustrations, including all those of most concern to cardiovascular patients. Defines relevant anatomical structures, functional terminology, and some widely used chemical compounds and drugs under generic names. An excellent resource for high school or college students.

Fishman, Alfred P., and Dickinson W. Richards, eds. *Circulation of the Blood: Men and Ideas*. 1964. Reprint. Baltimore: Williams & Wilkins, 1982. A historical account of cardiovascular physiology. Excellent reading for students in high school and college.

Sherwood, Lauralee. *Human Physiology: From Cells to Systems*. St. Paul, Minn.: West, 1989. A basic physiology textbook oriented toward an understanding of human function and disease. Superbly well written and offers excellent illustrations. Chapters 9 through 11 address cardiovascular function, with specific reference to heart failure and the cardiovascular abnormalities that precipitate it. The coverage includes a specific examination of how cardiovascular function is affected by exercise.

## HEARTBURN

**SYSTEM AFFECTED:** Gastrointestinal

**SPECIALISTS:** Family physicians, gastroenterologists, internists

**DEFINITION:** Also known as acid indigestion, heartburn is characterized by a burning sensation in the middle of the chest that may radiate upward to the throat; the term "heartburn" derives from its similarities to the pain of heart disease. It is caused by a reflux of stomach acids into the esophagus shortly after eating. Overeating, drinking alcohol, and consuming spicy or rich foods may precipitate an attack, as can lying down following a meal. Contributing factors include obesity, pregnancy, stress,

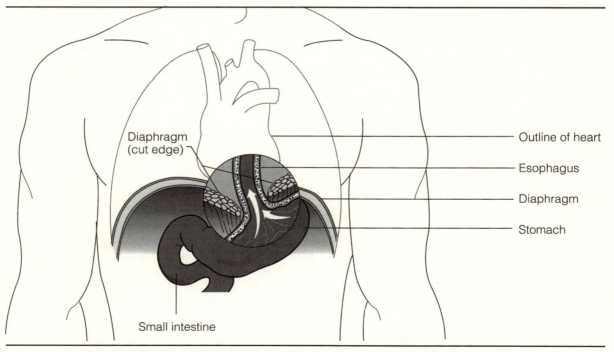

Diaphragm (cut edge)

Small intestine

Outline of heart

Esophagus

Diaphragm

Stomach

*Heartburn is caused by a reflux of stomach acid into the esophagus shortly after eating.*

emotional upset, the excessive swallowing of air, intestinal gas, congenital defects, and hiatal hernia. Antacids may be used to treat heartburn, and factors that trigger it should be avoided.

*See also* Abdominal disorders; Gastrointestinal disorders; Hernia; Indigestion; Obesity; Stress.

## HEAT EXHAUSTION AND HEAT STROKE

SYSTEMS AFFECTED: Skin, circulatory

SPECIALISTS: Emergency physicians, environmental medicine physicians, family physicians, internists, sports medicine physicians

DEFINITION: Heat-related illnesses in which the body temperature rises to dangerous levels and cannot be controlled through normal mechanisms, such as sweating.

### CAUSES AND SYMPTOMS

The human body is well equipped to maintain a nearly constant internal body temperature. In fact, the body temperature of human beings is usually controlled so closely that it rarely leaves a very narrow range of 36.1 to 37.8 degrees Celsius (97 to 100 degrees Fahrenheit) regardless of how much heat the body is producing or what the environmental temperature may be. Humans maintain a constant temperature so that the millions of biochemical reactions in the body remain at an optimal rate. An increase in body temperature of only 1 degree Celsius will cause these reactions to move about 10 percent faster. As internal temperatures rise, however, brain function becomes slower because important proteins and enzymes lose their ability to operate effectively. Most adults will go into convulsions when their temperature reaches 41 degrees Celsius (106 degrees Fahrenheit), and 43 degrees Celsius (110 degrees Fahrenheit) is usually fatal.

A special region of the brain known as the hypothalamus regulates body temperature. The hypothalamus detects the temperature of the blood much like a thermostat detects room temperature. When the body (and hence the blood) becomes too warm, the hypothalamus activates heat-loss mechanisms. Most excess heat is lost through the skin by the radiation of heat and the evaporation of sweat. To promote this heat loss, blood vessels in the skin dilate (open up) to carry more blood to the skin. Heat from the warm blood is then lost to the cooler air. If the increase in blood flow to the skin is not enough, then sweat glands are stimulated to produce and secrete large amounts of sweat. The process, called perspiration, is an efficient means of ridding the body of excess heat as long as the humidity is not too high. In fact, at 60 percent humidity, evaporation of sweat from the skin stops. When the body cannot dissipate enough heat, heat exhaustion and heat stroke may occur.

Heat exhaustion is the most prevalent heat-related illness. It commonly occurs in individuals who have exercised or worked in high temperatures for long periods of time. These people have usually not ingested adequate amounts of fluid.

Over time, the patient loses fluid through sweating and respiration, which decreases the amount of fluid in the blood. Because the body is trying to reduce its temperature, blood has been shunted to the skin and away from vital internal organs. This reaction, in combination with a reduced blood volume, causes the patient to go into a mild shock. Common signs and symptoms of heat exhaustion include cool, moist skin that may appear either red or pale; headache; nausea; dizziness; and exhaustion. If heat exhaustion is not recognized and treated, it can lead to life-threatening heat stroke.

Heat stroke occurs when the body is unable to eradicate the excess heat as rapidly as it develops. Thus, body temperature begins to rise. Sweating stops because the water content of the blood decreases. The loss of evaporative cooling causes the body temperature to rise rapidly, soon reaching a level that can cause organ damage. In particular, the brain, heart, and kidneys may begin to fail until the patient experiences convulsions, coma, and even death. Therefore, heat stroke is a serious medical emergency which must be recognized and treated immediately. The signs and symptoms of heat stroke include high body temperature (41 degrees Celsius or 106 degrees Fahrenheit); loss of consciousness; hot, dry skin; rapid pulse; and quick, shallow breathing.

### TREATMENT AND THERAPY

As with most illnesses, prevention is the best medicine for heat exhaustion and heat stroke. When exercising in hot weather, people should wear loose-fitting, lightweight clothing and drink plenty of fluids. When individuals are not prepared to avoid heat-related illness, however, rapid treatment may save their lives. When emergency medical personnel detect signs and symptoms of sudden heat-induced illness, they attempt to do three major things: cool the body, replace body fluids, and minimize shock.

For heat exhaustion, the initial treatment should be to place the patient in a cool place, such as a bathtub filled with cool (not cold) water. The conscious patient is given water or fruit drinks, sometimes containing salt, to replace body fluids. Occasionally, intravenous fluids must be given to return blood volume to normal in a more direct way. Hospitalization of the patient may be necessary to be sure that the body is able to regulate body heat appropriately. Almost all patients treated quickly and effectively will not advance to heat stroke. The activity that placed the patient in danger should be discontinued until one is sure all symptoms have disappeared and steps have been taken to prevent a future episode of heat exhaustion.

Heat stroke requires urgent medical attention, or the high body temperature will cause irreparable damage and often death. Reduction of body temperature must be done rapidly. With the patient in a cool environment, the clothing is removed and the skin sprinkled with water and cooled by fanning. Contrary to popular belief, rubbing alcohol should not be used, as it can cause closure of the skin's pores. Ice packs are often placed behind the neck and under the armpits and groin. At these sites, large blood vessels come close to the skin and are capable of carrying cool blood to the internal organs. Body fluid must be replaced quickly by intravenous administration because the patient is usually unable to drink as a result of convulsions or confusion and may even be unconscious. Once the body temperature has been brought back to normal, the patient is usually hospitalized and watched for complications. With early diagnosis and treatment, 80 to 90 percent of previously healthy people will survive. —*Matthew Berria*

*See also* Fever; Hyperthermia and hypothermia; Shock; Unconsciousness.

### FOR FURTHER INFORMATION:

*American Red Cross First Aid: Responding to Emergencies.* St. Louis: Mosby Year Book, 1991.

Clayman, Charles B., ed. *The American Medical Association Encyclopedia of Medicine.* New York: Random House, 1989.

Hales, Dianne. *An Invitation to Health.* 4th ed. Redwood City, Calif.: Benjamin/Cummings, 1989.

Marieb, Elaine N. *Human Anatomy and Physiology.* 2d ed. Redwood City, Calif.: Benjamin/Cummings, 1992.

## HEMIPLEGIA

**SYSTEMS AFFECTED:** Muscular, nervous

**SPECIALISTS:** Neurologists, physical therapists

**DEFINITION:** Hemiplegia is paralysis or weakness on one side of the body; it may affect the arm, leg, trunk, or face, or a combination of these. Spastic hemiplegia is characterized by stiff muscles, while flaccid hemiplegia is characterized by wasted, limp muscles. Unlike paraplegia (paralysis from the waist downward) or quadriplegia (paralysis from the neck downward), hemiplegia is attributable to brain injuries and diseases, rather than to spinal cord damage. Hemiplegia can result from a stroke, encephalitis, multiple sclerosis, meningitis, and hemorrhages or tumors in the brain. Physical therapy is used to aid in mobility, and treatment consists of addressing the underlying cause.

*See also* Brain disorders; Cerebral palsy; Encephalitis; Meningitis; Multiple sclerosis; Palsy; Paralysis; Paraplegia; Quadriplegia.

## HEMOPHILIA

**SYSTEM AFFECTED:** Blood

**SPECIALISTS:** Geneticists, hematologists

**DEFINITION:** A genetic disorder characterized by the blood's inability to form clots as a result of the lack or alteration of certain trace plasm proteins.

**KEY TERMS:**

*clotting factors:* substances present in plasma that are needed for the coagulation of blood

*hemophilia A:* a genetic blood disease characterized by a deficiency of clotting factor VIII

*hemophilia B:* a genetic blood disease characterized by a deficiency of clotting factor IX

*hemostasis:* the process of stopping the flow of blood at an injury site

*von Willebrand's disease:* a genetic blood disease characterized by a deficiency of the von Willebrand clotting factor

### CAUSES AND SYMPTOMS

The circulatory system must be self-healing; otherwise, continued blood loss from even the smallest injury would be life-threatening. Normally, all except the most catastrophic bleeding is rapidly stopped in a process known as hemostasis. Hemostasis takes place through several sequential steps or processes. First, an injury stimulates platelets (unpigmented blood cells) to adhere to the damaged blood vessels and then to one another, forming a plug that can stop minor bleeding. This association is mediated by what is called the von Willebrand factor, a protein that binds to the platelets. As the platelets aggregate, they release several substances that stimulate vasoconstriction, or a reduction in size of the blood vessels. This reduces the blood flow at the injury site. Finally, the aggregating platelets and damaged tissue initiate blood clotting, or coagulation. Once bleeding has stopped, the firmly adhering clot slowly contracts, drawing the edge of the wounds together so that tough scar tissue can form a permanent repair on the site.

Formation of a blood clot involves the participation of nearly twenty different substances, most of which are plasma-synthesized proteins. All but two of these substances, or factors, are designated by a roman numeral and a common name. A blood clot will be defective if one of the clotting factors is absent or deficient in the blood, and clotting time will be longer. The clotting factors, with some of their alternative names, are factor I (fibrinogen), factor II (prothrombin), factor III (tissue factor or thromboplastin), factor IV (calcium), factor V (proaccelerin), factor VII (proconvertin), factor VIII (antihemophilic factor), factor IX (Christmas factor), factor X (Stuart factor), factor XI (plasma thromboplastin antecedent), factor XII (Hageman factor), and factor XIII (fibrin stabilizing factor).

Several of the clotting factors have been discovered by the diagnosis of their deficiencies in various clotting disorders. The inherited coagulation disorders are uncommon conditions with an overall incidence probably of no more than 10 to 20 per 100,000 of the population. Hemophilia A, the most common or classic type of coagulation disorder, is caused by factor VIII deficiency. Hemophilia B (or Christmas disease) is the result of factor IX deficiency. It is quite common for severe hemophilia to manifest itself during the first year of life. Hazardous bleeding occurs in areas such as the central nervous system, the retropharyngeal area, and the retroperitoneal area. Bleeding in these areas requires mandatory admission to the hospital for observation and therapy. Joint lesions are very common in hemophilia because of acute spontaneous hemorrhage in the area, specially in weight-bearing joints such as ankles and knees. Urinary bleeding is often present at some time. The appearance of pseudotumors, caused by swelling involving muscle and bone produced by recurrent bleeding, is also common.

Hemophilia is transmitted entirely by unaffected females (carriers) to their sons in a sex-linked inheritance deficiency. Congenital deficiencies of the other coagulation factors are well recognized, even though bleeding episodes in these cases are uncommon. Deficiency of more than one factor is also possible, although documentation of such cases is very rare, perhaps because only patients with milder variations of the disease survive.

Von Willebrand's disease, unlike the hemophilias that mainly involve bleeding in joints and muscles, involves mainly bleeding of mucocutaneous tissues or skin. It affects both men and women. This disease shares clinical characteristics with hemophilia A, or classic hemophilia, including decreased levels of clotting factor VIII. This similarity made the differentiation between the two diseases very difficult to accomplish for a long time. It has now been established that there are two different factors involved in von Willebrand's disease, each with a different function. The von Willebrand factor is involved in the adhesion of platelets to the injured blood vessel wall and to one another, and together with factor VIII, circulates in plasma as a complex held by electrostatic and hydrophobic forces. The von Willebrand factor is a very large molecule, consisting of a series of possible multimeric structures. The bigger and heavier the multimer, the better it works against bleeding. Von Willebrand's disease is one of the least understood clotting disorders. Three types have been identified with at least twenty-seven variations. With type 1, all the multimers needed for successful clotting are present in the blood, but in lesser amounts than in healthy individuals. In type II, the larger multimers, which are more active in hemostasis, are lacking, and type III patients exhibit a severe lack of all multimers.

## TREATMENT AND THERAPY

The normal body is continually producing clotting factors in order to keep up with natural loss. Sometimes the production is stepped up to cover a real or anticipated increase in the need of these factors, such as in childbirth. Hemophiliacs, lacking some of these clotting factors, may lose large amounts of blood from even the smallest injury and sometimes hemorrhage without any apparent cause. The symptoms of their diseases may be alleviated by the intravenous administration of the deficient clotting factor. How this is done depends on the specific factor deficiency and the magnitude of the bleeding episode, the age and size of the patient, convenience, acceptability, cost of product, and method and place of delivery of care.

There are many sources for clotting factors. Fresh frozen plasma contains all the clotting factors, but since the concentration of the factors in plasma is relatively low, a large volume is required for treatment. Therefore, it can be used only when small amounts of clotting factor must be delivered. Its use is the only therapy for deficiencies of factors V, XI, and XII. Plasma is commonly harvested from single donor units to minimize the risk of infection by the hepatitis virus or human immunodeficiency virus (HIV), thus eliminating the risk involved in using pooled concentrates from many donors. Cryoprecipitates are the proteins that precipitate in fresh frozen plasma thawed at 4 degrees Celsius. The precipitate is rich in factors VIII and XIII and in fibrinogen, and carries less chance of infection with hepatitis. Its standardization is difficult, however, and is not required by the Food and Drug Administration. As a result, dosage calculation can be a problem. In addition, there is no method for the control of viral contamination. Therefore, cryoprecipitates are not commonly used unless harvested from a special known and tested donor pool. Clotting factor concentrates present many advantages. They are made from pooled plasma obtained from plasmapheresis or a program of total donor unit fractionation and are widely available. Factors VIII and IX can also be produced from plasma using monoclonal methods. Porcine factor VIII presents an alternative to patients with naturally occurring antibody to human factor VIII.

There are other substances that can replace missing clotting factors as well. The synthetic hormone desmopressin acetate (also known by the letters DDAVP) has been used to stimulate the release of factor VIII and von Willebrand factor from the endothelial cells lining blood vessels. It is commonly used for patients with mild hemophilia and von Willebrand's disease. DDAVP has no effect on the concentration of the other factors, and aside from the common side effect of water retention, it is a safe drug. Antifibrinolytic drugs prevent the natural breakdown of blood clots that are already formed. Although such drugs are not useful for the primary care of hemophiliacs, they are useful for use after dental extractions and in the treatment of other open wounds, after a clot has formed.

Between 10 and 15 percent of the patients affected with severe hemophilia develop factor VIII inhibitors (antibodies), which prevents their treatment with the usual methods. Newer therapeutic approaches have provided additional options for the management and control of bleeding episodes. The use of prothrombin complex concentrates or porcine factor VIII concentrates is indicated for low responders (those with a low amount of antibodies present in their system). An option for high responders is to try to eradicate the inhibitor present in their system. One way to do this is with a regimen of immunosuppressive drugs. These are very limited in value, however, and cannot be used with HIV-positive hemophiliacs. The drugs used in this approach include substances such as cyclophosphamide, vincristine, azathioprine, and corticosteroids. Another approach utilizes intravenous doses of gamma globulin to suppress, but not eradicate, the inhibitors. Yet another strategy is an immune tolerance regimen, in which factor VIII is administered daily in small amounts. This method causes the inhibitors to decrease and, in some cases, disappear. The regimen can also involve the prophylactic use of factor VIII (or factor VIII in combination with immunosuppressive drugs).

The introduction of plasma clotting factor concentrates has changed the treatment of patients with clotting factor deficiencies. It has brought about a remarkable change in the longevity of these patients and their quality of life. The availability of cryoprecipitates and concentrates of factors II, VII, VIII, IX, X, and XIII has made outpatient treatment for bleeding episodes routine and home infusion or self-infusion a possibility for many patients. Hospitalization for inpatient treatment is rare, and early outpatient therapy of bleeding episodes has decreased the severity of joint deformities.

Nevertheless, other problems are apparent in hemophiliac patients. Viral contamination of the factor concentrates has allowed the development of chronic illnesses, infection with HIV, immunologic diseases, liver and renal diseases, joint disorders, and cardiovascular diseases. While the use of heat for virus inactivation, beginning in 1983, resulted in a reduction in HIV infections, the majority of patients exposed to the virus had already been infected. The strategies to prevent contraction of hepatitis from these concentrates include vaccination against the contaminating viruses and the elimination of viruses from the factor replacement product. The non-A, non-B hepatitis virus is very difficult to remove, however, and the use of monoclonal factors seems to be the only solution to this problem. In general, difficulties associated with treatment have been largely eliminated through the production of the required clotting factors using recombinant DNA techniques, a process performed independent of human blood.

Treatment of von Willebrand's disease also includes pressure dressing, suturing, and oral contraceptives. A pasteurized antihemophiliac concentrate that contains substantial amounts of von Willebrand factor is used in severe cases.

Hematomas, or hemorrhages under the skin and within muscles, can frequently be controlled by application of elastic bandage pressure and ice. The ones that cannot be controlled easily within a few hours may cause muscle contraction and require factor replacement therapy. Exercise is recommended for joints after bleeding, as it helps protect joints by increasing muscle bulk and power and can also help relieve stress. Use of devices to protect joints, such as elastic bandages and splints, are commonly used. In extreme cases, orthopedic surgical procedures are readily available.

Analgesics, or painkillers, play an important part in the alleviation of chronic pain. Because patients cannot use products with aspirin and/or antihistamines, which inhibit platelet aggregation and prolong bleeding time, substances such as acetaminophen, codeine, and morphine are used. Chronic joint inflammation is reduced by the use of anti-inflammatory agents such as ibuprofen and of drugs used in rheumatoid arthritis patients.

The need for so many specialties and disciplines in the management of hemophilia has led to the development of multidisciplined hemophilia centers. Genetic education (information on how the disease is transmitted), genetic counseling (the discussion of an individual's genetic risks and reproductive options), and genetic testing have provided great help to patients and affected families. Early and prenatal diagnosis and carrier detection have provided options for family planning.

## Perspective and Prospects

Descriptions of hemophilia are among the oldest known accounts of genetic disease. References to a bleeding condition highly suggestive of hemophilia go back to the fifth century, in the Babylonian Talmud. The first significant report in the medical literature appeared in 1803 when John C. Otto, a Philadelphia physician, described several bleeder families with only males affected and with transmission through the mothers. The literature of the nineteenth century contains many descriptions of the disease, particularly the clinical characteristics of the hemorrhages and family histories. The disease was originally called haemorrhaphilia, or "love of hemorrhages," but the name was later contracted through usage to hemophilia ("love of blood"), the accepted name since around 1828.

Transfusion therapy was proposed as early as 1832, and the first successful transfusion for the treatment of a hemophiliac patient was reported in 1840 by Samuel Armstrong Lane. The use of blood from beef and pork in the transfusions was explored but abandoned because of the numerous side effects. It was not until the beginning of the twentieth century that serious studies on clotting in hemophilia were started. Attention was directed to the use of normal human serum for treatment of bleeding episodes. Some of the patients responded well, while others did not. This result is probably attributable to the fact that some had hemophilia A—these patients did not respond because factor VIII, in which they are deficient, is not present in serum—while some others had hemophilia B, for which the therapy worked. In 1923, harvested blood plasma was used in transfusion, and it was shown to work as well as whole blood. With blood banking becoming a reality in the 1930's, transfusions were performed more frequently as a treatment for hemophilia.

The history of the fractionation of plasma began around 1911 with Dr. Addis, who prepared a very crude fraction by acidification of plasma. In 1937, Drs. Patek and Taylor produced a crude fraction which on injection lowered the blood-clotting time in hemophiliacs. In the period from

1945 to 1960, a number of plasma fractions with antihemophiliac activity were developed. The use of fresh frozen plasma increased as a result of advances in the purification of the fractions. Some milestones can be identified in the production of the plasma fractions: the development of quantitative assays for antihemophiliac factors, the discovery of cryoprecipitation, and the development of glycine and polyethylene precipitation.

In 1952, four significant and independent publications indicated that there is a plasma-clotting activity separate from that concerned with classic hemophilia—in other words, that there are two types of hemophilia. One (hemophilia A) is characterized by a deficiency in factor VIII, while the other (hemophilia B) is characterized by deficiency in factor IX. Carriers of hemophilia A can have a mean factor VIII level that is 50 percent lower than that of normal females, while carriers of hemophilia B show levels of factor IX that are 60 percent below normal. The two diseases have the same pattern of inheritance, are similar in clinical appearance, and can be distinguished only by laboratory tests.

Hemophilias are caused by a disordered and complex biological mechanism that continues to be explored. Recombinant DNA techniques have now revealed the molecular defect in factor VIII or factor IX deficiencies in some families, demonstrating that a variety of gene defects can produce the classic phenotype of hemophilia. These techniques have also provided new tools for carrier detection and prenatal diagnosis.

Current treatment of hemophilia has converted the hemophiliac from an in-hospital patient to an individual with more independent status. Crucial in this development has been the creation of comprehensive care centers and of the National Hemophilia Foundation, which provide comprehensive treatment for the hemophilia patient. With the advancement of recombinant DNA technology, the future looks brighter for the sufferers of this disease.

—*Maria Pacheco*

**See also** Acquired immunodeficiency syndrome (AIDS); Bleeding; Genetic diseases.

### FOR FURTHER INFORMATION:

Brinkhous, K. M., and H. C. Hemker, eds. *Handbook of Hemophilia*. New York: Elsevier, 1975. The book consists of sixty-three chapters with eighty-nine authors representing the many disciplines that deal with the basic and clinical problems associated with hemophilia.

Bloom, Arthur L., ed. *The Hemophilias*. Methods in Hematology 5. New York: Churchill Livingstone, 1982. The series presents accounts of methods for the study of blood and its disorders. This book concentrates on hemophilia, presenting a description of available assay methods, purification methods, and prenatal diagnosis.

Hilgartner, Margaret W., and Carl Pochedly, eds. *Hemophilia in the Child and Adult*. 3d ed. New York: Raven Press, 1989. A compilation of the thoughts and experiences of clinicians who deal with hemophilia, as well as some practical approaches to patient care. A well-organized and informative book.

Jones, Peter. *Living with Haemophilia*. 2d ed. Lancaster, England: MTP Press, 1984. An excellent book for the layperson, it was written specifically for patients and their families. Explains the transmission of bleeding disorders through families, their manifestations, and their management in an easy-to-read, understandable format.

Voet, Donald, and Judith G. Voet. *Biochemistry*. New York: John Wiley & Sons, 1990. A comprehensive biochemistry textbook with an excellent section on blood and blood-clotting mechanism.

# HEMORRHOIDS

**SYSTEMS AFFECTED:** Gastrointestinal, circulatory

**SPECIALISTS:** Colorectal surgeons, gastroenterologists

**DEFINITION:** Blood-swollen enlargements of specialized tissues that help close the anus, as a result of intravenous pressure in the hemorrhoidal plexus; sometimes called piles.

**KEY TERMS:**

*anus:* the valve at the end of the rectum that prevents waste matter from leaking out until a person is ready to defecate

*cauterize:* to sear tissue with heat or a corrosive substance

*dentate line:* the junction in the anus where the external skin meets the internal mucosa

*gastroenterologist:* a physician who specializes in the gastrointestinal tract and related organs

*mucosa:* the mucus-secreting membrane that lines the surface of internal organs directly exposed to elements from outside the body, such as the lungs and intestines

*proctologist:* a physician who specializes in diseases of the rectum

*rectum:* the storage compartment at the end of the colon where wastes collect before defecation

*stool:* the excreted waste products of digestion

*thrombosis:* the condition of having a clot in a blood vessel

### CAUSES AND SYMPTOMS

Hemorrhoids, some physiologists suggest, are one of the prices that humans pay for walking upright. The vascular system—the veins and arteries that circulate blood—evolved in an animal that walked on all fours. Now that humans spend most of their time standing, gravity puts awkward pressure on the system, and at the bottom of major parts of the system, as in the tissue around the anus, the column of blood above weighs heavily on the network of small blood vessels there. It does not take much additional pressure to cause a vessel's wall to balloon out. When it does, the result is a hemorrhoid, a little pouch protruding on the surface of the anus, similar to a hernia or varicose vein. Most Americans have hemorrhoids, even if they do

## Hemorrhoids

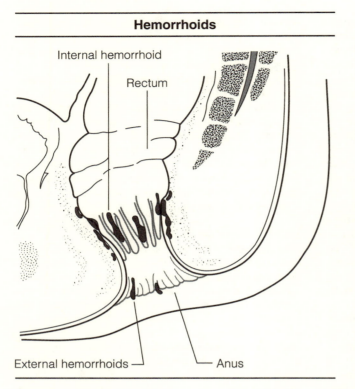

Internal hemorrhoid

Rectum

External hemorrhoids — Anus

ing place is a corrugated joint called the dentate line (or, alternatively, the anorectal juncture or pectinase line). It is in this area—between the skin covering the external (or lower) sphincter and the mucosa over the internal (or upper) sphincter—that hemorrhoids form. Those that bulge out from the dentate line or above are hidden from sight by the closed anus and are called internal hemorrhoids; those that protrude below the closed anus, and so can be seen or felt, are called external hemorrhoids.

External hemorrhoids are the ones famed for vexing people. When the skin is stretched over swelled hemorrhoids, its sense receptors are activated, making the hemorrhoids burn and itch, sometimes so intolerably that the urge to scratch them is uncontrollable. Scratching, especially with abrasive materials such as toilet paper, often scrapes and tears the tissue. The bright red blood from these lesions is easily noticeable on the toilet paper and may even drip into the toilet bowl or onto underclothes. Likewise, the passage of a hard, dry stool often abrades hemorrhoids to the point of bleeding.

Internal hemorrhoids do not itch or burn and rarely cause pain because the mucosal tissue over them has no nerve endings, but they can also bleed when a passing stool damages them. (Pain may be "referred," however, from a damaged internal hemorrhoid to the sciatic nerve, bladder, lower back, or genitals; that is, a person feels little or no pain in the anorectal area, but suddenly pain flares in one of these other areas.) An especially elongated internal hemorrhoid at times can protrude through the anus, a condition called prolapse. Usually, it spontaneously recedes or can be pushed back inside with a finger, but upon rare occasion a group of internal hemorrhoids prolapse, swelling and sending the internal sphincter into painful spasms. A doctor's help may then be required to reduce the pain and fit the hemorrhoids inside.

The blood vessels in the internal rectal plexus swell so easily because they lack valves. Without valves to regulate the local flow of blood, the walls are vulnerable to any sudden increase in pressure. Even a small, transient increase above the normal pressure of blood circulation can cause the vessels to bulge. Often, these bulges disappear when the excess pressure disappears or remain swollen only briefly afterward. If the increased pressure is high enough, however, a permanent protrusion results, drooping from the anal wall like lumps of melted wax on a candle. Even then, if the hemorrhoid is internal, the patient may feel no discomfort and may not realize that a hemorrhoid has formed.

Some people are more susceptible to chronic hemorrhoids than others because of a hereditary lack of elasticity in the blood vessels. In such people, standing for long periods of time can add enough pressure to make hemorrhoids swell. Nevertheless, anyone can get hemorrhoids; all that

not realize it, and the major symptoms are rarely dangerous, although they can be extremely annoying. Sometimes, however, hemorrhoids develop into or mask life-threatening diseases.

The term "hemorrhoid" derives from Greek words meaning "blood flowing," an apt description of the circulatory activity in the anal walls and an inadvertently apt warning of what most alarms people—hemorrhoids occasionally bleed. (The alternative, and now obsolescent, term "piles" comes from Latin *pila*, a ball, apparently a metaphor for the appearance of hemorrhoids.) Specifically, the "blood flowing" refers to the supple blood vessels of the internal rectal plexus, a series of pouches that act as cushions to help seal the anus shut. When these pouches become enlarged, they turn into hemorrhoids, which jut from the anus wall and swell up to 3 centimeters in length.

Because of the sphincter that controls defecation, not all hemorrhoids are visible without the aid of special instruments. The anus, an oval opening about three centimeters in front of the spine, is the valve ending the digestive tract. Like the mouth's lips, which begin the tract, the anus can purse shut, a state made possible by two concentric, circular sphincter muscles which act like drawstrings on a cloth bag. When sensors in the rectum signal the time to defecate, these muscles relax to pass stool and then immediately contract to close the anus again. As in the mouth, external skin meets the internal mucosal membrane in the anus; the meet-is needed is enough pressure in the lower abdomen. Straining on the toilet to pass stool is the most common cause. People strain when they are constipated or have diarrhea, and since a poor diet can lead to these conditions, hemorrhoids can be a secondary effect of poor eating habits. Those who like to sit on the toilet a long time, reading or watching television while waiting for a bowel movement, also increase pressure on the anus because of the posture and the compressing effect of the toilet ring; they are likely to develop hemorrhoids. People who regularly lift heavy weights as part of their jobs or for recreation are especially susceptible if they hold their breath while lifting: This action pushes the diaphragm downward on organs below it, including the anus, putting pressure on them. Similarly, during pregnancy women can develop hemorrhoids as the expanding womb crowds and increases pressure on nearby organs; these hemorrhoids are exacerbated by delivery, but they usually go away afterward. Psychologists add to these causes the guilt that some people feel about eating and excreting, guilt spawned by overindulgence in food or bad toilet training; they bear down on their bowels to defecate as quickly as possible and by doing so stress the hemorrhoidal vessels. Finally, hemorrhoids occasionally develop because of some serious diseases, such as heart failure and cirrhosis of the liver, which elevate pressure in the veins, and rectal cancer, which can create a false sense of fullness so that the person strains to pass a stool that is not really there.

Although they seldom do more than itch, external hemorrhoids can thrombose—develop clots of coagulated blood from a burst or swollen vessel under the skin—and grow as large as a grape. A doctor can relieve the pain by slicing open the hemorrhoid and squeezing out the clot. Left alone, a thrombosed hemorrhoid may rupture, causing a painful and bloody mess that is ripe for infection. Yet the greatest threat of hemorrhoids lies not in the symptoms themselves but in how they might be confused with those of other, deadly diseases. Colorectal cancer, inflammatory bowel disease, and sexually transmitted diseases such as syphilis, gonorrhea, and herpes can lead to discharges of blood, as can anal fissures (cracks in the anal canal), fistulas (tunnel-like passages between an infected gland and mucosa or skin), and abscesses (pus-filled sacs under the mucosa). A person who dismisses the bloody discharge as simply a flare-up of hemorrhoids may be delaying treatment for the real cause. In the case of colorectal cancer, one of the most common cancers in the United States, such a delay can be fatal. Only a doctor has the tools and vantage point to distinguish between the relatively benign hemorrhoids and a dangerous disorder.

### TREATMENT AND THERAPY

Since hemorrhoid-like symptoms can be produced by deadly diseases, a thorough checkup at the doctor's office includes an examination of the anus and rectum, especially if the patient has noticed bleeding. In addition to the visual inspection and "digital" examination, during which the doctor inserts a finger and feels around for enlarged hemorrhoids or other masses, patients provide clues by describing the color, amount, and time of bleeding. If the blood is bright red and occurs in small quantities during or just after defecation, hemorrhoids are most likely to blame. If dark red blood or clots appear in the stool or seep out randomly, however, the doctor will look for other causes, inspecting the anus, rectum, and colon with various types of endoscope, a fiber-optic-filled flexible tube that can also collect tissue samples. Once the doctor rules out other diseases, the patient has three basic choices: change habits, rely on therapy, or have the hemorrhoids removed.

If a person's hemorrhoids do not cause severe discomfort, the doctor will likely recommend a diet with high fiber and water intake. Fiber and water together make stools bulky and soft. They pass more easily during defecation than small, hard, dry stools. The patient does not have to strain, and so no further pressure is put on existing hemorrhoids. Furthermore, soft stools do not scrape hemorrhoids and cause them to bleed. The doctor will also suggest regular exercise, since this helps the bowels work more efficiently and reduces the chance of constipation. Finally, the patient may receive instructions on the proper way to breathe during heavy exertion so as to lessen the stress on the hemorrhoids. It is possible that with a better diet, more exercise, and less physical straining, patients may find that hemorrhoids have disappeared completely.

Until hemorrhoids shrink, they plague the patient, and to reduce the itching and burning a number of therapies prove effective, if only temporarily. An ice compress eases the discomfort, as does a sitz bath (sitting for at least fifteen minutes in shallow warm water), which also cleanses the site of potentially infecting wastes and promotes healing in damaged tissue. Should these relatively simple and cheap measures be impracticable, a variety of ointments, creams, medicated pads, and suppositories, either prescription or nonprescription, may provide relief. Some are inert, such as petroleum jelly, and coat and lubricate the hemorrhoids, protecting them from irritation. Some have an astringent effect, tightening and sealing tissue and thereby protecting it. Others have anesthetic ingredients, numbing the tissue, or anti-inflammatory effects, decreasing swelling. None of these medications has a proven capacity to make swelling go away entirely, and those with active ingredients may cause an allergic response. For patients with constipation, doctors may prescribe stool softeners to eliminate straining during defecation. Laxatives are usually to be avoided because the chemicals in them irritate hemorrhoids, and the resulting diarrhea often causes urgency and pressure in the rectal area.

When hemorrhoids become chronically and unusually swollen or the patient can no longer endure the discomfort, removing them is the last resort. This cure is certain, although not necessarily permanent, but it has its cost in pain and recovery time. There are seven basic methods, six that cause the target hemorrhoid to shrivel, to drop off on its own, or both, and one, surgery, that removes it directly.

The surgical removal of hemorrhoids, called hemorrhoidectomy, is a relatively simple operation; nevertheless, it is usually reserved for those patients who for one reason or another cannot undergo one of the other methods. The patient is given a local anesthetic to deaden the tissue in the anus, although some patients are rendered unconscious with a general anesthetic; the surgeon cuts off the hemorrhoid at its base and then sews the wound closed with absorbable sutures. The recovery period may require hospitalization for up to a week, during which pain medication, stool softeners, and anal pads are necessary until the tissues heal. Bed rest after hospitalization and sitz baths may also be necessary. Because of this recovery time—as much as a month all together—hemorrhoidectomies are not widely popular among patients or physicians. Moreover, urine retention and infection and hemorrhaging after the operation are possible complications.

The remaining methods avoid the trauma of cutting, and the first of them, ligation, is the oldest of all the methods, referred to in the writings of Hippocrates (c. 460-377 B.C.). Ancient Greek physicians tied a thread around a hemorrhoid to strangle its blood supply; modern gastroenterologists or proctologists use special rubber bands. The effect is the same: The hemorrhoid dries up, shrivels, and falls off. Little pain accompanies the procedure, which is done in the doctor's office. Ligation, however, can only be used for internal hemorrhoids.

Likewise, sclerotherapy, cryosurgery, and infrared coagulation are only for internal hemorrhoids because the pain would be too intense on external hemorrhoids. In sclerotherapy, the doctor injects a liquid—usually phenol in oil or quinine in urea—that seals closed the blood vessels at the base of the hemorrhoid. With no blood in them, the vessels eventually shrink to normal dimensions and, if stressing pressure on them is not resumed, the hemorrhoid disappears. In cryosurgery, super cold liquid nitrogen or nitrous oxide is applied to the hemorrhoid, freezing it and killing the tissue. The hemorrhoid slowly melts and, as it does, shrinks and finally sloughs off. Popular in the 1970's and early 1980's, cryosurgery lost favor because of the messy and extended recovery time. Useful for mild, small hemorrhoids, infrared coagulation involves a beam of infrared light that, aimed at the hemorrhoid, shrinks it by cauterizing the tissue. The heat of the beam can cause pain in other parts of the anus during the procedure.

The remaining methods, laser surgery and electric current coagulation, can be used on external hemorrhoids. Like infrared coagulation, laser surgery trains a beam of light—in this case intense visible light—that burns and shrinks the hemorrhoid to a stub. Since the laser cauterizes as it de-stroys tissue and therefore seals off blood vessels, its main advantage over regular surgery lies in reduced bleeding. Recovery time is shorter, about a week, and hospitalization is usually not necessary. This procedure is much more expensive that a hemorrhoidectomy or ligation, however, because of the cost of laser technology. In electric current coagulation, electrodes pass either direct or alternating current through the hemorrhoids. Because tissue is a poor conductor, the resistance to the current creates heat, which cooks the hemorrhoid, coagulating and shrinking it.

Which method the surgeon, gastroenterologist, or proctologist uses depends partly upon the physician's and patient's preferences and partly upon the size and location of the hemorrhoid. Ligation remains the most frequently used method because it is relatively cheap and fast.

## PERSPECTIVE AND PROSPECTS

According to Napoleon's personal physician, piles cost the emperor the Battle of Waterloo, which ended his reign. His hemorrhoids were so inflamed and painful on the morning of the battle that he could not get out of bed, much less sit on his horse. Without his personal direction, the French lost. Popular writers often cite this dramatic example, sometimes with humorous overtones, to demonstrate how seriously hemorrhoids can interfere with even the lives of the great.

Certainly, hemorrhoids are no laughing matter. Yet the long-standing taboo in the United States about excretion and the anus has prompted many Americans either to laugh nervously about their hemorrhoids or to keep silent, preferring to suffer stoically rather than to risk becoming the target of jokes. For this reason, it is nearly impossible to say how many sufferers there are in the United States. Estimates vary from several million people to the entire population over the age of thirty.

Whatever the exact statistic, clearly many people share a problem that embarrasses them too much to discuss openly or that they believe is too trivial for medical attention. If they need relief from the itching and pain, they treat themselves. A large industry in home remedies and over-the-counter medications serves them: Medications alone earned drug companies $117.1 million in 1986, according to the Non-Prescription Drug Manufacturers Association. The benefits of such medications are difficult to assess, and some authorities claim that petroleum jelly eases the itching and burning as much as any preparation specifically intended for hemorrhoids. Folk remedies, such as suppositories made of tobacco or compresses soaked in papaya juice, can damage tissue outright, making the problem worse. Moreover, throughout the United States specialized clinics offer surgical cures for hemorrhoids, promising patients quick relief on an outpatient basis and using expensive methods, particularly laser surgery.

Therefore, many people spend a considerable amount of money and time, often wasting both, to tend a chronic discomfort that can as readily be prevented or palliated by a change in habits, doctors claim. Like colon cancer and many other intestinal ailments, hemorrhoids are most common in populations whose diet includes a high number of processed foods, which are low in fiber. While fiber is no panacea, people in cultures whose diet contains significant fiber have larger stools and fewer intestinal complaints in general.

Because hemorrhoids are in most cases preventable or controllable without treatment, they have been cited, along with deadly maladies such as colon cancer and inflammatory bowel disease, in criticisms of both the American diet and Americans' eagerness to rely on medical intervention to save them from their own unhealthy habits. In the case of hemorrhoids—while they are not exclusively a malady of Western civilization—the fast pace and pressures of life, the attitudes about defecation, and the eating habits of industrial cultures help give them a distracting prominence.
—*Roger Smith*

**See also** Colon cancer; Hernia; Intestinal disorders; Thrombosis and thrombus.

**FOR FURTHER INFORMATION:**

Becker, Barbara. *Relief from Chronic Hemorrhoids*. New York: Dell, 1992. An excellent book for general readers, it gives advice on every aspect of diagnosis, treatment, removal procedures, and alternative therapies. Special attention is given to improving the patient's diet, and extensive, very specific tables on proper foods accompany the argument for this self-help approach. A handy glossary of key medical terms concludes the text.

*The Hemorrhoid Book: A Look at Hemorrhoids—How They're Treated and How You Can Prevent Them from Coming Back.* San Bruno, Calif.: Krames Communications, 1991. Available through doctors' offices, this pamphlet is well worth the trouble to find it. It is fully illustrated and each illustration is captioned, thereby making the major anatomical features of hemorrhoids clear and memorable, as are the aspects of medical examinations and surgical treatment.

Holt, Robert Lawrence. *Hemorrhoids: A Cure and Preventive*. New York: William Morrow, 1980. Somewhat out of date and often cranky in tone, this book nevertheless contains clear descriptions of causes, misconceptions, and treatments of hemorrhoids. The author champions cryosurgery, which has since lost popularity. Illustrations accompany the anatomical explanations.

Sachar, David B., Jerome D. Waye, and Blair S. Lewis, eds. *Pocket Guide to Gastroenterology*. Baltimore: Williams & Wilkins, 1991. This diagnosis-oriented handbook gives information on all gastroenterological ailments in outline form, making it valuable for quick studies on major problems. The section on hemorrhoids, though superficial, lays out the basic symptoms and treatments. The book identifies and describes all related prob-

lems, expanding the scope of its usefulness far beyond that of a book dedicated to hemorrhoids alone.

Wanderman, Sidney E., with Betty Rothbart and the editors of Consumer Reports Books. *Hemorrhoids*. Yonkers, N.Y.: Consumer Reports Books, 1991. Providing a simple but thorough overview of anatomical problems, causes, medications, therapies, and removal methods, this short book also discusses related complaints, such as fissures and fistulas, and dangerous diseases whose symptoms can be mistaken for those of hemorrhoids. The authors' intent is to help sufferers find the best way to cope with their hemorrhoids.

# HEPATITIS

**SYSTEM AFFECTED:** Liver

**SPECIALISTS:** Epidemiologists, infectious disease physicians, internists, toxicologists

**DEFINITION:** An inflammatory condition of the liver, characterized by discomfort, jaundice, and enlargement of the organ and bacterial, viral, or immunological in origin; may also result from use of alcohol and other toxic drugs.

**KEY TERMS:**

*alanine aminotransferase:* a liver enzyme associated with the metabolism of the amino acid alanine; elevated levels are an indication of liver damage

*aspartate aminotransferase:* a liver enzyme associated with metabolism of the amino acid aspartate; elevated levels are an indication of liver damage

*cirrhosis:* chronic degeneration of the liver, in which normal tissue is replaced with fibroid tissue and fat; commonly associated with alcohol abuse but can also result from hepatitis

*hepatitis A virus:* the virus associated with certain forms of hepatitis; generally contracted through fecal contamination of food and water

*hepatitis B virus:* the agent associated with severe forms of viral hepatitis; contracted through contaminated blood or hypodermic needles or through contaminated body fluids, and sometimes found in association with hepatitis D virus

*hepatitis C virus:* formerly referred to as the etiological agent for non-A, non-B viral hepatitis; most often passed in contaminated blood

*hepato:* a prefix denoting anything associated with the liver—for example, a hepatocyte is a liver cell

*jaundice:* a symptom of a variety of liver disorders which manifests as yellowish discoloration of the skin, the whites of the eyes, and other tissues; hepatocellular jaundice results from hepatitis

## CAUSES AND SYMPTOMS

Hepatitis, a pathology referring to inflammation of the liver, may result from any of a variety of causes but commonly follows bacterial or viral infection. Hepatitis may also be associated with an autoimmune phenomenon in which the body produces antibodies against liver tissue. Liver inflammation may also be an aftereffect of the use of alcohol or various hepatotoxic chemicals, either through the taking of illegal drugs or as a side effect of the legal use of pharmacological agents. Among the pharmaceuticals that can cause liver damage are antibiotics such as isoniazid and rifampin and the painkiller acetaminophen.

Symptoms associated with hepatitis are a reflection of the function of the liver. The liver is arguably the most complex organ in the body. More than five hundred different functions have been associated with the organ, including the production of bile for emulsification of fats and the secretion of glucose, proteins, or vitamins for use elsewhere in the body. The liver also plays a major role in the detoxification of the blood, removing alcohol, nicotine, and other potentially poisonous substances. The Kupffer cells in the liver function in the removal of infectious agents or foreign material from the blood. More than 10 percent of the blood supply in the body is found within the liver at any time.

Among the functions of the liver is the removal of hemoglobin in the blood, released as a result of the lysis (disintegration) of red blood cells. A breakdown product of hemoglobin is the yellowish compound bilirubin. It is the buildup of bilirubin in blood that results in the appearance of jaundice in cases of inadequate liver function, such as during hepatitis.

Though hepatitis may develop from a variety of causes, it most commonly results from infection of the liver. Nearly any infectious agent may potentially damage the liver, but generally these involve one of several types of viruses, bacteria, fungi, or amoebas. Liver disease may also be significantly exacerbated by alcohol abuse, as is seen in patients with cirrhosis. Regardless of the specific cause, symptoms of liver disease remain similar in most cases. The liver is often enlarged and tender to physical examination. The person may feel tired and run a low-grade fever. It is not un-

**Hepatitis**

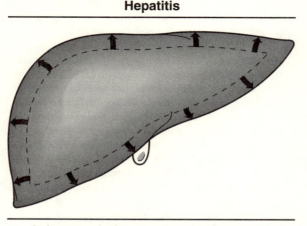

*In hepatitis, the liver is enlarged and congested.*

usual for the person to feel nauseous and lose weight. Jaundice is common in most patients, and the levels of the enzymes alanine aminotransferase (ALT) and aspartate amino transferase (AST) may rise. Levels of these enzymes, however, are not necessarily indications of the severity of liver disease; in any event, their levels often fall over the course of the disease.

Three particular viruses have been associated with most forms of viral hepatitis (types A, B, and C), while a fourth (type D) appears as a passenger during some cases of hepatitis B. Hepatitis A results from infection with hepatitis A virus (HAV), a virus classified in the same group as the poliovirus and rhinoviruses (cold viruses). The disease is transmitted through a fecal-to-oral method and is self-limited (running a definite and limited course). Often the disease is subclinical (undetectable), particularly as seen in children. Replication of the virus occurs in hepatocytes (liver cells); the virus then passes into the intestine and is eliminated with the feces. A long incubation period following ingestion may occur, sometimes as long as a month, and during much of this period the person is capable of transmitting the disease. In otherwise healthy individuals, recovery is complete and occurs over several weeks. Anti-HAV antibodies are present in the blood of about 30 to 40 percent of the general population, reflecting the widespread nature of the disease.

Hepatitis B (HBV), formerly called serum hepatitis, is a potentially much more severe form of the disease. The disease in young children is frequently asymptomatic, with appearance of symptoms in older individuals being more common. In general, however, the most frequent result of primary infection with HBV is a mild or subclinical course of infection. The disease is most commonly seen in the fifteen-to-thirty-five age group, in part reflecting its method of transmission (through blood or body fluids).

Persistent infection with HBV, occurring in approximately 1 to 3 percent of patients, can be associated with either an asymptomatic carrier state or chronic hepatitis. The chronic state may be severe, with progression to cirrhosis and cellular degeneration or inflammation. In fact, it is the immune response to the presence of HBV that may contribute to liver degeneration. HBV infection results in the expression of viral antigens, which stimulate an immune response, on the surface of liver cells. Among the inflammatory cells present at the sites of infection are a large proportion of lymphocytes. These include cytotoxic T cells, lymphocytes associated with the killing of viral infected cells. Because immunologically impaired individuals infected with HBV often suffer a mild form of the disease, the possibility exists that it is the immune response itself that contributes to the ensuing liver damage.

Hepatitis B transmission occurs through blood or bodily fluids, including semen and vaginal secretions. Because HBV is also found in saliva, the disease may be transmitted among family members through nonsexual contact. Maternal-neonatal transmission may occur, occasionally while the fetus is in the uterus but more likely during the labor or birth process. There is, however, no evidence for transmission through food or water or by an airborne means.

Clinical features of HBV infections are similar to those associated with other forms of hepatitis. In the asymptomatic form of type B disease, AST or ALT levels may be elevated, but jaundice is absent. Adults with symptomatic hepatitis B may suffer jaundice (icteric hepatitis), or they may not (nonicteric hepatitis). There is generally a mild fever, fatigue, and weakness.

Accompanying an indeterminant number of HBV infections is a second virus, designated the hepatitis D virus (HDV). HDV is a defective virus, capable of replication only in the presence of HBV. Not surprisingly, its geographic distribution and mode of transmission are similar to those of HBV. The prevalence of HDV has been found to be as high as 70 percent in some outbreaks of HBV and nonexistent in others. In most cases, HDV infection results in subclinical or mild hepatitis. In about 15 percent of cases, the disease may progress to a more severe form. HDV may itself be cytopathic (causing pathological changes) for hepatocytes, but this remains to be established firmly.

Based on the exclusion of other types of etiologic agents, including HAV, HBV, Epstein-Barr virus, and cytomegalovirus, non-A, non-B (NANB) hepatitis was considered a clinical entity. During the late 1980's, NANB hepatitis was determined to be caused by a newly isolated infectious agent, designated hepatitis C virus (HCV). In the United States, approximately 25 percent of hepatitis is associated with HCV. HCV is recognized as the major complication of blood transfusions or transfusions of blood products, with nearly all cases associated with such transfusions. About 70 percent of cases are asymptomatic, based on measurements of AST or ALT levels. Most cases are mild, with a temporary carrier state established in a large proportion of infected individuals.

Outbreaks of an enterically transmitted NANB hepatitis (NANB hepatitis transmitted through the intestines), designated hepatitis E, have also been found in some parts of the world. Though hepatitis E has been around at least since 1955 (and no doubt earlier, but undocumented), it was only in the late 1980's that it was determined to be a unique form of the disease. Transmission occurs through eating or drinking contaminated food or water, though there is evidence that household contact with infected persons may also transmit the disease. Hepatitis E is most common in the poor countries of Asia, with sporadic outbreaks elsewhere. The few cases found in the United States have involved travelers to these areas.

Acute hepatitis is less commonly associated with infection by other viruses. These include the herpes family of viruses, such as herpes simplex, cytomegalovirus, and Epstein-

Barr virus. Because the prevalence of these viruses is quite high, immunosuppressed or immunodeficient patients may be at particular risk.

Certain forms of hepatitis are associated with an autoimmune response. In these cases, the cause is not an infectious agent but rather a form of rejection by the body of its own liver tissue. Autoimmune hepatitis is suspected in individuals in which the disease persists for at least six months with no evidence of exposure to an infectious agent or hepatotoxin. In nearly one-third of these individuals, other immunological diseases such as lupus or arthritis may be present. The clinical manifestations of autoimmune hepatitis are similar to those of other forms of the disease. Most patients exhibit jaundice, a mild fever, weakness, and weight loss. The liver is often enlarged and tender. Unlike other forms of hepatitis, found equally in men and women, autoimmune hepatitis is most commonly found in women. Prognosis of the disease is unclear, as an unknown percentage of cases are subclinical. Severe forms have a high fatality rate.

### TREATMENT AND THERAPY

No specific treatments exist for the various forms of viral hepatitis; hence, treatment is for the most part symptomatic and supportive. Hospitalization may be required in severe cases, but, in general, any restriction of activity is left to the desire of the patient. This is particularly convenient, since recovery often involves a long convalescence. As long as a healthy diet is maintained, no special dietary requirements exist, but a high-calorie diet is often preferable. Drugs or chemicals that are potentially damaging to the liver, including alcohol and certain antibiotics or painkillers, should be avoided.

Hepatitis induced by other forms of infectious agents such as bacteria or fungi may be treated using an appropriate course of antibiotic therapy. In cases of drug-induced disease, avoidance of the chemical is a key to recovery. Bacterial infections of the liver are often associated with patients who are malnourished, such as the elderly or alcoholics, or who may be immunosuppressed. These problems must also be addressed during the course of treatment.

Prevention of the disease is preferable, however, and because the means of viral spread has been well established in most cases, appropriate measures can often be taken. For the most part, the viruses associated with hepatitis have little in common with one another aside from their predilection for hepatocytes. Thus, preventing their spread involves different strategies.

HAV is almost always spread through a fecal-oral means of transmission. Often the source is an infected person involved in the preparation of uncooked foods. Common sense dictates that the person should wash after every use of a toilet, but this is often not the case. Not surprisingly, children attending day care centers frequently become infected. Contaminated groundwater is also a potential source of outbreaks in areas in which proper sewage treatment does not take place. Less commonly, HAV is spread directly from person to person through sexual contact. A method called immunoprophylaxis can prevent the development of symptoms in individuals exposed to hepatitis A by utilizing a form of passive immunity. Developed during World War II, the procedure involves the pooling of serum from immune individuals. Inoculation of the serum into exposed persons is effective in prevention of the disease in most cases.

The transmission of HBV generally involves passage via contaminated blood or body secretions. In the period prior to the screening of blood, transfusions were the most common means of spreading the disease—hence the designation "serum hepatitis." Since the 1980's, the most common means of documented spread has been through either sexual contact or the sharing of contaminated hypodermic needles. Semen, vaginal secretions, and saliva from infected individuals all contain the active virus, and limiting exchange of these fluids is key to prevention of transmission. Even so, the means of infection in nearly one-third of symptomatic cases remains unknown.

An effective vaccine for prevention of HBV infection was first developed during the 1970's and early 1980's. The vaccination procedure was subsequently modified to create an effective combined active-passive vaccine. Passive immunization utilizes antibodies purified from the blood of donors who have recovered from HBV infection. This hepatitis B immune globulin (HBIG) is combined with a recombinant yeast vaccine that contains hepatitis virus proteins but lacks the genetic material necessary for the virus to replicate. Because HBIG already contains a high level of anti-HBV antibody, it is effective as a postexposure preventive for an individual who has come in contact with the disease. For example, a person exposed to the virus through an accidental needle stick, such as an unimmunized health care worker, may not have time to proceed through the regimen of treatment. The use of HBIG provides a short-term means of protection. The combined vaccine is used as a method of pre-exposure immunization. In the early 1990's, vaccination was recommended to only those persons at high risk for exposure to HBV. This group is composed of homosexual or bisexual men, health care workers (including physicians and dentists), and persons dealing with individuals in whom the disease is commonly found.

Because hepatitis D virus is defective in replication, requiring the presence of HBV, no specific measures of prevention are necessary. Immunization against HBV is sufficient to prevent the spread of HDV.

Treatment of NANB hepatitis consists primarily of allowing the disease to run its course. Because this form of hepatitis is almost exclusively blood-borne and no vaccine exists, prevention requires the exclusion of blood from contaminated individuals in the blood pool available for transfusions. Routine screening of blood for anti-HCV antibodies was begun in 1990. The use of surrogate markers has also proven helpful. For example, elevated levels of ALT and anti-HBV antibodies in the serum of blood donors have been shown to predispose the recipient to NANB hepatitis; hence the exclusion of such blood has been particularly useful in limiting the transmission of the disease. Sharing of contaminated needles is also a means of transmission, requiring increased individual responsibility in order to prevent the spread of the virus. The use of immunoprophylaxis, so useful in the prevention of transmission of HBV, has not proven effective in the case of HCV.

The transmission of hepatitis E virus is also through a fecal-oral route. The drinking of sewage-contaminated water has been the most common source of transmission. Because no active means of prevention has been developed, prevention of exposure requires that the individual avoid any food or water potentially contaminated with sewage. This is particularly true in areas of the world in which hepatitis E is found. Though the precaution may seem obvious, the safety of the water, as well as any object washed in the water, is not always readily apparent.

Autoimmune hepatitis results from an aberrant immune system rather than from an infectious agent. Treatment generally involves the use of immunosuppressive drugs to limit the immune response. Corticosteroids such as prednisone, sometimes in combination with azathioprine, have proven effective in the therapy of many patients. Still, in some cases the disease progresses to cirrhosis and results in death. Treatment generally is carried out over a long period of time, at least a year, and relapses are common. Often, the patient requires lifetime therapy. The immunosuppressive activity of the therapy may also leave the patient more susceptible to infection. In some cases, liver transplantation has proven effective, at least in the short term. Because the liver rejection was caused by an autoimmune response in the first place, the transplant may also be subject to the same phenomenon.

## PERSPECTIVE AND PROSPECTS

Inflammation of the liver resulting in hepatitis can develop from a variety of mechanisms. Most often, these mechanisms are associated with either a chemical injury or infection by a microbiological agent.

Infections of the liver generally involve one of several viral agents. The association of liver disease, or at least jaundice, with an infectious agent was suspected as early as the time of Hippocrates (the fifth century B.C.). Hippocrates described a syndrome which was undoubtedly viral hepatitis. The disease was also described in the Babylonian Talmud about eight hundred years later. Epidemics of the disease have been reported since the Middle Ages, which most likely involved outbreaks of hepatitis A. The spread of this disease through personal contact was confirmed in the 1930's.

Type B, or serum hepatitis, was described as a clinical entity by A. Lurman in 1855. Lurman observed that 15 percent of shipyard workers in Bremen, Germany, who received a smallpox vaccine containing human lymph developed jaundice within the following six months. In the early years of the twentieth century, jaundice frequently developed among patients who received vaccines prepared from convalescent serums or who underwent procedures such as venipuncture using instruments which had not been properly sterilized. By 1926, the blood-borne nature of the disease was confirmed. In 1942, more than twenty-eight thousand American soldiers developed jaundice after vaccination with a yellow fever vaccine prepared from pooled human serums. By then it had become obvious that at least two forms of infectious agents were associated with viral hepatitis.

The isolation of HBV occurred as a result of studies initiated by Baruch Blumberg in 1963. Blumberg was actually attempting to correlate the development of diseases such as cancer with particular patterns of proteins found in the serum of individuals. His approach was to collect blood from persons in various parts of the world and then analyze their serum proteins. Blumberg found an antigen, a protein, in the blood of Australian aborigines which reacted with antibodies in the blood of an American hemophiliac. Blumberg called the protein the Australia (Au) antigen. It later became apparent that the Au antigen could be isolated from the blood of patients with serum hepatitis. By 1970, it was established that what Blumberg had referred to as the Au antigen was in fact the HBV particle.

HBV is associated with more than simply viral hepatitis. Chronic hepatitis associated with HBV can often develop into hepatocellular carcinoma, or cancer of the liver. The precise reason is unclear; the cancer may result from the chronic damage to liver tissue associated with long-term infection by HBV.

Because an effective vaccine exists only against HBV, much research continues in this area. A vaccine directed against HAV may become available, and the efficacy of early vaccination against HBV in children may soon be established. If early vaccination proves effective, the prevalence of both hepatitis B and hepatocellular carcinoma should decrease.   —*Richard Adler*

*See also* Addiction; Alcoholism; Autoimmune disorders; Cirrhosis; Jaundice; Liver cancer; Liver disorders.

**FOR FURTHER INFORMATION:**

Gorbach, Sherwood L., John G. Bartlett, and Neil R. Blacklow, eds. *Infectious Diseases*. Philadelphia: W. B. Saunders, 1992. A thorough discussion of infectious diseases. Included is a brief history, an account of the mechanisms of disease and immunity, and a concise discussion of a broad range of infectious agents. The section on hepatitis viruses is well written and not particularly detailed. Also addresses methods of prevention, diagnosis, and therapy.

Johnson, P. J., and I. G. McFarlane. *The Laboratory Investigation of Liver Disease*. Philadelphia: W. B. Saunders, 1989. An introduction to liver function and disease. Also included are chapters on virology, immunology, and the effects of drugs on the liver. A broad range of subjects are covered. Particularly useful are the sections dealing with measurements of liver functions.

Kelley, William, ed. *Textbook of Internal Medicine*. 2d ed. New York: J. B. Lippincott, 1992. A medical textbook on the subject. The book contains an extensive section on liver diseases, including a concise description of viral hepatitis. The discussion on hepatitis viruses is thorough, clear, but not overly detailed.

Leevy, Carroll. *Liver Regeneration in Man*. Springfield, Ill.: Charles C Thomas, 1973. A concise description of the liver and its function. Emphasized are the recuperative powers of the organ. The text is not overly clinical and is within the reach of persons with some knowledge of biology.

Levine, Arnold. *Viruses*. New York: W. H. Freeman, 1992. A well-written outline of viruses and their history. Some basic knowledge of biology is helpful in certain areas of the book, but overall the format and style should reach nearly all general readers. The book is profusely and colorfully illustrated. Several sections deal specifically with viral hepatitis.

Zakim, David, and Thomas Boyer, eds. *Hepatology: A Textbook of Liver Disease*. Philadelphia: W. B. Saunders, 1982. A thorough compendium on most aspects of liver disease. The book provides extensive discussion on the subject, with numerous diagrams and pictures. The section on hepatitis contains a complete clinical description of the disease and of the biology of the hepatitis viruses.

# HERNIA

**SYSTEMS AFFECTED:** Gastrointestinal, reproductive (male)
**SPECIALISTS:** General surgeons, internists
**DEFINITION:** A pouchlike mass consisting of visceral material encased in properitoneal tissue (the hernial sac) protruding through an aperture in the abdomen—a result of a weakening in the abdominal wall.

**KEY TERMS:**

*Bassini technique:* the most widely accepted surgical method for treating hernias; named after the Italian surgeon Edoardo Bassini

*hernioplasty:* the surgery performed to tread hernia patients

*incarceration:* an advanced and dangerous hernial stage which occurs when the hernial sac protrudes well beyond the abdominal sperture and is constricted at the neck

*inguinal hernia:* the most common form of hernia, in which the hernial sac protrudes into the lower groin area

*reducible hernia:* a hernia that has not advanced significantly beyond the weakened aperture in the abdomen; such hernias were formerly treated by means of the externally applied pressure of a truss

## Causes and Symptoms

A hernia condition exists when either tissues from, or actual portions of, vital internal organs protrude beyond the enclosure of the abdomen as a result of an abnormal opening in several possible areas of the abdominal wall. In most hernias, the protruding material remains encased in the tissue of the peritoneum. This saclike extension forces itself into whatever space can be ceded by neighboring tissues outside the abdomen. Because of the swelling effect produced, the hernia is usually visible as a lump on the surface of the body. As there are several types of hernias that may occur in different areas of the abdomen, the place of noticeable swelling and the internal organs affected may vary. With the single exception of the pancreas, hernia cases have been recorded involving all other organs contained in the abdomen. The most common hernial protrusions, however, involve the small intestine and/or the omenta, folds of the peritoneum. Another category of hernia, referred to as hernia adipose, consists of a protrusion of peritoneal fat beyond the abdominal wall.

Generally speaking, the cause of hernial conditions involves not only an internal pressure pushing portions of the viscera against the abdominal wall (hence the danger of bringing on a hernia through heavy physical exertion in work or athletics) but also a point of weakness in the abdominal wall itself. Two such points of potential weakness exist in all normal, healthy individuals: the original umbilical ring, which should normally "heal" over after the um-

### Hiatal Hernia

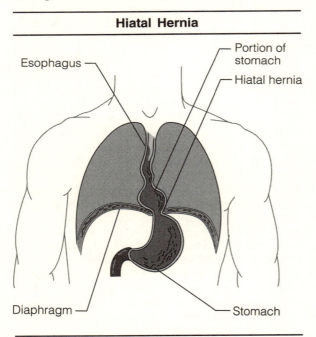

*A portion of the stomach has pushed through the weakened abdominal wall.*

bilical cord is severed; and the groin tissues in the lower portion of the abdomen—the region where the most common hernia, the inguinal hernia, occurs. Another possible source of vulnerability to hernia protrusions is connected to the individual's prior surgical history: Scar tissue may prove to be the weakest point of resistance to pressures originating anywhere in the abdominal region.

It should be noted that, because the abdominal tissues of infants and young children are particularly delicate, there is a proportionately higher occurrence of hernial conditions among babies and toddlers. If the hernia is diagnosed and treated early enough, complete healing is almost certain in such cases, most of which do not develop beyond the preliminary, or reducible, stage.

The several stages, or degrees, of hernial development usually begin with what doctors call a reducible hernia condition. At this stage, a patient suffering from hernia, sensing the onset of the disorder, may be able to obtain temporary relief from a developing protrusion by changing posture angle when upright or by lying down. Until the late twentieth century, some physicians preferred to treat reducible hernias by means of an externally attached pressure device, or truss, rather than resorting to surgical intervention. This form of treatment was gradually dropped in favor of increasingly effective hernioplasty operations.

When a hernial condition enters what is called the stage of incarceration, the advanced protrusion of the sac containing portions of viscera through the opening, or ring, in the abdominal wall can cause very severe complications. If, as is frequently the case, the protruding hernia sac passes through the ring as a fingerlike tube and then assumes a globular form outside the abdominal wall, a state of incarceration exists. As this state advances, the patient runs the risk of hernial strangulation. The constricting pressure of the ring's edges on the hernial sac interferes with circulatory functions in the herniated organ, causing destruction of tissues and, unless surgical intervention occurs, rapid spread of gangrene throughout the affected organ. It was the sixteenth century French surgeon Pierre Franco who carried out the first operation to release a strangulated hernia by inserting a thin instrument between the incarcerated bowel and the herniated sac, then incising the latter without touching the extruded vital organ.

A surprisingly wide range of hernial conditions have been noted and studied. These include hernias in the umbilical, epigastric (upper abdominal), spigelian (transversus abdominal muscle), interparietal, and groin regions. Hernias in the groin can be either femoral or inguinal. Inguinal hernias affecting the groin area have always been by far the most common, accounting for more than three-quarters of hernial cases, particularly among males.

Inguinal hernias share a number of common characteristics with one another and with the other closely associated form of groin hernia, the femoral hernia. Inguinal hernias are all caused by the abnormal introduction of a hernial sac into one of the 4 centimeter-long inguinal canals located on the sides of the abdomen. These canals originate in the lower portion of the abdomen at an aperture called the inguinal ring. They have an external exit point in the rectus abdominal tissue. Located inside each inguinal canal are the ilioinguinal nerve, the genital branch of the genitofemoral nerve, and the spermatic cord. A comparable passageway from the abdomen into the groin area is found at the femoral ring, through which both the femoral artery and the femoral vein pass.

It may take a long period, sometimes years, for the sac to engage itself fully in the inguinal or femoral ring. Once the ring is passed, however, pressures from inside the abdomen help it descend through the canal rather quickly. If the external inguinal ring is firm in structure, and particularly if the narrow passageway is largely filled with the thickness of the spermatic cord, the inguinal hernia may be partially arrested at this point. In men, once it passes beyond the external inguinal ring, however, it quickly descends into the scrotum. In women, the inguinal canal contains the round ligament, which may also temporarily impede the further descent of the hernial sac beyond the external inguinal opening.

### TREATMENT AND THERAPY

Given the widespread occurrence of hernia conditions at all age levels in most societies, physicians receive extensive training in the diagnosis and, among those with surgical training, the treatment of hernia patients. Near-total consensus among doctors now demands surgery (external trusses having been largely abandoned), but different schools support different surgical methods. With the exception of operations involving the insertion of prosthetic devices to block the extension of hernia damage, most recent inguinal hernioplasty methods derive from the model finalized by the Italian Edoardo Bassini in the late nineteenth century.

Bassini believed that the surgical methods of his time fell short of the goal of complete hernial repair, since most postoperational patients were required to wear a truss to guard against recurring problems. In the simplest of surgical terms, his solution involved the physiological reconstruction of the inguinal canal. The operation provided for a new internal passageway to an external opening, as well as strengthened anterior and posterior inguinal walls. After initial incisions and ligation of the hernial sac, Bassini's method involved a separation of tissues between the internal inguinal ring and the pubis. A tissue section referred to as the "triple layer" (containing the internal oblique, the transversus abdominal, and the transversalis fascia tissue layers) was then attached by a line of sutures to the Poupart ligament, with a lowermost suture at the edge of the rectus abdominal muscle. Such local reconstruction of the inguinal canal proved to strengthen the entire zone against the recurrence of ruptures.

Physicians operating on indirect, as opposed to direct, inguinal hernias confront a relatively uncomplicated set of procedures. In the former case, a high ligation of the peritoneal sac (a circular incision of the peritoneum at a point well inside the abdominal inguinal ring) usually makes it possible to remove the sac entirely. Complications can occur if the patient is obese, since a large mass of peritoneal fatty material may be joined to the sac, obstructing access to the inguinal ring. For normal indirect inguinal hernias, the next basic step, after ensuring that no damage has occurred to the viscera either during formation of the hernia or in the process of replacing the contents of the hernial sac inside the abdomen, is to use one of several surgical methods to reduce the opening of the inguinal ring to its normal size. The physician must also ensure that no damage to the posterior inguinal wall has occurred and that its essential attachment to Cooper's ligament does not require additional surgical attention.

One must contrast the relative simplicity of indirect inguinal hernia surgery to treatment of direct inguinal hernias. In these cases, the hernia does not protrude through the existing inguinal aperture, but, as a result of a weakening of local tissues, passes directly through the posterior inguinal wall. The direct inguinal hernia is usually characterized by a broad base at the point of protrusion and a relatively short hernial sac. When a physician recommends surgical treatment of such hernias, the surgeon must be prepared for the extensive task of surgical reconstruction of the posterior inguinal wall as part of the operation.

Two additional reasons tend to discourage an immediate decision to operate on direct inguinal hernias. First, this form of hernia rarely strangulates the affected viscera, since the aperture stretches to allow protrusion of the hernial sac. Second, once physicians find obvious symptoms of a direct inguinal hernia (a ceding of the weakened posterior inguinal wall to pressures originating in the abdomen), they may decide to examine the patient more thoroughly to determine if the cause behind the symptoms demands an entirely different prognosis. Such causes of abdominal pressures may range from the effects of a chronic cough to much more serious problems, including inflammation of the prostate gland or other forms of obstruction in the colon itself.

### PERSPECTIVE AND PROSPECTS

Because the phenomenon of hernias has been the subject of scientific observation since the onset of formal medical writing itself, there was a stage-by-stage development of prognoses associated with this condition. A main dividing line appears between the mid-eighteenth and mid-nineteenth centuries, however, between the extremely rudimentary surgical treatments of the late Middle Ages and Renaissance and what can be called modern prognoses.

No doubt the surgical contribution of the sixteenth century Frenchman Pierre Franco, who performed the first operation to release an incarcerated hernia, must be considered a landmark. The major general cause for advancement in knowledge of hernias, however, is tied to the birth of a new era in medical science, characterized by the use, from about 1750 onward, of anatomical dissection to investigate the essential characteristics of a number of common diseases.

Before the relatively long line of contributions that led to general adoption of the Bassini technique of operating on hernias, surgeons tended to follow the so-called Langenbeck method, named after the German physician who pioneered modern hernioplasty. This method held that simple removal of a hernial sac at the point of its protrusion from the abdomen and closing the external aperture would lead to a closing of the sac by "adhesive inflammation." Such spontaneous closing occurs when a severed artery "recedes" to the first branching off point.

It took contributions by at least two lesser-known late nineteenth century forerunners to Edoardo Bassini to convince the surgical world that hernia operations must involve a high incision of the hernial sac. Both the American H. O. Marcy (1837-1924) and the Frenchman Just Marie Marcellin Lucas-Championnière (1843-1913) have been recognized for their insistence on the necessity of high-incision operations. Their hernia operations, by incising the external oblique fascia, were the first to penetrate well beyond the external ring to expose the entire hernial sac. Following removal of the sac, it was then possible for surgeons to close the transversalis fascia and to repair the higher interior tissues that might have been damaged by the swollen hernia.

Following initial acceptance of the technique of high-incision hernial operations, a number of physicians recommended a variety of methods that might be used to repair internal tissue damage. These methods ranged from simple ligation of the sac at the internal ring, without more extensive surgery involving either the abdominal wall or the spermatic cord, to the much more extensive method practiced by Bassini. Even after the Bassini method succeeded in gaining almost universal recognition, other adaptations (but nothing that represented a full innovation) would be added during the middle decades of the twentieth century. One such method, which borrowed from the German physician Georg Lotheissen's use of Cooper's ligament to serve as a foundation for suturing damaged layers of lower abdominal tissues, earned its proponent, the American Chester McVay, the honor of having the operation named after him.

Finally, one should note that, although few significant changes have occurred in most doctors' view of what must be done surgically to treat hernia patients, surgical use of laser beams in the 1990's began to affect the techniques of hernioplasty, particularly in terms of recovery time.

—*Byron D. Cannon*

**See also** Abdominal disorders; Gastrointestinal disorders; Hemorrhoids; Intestinal disorders.

## FOR FURTHER INFORMATION:

Gaster, Joseph. *Hernia: One Day Repair*. Darien, Conn.: Hafner, 1970. Intended to provide a practical surgical guide to the various methods of operating on different forms of hernias. Also contains a very useful review of the historical evolution of anatomical science relating to hernial problems.

McVay, Chester Bidwell. *Hernia: The Pathologic Anatomy of the More Common Hernias and Their Anatomic Repair*. Springfield, Ill.: Charles C Thomas, 1954. Despite the somewhat dated nature of the technical material in this manual, the style of presentation makes it very readable for the layperson.

Nyhus, Lloyd M., and Robert E. Condon, eds. *Hernia*. 3d ed. Philadelphia: J. B. Lippincott, 1989. Widely recognized and updated joint contribution by a large number of specialized physicians.

Ponka, Joseph L. *Hernias of the Abdominal Wall*. Philadelphia: W. B. Saunders, 1980. A general medical textbook containing excellent illustrative plates.

Zimmerman, Leo M., and Barry J. Anson. *Anatomy and Surgery of Hernia*. 2d ed. Baltimore: Williams & Wilkins, 1967. The most readable medically technical account, although less current than the Nyhus and Condon textbook listed above.

# HERNIATED DISK. *See* SLIPPED DISK.

# HERPES

**SYSTEMS AFFECTED:** Reproductive, mucous membranes

**SPECIALISTS:** Family physicians, gynecologists, internists

**DEFINITION:** A family of viruses that cause several diseases, including infectious mononucleosis, cold sores, genital herpes, and chickenpox; for most individuals, these widespread diseases are mild and of brief duration, but they may be fatal to those with impaired immune systems.

**KEY TERMS:**

*antibody:* a protein found in the blood and produced by the immune system in response to bodily contact with a foreign substance, such as a virus

*congenital disease:* a disease resulting from heredity or acquired while in the womb

*disseminated:* spread throughout the body

*immune system:* the body system that is responsible for fighting off infectious disease

*immunocompromised:* a condition in which the immune system is impaired in some way, such as being not fully developed, deficient, or suppressed

*latent:* lying hidden or concealed

*primary infection:* a person's first infection with a particular virus

*recurrent infection:* an infection caused by the reactivation of a latent virus

*vaccine:* a substance given in order to prevent or ameliorate the effect of some disease

*virus:* the simplest entity that can reproduce; viruses are essentially made of some genetic material in a protective coating; viruses can reproduce only inside a living cell

### TYPES OF HERPESVIRUS

Herpesviruses that affect humans include herpes simplex virus types 1 and 2, Epstein-Barr virus, varicella-zoster virus, and cytomegalovirus. Herpesviruses cause three types of infections: primary, latent, and recurrent. Most first-time, or primary, infections with herpesviruses cause few or no symptoms in the victim. Following the primary infection, herpesviruses have the unique ability to become latent, or hidden, in the body. Latent infections may persist for the life of the individual with no further symptoms, or the virus may reactivate (come out of hiding) and cause a recurrent infection. Although herpesvirus infections are often mild in healthy persons, they can cause potentially fatal infections in immunocompromised patients. Persons in this group include infants, whose immune systems are not fully developed; immunodeficient persons, whose immune systems are lacking some important component; and immunosuppressed patients, such as cancer or transplant patients, whose immune systems are being suppressed by immunosuppressive drugs or radiation. Herpesviruses have also been implicated in the causes of certain types of cancer.

Herpes simplex viruses exist in two forms: type 1 (HSV1) and type 2 (HSV2). HSV1 and HSV2 infections cause the formation of painful or itchy vesicular (blister-like) lesions, which ulcerate, crust over, and heal within a few weeks. The virus is transmitted from one person to another by direct contact with infected lesions, and the virus enters the recipient through broken skin or mucous membranes. HSV1 usually causes infections above the waist; for example, in the mouth, throat, eye, skin, and brain. Gingivostomatitis, the most common form of primary HSV1 infection, is seen mostly in small children and is characterized by ulcerative lesions inside the mouth. Herpes labialis, or cold sores, the most common recurrent disease caused by HSV1, is characterized by blisters on the outer portion of the lips. HSV1 can also cause infection in any area of the skin where trauma (for example, a burn, scrape, or eczema) gives the virus an opening to get in. HSV1 infection of the eye can lead to scarring and blindness, and HSV1 infection of the brain can lead to death. Genital herpes, a disease transmitted by sexual contact, is most often caused by HSV2. The virus infects the penis in males and the cervix, vulva, vagina, or perineum in females. Two to seven days after infection, painful blisters appear in the genital area that ulcerate, crust over, and disappear in a few weeks. Fever, stress, sunlight, or local trauma may trigger the virus to come out of hiding and cause a recurrent infection, and about 88 percent of persons with a HSV2 genital infection will have recurrences at a frequency of up to

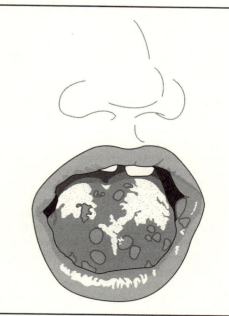

*The herpesvirus is responsible for the common cold sore.*

five to eight times per year. A severe form of HSV2 infection, neonatal herpes, occurs when a mother suffering from genital herpes passes the virus to her baby as it travels through the birth canal during delivery. This type of infection is usually disseminated, its death rate is high, and its survivors suffer from severe neurological damage.

Varicella-zoster virus (VZV) causes two diseases: Chickenpox (varicella) and shingles (zoster). Chickenpox is a highly contagious common childhood disease caused by a primary infection with VZV. The virus is transmitted during close personal contact with an infected patient via airborne droplets that enter the respiratory tract or direct contact with skin lesions. Once inside a person, the virus travels from the respiratory tract to the blood, and then to the skin. Ten to twenty-one days after infection, a typical rash appears on the skin and mucous membranes. On skin, the rash begins as red spots that develop into clear, fluid-filled vesicles that become cloudy, ulcerate, scab over, and fall off in a few days. Mucous membrane lesions in the mouth, eyelid, rectum, and vagina rupture easily and appear as ulcers. Fever, headache, tiredness, and itching may accompany the rash. Recovery from chickenpox confers lifelong immunity to reinfection but not latency. Reye's syndrome, an occasional severe complication of chickenpox, is associated with the use of aspirin. A few days after the initial infection has receded, the patient persistently vomits and exhibits signs of brain dysfunction. Coma and death can follow if the syndrome is not treated. Chickenpox infection in adults is often more severe than in children, and adults run the risk of developing a fatal lung or brain infection.

Individuals with prior varicella infection may later develop shingles, which is caused by the reactivation of latent VZV. More than 65 percent of cases of shingles appear in adults older than forty-five years of age. The mechanism of reactivation is unknown, but recurrence is often associated with physical and emotional stress or a suppressed immune system. Shingles is usually localized to one area of the skin; it begins with pain in the nerves, and then a chickenpox-like rash appears on the skin over the nerves. The pain may be severe for one to four weeks, and recovery occurs in two to five weeks, with pain persisting longer in some elderly patients.

Epstein-Barr virus (EBV) causes infectious mononucleosis, an infection of the lymphatic system. In infected persons, the virus is present in saliva and blood, and thus it is transmitted by intimate oral contact (for example, kissing), sharing food or drinks, or by blood transfusions. Primary infection early in life usually causes no symptoms of disease, whereas primary infection later in life usually causes symptoms of infectious mononucleosis. In countries where sanitation is poor, most people have been infected by the age of five, without symptoms. In contrast, in countries where sanitation is good, primary infection is delayed until adolescence or young adulthood, and thus more than half the people in this age group develop symptoms. Once the infection begins, the virus grows in the throat and spreads to blood and lymph, invading white blood cells called B lymphocytes. The typical symptoms of infectious mononucleosis are extreme exhaustion, sore throat, fever, swollen lymph nodes, and sometimes an enlarged liver and spleen. The disease is self-limiting, and recovery takes place in four to eight weeks. The virus remains latent in the blood, lymphoid tissue, and throat and can continue to be transmitted to others even when no signs of active infection are present. EBV infection has also been associated with chronic fatigue syndrome and several types of cancer.

The widespread cytomegalovirus (CMV) is responsible for a broad spectrum of diseases. As is the case with EBV infection, primary infection by CMV early in life usually results in no symptoms, while primary infection as an adult yields mononucleosis-like symptoms. CMV also causes congenital cytomegalic inclusion disease and is a significant danger to bone marrow transplant patients. The virus is found in body secretions such as saliva, urine, semen, cervical secretions and breast milk. Babies may acquire the virus from infected mothers congenitally, during birth while passing through the birth canal, or through breast milk. Children in day care may acquire CMV from other children who orally excrete the virus, and parents may get it from their children. CMV may be acquired through sexual transmission and blood transfusions. Patients undergoing transplants, especially bone marrow transplants, are at higher risk for CMV infection, since the virus may be present in the transplanted organs. The mononucleosis-like disease caused by CMV has the same symptoms as EBV-induced mononucleosis except the sore throat, swollen lymph nodes, and enlarged spleen. Congenital cytomegalic inclusion disease causes severe neurological damage, mental retardation, and death in infants; it is a result of primary CMV infection of the mother during pregnancy.

## CAUSES, SYMPTOMS, AND TREATMENTS

A physician can often tell whether a person has an HSV infection based on the presence of the characteristic lesions and a history of exposure or previous lesions. For more severe HSV infections, the virus can be isolated and identified from infected tissue to confirm HSV as the causative agent. The major treatment procedure for most mild HSV infections is supportive care. These measures, such as bed rest and anti-itch or anti-pain medication, treat the symptoms but not the infection. For most infections, the symptoms eventually go away by themselves. For more severe HSV infections, several antiviral drugs have been used. Idoxuridine and trifluridine have been used to treat eye infections. Vidarabine and acyclovir are used to treat encephalitis and disseminated disease; both reduce the severity of the infection but do not reverse any neurological damage or prevent recurrent infections. Acyclovir has also been useful in reducing the duration of primary genital herpes, but not recurrent infection. The use of oral acyclovir to suppress recurrent infection may cause more severe and more frequent infections once the therapy has stopped. The best way to prevent infection with HSV is to avoid contact with a person with active lesions. Victims of genital herpes should avoid all sexual contact during episodes of lesions, to avoid transmitting the virus to someone else. Using condoms may be somewhat helpful in preventing the sexual transmission of HSV2. Newborns, children with eczema or other skin problems, burn patients, and immunocompromised patients should avoid persons with active HSV lesions. Pregnant females with active genital lesions must be delivered by cesarean section, in order to prevent the infection of their infants.

A diagnosis of chickenpox or shingles is based mainly on the symptoms of the patient, since they are so characteristic. It is possible to grow the virus from tissue samples or test the person for antibodies to VZV if necessary. Chickenpox takes care of itself and disappears after a few weeks; therefore, the only treatment needed is supportive care for the patient during that time. Often, drying lotions such as calamine help relieve the itching. It is important to cut the fingernails of especially young children so that they cannot scratch hard enough to break through the skin and leave themselves susceptible to secondary bacterial infection. It is extremely important not to give a child aspirin for the fever, because of the association between the use of aspirin during chickenpox and the development of Reye's syndrome. A child may be given acetaminophen if necessary. Zoster is treated mostly with pain medication to control the pain. Steroids given early in the infection help reduce the severity of the infection, and acyclovir increases the rate of recovery. Antiviral drugs such as acyclovir, interferon, and vidarabine have been used in the treatment of immunocompromised patients with chickenpox to help reduce the potential severe complications of the disease. For most healthy persons, it is not necessary to prevent chickenpox, since it is a mild disease. It is important for newborns and immunocompromised patients to avoid exposure to persons with chickenpox because of threats such as pneumonia, encephalitis, and death. Since 1981, varicella-zoster immune globin (VZIG) has been available for the prevention and treatment of chickenpox in these patients. VZIG provides a short time of immunity, can lessen symptoms, and is recommended for immunocompromised children exposed to chickenpox, but it has no value once chickenpox has started. A VZV vaccine has been developed and shown to provide temporary protection from severe infection in immunocompromised children. This vaccine is not useful for the general population because the immunity gained is short-term and might result in more persons getting the disease later in life, which is a more dangerous time to get chickenpox.

Unlike diagnoses of most VZV or HSV infections, the diagnosis of an EBV infection cannot be made based on the symptoms alone, because the virus causes a wide range of symptoms that could be caused by many other disease-causing agents. The diagnosis of EBV infection is made, therefore, based on laboratory tests. One test is a blood test in which technicians count the number of and kinds of white blood cells present in a patient. Persons with infectious mononucleosis have an abnormally large number of lymphocytes (one type of white blood cell) in their blood, and many of these lymphocytes have an odd appearance. A second test involves mixing the patients' blood serum (the fluid portion from their blood) with the red blood cells of sheep. The serum from 90 percent of persons with infectious mononucleosis will cause the sheep cells to clump. It is unknown why serum from infectious mononucleosis patients has this odd property (referred to as heterophil-positive). Persons suspected of having EBV but who give a heterophil-negative test are tested more rigorously for antibodies in their blood that are specific for the EBV virus. The isolation of EBV from patients is not routinely performed to confirm a diagnosis of EBV infection, because the techniques needed are too complex for most laboratories. Infectious mononucleosis is a self-limiting disease, which means that it will eventually run its course and go away. Therefore, treatment involves mostly supportive care, such as bed rest and aspirin or acetaminophen for the fever and sore throat. It is also recommended that mononucleosis patients avoid contact sports, to prevent possible rupture of an enlarged spleen. In some severe cases, steroids are administered, and antiviral drugs are in the process of being

tested to determine whether they are of any therapeutic value. The best way to prevent an EBV infection is to avoid intimate contact (for example, kissing) with an infected individual. Unfortunately, many persons shed EBV virus in their saliva without exhibiting any symptoms, so one cannot always tell who is infected and who is not.

Like EBV infection, CMV infection causes vague symptoms, and therefore diagnosis depends on laboratory tests. The virus can be grown from tissue samples, tissue can be examined to look for typical infected cells or the presence of virus, or the blood can be tested to look for antibodies to CMV. Mild cases of CMV need no treatment except supportive measures. Antiviral drugs such as interferon, vidarabine, idoxuridine, and cytosine arabinoside as well as CMV immune globin have all been tested for their benefit in severe cases of CMV infections, but none has been successful. The drug ganciclovir has been shown to have some therapeutic value. Most preventive measures have been aimed at developing a vaccine to prevent congenital CMV and CMV infection in immunosuppressed patients. A CMV vaccine has been developed, but further work is needed. Until better measures are available, it is important to try to avoid infection in immunocompromised patients, especially transplant recipients. The screening of organ donors for the presence of CMV may be helpful in accomplishing this goal. In addition, to prevent congenital CMV, pregnant females need to avoid primary CMV infection during their pregnancies. All pregnant females should be tested for CMV antibodies to determine whether they have already been infected; if not, they should avoid contact with small children who might carry CMV.

## PERSPECTIVE AND PROSPECTS

Between 20 and 40 percent of the people in the United States suffer from cold sores, and more than 20 million persons suffer from genital herpes. In addition, HSV1 infection of the eye is the most common cause of corneal blindness in the United States, and HSV2 infection is associated with an increased risk of cervical cancer, which strikes some 15,000 women each year. Two hundred babies in the United States die each year, and 200 more suffer physical or mental impairment caused by HSV infection.

Chickenpox is the second most reported disease in the United States, with more than 200,000 cases per year. This number is probably too low, since many cases go unreported. About 100 deaths per year are attributed to chickenpox.

EBV infection is worldwide, and EBV antibodies can be found in more than 90 percent of most adult populations. EBV infection has been shown to be an important factor in the development of Burkitt's lymphoma (a cancer of the jaw) in Africa and nasopharyngeal carcinoma (a fatal cancer of the nose) in China. EBV has also been linked to chronic fatigue syndrome, but the relationship is not conclusive.

CMV infection is worldwide, with 40 to 100 percent of a population possessing antibodies to CMV. Almost all kidney transplant recipients and half of bone marrow recipients get CMV infection. Congenital CMV infection is the cause of severe neurological damage in more than 5,000 children born each year in the United States.

It is clear from these facts that infections with herpesviruses are a very important public health problem. The infections are widespread, and they cause a significant amount of distress, sickness, and death. The development of vaccines and other drugs to treat these diseases is important for infants and other immunocompromised persons whose lives can be threatened by acquiring a herpesvirus infection. The viruses' ability to become latent and the lack of drugs to destroy the latent viruses, however, make it virtually impossible to eradicate these diseases from the human population. Persons are infected for life, and they may continue to transmit the infection to other persons. Many other viral diseases, such as smallpox, measles, and polio, have been controlled by the use of vaccines that prevent a person from getting the disease, but the development of vaccines for herpesviruses is a complex problem. First, most of the diseases they cause are mild and self-limiting, so there is no pressing need to develop a vaccine quickly. Second, the association of the viruses with cancer causes scientists to proceed with caution in the development of a vaccine. Third, even if a vaccine does become available, it will be a long time before the viruses will be gone from the human population. Since herpesviruses can remain hidden in a person and stay there for life, they will not disappear until all currently infected persons die.

—*Vicki J. Isola*

*See also* Cervical, ovarian, and uterine cancers; Chickenpox; Chronic fatigue syndrome; Mononucleosis; Reye's syndrome; Sexually transmitted diseases; Shingles; Viral infections; Warts.

**For Further Information:**

Langston, D. P. *Living with Herpes*. Garden City, N.Y.: Doubleday, 1983. Written to help patients suffering from herpesvirus infections to understand the disease better. Discusses all types of herpesvirus infections, with a particular emphasis on genital herpes.

Nourse, A. E. *Herpes*. New York: Franklin Watts, 1985. A well-written, informative, and easy-to-read book. Focuses mostly on genital herpes but also includes information on other sexually transmitted diseases and the other herpesvirus infections.

Radetsky, Peter. *The Invisible Invaders*. Boston: Little, Brown, 1991. Discusses viruses in general, how they were discovered, and the diseases they cause. Chapter 10 gives an interesting account of the discovery of the links between EBV infection and chronic fatigue syndrome, infectious mononucleosis, and Burkitt's lymphoma.

Stoff, J. A., and C. R. Pellegrino. *Chronic Fatigue Syndrome*. New York: Random House, 1988. Discusses EBV and its relationship to chronic fatigue syndrome.

Wickett, W. H. *Herpes: Cause and Control*. New York: Pinnacle Books, 1982. Written for the intelligent layperson. Includes descriptions of all forms of HSV infection, other viral infections, and sexually transmitted diseases. Much of the book tells how to take care of oneself if one is infected with a herpesvirus.

Zinsser, Hans. *Zinsser Microbiology*. 19th ed. Edited by W. K. Joklik et al. Norwalk, Conn.: Appleton and Lange, 1988. The information presented in this textbook is thorough, logical, and supplemented by interesting diagrams, photographs, and charts. Chapter 66, "Herpesviruses," gives a complete description of infections with HSV, VZV, EBV, and CMV.

## HIV. *See* Human immunodeficiency virus (HIV).

## Hodgkin's disease

**System affected:** Lymphatic

**Specialists:** Hematologists, internists, oncologists

**Definition:** A neoplastic disorder originating in the tissues of the lymphatic system, recognized by distinctive histologic changes and defined by the presence of Reed-Sternberg cells.

**Key terms:**

*chemotherapy:* a modality of cancer treatment consisting of the administration of cytotoxic drugs

*combination chemotherapy:* the use of multiple chemical agents in the treatment of cancer, each in a lower dosage so that the overall toxicity, but not the effectiveness, is reduced

*neoplastic:* pertaining to cancerous growths

*prognosis:* a prediction of the outcome of treatment for a disease on the basis of clinical and pathologic parameters, such as pathology, clinical stage, and presence or absence of symptoms such as fever, night sweats, and unexplained weight loss

*radiotherapy:* the use of radiation to kill cancer cells or shrink cancerous growth; when high and full doses of radiation (measured in units called rads) are used, the patient is said to be given a "megavoltage"

### Causes and Symptoms

Malignant lymphomas are neoplasms of lymphoid tissues and are of two general categories: those related to Hodgkin's disease and others that are collectively called non-Hodgkin's lymphomas. The lymphoid tissues represent the structural expressions of the immune system, which defends the body against microbes. This system is widely spread throughout the body, is highly complex, and interacts closely with other physiologic systems of the body—especially the mucosa that lines the airways and digestive tract, where there is direct exposure to environmental microbes and other foreign substances. The components of this system are aggregations of lymphocytes in the mucosal linings (such as tonsils and adenoids), lymph nodes, and the spleen. The components of the lymphatic system connect with one another via small lymphatic vessels. The lymph nodes, which are situated in anatomical regions all over the body, interconnect and drain centrally toward the great veins of the body. The cellular components of the immune system are the lymphocytes, also called immunocytes. These account for about 20 percent of blood cells; lymphocytes make up the bulk of the lymphoid tissue that makes up the lymphatic system. The blood cells have a finite life and are disposed of in the spleen, which is the largest lymphoid organ in the body.

There are two major functional immunologic classes of lymphocytes and several other subclasses. Nevertheless, all share similar morphologic appearance, being small round cells almost completely occupied by a round nucleus. The B lymphocyte (the B refers to its bone-marrow derivation) can, under proper antigenic stimulation, transform and mature into a plasma cell, which is the cell in charge of producing antibodies. Antibodies are the protein products of the immune system that act by capturing and removing foreign substances, called antigens. The other major class of lymphocytes is the T lymphocyte (the T refers to its thymus derivation). T lymphocytes are of at least two major functional subclasses, which either help or suppress the B lymphocyte in its transformation into plasma cell; thus they are termed helper and suppressor T cells, respectively. Other cellular components of the immune system, cellular monocytes and macrophages, play an important role in carrying and transferring specific immunologic information between the various cellular components of the immune-lymphatic system. This, then, is a highly organized and complex system, with positive and negative biofeedbacks that maintain optimal, balanced proportions of all the cellular components that make up the system.

Hodgkin's disease is a neoplasm of the lymphoid tissues that usually arises in lymph nodes, often in the neck, and has varied histologic appearance characterized by the presence of Reed-Sternberg cells. The Reed-Sternberg cell is a giant cell having two nuclei that are situated in a mirror-image fashion. Treatment and prognosis in Hodgkin's disease are determined by two parameters: the histopathologic classification, whereby the morphologic appearance is evaluated by the pathologist, and the clinical staging classification, whereby the extent of spread of the disease and its localization are determined by clinical studies. The pathology is studied by reviewing thinly cut sections of diseased lymph nodes removed from the patient. This study is most important for establishing a diagnosis of Hodgkin's disease and ruling out other conditions that may closely simulate its clinical and/or pathologic features. At times, peer consultations are used to confirm the diagnosis.

Reed-Sternberg cells have a characteristic appearance and must be identified to make a diagnosis of Hodgkin's disease. The pathologic classification of this disease, based on microscopic study, recognizes four different types, each with its own clinical implications regarding survival and prognosis. The classification is based on the relative dominance of lymphocytes when compared to the number of the neoplastic Reed-Sternberg cells. In the most favorable type, the lymphocytes predominate and Reed-Sternberg cells are sparse; this type is called lymphocyte predominance. In the worst type, the lymphocytes are very sparse and there are many more Reed-Sternberg cells and their variants; this type is called lymphocyte depletion. In between these two extremes are the mixed-cellularity type, in which there is an even mixture of lymphocytes and Reed-Sternberg cells, and nodular sclerosis, which forms nodules of fibrous scar tissue that surround the mixture of lymphocytes and Reed-Sternberg cells.

This classification has important prognostic implications. It correctly presumes that the neoplastic cell is the Reed-Sternberg cell and its variants, and that the lymphocytes are induced by the immune system to multiply and to fight the spread of the neoplastic cells. It follows that the more the process is successful, the better is the prognosis. Hence lymphocyte predominance carries a more favorable outlook than lymphocyte depletion, with mixed-cellularity type somewhere in between. Nodular sclerosis also carries a good prognosis. Other inflammatory cells are invariably mixed with the lymphocytes and Reed-Sternberg cells; these cells are also part of the body's immune response against cancer cells.

The clinical staging classification of Hodgkin's disease was formulated by a group of experts who met at a workshop in Ann Arbor, Michigan, in 1971. It is based on the proposition that the disease begins in a single group of lymph nodes (usually in the neck) and then spreads to the next adjacent group of lymph nodes, on the same side, before it crosses over to the other side of the body. The disease then advances further across the diaphragm muscle, which separates the thorax from the abdominal cavity, and finally disseminates into the blood to involve the bone marrow and other distant sites. In this schema, stage I represents early stage, with involvement of only a single lymph node region, and stage II is when two or more such regions are involved on the same side of the diaphragm (that is, either above or below the diaphragm).

In the United States, Hodgkin's disease is an uncommon neoplasm accounting for 7,900 cases, or fewer than 1 percent of all new cases of cancer, and 1,500 deaths, according to the 1993 American Cancer Society's statistics. This represents an incidence in the United States of 3.2 per 100,000 population overall, with slightly higher incidence in males than females, and in whites than blacks. Incidence trends show a mild rise for the nodular sclerosis type in young adults and a mild decrease of Hodgkin's disease over the age of forty.

## Staging of Hodgkin's Disease

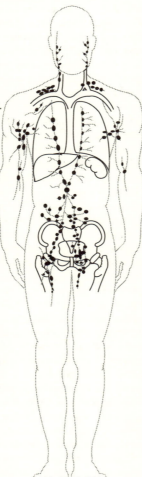

**Stage I**
Disease involves only a
single lymph node region.

**Stage II**
All lesions are on one
side of the diaphragm.

**Stage III**
Disease is on both
sides of diaphragm.

**Stage IV**
Widespread involvement
of extralymphoid sites:
spleen, marrow, liver, etc.

Hodgkin's disease can occur at any age, although the highest peak incidence occurs in adolescents and young adults and smaller peaks occur in the fifth and sixth decades of life. Most patients come to clinical attention because of painless, nontender, enlarged lymph nodes in the neck or armpits (above the diaphragm) or, less commonly, in the groin. In the young adult or adolescent, a mass in the chest may press against the airways to produce a dry, hacking cough and shortness of breath, which may be the patient's first symptoms. Some patients may have anemia or severe itching. At times, especially when the disease is aggressive and extensive, the patient may have a fever, which may run for a few days and then disappear, only to recur after a week or two; there can also be night sweats and weight loss. These symptoms—fever, night sweats, and weight loss—indicate a less favorable prognosis. Younger patients

and those with lymphocyte predominance and nodular sclerosis histologic types (favorable histologic types) tend to have limited disease—that is, stages I and II—found primarily above the diaphragm. Older patients and those with mixed-cellularity or lymphocyte depletion types are more likely to have extensive disease involving lymph nodes on both sides of the diaphragm (stage III) or even involving the liver, spleen, and bone marrow (Stage IV).

When a patient with persistent lymph node enlargement seeks medical attention, a lymph node biopsy is usually made to make sure of the diagnosis. There is a long list of benign conditions that may simulate Hodgkin's disease and must be excluded, such as infectious mononucleosis and tuberculosis, as well as other cancers. A series of blood tests, X-ray and other imaging studies, and a bone marrow biopsy are done in order to evaluate the spread of disease and to assign the proper clinical stage. At times, even surgical exploration of the abdomen, with biopsies of abdominal lymph nodes, the liver, and the spleen, is done to assign an accurate stage of Hodgkin's disease; this procedure is called staging laparotomy.

### TREATMENT AND THERAPY

Modern cancer therapy has achieved its greatest triumph in the treatment of Hodgkin's disease. The advent of a generally acceptable histopathologic classification, accurate staging, improved radiotherapy, effective chemotherapy, and supportive care, such as antibiotics and the transfusion of platelets, has contributed to the impressive 75 percent overall cure rate. The therapy is enhanced by an effective teamwork of medical experts in oncology, radiation therapy, surgery, pathology, and diagnostic radiology.

Because Hodgkin's disease spreads in an orderly fashion through adjacent lymph node groups, effective high-dose radiation can be directed at affected lymph nodes and at their neighboring, uninvolved nodes. Irradiation, with a full dose of 3,500 to 4,000 rads in three to four weeks, can eradicate Hodgkin's disease in involved nodes within the treatment field more than 95 percent of the time. In addition, extended-field irradiation of the adjacent uninvolved nodes is a standard practice used to eradicate minimal or early disease in these lymph nodes.

Stages I and II can be treated with radiotherapy alone by an extended field to include all lymph-node-bearing areas above the diaphragm (the axilla, neck, and chest), and in most cases the lymph nodes in the abdomen. Such treatment cures about 90 percent of patients. For patients in which the disease is found extensively in the chest, chemotherapy is added to the radiotherapy and results in prolonged, relapse-free survival in 85 percent of patients.

A variety of cytotoxic drugs (those that kill cells) are available to treat Hodgkin's disease. Such drugs are similar to nitrogen mustard (which was once used in war) and are toxic to the body. It has been found that when more than one drug is used, each with a smaller dose, the toxicity can be reduced without diminishing effectiveness. Thus combination chemotherapy has evolved. There are many effective regimens of combination chemotherapy that are called by the initials of the individual components; the most widely used of these is called MOPP (mechlorethamine, Oncovin, procarbazine, and prednisone). In stage III, chemotherapy with or without radiotherapy is used, depending upon specific variations within the stage, with cure rates achieved in 75 to 80 percent of patients. Even in stage IV disease, combination chemotherapy (particularly with MOPP) has produced a complete remission in about 75 percent of patients, with a cure rate of more than 50 percent.

Bone marrow transplantation, which is the intravenous infusion of normal marrow cells into the patient shortly after treatment in order to protect the patient from toxicity, has permitted the use of much higher doses of certain drugs. It allows the therapist to irradiate all the patient's bone marrow, eradicating both "good" and "bad" cells, with the hope that the normal marrow cells that are infused will populate the bone marrow and grow there. Bone marrow transplantation has been successfully used mainly in young patients who were resistent to conventional chemotherapy.

## PERSPECTIVE AND PROSPECTS

Thomas Hodgkin of Guy's Hospital in London was the first to recognize the disease that would bear his name. In 1832, he described the gross autopsy findings and clinical features of seven patients who had simultaneous enlargement of grossly diseased lymph nodes and spleens, and he considered the condition to be a primary affection of these organs. This condition, he himself records, was vaguely outlined by Marcello Malpighi in 1665. Four years earlier than Hodgkin, David Craige had described the autopsy findings of a similar case. Subsequent histologic examination of tissues from Hodgkin's original cases confirmed the disease in three of them. In 1865, Sir Samuel Wilks elaborated on the autopsy studies of similar cases and published the findings on fifteen patients, calling the condition Hodgkin's disease.

Important histopathologic observations were contributed by William Greenfield in 1878 and E. Goldman in 1892. George Sternberg described the giant cells but believed the condition to be a peculiar form of tuberculosis. The recognition that these cells were an integral part of the disease awaited the careful pathologic observation of Dorothy Reed of The Johns Hopkins Hospital in Baltimore. These cells, appropriately named Reed-Sternberg cells, are the hallmark of Hodgkin's disease.

Controversy as to the nature of this disease led early investigators to study infectious agents as possible etiologic causes, especially the tuberculosis bacillus, but to no avail. More recent studies have examined the roles of other viral infectious agents, especially the agent of infectious mononucleosis, but with no consistent results. At present, the condition is accepted as neoplastic, probably triggered by some unknown environmental agent or agents.

Between 1930 and 1950, major advances included the recognition of meaningful histologic subtypes of Hodgkin's disease correlating with prognosis, and the development by Vera Peters of a clinical staging system. Impressive responses to X-ray therapy were reported at the beginning of the twentieth century, and treatment with megavoltage therapy was further developed. By World War II, it became realistic to speak of curing some patients with early Hodgkin's disease. The potential for a cure meant that accurate histologic diagnosis and estimation of the extent and localization of disease was imperative in planning treatment; a multidisciplinary approach to the diagnosis and treatment was developed. Modern concepts of histologic classification became codified at a conference held in Rye, New York, in 1965, and the clinical staging system was refined into its present form at a workshop held at Ann Arbor, Michigan, in 1971.

Modern effective chemotherapy was developed concurrently with these advances in classification, staging, and radiotherapy. The alkylating agents, created as an outgrowth of studies on nitrogen mustard gas during World War II, provided the first drugs to produce impressive shrinkage of the tumor and significant palliation of the disease. The subsequent developments in modern pharmacology and therapeutics enabled Vince DeVita and his coworkers, in 1970, to design the first effective combination chemotherapy regimen, MOPP.

Today, many more such regimens are being tested; the possibility for cure has become a realistic hope for every patient with Hodgkin's disease. This is the case because of the refinement of ancillary therapies with antibiotics (for infections that may occur during the necessary phases of suppression of the immune system by these powerful toxic drugs) and platelet transfusion technology. Bone marrow transplantation technology also offers strong hope for the possibility of curing of patients with advanced cases who are resistant. The bone marrow is harvested and then reintroduced into a patient whose marrow has been effectively disabled. Immunotherapy is also being investigated. It can boost the patient's ability to combat disease by modulating the body's responses. The drawback to aggressive combinations of chemotherapy and radiotherapy, however, is the emergence of therapy-related leukemia and leukemia-like malignancies several years after the completion of successful therapy for Hodgkin's disease.

—*Victor H. Nassar*

*See also* Cancer; Lymphadenopathy and lymphoma; Malignancy and metastasis.

## FOR FURTHER INFORMATION:

*CA: A Cancer Journal for Clinicians* 43, no. 1. January/ February, 1993. A journal published by the American Cancer Society. This special issue is devoted to a discussion of cancer statistics, including those regarding Hodgkin's disease.

Garrison, Fielding H. *History of Medicine*. 4th ed. Philadelphia: W. B. Saunders, 1960. A textbook that contains a review of the life and times of Thomas Hodgkin, the British physician who first described Hodgkin's disease.

Kampe, W. A., G. B. Humphrey, and S. Poppema. *Hodgkin's Disease in Children: Controversies and Current Practice*. Boston: Kluwer Academic Publishers, 1989. This volume in a series on cancer treatment and research discusses the evaluation and treatment of Hodgkin's disease in infants and children. Bibliographies and an index are included.

Lacher, Mortimer J., and John R. Redman, eds. *Hodgkin's Disease: The Consequences of Survival*. Philadelphia: Lea & Febiger, 1990. Discusses the treatment of and the complications associated with this disease. Therapy options are analyzed, including chemotherapy, radiotherapy, and the adverse effects of both methods of treatment. Bibliographies and an index are provided.

Williams, Stephanie F., Ramez Farah, and Harvey M. Golomb, eds. *Hodgkin's Disease*. A volume in the series Hematology/Oncology Clinics of North America. A thorough review of this disease—its diagnosis, pathology, and treatment. Includes bibliographical references and an index.

Williams, W. J., E. Beuter, A. J. Erslev, and M. A. Lichtman, eds. *Hematology*. 4th ed. New York: McGraw-Hill, 1990. An up-to-date textbook that offers an authoritative review of all aspects of Hodgkin's disease.

Wintrobe, Maxwell M., ed. *Clinical Hematology*. 8th ed. Philadelphia: Lea & Febiger, 1981. A textbook of hematologic disorders, with an excellent review of Hodgkin's disease. Written for clinicians and students of medicine.

# HUMAN IMMUNODEFICIENCY VIRUS (HIV)

**SYSTEM AFFECTED:** Immune

**SPECIALISTS:** Immunologists, internists, public health specialists

**DEFINITION:** HIV is the virus responsible for acquired immunodeficiency syndrome (AIDS) and AIDS-related complex (ARC). Although the virus has been found in various body fluids—such as saliva, tears, and breast milk—only blood and semen have been associated with its transmission. Therefore, any activities involving blood or semen can spread HIV, including sexual intercourse, the sharing of needles, blood transfusions, kidney transplantations, and artificial insemination; the risk of transmission from the last three activities has been virtually eliminated through testing procedures. There is an unpredictable lag between exposure to HIV and a positive test result for HIV antibodies (although it is usually within one year), and another lag until the HIV-positive individual develops AIDS (which may range from eighteen months to many years). Infection with HIV increases the chances of developing dermatitis, thrush, shingles, herpes simplex infection, and tuberculosis.

*See also* Acquired immunodeficiency syndrome (AIDS); Autoimmune disorders; Immunodeficiency disorders; Sexually transmitted diseases.

# HUNTINGTON'S DISEASE. *See* BRAIN DISORDERS.

# HYDROCEPHALUS

**SYSTEM AFFECTED:** Brain

**SPECIALISTS:** Neonatologists, pediatricians

**DEFINITION:** An excessive collection of cerebrospinal fluid in the brain.

### CAUSES AND SYMPTOMS

Hydrocephalus is commonly called "water on the brain." This water is actually cerebrospinal fluid (CSF), which is normally found in cavities in the brain and surrounding the brain and is continuous through the spinal canal. Excessive collection of CSF can cause swelling and pressure against the brain. Too much fluid may result from overproduction or inefficient drainage. Drainage can be prevented by either an inflammation or a tumor that blocks the drainage canal.

There are several causes of hydrocephalus. It may be inherited, or it may follow illnesses such as meningitis or brain hemorrhages into the ventricles. The patient may develop symptoms fairly quickly as intracranial pressure increases. In adults especially, symptoms and signs may be arrested because some fluid may be reabsorbed or some

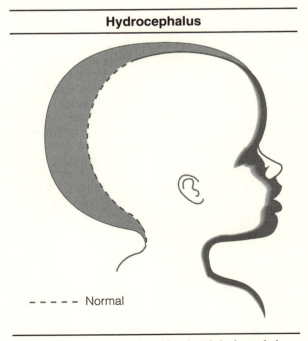

**Hydrocephalus**

- - - - - Normal

*Normal head size vs. size of head with hydrocephalus.*

nerve cells may be destroyed and their vacancy filled by the fluid.

Malformations associated with congenital hydrocephalus include symmetric dilation of the ventricles accompanying atrophy of the brain. Additionally, such infants may suffer from a variety of brain deformities and spina bifida, as well as other abnormalities. The collection of fluid pushes against the skull bones and causes separation of the bones at their sutures. The fontanelles may be easily seen, and the scalp looks thin and stretched. The upper head dwarfs the lower face. Optic atrophy, mental deficiency, and spastic elasticity of arms and legs are often apparent.

### TREATMENT AND THERAPY

The presence or absence of free-flowing CSF from the ventricles can be detected by a test in which dye is injected into a ventricle; its absence or presence in the drainage area determines if drainage has occurred.

Prognosis for the child with hydrocephalus is poor. Death typically occurs in the first or second year of life, usually as a result of infection. Many cases of hydrocephalus can be successfully treated with medication or surgery. If hydrocephalus is a result of hemorrhage, for example, the drugs furosemide (Lasix) and acetazolamide (Diamox) can reduce swelling because they decrease the amount of CSF produced. Surgical treatment may include cutting new routes or building shunts to carry CSF to the abdominal cavity for elimination. —*Iona C. Baldridge*

*See also* Birth defects; Brain disorders.

# HYPERLIPIDEMIA

**SYSTEM AFFECTED:** Blood
**SPECIALISTS:** Family physicians, hematologists, internists
**DEFINITION:** The presence of abnormally large amounts of lipids (fats) in the blood.

### CAUSES AND SYMPTOMS

Although elevated triglyceride levels have been implicated in clinical ischemic diseases, most investigators believe that cholesterol-rich lipids are a more significant risk factor. Although measurements of both cholesterol and triglyceride levels have been used to predict coronary disease, studies suggest that the determination of the alpha-lipoprotein/beta-lipoprotein ratio is a more reliable predictor. Because the alpha-lipoprotein has a higher density than the beta-lipoprotein, they are more often designated as high-density lipoprotein (HDL) and low-density lipoprotein (LDL), respectively. HDL is often referred to as "good cholesterol," and LDL is referred to as "bad cholesterol." The latter is implicated in the development of atherosclerosis.

Atherosclerosis is a disease that begins in the innermost lining of the arterial wall. Its lesions occur predominantly at arterial forks and branch openings, but they can also occur at sites where there is injury to the arterial lining. The initial lesion usually appears as fatty streaks or spots,

which have been detected even at birth. With passing years, more of these lesions appear, and they may develop into elevated plaques that obstruct the flow of blood in the artery. The lesions are rich in cholesterol derived from beta-lipoproteins in the plasma. In addition to elevated blood lipids, other risk factors associated with atherosclerosis include hypertension, faulty arterial structure, obesity, smoking, and stress.

### TREATMENT AND THERAPY

The treatment of hyperlipidemia involves both dietary and drug therapies. Although studies in nonhuman primates indicate that the reduction of hyperlipidemia results in decreased morbidity and mortality rate from arterial vascular disease, studies in humans are less conclusive. Initial treatment involves restricting the dietary intake of cholesterol and saturated fat. Drug therapy is instituted when further lowering of the serum lipids is desired. Among the drugs that have been used as antihyperlipidemic agents are lovastatin and its analogs, clofibrate and its analogs (particularly gemfibrozil), nicotinic acid, D-thyroxine, cholestyramine, probucol, and heparin. A simplified diagram of the endogenous biosynthesis and biotransformation of cholesterol is given below.

acetate $\longrightarrow$ acetyl SCoA $\longrightarrow$ HMGCoA $\longrightarrow$ MVA $\longrightarrow$ squalene $\longrightarrow$ desmosterol $\longrightarrow$ cholesterol $\longrightarrow$ bile acids

Lovastatin blocks the synthesis of cholesterol by inhibiting the enzyme (HMGCoA reductase) that catalyzes the conversion of beta-hydroxy-beta-methyl glutaryl coenzyme A (HMGCoA) to mevalonic acid (MVA), the regulatory step in the biosynthesis of cholesterol. Both lovastatin and MVA are beta, delta-dihydroxy acids, but lovastatin has a much more lipophilic (fat-soluble) group attached to it. Clofibrate and gemfibrozil block the synthesis of cholesterol prior to the HMGCoA stage. For this reason, they are likely to inhibit triglyceride formation as well. Nicotinic acid inhibits the synthesis of acetyl coenzyme A (acetyl SCoA) and thus would be expected to block the synthesis of both cholesterol and the triglycerides. To be effective in lowering the serum level of lipids, nicotinic acid must be taken in large amounts, which often produces an unpleasant flushing sensation in the patient. A way to inhibit the synthesis of cholesterol at the post-MVA stages has also been sought. Agents such as triparanol, which inhibit biosynthesis near the end of the synthetic sequence, have been developed. Although they are effective in lowering serum cholesterol, they had to be withdrawn from clinical use because of their adverse side effects on the muscles and eyes. Moreover, the penultimate product in the biosynthesis of cholesterol proved to be atherogenic. Investigations are being conducted on the inhibition of cholesterol synthesis at both the immediate pre-squalene and immediate post-squalene stages. The effects of such inhibitors on the production of steroid hormones and ubiquinones, as well as on cholesterol and triglycerides, are expected to be of considerable interest.

D-thyroxine promotes the metabolism of cholesterol in the liver, transforming it into the more hydrophilic (water-soluble) bile acids, thereby facilitating its elimination from the body. An approach to reducing the serum level of cholesterol by a process involving the sequestering of the bile acids utilizes the resin cholestyramine as the sequestrant. The sequestered bile acids cannot be reabsorbed into the enterohepatic system and are eliminated in the feces. Consequently, more cholesterol is oxidized to the bile acids, resulting in the reduction of the serum level of cholesterol. Unfortunately, a large quantity of cholestyramine is required. Sequestration of cholesterol with beta-sitosterol prevents both the absorption of dietary cholesterol and the reabsorption of endogenous cholesterol in the intestines. Here, too, a large quantity of the sequestrant needs to be administered.

Probucol is an antioxidant. Because, structurally, it is a sulfur analog of a hindered hydroquinone, it acts as a free radical scavenger. Evidence suggests that the antihyperlipidemic effect of probucol is attributable to its ability to inhibit the oxygenation of LDL. The oxygenated LDL is believed to be the atherogenic form of LDL. Heparin promotes the hydrolysis of triglycerides as it activates lipoprotein lipase, thereby reducing lipidemia. Because of its potent anticoagulant properties, however, its use in therapy must be closely monitored. Cholesterol that is present in atherosclerotic plaques is acylated, generally by the more saturated fatty acids. The enzyme catalyzing the acylation process is acyl-CoA cholesterol acyl transferase (ACAT). The development of regulators of ACAT and the desirability of reducing the dietary intake of saturated fatty acids are based on this rationale.

Cholesterol within the cell is able to inhibit further synthesis of cholesterol by a feedback mechanism. Cholesterol that is associated with LDL is transported into the hepatic cell by means of the LDL receptor on the surface of the cell. In individuals who are afflicted with familial hypercholesterolemia, an inherited disorder that causes death at an early age, the gene that is responsible for the production of the LDL receptor is either absent or defective. Studies in gene therapy have shown that transplant of the normal LDL receptor gene to such an individual results in a dramatic decrease in the level of the "bad cholesterol" in the serum. Cholesterol derivatives that are oxygenated at various positions have also been found to regulate the serum level of cholesterol by either inhibiting its synthesis or promoting its catabolism. More studies need to be done, however, in order to demonstrate their effectiveness in humans and to establish that they themselves do not induce atherosclerosis. —*Leland J. Chinn*

*See also* Atherosclerotic disease; Cholesterol; Hypertension; Obesity.

**FOR FURTHER INFORMATION:**
Larsen, Scott D., and Charles H. Spilman. "New Potential Therapies for the Treatment of Atherosclerosis." *Annual Reports in Medicinal Chemistry* 28 (1993): 217.
Motulsky, A. G. "The 1985 Nobel Prize in Physiology or Medicine." *Science* 231 (January 10, 1986): 126-129.
Rifkind, Basil M., ed. *Drug Treatment of Hyperlipidemia.* New York: Marcel Dekker, 1991.
Witiak, D. T., H. A. I. Newman, and D. R. Feller, eds. *Antilipidemic Drugs.* Amsterdam: Elsevier, 1991.

# HYPERPARATHYROIDISM AND HYPOPARATHYROIDISM

**SYSTEMS AFFECTED:** Endocrine, skeletal
**SPECIALISTS:** Endocrinologists
**DEFINITION:** Excessive, uncontrolled secretion (hyperparathyroidism) or reduced secretion (hypoparathyroidism) of parathyroid hormone.

## CAUSES AND SYMPTOMS

The precise regulation of calcium is vital to the survival and well-being of all animals. Approximately 99 percent of the calcium in the body is found in bones and teeth. Of the remaining 1 percent, about 0.9 percent is packaged within specialized organelles inside the cell. This leaves only 0.1 percent of the total body calcium in blood. Approximately half of this calcium is either bound to proteins or complexed with phosphate. The other half of blood calcium is free to be utilized by cells. For this reason, it is critical that the concentration of calcium inside the cell be rigorously maintained at extremely low concentrations. Even a slight change in calcium outside the cell can have dramatic consequences.

*The function and regulation of calcium.* Calcium plays a vital role in many different areas of the body. For example, the entry of calcium into secretory cells, such as a nerve cell, triggers the release of neurotransmitters into the synapse. A fall in blood calcium results in the overexcitability of nerves, which can be felt as a tingling sensation and numbness in the extremities. Similarly, calcium entry into cells is essential for muscle contraction in both heart and skeletal muscle.

Free calcium is thus one of the most tightly regulated substances in the body. The key player in the moment-to-moment regulation of calcium is parathyroid hormone (PTH). PTH is synthesized in the parathyroid glands, a paired gland located in the neck, and released in response to a fall in blood calcium. PTH serves several functions: to increase blood calcium, to decrease blood phosphate, and to stimulate the conversion of vitamin D into its active form, which can then stimulate the uptake of calcium across the digestive tract. Together these actions result in an increase in free calcium, which returns calcium concentrations in the blood to normal.

PTH binds to specific receptors located primarily in bone and kidney tissue. Since most calcium is stored in bone, it serves as a bank for withdrawal of calcium in times of need. Activation of a PTH receptor on osteoclasts, or bone-cutting cells, results in the production of concentrated acids that dissolve calcium from bone, thereby making more free calcium available to the blood supply. PTH also acts on the kidney, where it stimulates calcium uptake from the urine while promoting phosphate elimination. As a result, more calcium is made available to the blood and less phosphate is available to form complexes with the free calcium.

By exerting these effects on its target organs, PTH can restore low calcium concentrations in the blood to normal. Once calcium has returned to a particular set point, PTH secretion is slowed dramatically. If PTH release is not controlled, however, the imbalance in calcium can lead to life-threatening situations. These conditions are termed hyperparathyroidism and hypoparathyroidism.

*Hyperparathyroidism.* This disorder is defined as the excessive and uncontrolled secretion of PTH. The release of a closely related substance, PTH-related protein, from cancer cells can also cause this condition. Hyperparathyroidism is found in 0.1 percent of the population and is more com-

mon in the elderly, who have an incident rate of approximately 2 percent.

There are two types of hyperparathyroidism, primary and secondary. Primary hyperparathyroidism is caused by disease or damage to the parathyroid glands. For example, cancer of the parathyroid gland can result in the uncontrolled release of PTH and is characterized by an increase in blood calcium. The symptoms associated with primary hyperparathyroidism include osteoporosis, muscle weakness, nausea, and increased incidence of kidney stones and peptic ulcers. These symptoms can all be linked to the presence of excess calcium, which is a result of the overexcretion of PTH.

Secondary hyperparathyroidism often results when PTH cannot function normally, such as in kidney failure or insensitivity of target tissues to PTH. Secondary hyperparathyroidism is usually characterized by an overall decrease in blood calcium levels, even though there is a marked increase in the amount of PTH being released. Its symptoms may include muscle cramps, seizures, paranoia, depression, and in severe cases, tetany (the tonic spasm of muscles).

## Hyperparathyroidism

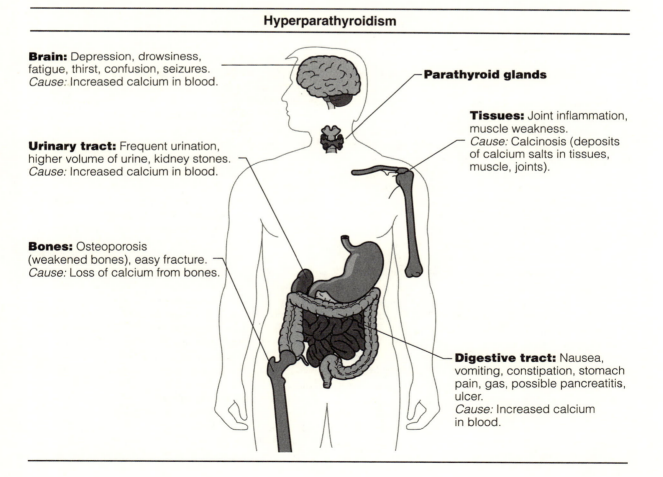

**Brain:** Depression, drowsiness, fatigue, thirst, confusion, seizures. *Cause:* Increased calcium in blood.

**Parathyroid glands**

**Tissues:** Joint inflammation, muscle weakness. *Cause:* Calcinosis (deposits of calcium salts in tissues, muscle, joints).

**Urinary tract:** Frequent urination, higher volume of urine, kidney stones. *Cause:* Increased calcium in blood.

**Bones:** Osteoporosis (weakened bones), easy fracture. *Cause:* Loss of calcium from bones.

**Digestive tract:** Nausea, vomiting, constipation, stomach pain, gas, possible pancreatitis, ulcer. *Cause:* Increased calcium in blood.

## Hypoparathyroidism

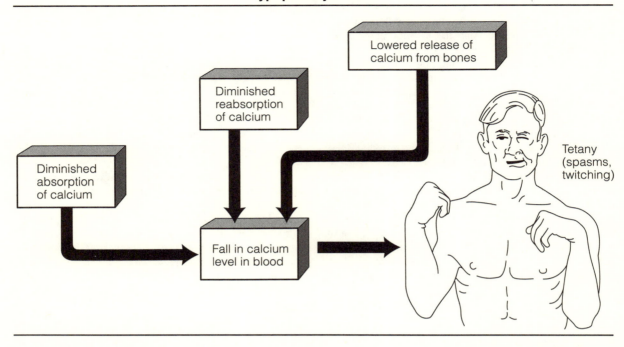

These symptoms are a direct result of the decline in available calcium.

*Hypoparathyroidism.* Less common than hyperparathyroidism, hypoparathyroidism is defined by a reduction in the secretion of PTH. This condition is normally characterized by low calcium levels and elevated phosphate levels in response to the lack of PTH. Not only are calcium levels unusually low, but phosphate levels are unusually high as well, which complicates this condition because phosphate ties up some of the free calcium.

Hypoparathyroidism can also have primary and secondary causes. Primary hypoparathyroidism is known to have two separate origins. The most common is a decrease in PTH release caused by accidental removal of the parathyroid gland. The other is damage of the blood supply around the parathyroid glands. Both occur after there has been some type of surgery or other medical procedure in the neck area. Consequently, the decline in PTH results in low calcium and elevated phosphate concentrations.

Secondary hypoparathyroidism is a frequent complication of cirrhosis (alcoholic liver disease) and is characterized by a decrease in both calcium and magnesium concentration. Because magnesium is essential for the release of PTH, this condition can be corrected with magnesium replacement.

Complications associated with all types of hypoparathyroidism include hyperventilation, convulsions, and in some cases tetany of the muscle cells.

### TREATMENT AND THERAPY

The treatments for primary hyperparathyroidism vary and are dependent on the severity of the condition. Specific drugs can be prescribed that lower elevated blood calcium. Hormone therapy, which includes the administration of estrogen, also acts to restore calcium to normal. Other treatments include dietary calcium restriction and/or surgery to remove the abnormal parathyroid tissue.

Treatment of secondary hyperparathyroidism is often achieved by correcting the problems associated with kidney failure. This can be done by administration of a dietary calcium supplement to restore plasma calcium levels or, in more severe cases, by kidney transplantation. Vitamin D therapy has also been attempted for those patients diagnosed in the early stages of renal failure.

Hypoparathyroidism is usually treated with dietary calcium and vitamin D supplementation. Both of these treatments promote calcium absorption and decrease calcium loss. The duration of the treatment depends on the severity of the condition and may last a lifetime.

—*Jeffrey A. McGowan and Hillar Klandorf*

*See also* Endocrine disorders; Osteoporosis; Stones; Vitamin and mineral deficiencies.

### FOR FURTHER INFORMATION:

Burch, Warner M. *Endocrinology.* 3d ed. Baltimore: Williams & Wilkins, 1994.

Paloyan, Edward, Ann M. Lawrence, and Francis H. Straus. *Hyperparathyroidism.* New York: Grune & Stratton, 1973.

Parsons, John A., ed. *Endocrinology of Calcium Metabolism*. New York: Raven Press, 1982.

# HYPERTENSION

**SYSTEMS AFFECTED:** Heart, circulatory, kidneys

**SPECIALISTS:** Cardiologists, family physicians, internists, nephrologists

**DEFINITION:** An abnormally high blood pressure, an often silent cardiovascular condition that may lead to heart attack, stroke, and major organ failures.

**KEY TERMS:**

*cardiovascular:* of, relating to, or involving the heart and blood vessels

*cerebrovascular:* of or involving the cerebrum (brain) and the blood vessels supplying it

*diastolic blood pressure:* the pressure of the blood within the artery while the heart is at rest

*hypertension:* abnormal blood pressure, especially high arterial blood pressure; also the systemic condition accompanying high blood pressure

*peripheral vascular:* of, relating to, involving, or forming the vasculature in the periphery (the external boundary or surface of a body); usually referring to circulation not involving cardiovascular, cerebrovascular, or major organ systems

*side effect:* a secondary and usually adverse effect (as of a drug); also known as an adverse effect or reaction

*sphygmomanometer:* a device that uses a column of mercury to measure blood-pressure force; pressure is measured in millimeters of mercury

## Blood Pressure

|   Systolic   |   Diastolic   |

*Blood pressure is measured in two numbers:* systolic *pressure (the pressure of the blood as it flows out when the heart contracts) over* diastolic *pressure (the pressure of the blood within the artery as it flows in when the heart is at rest). Readings greater than 140 systolic over 90 diastolic indicate the presence of hypertension.*

*systolic blood pressure:* the pressure of the blood within the artery while the heart is contracting

### CAUSES AND SYMPTOMS

Hypertension is a higher-than-normal blood pressure (either systolic or diastolic). Blood pressure is usually measured using a sphygmomanometer and a stethoscope. The stethoscope is used to hear when the air pressure within the cuff of the sphygmomanometer is equal to that in the artery. When taking a blood pressure, the cuff is pumped to inflate an air bladder secured around the arm; the pressure produced will collapse the blood vessels within. As cuff pressure decreases, a slight thump is heard as the artery snaps open to allow blood to flow. At this point, the cuff pressure equals the systolic blood pressure. As the cuff pressure continues to fall, the sound of blood being pumped will continue but become progressively softer. At the point where the last sound is heard, the cuff pressure equals the diastolic blood pressure.

### Blood Pressure and Hypertension

| Status | Systolic/Diastolic |
|---|---|
| Normal (maximum) | 130/85 |
| High normal | 131-139/86-89 |
| Stage I hypertension (mild) | 140-159/90-99 |
| Stage II (moderate) | 160-179/100-109 |
| Stage III (severe) | 180-209/110-119 |
| Stage IV (very severe) | 210/120+ |

In hypertension, both systolic and diastolic blood pressures are usually elevated. Blood pressures are reported as the systolic pressure over the diastolic pressure, such as 130/80 millimeters of mercury. It is important to recognize there are degrees of seriousness for hypertension (see table). The higher the blood pressure, the more rigorous the treatment may be. When systolic pressures are in the high normal range, the individual should be closely monitored with annual blood pressure checks. Persistently high blood pressures (greater than 140-159/90-99 millimeters of mercury) require closer monitoring and may result in a decision to treat the condition with medication or other types of intervention.

The blood pressure in an artery is determined by the relationship among three important controlling factors: the blood volume, the amount of blood pumped by the heart (cardiac output), and the contraction of smooth muscle within blood vessels (arterial tone). To illustrate the first point, if blood volume decreases, the result will be a fall in blood pressure. Conversely, the body cannot itself increase blood pressure by rapidly adding blood volume; fluid must be injected into the circulation to do so.

A second controlling factor of blood pressure is cardiac output (the volume of blood pumped by the heart in a given unit of time, usually reported as liters per minute). This output is determined by two factors: stroke volume (the volume of blood pumped with each heartbeat) and the heart rate (beats per minute). As heart rate increases, output generally increases and blood pressure may rise as well. If blood volume is low, such as with excessive bleeding, the blood returning to the heart per beat is lower and could lead to decreased output. To compensate, the heart rate increases to prevent a drop in blood pressure. Therefore, as cardiac output changes, blood pressure does not necessarily change.

Lastly, a major controlling factor of blood pressure is arterial tone. Arteries are largely tubular, smooth muscles that can change their diameter based on the extent of contraction (tone). This contraction is largely under the control of a specialized branch of the nervous system called the sympathetic nervous system. An artery with high arterial tone (contracted) will squeeze the blood within and increase the pressure inside. There is also a relaxation phase that will allow expansion and a decrease in blood pressure. Along with relaxation, arteries are elastic to allow some stretching, which may further help reduce pressure or, more important, help prevent blood pressure from rising.

There are two general types of hypertension: essential and secondary. Secondary hypertension is attributable to some underlying identifiable cause, such as a tumor or kidney disease, while essential hypertension has no identifiable cause. Therefore, essential hypertension is a defect that results in excessive arterial pressure secondary to poor regulation by any one of the three controlling factors discussed above. Each factor can serve as a focal point for treatment with medications.

The negative consequences of hypertension are mainly manifested in the deteriorating effect that this condition has on coronary heart disease (CHD). Cardiovascular risk factors for CHD are described as two types; unmodifiable and modifiable. Unmodifiable risk factors cannot be changed; this group includes gender, race, advanced age, and a family history of heart disease (hypertensive traits can be inherited). The modifiable risk factors are cigarette smoking (or other forms of tobacco abuse), high blood cholesterol levels, control over diabetes, and perhaps other factors not yet discovered. For example, additional factors are now recognized for their adverse effects on hypertension, including obesity, a lack of physical activity, and psychological factors.

There is no definitive blood pressure level at which a person is no longer at risk for CHD. While any elevation above the normal range places the person at increased risk for CHD, what are considered high normal blood pressures were previously defined as normal. (Looking back at older data, researchers noted that persons able to maintain pressures at or below 139/89 millimeters of mercury had less severe CHD.) The definition of "normal" blood pressure may change again in the future as new information is discovered. There is a practical limit as to how low pressure can be while maintaining day-to-day function.

In coronary heart disease, the blood supply to the heart is reduced and the heart cannot function well. The common term for arteriosclerosis, "hardening of the arteries," indicates the symptom of reduced blood flow, which is a major component of CHD. When the heart cannot supply itself with the necessary amount of blood (a condition known as ischemia), a characteristic chest pain called angina may be produced. The hardening aspect of this disease is the result of cholesterol deposits in the vessel, which decreases elasticity and makes the vessel wall stiff. This stiffness will force pressures in the vessel to increase if cardiac output rises. As pressures advance, the vessel may develop weak spots. These areas may rupture or lead to the development of small blood clots that may clog the vessel; either problem will disrupt blood flow, making the underlying CHD worse. Eventually, if the blood supply is significantly reduced, a myocardial infarction (heart attack) may occur. Where the blood supply to the heart muscle itself is functionally blocked, that part of the heart will die.

Besides contributing to an increased risk of heart attack and coronary heart disease, hypertension is a major risk for other vascular problems, such as stroke, kidney failure, heart failure, and visual disturbances secondary to the effects on the blood vessels within the eye. It is a major source of premature death in the United States, and by all estimates affects more than 60 million Americans. Forty percent of all African Americans and more than half of those over the age of sixty are affected. Public awareness of hypertension is increasing, yet less than half of all patients diagnosed are treated. More important, only one in five identified hypertensives have the condition under control. This lack of control is particularly important when one considers the organs influenced by hypertension, most notably the brain, eyes, kidneys, and heart.

Although causative factors of hypertension cannot be identified, many physiological factors contribute to hypertension. They include increased sympathetic nervous activity (part of the autonomic nervous system), which promotes arterial contraction; overproduction of an unidentified sodium-retaining hormone or chronic high sodium intake; inadequate dietary intake of potassium or calcium; an increased or inappropriate secretion of renin, a chemical made by the kidney; deficiencies of arterial dilators, such as prostaglandins; congenital abnormalities (birth defects) of resistance vessels; diabetes mellitus or resistance to the effects of insulin; obesity; increased activity of vascular growth factors; and altered cellular ion transport of electrolytes, such as potassium, sodium, chloride, and bicarbonate.

The kidneys are greatly responsible for blood pressure control. They have a key role in maintaining both blood volume and blood pressure. When kidney function declines, secondary to problems such as a decrease in renal blood flow, the kidney will release renin. High renin levels result in activation of the renin-angiotensin-aldosterone system. The resulting chemical cascade produces angiotensin II, a potent arterial constrictor. Another chemical released is aldosterone, an adrenal hormone which causes the kidney to retain water and sodium. These two actions add to blood volume and increase arterial tone, resulting in higher blood pressure. Normally, the renin-angiotensin-aldosterone system protects kidney function by raising blood pressure when it is low. In hypertensives, the controlling forces seem to be out of balance, so that the system does not respond appropriately. The renin-angiotensin-aldosterone system has a negative effect on bradykinin, a chemical which protects renal function by producing vasodilating prostaglandins that help maintain adequate renal blood flow. This protection is especially important in elderly individuals, who may depend on this system to maintain renal function. The system can be inhibited by medications such as aspirin or ibuprofen, resulting in a recurrence of hypertension or less control over the existing disease.

Arteries are largely smooth muscles under the control of the autonomic nervous system, which is responsible for organ function. Yet there is often no conscious control of organs; for example, one can "tell" the lungs to take a breath, but one cannot "tell" the heart to beat. The autonomic nervous system has two branches, sympathetic and parasympathetic, that essentially work against each other. The sympathetic system exerts much control over blood pressure. Many chemicals and medicines, such as caffeine, decongestants, and amphetamines, affect blood pressure by mimicking the effects of increased sympathetic stimulation of arteries.

Numerous factors associated with blood-pressure elevations will affect one or more of the key determinants of blood pressure; they affect one another as well. An example will show the extent of their relationship. Sodium and water retention will increase blood volume returning to the heart. As this return increases, the heart will increase output (to a point) to prevent heart failure. This higher cardiac output may also raise blood pressure. If arterial vessels are constricted, pressures may be even higher. This elevated pressure (resistance) will force the heart to try to increase output to maintain blood flow to vital organs. Thus, a vicious cycle is started; hypertension can be perceived as a merry-go-round ride with no exit.

## TREATMENT AND THERAPY

Blood pressure reduction has a protective effect against cardiovascular disease. Generally, as blood pressure decreases, arteries are less contracted and are able to deliver more blood to the tissues, maintaining their function. Further, this decreased blood pressure will help reduce the risk of heart attack in the patient with heart disease. With lower pressures, the heart does not need to work as hard supplying blood to itself or the rest of the body. Therefore, the demand

for cardiac output to supply blood flow is less. This reduced workload lowers the incidence of angina.

Treatment of hypertensive patients may involve using one to four different medications to achieve this goal. There are many types of medications from which to choose: diuretics, sympatholytic agents (also known as antiadrenergic drugs), beta-blockers (along with one combined-action alpha-beta blocker), calcium-channel blockers, peripheral vasodilators, and angiotensin-converting enzyme inhibitors. The list of available drugs is extensive; for example, there are fourteen different thiazide-type diuretics and another six diuretics with different mechanisms of action. So many choices may present the physician with a confusing set of alternatives.

Patients prone to sodium and water retention are treated with diuretics, agents that prevent the kidney from reabsorbing sodium and water from the urine. Diuretics are usually added to other medications to enhance those medications' activity. Research into thiazide-type diuretics has shown that these agents possess mild calcium-channel blocking activity, aiding their ability to reduce hypertension.

Beta-blocking agents are used less often than when they were first developed. They work by decreasing cardiac output through reducing the heart rate. Although they are highly effective, the heart-rate reduction tends to produce side effects. Most commonly, patients complain of fatigue, sleepiness, and reduced exercise tolerance (the heart rate cannot increase to adapt to the increasing demand for blood in tissues and the heart itself). These agents are still a good choice for hypertensive patients who have suffered a heart attack. Their benefit is that they reduce the risk of a second heart attack by preventing the heart from overworking.

Calcium-channel blockers were originally intended to treat angina. These agents act primarily by decreasing arterial smooth muscle contraction. Relaxed coronary blood vessels can carry more blood, helping prevent the pain of angina. When calcium ion enters the smooth muscle, a more sustained contraction is produced; therefore, blocking this effect will produce relaxation. Physicians noted that this relaxation also produced lower blood pressures. The distinct advantage to these agents is that they are well tolerated; however, some patients may require increasing their fiber intake to prevent some constipating effects.

Peripheral vasodilators have been a disappointment. Theoretically, they should be ideal since they work directly to cause arterial dilation. Unfortunately, blood pressure has many determinants and patients seem to become "immune" to direct vasodilator effects. They are useful, however, when added to other treatments such as beta-blockers or sympatholytic medications.

The sympatholytic agents are divided into two broad categories. The first group works within the brain to decrease the effects of nerves that would send signals to blood vessels to constrict (so-called constrict messages). They do this by increasing the relax signals coming out of the brain to offset the constrict messages. The net effect is that blood vessels dilate, reducing blood pressure. Many of these agents have fallen into disfavor because of adverse effects similar to those of beta-blockers. The second group of sympatholytics works directly at the nerve-muscle connection. These agents block the constrict messages of the nerve that would increase arterial smooth muscle tone. Overall, these agents are well tolerated. Some patients, especially the elderly, may be very susceptible to their effect and have problems with low blood pressure; this issue usually resolves itself shortly after the first dose.

The renin-angiotensin-aldosterone system is a key determinant of blood pressure. Angiotensin-converting enzyme inhibitors (ACE inhibitors) work by blocking angiotensin II and aldosterone and preserving bradykinin. They have been found quite effective for reducing blood pressure and are usually well tolerated. Some patients will experience a first-dose effect, while others may develop a dry cough that can be corrected by dose reductions or discontinuation of the medication.

Unfortunately, and contrary to popular belief, no one can reliably tell when his or her own blood pressure is elevated. Consequently, hypertension is called a "silent killer." It is extremely important to have regular blood-pressure evaluations and, if diagnosed with hypertension, to receive treatment.

From 1950 through 1987, as advances in understanding and treating hypertension were made, the United States population enjoyed a 40 percent reduction in coronary heart disease and a more than 65 percent reduction in stroke deaths. (By comparison, noncardiovascular deaths during the same period were reduced little more than 20 percent.)

It is evident that blood pressure can be reduced without medications. Research in the 1980's led to a nonpharmacologic approach in the initial management of hypertension. This strategy includes weight reduction, alcohol restriction, regular exercise, dietary sodium restriction, dietary potassium and calcium supplementation, stopping of tobacco use (in any form), and caffeine restriction. Often, these methods can produce benefits without medication being prescribed. Using this approach, medication is added to the therapy if blood pressure remains elevated despite good efforts at non-pharmacologic control.

Other aspects of hypertension and hypertensive patients have been identified to help guide the clinician to the proper choice of medication. With this approach, the clinician can focus therapy at the most likely cause of the hypertension: sodium and water retention, high cardiac output, or high vascular resistance. This pathophysiological approach led to the abandonment of the rigid step-care approach described in many tests covering hypertension. The pathophysiological approach to hypertension management is based on a series of steps that are taken if inadequate responses are seen (see figure).

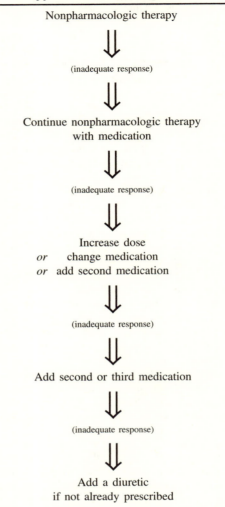

**Hypertension Management**

Nonpharmacologic therapy

⇓

(inadequate response)

⇓

Continue nonpharmacologic therapy
with medication

⇓

(inadequate response)

⇓

Increase dose
*or*    change medication
*or*  add second medication

⇓

(inadequate response)

⇓

Add second or third medication

⇓

(inadequate response)

⇓

Add a diuretic
if not already prescribed

By far, the best strategy for controlling hypertension is to be informed. Each person needs to be aware of his or her personal risk for developing hypertension. One should have regular blood pressure evaluations, avoid eating excessive salt and sodium, increase exercise, and reduce fats in the diet. Maintaining ideal body weight may be a key control factor. Studies have shown that patients who have been successful at losing weight will require less stringent treatment. The benefits could be a need for fewer medications, reduced doses of medications, or both.

—*Charles C. Marsh*

***See also*** Atherosclerotic disease; Cholesterol; Claudication; Embolism; Heart attack; Heart disease; Hyperlipidemia; Kidney disorders; Phlebitis; Strokes and TIAs; Thrombosis and thrombus.

**FOR FURTHER INFORMATION:**

The American Heart Association. *Heartbook.* New York: E. P. Dutton, 1980. This landmark reference work is a concise overview of all cardiovascular diseases. Offers specific chapters covering such topics as hypertension, diet and nutrition, exercise, quality-of-life issues, and smoking. The American Heart Association makes a wealth of printed educational materials available to the public.

Davis, Goode P. *The Heart: The Living Pump.* Washington, D.C.: U.S. News Books, 1981. A wonderfully illustrated basic anatomy reference containing unique photographs of blood circulation within the heart and lungs. Describes the early work in developing methods for blood-pressure measurement. A helpful overview of coronary heart disease is included.

Dorland, W. A. Newman. *Dorland's Illustrated Medical Dictionary.* 27th ed. Philadelphia: W. B. Saunders, 1988. A standard work for the explanation of medical terms. It is well illustrated and should help any reader gain more understanding of complex medical terms. Reviewing this reference is an educational experience in itself.

Messerli, Franz H., ed. *Cardiovascular Disease in the Elderly.* 3d ed. Boston: Kluwer Academic Publishers, 1993. An excellent book for detailed discussions regarding cardiovascular disease in older persons. Issues such as aging, multiple illnesses, and the social challenges seen in the elderly are discussed.

_____. *The Heart and Hypertension.* New York: Yorke Medical Books, 1987. An excellent reference work written by one of the most distinguished clinicians and researchers in hypertension. This text's strength is its discussion of the pathophysiology of hypertension.

Rees, Michael K. *The Complete Family Guide to Living with High Blood Pressure.* Englewood Cliffs, N.J.: Prentice Hall, 1980. The author does an excellent job of describing blood pressure itself, as well as the methods and importance of blood-pressure measurement (including by the patient). Quality of life and how hypertension affects the family are discussed.

Seeley, Rod R. *Anatomy and Physiology.* St. Louis: Times Mirror/Mosby, 1989. A well-illustrated, easy-to-read basic reference text for the general reader. The text's obvious strengths are its discussions of the heart, arteries, and veins and their roles in cardiovascular function.

# HYPERTHERMIA AND HYPOTHERMIA

**SYSTEMS AFFECTED:** All

**SPECIALISTS:** Anesthesiologists, emergency physicians, environmental medicine physicians, general surgeons, internists, thoracic surgeons

**DEFINITION:** Hyperthermia is the elevation of the body core temperature of an organism, while hypothermia is a decrease in that temperature; both conditions are medical emergencies when not intentionally induced, and both can be useful when applied to surgical and treatment techniques.

**KEY TERMS:**

*ambient temperature:* the temperature of the surrounding environment

*body temperature:* the temperature that reflects the level of heat energy in an animal's body; a consequence of the balance between the heat produced by metabolism and the body's exchange of heat with the surrounding environment

*frostbite:* injury that results from exposure of skin to extreme cold, most commonly affecting the ears, nose, hands, and feet

*hibernation:* a condition of dormancy and torpor that occurs in poikilotherm vertebrates and invertebrates; as the environmental temperatures drop, the inner core temperature of such animals also drops to decrease the metabolic rate and physiological functions

*homeotherms:* animals, such as birds and mammals, that have the ability to maintain a high body core temperature despite large variations in environmental temperatures

*hyperthermia:* an abnormally elevated body temperature that leads to fever and muscle rigidity

*hypothermia:* an abnormally low body temperature that leads to drastic metabolic changes and eventual death

## CAUSES AND SYMPTOMS

Body temperature reflects the level of heat energy in the body of an animal or human being. It is the consequence of the balance between the heat generated by metabolism and the body's heat exchange with the surrounding environment (ambient temperature). Generally, animal life can be sustained in the temperature range of 0 degrees Celsius (32 degrees Fahrenheit) to 45 degrees Celsius (113 degrees Fahrenheit), but appropriate processes can store animal tissues at much lower temperature. Homeotherms, such as birds and most mammals, have the ability to maintain their high body core temperature despite large variations in environmental temperatures. Poikilotherms have slow metabolic rates at rest and, as a result, difficulty in maintaining their inner core temperatures. Such a form of thermal regulation is called ectothermic ("outer heated") and is directly affected by the uptake of heat from the environment; such organisms are often termed cold-blooded. On the other hand, homeotherms are endothermic ("inner heated") and depend largely on their fast and controlled rates of heat production; such organisms are termed warm-blooded. Thus, the lizard, an example of ectotherm, maintains its body temperature by staying in or out of shade and by assuming a posture toward the sun that would maximize the adjustment for its body heat. At night, the lizard burrows, but its body temperature still drops considerably until the next morning, when it increases with the rising sun.

Body core temperatures vary considerably among mammals and birds. For example, the sparrow's inner core temperature is about 43.5 degrees Celsius (110.3 degrees Fahrenheit), the turkey's 41.2 degrees Celsius (106.2 degrees Fahrenheit), the cat's 36.4 degrees Celsius (97.5 degrees Fahrenheit), and the opossum's 34.7 degrees Celsius (94.5 degrees Fahrenheit). In humans, although the temperature of the inner organs varies by only 1 to 2 degrees Celsius (1.8 to 3.6 degrees Fahrenheit), the skin temperature may vary 10 to 20 degrees Celsius (18 to 36 degrees Fahrenheit) below the core temperature of 37 degrees Celsius (98.6 degrees Fahrenheit), depending on the ambient temperature. This is possible because the cells of the skin, muscles, and blood vessels are not as sensitive as are those of the vital organs.

An elevation in core temperature of homeotherms above the normal range is called hyperthermia, while a corresponding decrease is called hypothermia. Both can be brought about by extremes in the environment. Although the human body can withstand a lack of food for a number of weeks and that of water for several days, it cannot survive a lack of thermoregulation, which is the maintaining of the inner core temperature. The core temperature has to be kept within strict limits; otherwise, the brain and heart will be compromised and death will result. Clinically, the inner core temperature can be monitored by recording the temperature of the rectum, the eardrum, the mouth, and the esophagus. In elderly people, the body's ability to cope with extreme temperatures may be impaired. Exposure to even mildly cold temperatures may lead to accidental hypothermia that can be fatal if not detected and treated properly.

All animals produce heat by oxidation of substrates to carbon dioxide. On the average, about 75 percent of food energy is converted to heat during adenosine triphosphate (ATP) formation and its transfer to the functional systems of the cells. In defense against heat, sweating is the primary physiological mechanism in mammals. Dogs, cats, and other furred carnivores increase evaporative heat loss by panting, while small rodents spread saliva. Human beings have two to three million glands that can produce up to 23 liters of sweat per hour for a short period of time. At the same time, the blood volume may increase by 10 percent within twenty-four hours.

Fever may occur for at least four main reasons. Infection by microorganisms is the most well known because of its large variety of causes. Such an infection may be bacterial (as with septicemia and abscesses), viral (in measles, mumps, and influenza), protozoal (in malaria), or spichaetal (in syphilis). Fever can also take place because of immunological conditions, such as drug allergies and incompatible blood transfusions. The last two reasons are malignancy, which can lead to Hodgkin's disease and leukemia, and noninfective inflammation, which results in gout and thrombophlebitis.

Antipyretics are medicines whose consumption results in the lowering of fever. The bark of trees provides antipyretics such as spiraeic acid and its derivatives (aspirin). The mechanism of action of the non-narcotic antipyretics remains a subject of research. Two hypotheses are considered to justify the suppression of fever. One involves inhibition of the formation of arachidonic acid metabolites, which leads to the formation of pain-reducing substances. The other postulates that a modification of the physiological membrane properties takes place, with subsequent incorporation of drug molecules into the tertiary structure of proteins.

Temperature regulation involves the brain and spinal cord, which monitor the difference between the internal and peripheral (skin and muscle) temperature, with physiological and psychological adjustments to maintain a constant internal temperature. The brain records the various body temperatures via specialized nerve endings called thermal receptors. Heat transfer occurs between the skin surface and the environment via conduction (which takes place by means of physical contact) or convection (which occurs through the movement of air).

During cold weather, hikers and climbers are particularly at risk for hypothermia; in extreme cases, body functions are depressed to the extent that victims may be mistaken for dead. Injuries that result from skin exposure to extreme cold are described as frostbite. Frostbite most commonly affects outer organs such as the nose, ears, hands (especially the fingertips), and feet, which first turn unusually red and then unnaturally white. Early symptoms include feelings of coldness, tingling, pain, and numbness. Frostbite takes place when ice crystals form in the skin and (in the most serious cases) in the tissue beneath the skin. If not treated, frostbite may lead to gangrene, the medical term for tissue death. The freezing-thawing process causes mechanical disruption (from ice), intracellular and extracellular biochemical changes, and the disruption of the blood corpuscles. Frostbite treatment involves the use of warm water to restore blood circulation and heat to the affected body part.

There are several types of hypothermia. Immersion hypothermia occurs when a person falls into cold water. Any movement of the body leads to loss of heat, and the drastic temperature change may trigger a heart attack. Generally, a person can withstand immersion in water that is 10 degrees Celsius (50 degrees Fahrenheit) for about ten minutes before succumbing to death. Divers are equipped with wet suits to minimize heat loss, but they cool themselves rapidly when they move in cold water and, at the same time, breathe dry air mixtures. Submersion hypothermia is actual drowning in cold water. Although a person cannot last more than a few minutes without oxygen, drowning in cold water is more survivable than in water of other temperatures. As the cold water enters the lungs and bathes the skin, the body's metabolic rate decreases, which allows the individual (especially a child) up to forty-five minutes of oxygen debt before death occurs.

Clinical reports also indicate hypothermia in alcohol-intoxicated individuals. Shivering, which is common to people suffering from hypothermia, is a sequence of skeletal muscle contractions which lead to coordinated movements and produce a maximum amount of heat. Other conditions of heat loss that deteriorate the already hypothermic person include tight and wet clothing, injury causing hemorrhage, fatigue, and even psychosis.

### TREATMENT AND THERAPY

Nature protects poikilotherm vertebrates and invertebrates in winter by means of hibernation. Hibernation, which is a condition of dormancy and torpor, occurs when the body temperatures of such animals drop when the environmental temperatures decrease. Animals such as bears, raccoons, badgers, and some birds become drowsy in winter because ambient temperature drops of a few degrees considerably decrease their metabolic rates and physiological functions. For example, the body temperature of a bear is 35.5 degrees Celsius (96 degrees Fahrenheit) at an air temperature of 4.4 degrees Celsius (40 degrees Fahrenheit) and only 31.2 degrees Celsius (88 degrees Fahrenheit) at an air temperature of 31.2 degrees Celsius (25 degrees Fahrenheit).

In humans, however, a significant decrease in body temperature is always a medical emergency requiring immediate attention. The treatment for mild cases of hypothermia may consist only of covering the head and offering the victim a warm drink. More serious cases may involve immersing the victim in a warm bath. Severe hypothermia requires hospitalization in an intensive care unit, where the body temperature is returned to normal by placing the patient under special heat-reflecting blankets, by injecting warm fluid into the abdominal cavity, or by bypassing the circulating blood through a machine to heat it.

Hyperthermia is often termed heat stroke, while mild elevations in temperature can produce heat exhaustion. Heat stroke is a serious condition treated with emergency procedures. The victim is wrapped naked in a cold, wet sheet or blanket or sponged with cold water and fanned constantly. Salt tablets or a weak salt solution is given to conscious patients.

Both hyperthermia and hypothermia can be used medically. Although cancer treatment consists primarily of radiation therapy, surgery, and chemotherapy, experimental approaches include immunotherapy and hyperthermia. In the latter case, heat is used to destroy cancer cells. In all cases, except surgery, the tumor cells have to be killed in situ, meaning that their reproductive ability has to be inhibited without affecting irreversibly the normal tissues.

A study of cell exposure to high temperatures has demonstrated that the circulation of blood decreased as temperature treatment at 42.5 degrees Celsius continued. The electron microscope showed that after about three hours, a vascular collapse (seen as cloudiness) took place in most of the located vessels. At that point, the high-temperature

## First Aid for Hypothermia

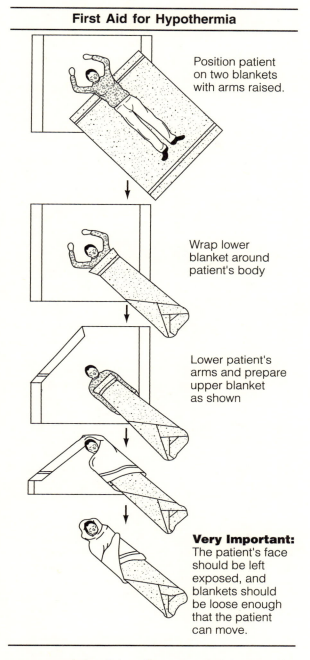

Position patient on two blankets with arms raised.

Wrap lower blanket around patient's body

Lower patient's arms and prepare upper blanket as shown

**Very Important:** The patient's face should be left exposed, and blankets should be loose enough that the patient can move.

treatment ended and the cells were cooled down to 33.5 degrees Celsius. Two days later, the central areas displayed an extensive degree of necrosis, while the periphery was largely unaffected.

There are indications that malignant tumor cells are more thermosensitive than the surrounding normal cells from which the malignant cells have probably developed. Although some scientists believe that brain neurons are damaged by temperature greater then 42 degrees Celsius, in most cases neurons can tolerate temperatures in the range of 42.5 to 43 degrees Celsius for up to thirty minutes. Chemotherapy has been found to be much more potent upon exposure of the tumor cells to higher temperatures. Although the mechanisms responsible are not fully understood, there are several possible explanations. Some scientists believe that hyperthermia may increase the drug uptake by cancer cells, alter the intracellular distribution of the drug, or even alter the metabolism of the drug.

In brain cancer patients, it was common practice to induce brain hyperthermia by means of whole body hyperthermia, but this method has been substituted by several others. Isolated perfusion of the appropriate artery and vein has produced excellent results. Radiofrequency capacitive heating (in which paddle-shaped transmitters are placed next to the exposed brain) and interstitial radiofrequency (in which a gold-plated brass electrode provides tumor temperatures of 44 degrees Celsius while holding the surroundings at 42 degrees Celsius) are also extensively used. Microwave hyperthermia, magnetic loop induction, and ferromagnetic seeds (which are surgically implanted into the tumor and later heated by external radiofrequency of 300 to 3,000 megahertz) are also applied to brain cancer patients.

Ultrasonic irradiation, which uses a thin, stainless steel tube to induce hyperthermia, is believed to be the promising technique of the future. The heat generated by the energy produced improves the local blood supply by dilating the blood vessels. This dilation, together with an acceleration of enzyme activity, helps cells to obtain fresh nutrients and, at the same time, rid themselves of waste products. The other advantage of ultrasonic irradiation is the vibrations that it creates. In a hardened and calcified brain tumor, for example, these vibrations can crush the tumor, which can then be removed via vacuum.

Hypothermia began to be used extensively in modern surgery in the 1970's and 1980's. In certain operations, the patient's body temperature is lowered by wrapping the already anesthetized patient in a rubber blanket that contains coils through which cold water is circulated. When the temperature is sufficiently low, as determined by an electrical rectal thermometer, general anesthesia is discontinued. As a result, much less bleeding occurs in both brain and heart surgery. Under conditions of hypothermia, breathing is slower and shallower, and the brain requirements for blood and oxygen are drastically reduced. This situation allows an intentional stoppage of the heart for prolonged periods of time in order to complete the surgical repairs of that organ.

There is a point, however, below which the human body temperature cannot be lowered. In cold-blooded animals, the loading and unloading of oxygen can be carried out adequately only within a certain temperature range; thus an octopus' blood becomes fully saturated with oxygen at 0 degrees Celsius but little oxygen is unloaded by hemoglobin, which results in the animal's oxygen starvation. In humans, little oxygen is delivered to the tissues at 20 degrees Celsius, which sets a natural limit to the possibility of lowering body temperature during surgical procedures. The lack of dissociation of oxyhemoglobin at low temperature accounts for the red color of ears and noses on cold days.

## Perspective and Prospects

Both hypothermia and hyperthermia have had a commanding role in medicine. An Egyptian papyrus roll which can be dated back to 3,000 B.C. describes the treatment of a breast tumor with hyperthermia. Heat has been used as a therapeutic agent since the days of Hippocrates (c. 460-377 B.C.), who stated that a patient who could not be cured by heat was actually incurable. In the seventeenth century, the Japanese performed hyperthermia to treat syphilis, arthritis, and gout, using hot water to increase the body temperature to about 39 degrees Celsius.

The medical use of hyperthermia owes much of its modern-era development to Georges Lakhovsky (1880-1942), a Russian Jew who had a brilliant physics background and did most of his work in Paris, France. Although he is not generally given the credit for it, he was the first person to design and build a "short wave diathermy" machine, which created artificial fever for the first time in 1923. His work was done primarily on patients with malignant tumors at the Hospital de la Salpetriere and the Hospital Saint-Louis. The first machine that he developed used frequencies from 0.75 megahertz to 3,000 megahertz, a range very much in use in today's clinical hyperthermia. In 1931, he started using a new machine that emitted radio waves of multiple, different wavelengths. He had partial success with his treatment, as reported to the Pasteur Institute and the French Academy of Sciences. Other scientists in this field include the German physician W. Busch and the English physician Bruns, who applied it to erysipelas infection in 1886, and the Swedish gynecologist N. Westermark, who applied it with partial success to nonoperable carcinomas of the cervix uteri in 1898. The combination of hyperthermia and immunotherapy was applied by W. B. Coley, a New York surgeon who managed to cause complete regression of malignant melanoma in patients by inducing artificial fever created by inoculation of infected erysipelas cells.

The application of hyperthermia to serious cases of cancer will take a gigantic leap once it is firmly established that the cancer cells have a greater thermosensitivity than normal cells. At this time, it is generally used in combination with surgery and radiation. Hyperthermia is applied to the cancer cells left behind following surgery, and it can kill those cells that tend to be radioresistant. Unlike radiation, hyperthermia has no known cumulative toxicity, and it can be safely reapplied to recurrent lesions. Ultrasound-induced hyperthermia has produced encouraging results, and it is hoped to be as useful as ultrasound is to the removal of kidney stones.

The application of hyperthermia in cases of acquired immunodeficiency syndrome (AIDS) has not yet provided decisively positive results. The process has involved circulating the patient's blood through a chamber heated to approximately 10 degrees Fahrenheit higher than the body temperature. Although the AIDS virus is killed, many of the patients' other enzymes are found to lose their activity, resulting in their subsequent death. Consequently, United States health officials have opposed and criticized blood-heating therapy for this disease until more convincing results are produced.

The role of hyperthermia in treating metastatic cancer, in combination with radiation and drugs that are heat and radiation cell sensitizers, is increasing. This technique has been made feasible by the technological advancements in deep-heating machines, such as the Magnetrode and the BSO annular array, which allow the sequential regional hyperthermia of large body regions such as the thorax and the abdomen.

Hypothermic brain operations have the great advantage of reduced swelling. As a result, during the surgery the brain rarely bulges out of the opening in the skull, which is not the case when the operation is performed at room temperature. This advantage has led to reduced hospital stays and faster recovery times. The requirements of the tissues for oxygen and the rate at which they produce waste products fall as temperature drops.

—*Soraya Ghayourmanesh*

*See also* Fever; Frostbite; Gangrene; Heat exhaustion and heat stroke.

## FOR FURTHER INFORMATION:

Bicher, Haim I., J. R. McLaren, and G. M. Pigliucci, eds. *Consensus on Hyperthermia for the 1990s.* New York: Plenum Press, 1989. A series of research papers presented at the Twelfth International Symposium on Clinical Hyperthermia in Rome in 1989. Topics include the clinical use and instrumentation for hyperthermia types (including ultrasound) and applications in liver, brain, and ovarian cancer.

Bloomfield, Molly M. *Chemistry and the Living Organism.* 5th ed. New York: John Wiley & Sons, 1992. An excellent health-allied text. Perspective 9-2 discusses hypothermia and death.

Farrell, K. "Hyperthermia in Malignant Disease—A History of Medicine Note—The Work of Georges Lakhovsky." In *Hyperthermia,* edited by Haim I. Bicher and D. F. Bruley. New York: Plenum Press, 1982. A short description of the history of hyperthermia that depicts the significance of Lakhovsky's contributions. A complete bibliography of Lakhovsky's work is offered.

Gautherie, Michel, ed. *Biological Basis of Oncologic Thermotherapy.* Berlin: Springer-Verlag, 1990. An advanced treatise on cancer thermotherapy that discusses heat transfer to tissues, types of hyperthermia treatment, mechanisms of heat and radiosensitization action in the killing of cells, and temperature distribution in tumors.

Issels, Rolf D., and Wolfgang Wilmanns, eds. *Application of Hyperthermia in the Treatment of Cancer.* Berlin: Springer-Verlag, 1988. Offers a series of articles on the effect of hyperthermia and its combination with radiation and chemotherapy. The discussion analyzes both biological and clinical studies results.

Storm, F. Kristian, ed. *Hyperthermia in Cancer Therapy.* Boston: G. K. Hall, 1983. A collection of articles that cover the thermosensitivity of cancer cells in vitro and in vivo, blood flow in tumors and normal tissues in hyperthermia, hyperthermia techniques and instrumentation, and clinical studies with microwave and radiowave hyperthermia.

# HYPERTROPHY

**SYSTEMS AFFECTED:** All

**SPECIALISTS:** Endocrinologists, family physicians, internists

**DEFINITION:** The growth of a tissue or organ as the result of an increase in the size of the existing cells within that tissue or organ; this process is responsible for the growth of the body as well as for increases in organ size caused by increased workloads on particular organs.

**KEY TERMS:**

*atrophy:* the wasting of tissue, an organ, or an entire body as the result of a decrease in the size and/or number of the cells within that tissue, organ, or body

*compensatory hypertrophy:* an increase in the size of a tissue or an organ in response to an increased workload placed upon it

*growth:* the increase in size of an organism or any of its parts during the developmental process; caused by increases in both cell numbers and cell size

*hyperplasia:* the increase in size or growth of a tissue or an organ as a result of an increase in cell numbers, with the size of the cells remaining constant

## PROCESS AND EFFECTS

The growth and development of the human body and all its parts requires not only an increase in the number of body cells as the body grows, a process known as hyperplasia, but also an increase in the size of the existing cells, a process known as hypertrophy. It is true that as humans grow, they increase the number of cells in their bodies, resulting in an increase in the size of tissues, organs, systems, and the body. For some tissues, organs, and systems, however, the number of cells is genetically set; therefore, the number of cells will increase minimally if at all after birth. Thus, if growth is to occur in those tissues, organs, and systems, it must take place by means of an increase in the size of the existing cells.

The process of hypertrophy occurs in nearly all tissues in the body but is most common in those tissues in which the number of cells is set at the time of birth. Among such tissues are adipose tissue, which is composed of fat cells, and nervous tissue, which is found in the brain, in the spinal cord, and in skeletal muscle tissue. Other tissues, such as cardiac tissue and smooth muscle tissue, also show the ability to undergo hypertrophy.

It is generally true that the number of fat cells within the human body is set at birth. Therefore, an increase in body fat is thought to result primarily from an increase in the amount of fat stored within the fat cells. An increase in the amount of fat consumed in the diet increases the amount of fat that is placed inside a fat cell, resulting in an increase in the fat cell's size.

The number of nerve cells within the brain and spinal cord also is set at birth. The cerebellum of the human brain, however, increases in size about twentyfold from birth to adulthood. This increase is brought about by an increase in the size of the existing nerve cells, and particularly by an increase in the number of extensions protruding from each nerve cell and the length to which the extensions grow. Furthermore, there is an increase in the number of the components within the cell. Specifically, there is an increase in the number of mitochondria within the cell, which provide a usable form of energy so that the cell can grow.

The number of skeletal muscle cells is also, in general, preset at the time of birth. The skeletal muscle mass of the human body increases dramatically from birth to adulthood. This increase is accomplished primarily by means of individual skeletal muscle cell hypertrophy. This increase in the diameter of the individual muscle cells is brought about by increases in the amounts of the contractile proteins, myosin and actin, as well as increases in the amount of glycogen and the number of mitochondria within individual cells. As each muscle cell increases in size, it causes an increase in the size of the entire muscle of which it is a part.

Each of the above-mentioned examples occurs naturally as part of the growth process of the human body. Some tissues, however, are capable of increasing in size as the result of an increased load or demand being placed upon them. This increased load or demand is usually brought about by an increased use of the muscle. This increase in the size of cells in response to an increased demand or use is called compensatory hypertrophy. The most common tissues that show the phenomenon of compensatory hypertrophy are the skeletal, cardiac, and smooth muscles.

Skeletal muscle is particularly responsive to being utilized. This response, however, is dependent upon the way in which the skeletal muscle is used. It is well known that an increase in the size of skeletal muscle can be brought about by such exercises as weight lifting. Lifting heavy weights or objects requires strong contractions of the skeletal muscle that is doing the lifting. If this lifting continues over a long period of time, it eventually results in an increase in the size of the existing muscle fibers, leading to an increase in the size of the exercised muscle. Because the strength of a muscle is dependent upon its size, the increase in the muscle's size results in an increase in its strength. The extent to which the size of the muscle increases is dependent upon the amount of time spent lifting the objects and the weight of the objects. The size that a muscle can reach is, however, limited.

Unlike exercises such as weight lifting, endurance types of exercise, such as walking, jogging, and aerobics, do not result in larger skeletal muscles. These types of exercise do not force the skeletal muscles to contract forcibly enough to produce muscle hypertrophy.

In the same way that an increased load or use will cause compensatory hypertrophy in skeletal muscle, a decreased use of skeletal muscle will result in its shrinking or wasting away. This process is referred to as muscle atrophy. This type of atrophy commonly occurs when limbs are broken or injured and must be immobilized. After six weeks of the limb being immobilized, there is a marked decrease in muscle size. A similar type of atrophy occurs in the limb muscles of astronauts, since there is no gravity present in space to provide resistance against which the muscles must work. If the muscles remain unused for more than a few months, there can be a loss of about one-half of the muscle mass of the unused muscle.

Cardiac muscle, like skeletal muscle, can also be caused to hypertrophy by increasing the resistance against which

## Hypertrophy

*Weight lifters and body builders take advantage of the process of hypertrophy to increase the size of their muscles.*

it works. Although endurance exercise does not cause hypertrophy in skeletal muscle, it does result in an increased size of the heart because of the hypertrophy of the existing cardiac muscle cells in this organ. In fact, the heart mass of marathon runners enlarges by about 40 percent as a result of the increase in endurance training. This increase occurs because the heart must work harder to pump more blood to the rest of the body when the body is endurance exercising. Only endurance forms of exercise result in the hypertrophy of the cardiac muscle. Weight lifting, which causes hypertrophy of skeletal muscle, has no effect on the cardiac muscle.

Smooth muscle also is capable of compensatory hypertrophy. Increased pressure or loads on the smooth muscle within arteries can result in the hypertrophy of the muscle cells. This in turn causes a thickening of the arterial wall. Smooth muscle, however, unlike skeletal and cardiac muscle, is capable of hyperplasia as well as hypertrophy.

## COMPLICATIONS AND DISORDERS

Hypertrophy also occurs as a result of some pathological and abnormal conditions. The most common pathological hypertrophy is enlargement of the heart as a result of cardiovascular disease. Most cardiovascular diseases put an increased workload on the heart, making it work harder to pump the blood throughout the body. In response to the increased workload, the heart increases its size, a form of compensatory hypertrophy.

The left ventricle of the heart is capable of hypertrophying to such an extent that its muscle mass may increase four- or fivefold. This increase is the result of improper functioning of the valves of the left heart. The valves of the heart work to prevent the backflow of blood from one chamber to another or from the arteries back to the heart. If the valves in the left heart are not working properly, the left ventricle contracts and blood that should leave the ventricle to go out to the body instead returns to the left ventricle. The enlargement of the left ventricle increases the force with which it can pump the blood out to the body, thus reducing the amount of blood that comes back to the left ventricle despite the damaged heart valves. There is, however, a point at which the enlargement of the left ventricle can no longer continue or help keep the needed amount of blood flowing through the body. At that point, the left ventricle finally tires out and left heart failure occurs.

The same type of hypertrophy can and does occur in the right side of the heart as well. Again, this is the result of damaged valves that are supposed to prevent the backflow of blood into the heart. Should the valves of both sides of the heart be damaged, hypertrophy can occur on both sides of the heart.

High blood pressure, also known as hypertension, may also lead to hypertrophy of the ventricles of the heart. With high blood pressure, the heart must work harder to deliver blood throughout the body because it must pump blood against an increased pressure. As a result of the increased demand upon the heart, the heart muscle hypertrophies in order to pump more blood.

The hypertrophy of the heart muscle is beneficial in the pumping of blood to the body in individuals who have valvular disease and hypertension; however, an extreme hypertrophy sometimes leads to heart failure. One of the reasons this may occur is the inability of the blood supply of the heart to keep up with the growth of the cardiac muscle. As a result, the cardiac cells outgrow their blood supply, resulting in the loss of blood and thus a loss of oxygen and nutrients needed for the cardiac cells to survive.

Smooth muscle, like cardiac muscle, may also hypertrophy under the condition of high blood pressure. Smooth muscle makes up the bulk of many of the arteries and smaller arterioles found in the body. The increased pressure on the arterial walls as a result of high blood pressure may cause the hypertrophy of the smooth muscles within the walls of the arteries and arterioles. This increases the thickness of the walls of the arteries and arterioles but also decreases the size of the hollow spaces within those vessels, which are known as the lumina. In the kidneys, the narrowing of the lumina of the arterioles may result in a decreased blood supply to these organs. The reduced blood flow to the kidneys may eventually cause the kidneys to shut down, leading to renal failure.

Smooth muscle may also hypertrophy under some unique conditions. During pregnancy, the uterus will undergo a dramatic hypertrophy. Recall that the uterus is a smooth muscle organ that is involved in the housing and nurturing of the developing fetus during pregnancy. Immediately prior to the birth of the fetus, there is marked hypertrophy of the smooth muscle within this organ. This increase in the size of the uterus is beneficial in providing the strong contractions of this organ that are needed for childbirth.

Skeletal muscle also may be caused to hypertrophy in some diseases in which there is an increase in the secretion of male sex hormones, particularly testosterone. Men's higher levels of testosterone, a potent stimulator of muscle growth, are responsible for the fact that males have a larger muscle mass than do females. Furthermore, synthetic testosterone-like hormones have been used by some athletes to increase muscle size. These synthetic hormones are called anabolic steroids. The use of these steroids does result in the hypertrophy of skeletal muscle, but these steroids have been shown to have harmful side effects.

Obesity is another condition that results largely from the hypertrophy of existing fat cells. In children, however, obesity is thought to result not only from an increase in the size of fat cells but also from an increase in their number. In adults, when weight is lost, it is the result of a decrease in the size of the existing fat cells; the number of fat cells remains constant. Thus, it is important to prevent further weight increases in overweight children to prevent the creation of fat cells that will never be lost.

In the onset of diseases that result in muscle degeneration, such as muscular dystrophy, there is a hypertrophy of the affected muscles. This hypertrophy differs from other forms of muscle hypertrophy in that the muscle cells do not increase in size because of an increase in the contractile protein, mitochondria, or glycogen, but because the muscle cells are being filled with fat. As a result of the contractile protein being replaced with fat, the affected muscles are no longer useful.

## PERSPECTIVE AND PROSPECTS

The exact mechanisms that bring about and control the hypertrophy of cells and tissues are not well understood. During the growth and developmental periods, however, the hypertrophy of many tissues is thought to be under the control of blood-borne chemicals known as hormones. Among these hormones is one that promotes growth and is thus called growth hormone. Growth hormone brings about an increase in the number and size of cells. Growth hormone causes the hypertrophy of existing cells by increasing the protein-making capability of these cells. Thus, there is an increase in the number of organelles, such as mitochondria, within the cell, which leads to an increase in cell size.

Growth hormone also causes the release of chemicals known as growth factors. There are several different growth factors, but one of particular importance is nerve growth factor. Nerve growth factor is involved with the increase in number of cell processes of single nerve cells. Such chemicals have been shown to enhance the growth of damaged nerve cells in the brains of animals. As a result, it is possible that nerve growth factor could be used in the treatment of nerve damage in humans by causing the nerves to grow new cell processes and form new connections to replace those that were damaged. This may be of great importance for the treatment of those suffering from brain or spinal cord damage.

Other hormones may have similar effects on tissues other than nervous tissue. For example, the hypertrophy of the smooth muscle in the uterus is thought to be brought about hormonally. Immediately prior to birth, when the hypertrophy of the uterus is occurring, there is an increased amount of estrogen, the primary female hormone, in the blood. It is this increase in estrogen that is thought to lead to the great enlargement of the uterus during this time. Some hormones have the effect of preventing or inhibiting the hypertrophy of body tissues. The enlargement of the uterus prior to birth is brought about not only by an increase in estrogen but also as a result of a decrease in another hormone known as progesterone. Progesterone levels are high in the blood throughout pregnancy. Immediately prior to birth, however, there is a dramatic decrease in the level of progesterone in the blood. Thus, it is believed that the high level of progesterone prevents or inhibits the hypertrophy

of the smooth muscle cells in the uterus, since the hypertrophy of this organ will not occur until estrogen levels are high and progesterone levels are low.

It has been suggested that compensatory hypertrophy, such as that which occurs in skeletal, smooth, and cardiac muscle, occurs as a result of the stretching of muscle. Some studies have shown that the stretching of skeletal, cardiac, and smooth muscle does lead to hypertrophy. American astronauts and Russian cosmonauts, however, showed a loss in muscle mass even though they exercised and stretched their muscles as much as three hours per day, seven days per week. This suggests that mechanisms other than the stretching of muscles may be involved in compensatory muscle hypertrophy.

Through an understanding of the mechanisms involved in muscle hypertrophy, it may one day be possible to prevent the atrophy that occurs during space flights, prolonged bed rest, and immobilization necessitated by the injury of limbs. Furthermore, the understanding of the mechanisms that control hypertrophy may help to alleviate the effects of disabling diseases such as muscular dystrophy by reversing the effects of muscle atrophy. —*David K. Saunders*

*See also* Growth; Muscular dystrophy; Obesity; Pregnancy and gestation.

## FOR FURTHER INFORMATION:

Guyton, Arthur C. *Textbook of Medical Physiology.* 7th ed. Philadelphia: W. B. Saunders, 1986. An easily read textbook that provides much information on compensatory hypertrophy and other forms of hypertrophy. Provides an in-depth look at hypertrophy and the mechanisms that bring it about, particularly the effects of exercise on the hypertrophy of skeletal and cardiac muscle. Also provides many examples of diseases and abnormal processes that cause hypertrophy.

Hatfield, Frederick C. *Power: A Scientific Approach.* Chicago Contemporary Books, 1989. This book was written for body builders so that they might better understand the science behind body building. The author provides an in-depth but easily read view of skeletal muscle hypertrophy caused by weight lifting. He also provides information on the effects of anabolic steroids on skeletal muscle hypertrophy and on the other organs of the body.

Hole, John W., Jr. *Human Anatomy and Physiology.* 6th ed. Dubuque, Iowa: Wm. C. Brown, 1993. An introductory college anatomy and physiology text that is easily read and understood. Provides a good general overview of the processes of hypertrophy and atrophy. Also provides a close look at the effects of muscle use and disuse on skeletal muscle hypertrophy and atrophy.

Marieb, Elaine N. *Human Anatomy and Physiology.* 2d ed. Redwood City, Calif.: Benjamin/Cummings, 1992. Provides an in-depth look at how obesity occurs as a result of both hypertrophy and hyperplasia. Also provides an overview of the hormones that can cause hypertrophy and the mechanisms by which they bring about changes in size.

Shostak, Stanley. *Embryology: An Introduction to Developmental Biology.* New York: HarperCollins, 1991. Provides an introduction to the growth and development of the human body. It provides a good discussion of the role that hypertrophy plays in the development of the human body. It also points out those tissues that grow primarily by hypertrophy rather than by hyperplasia.

Tortora, Gerard J., and Nicholas P. Anagnostakos. *Principles of Anatomy and Physiology.* 6th ed. New York: Harper & Row, 1990. This textbook does a good job of explaining hypertrophy in skeletal, cardiac, and smooth muscle. It provides several examples of pathological conditions in which hypertrophy occurs and may be harmful.

# HYPOCHONDRIASIS

**SYSTEMS AFFECTED:** Psychic-emotional, all bodily systems

**SPECIALISTS:** Psychiatrists, psychologists

**DEFINITION:** Unwarranted belief about or anxiety over having a serious disease which is based on one's subjective interpretation of physical symptoms or sensations; the belief or anxiety is maintained in spite of appropriate medical assurances that there is no serious disease.

**KEY TERMS:**

*defense mechanisms:* automatic, unconscious mental processes that become activated in the presence of emotional distress and anxiety; these processes work to maintain inner harmony by preventing mental awareness of that which would be otherwise too emotionally painful to endure

*hypochondria:* an earlier term for hypochondriasis; from classical Greek, it means the abdominal region of the body below the rib cage, from which black bile was believed to cause melancholy and yellow bile was believed to cause ill-temper

*hypochondriacal neurosis:* an earlier, but still-used term for hypochondriasis; because experts have disagreed about what "neurosis" means precisely, the term is considered less descriptive than "hypochondriasis"

*hypochondriacal reaction:* another earlier term for hypochondriasis; experts who still prefer this term view hypochondriasis as a transient reaction to life stress and tend not to see it as a mental-emotional disorder in its own right

*primary hypochondriasis:* hypochondriasis as a disorder in its own right, and not accompanied by another psychiatric disorder such as generalized anxiety or panic

*secondary hypochondriasis:* the experience of hypochondriacal symptoms as part of an underlying, causal condition such as panic disorder, generalized anxiety disorder, schizophrenia, or major depression with psychotic features

*somatization disorder:* the somatoform disorder most similar to hypochondriasis; in somatization, the preoccupation is primarily with symptoms that one experiences and not with a disease that one is fearful of getting, an important distinction when these conditions are treated

*somatoform disorders:* the grouping of disorders that includes hypochondriasis; these disorders feature symptoms that suggest physical disease but that are actually caused by psychological upset

## CAUSES AND SYMPTOMS

With hypochondriasis, the real problem is the patient's excessive worry and mental preoccupation with having or developing a disease, not the disease about which the patient is so worried. While concern about contracting a serious disease is common, normal, and may even make one more prudent, excessive worry, endless rumination, and obsessive interpretation of every symptom and sensation can disable and prevent effective functioning. A diagnosis of hypochondriasis is made when the patient's dread about the disease or diseases impairs normal activity and persists despite appropriate medical reassurances and evidence to the contrary. Even though hypochondriacs can acknowledge intellectually the possibility that their fears might be without rational foundation, the acknowledgment itself fails to bring any relief.

Researchers estimate that a low of 3 percent to a high of 14 percent of all medical (versus psychiatric) patients have hypochondriasis. Just how prevalent it is in the population as a whole is unknown. What is known is that the disorder shows up slightly more in men than in women, starts at any age but most often between twenty and thirty, shows up most often in physicians' offices with patients who are in their forties and fifties, and tends to run in families.

Most clinicians believe that hypochondriasis has a primary psychological cause or causes but that, in general, hypochondriacs have only a vague awareness that they are doing something that perpetuates and worsens their hypochondriacal symptoms. Hypochondriacs do not feign illness; they genuinely believe themselves to be sick, or about to become so.

Clinicians usually favor one of four hypotheses about how hypochondriasis starts. The hypotheses are based on anecdotal, clinical experience with patients who have gotten better when treated specifically for hypochondriasis. Researchers have rarely studied hypochondriasis using strict experimental methods. Nevertheless, the anecdotal evidence is important, because it gives clinicians a way to think about how to treat the condition.

The most popular view among mental health professionals sees hypochondriacs as essentially angry, but deep down inside. Because their life experience is of hurt, disappointment, rejection, and loss, they engage in a two-stage process to make up for their sad state of affairs. Though they believe themselves unlovable and unacceptable as they are, they solicit attention and caring by presenting themselves either as ill or as dangerously close to becoming ill. Their fundamental anger fosters their development of an interpersonal pattern in which they bite the emotional hands which seek to feed them. Endless worry and rumination soon render ineffective others' concern. No amount of reassurance allays their preoccupation and anxiety. In this way, those moved to show concern tire, grow impatient, and finally give up their efforts to help, proving to the worried hypochondriacs that no one really does care about them after all. Meanwhile, the hypochondriacs remain sad and angry.

This view often assumes that hypochondriasis is actually a form of defense mechanism which transfers angry, hostile, and critical feelings felt toward others into physical symptoms and signs of disease. Because hypochondriacs find it too difficult to admit that they feel angry, isolated, and unloved, they hide from the emotional energy associated with these powerful feelings and transfer them into bodily symptoms. This process seems to occur most often when hypochondriacal people harbor feelings of reproach because they are bereaved and lonely. In effect, they are angry at being left alone and left uncared for, and they redirect the emotion inwardly as self-reproach manifested in physical complaints.

Others hypothesize that hypochondriasis enables those who either believe themselves to be basically bad and unworthy of happiness or feel guilty for being alive ("existential guilt") to atone for their wrongdoings and, thereby, undo the guilt that they are always fighting not to feel. The mental anguish, emotional sadness, and physical pain so prevalent in hypochondriasis make reparation for the patients' real, exaggerated, or imagined badness.

A third view is sociological in orientation. Health providers who endorse it see hypochondriasis as society's way of letting people who feel frightened and overwhelmed by life's challenges escape from having to face those challenges, even if temporarily. Hypochondriacs take on a "sick role" which removes societal expectations that they will face responsibilities. In presenting themselves to the world as too sick to function, they also present themselves as excused from doing so. A schoolchild's stomachache on the day of a big test provides a relatively common and potentially harmless example of this role at work. Non-physically disabled adults who seek refuge from life stress by staying in bed, and who find themselves with true physical paralysis years later, provide a more serious and regrettable example.

A fourth view utilizes some experimental data which suggest that hypochondriacal people may have lower thresholds for (and lower tolerances of) emotional and physical pain. The data suggest that hypochondriacs experience physical and/or emotional sensations that are a magnification of what is normal experience. Thus, sensation that what would be sinus pressure for most people would be experienced as severe sinus headache in the hypochondriac. Hypersensitivity (lower threshold) to bodily sensations keeps hypochondriacs ever on watch for these upsetting, intense sensations because of how amplified the physical and emotional experiences are. What seems to most people an exaggerated concern with symptoms is simply prudent, self-protective vigilance to hypochondriacs.

Regardless of why the disorder develops, the majority of hypochondriacs go to their physicians with concerns about stomach and intestinal problems or heart and blood circulation problems. These complaints are usually only part of broader concerns about other organ systems and other anatomical locations. The key clinical feature of the disorder of hypochondriasis, however, is not where and how many bodily complaints there are but the patients' belief that they are seriously sick, or are just about to become so, and that the disease has yet to be detected. Laboratory tests that reveal healthy organs, physician reassurances that they are well, and long periods in which the dreaded disease fails to manifest itself are not reassuring at all. In fact, before the hypochondriasis itself is treated psychologically, it seems that nothing can stop the frantic rumination and accompanying nervousness, even the patients' acknowledgment that they may be exaggerating their reaction to their heartbeat, headache, diarrhea, morning cough, or perspiration. Hypochondriacs seem genuinely unable not to worry.

Hypochondriacs typically present their medical history in great detail and at great length. Often, they have an elaborate, exotic, and complex pathophysiological theory to explain how they acquired the disease and what it is doing, or will soon do, to them. At times, they cite recent research and give great importance to other causes, tests, or treatments that they and their health providers have not yet tried. Because their actual problem is not, strictly speaking, medical (or not only medical) and because they usually frustrate professional caretakers such as physicians, as well as nonprofessional caretakers such as family and friends, breakdown in the helping process is common. Worried patients tax physicians' time and resources, while busy physicians feel increasingly drained for what they believe is no good reason. The hypochondriacal patients sense that their concerns are not respected or taken seriously; they start to sense resentment. Phone calls to physicians' offices go unreturned for longer and longer periods. The perceived lack of access to their health providers makes the hypochondriac worry even more frenetically. The physicians increasingly believe that these patients are unappreciative—that they are, in fact, healthy and that they are not cooperating with treatment goals. Instead, these hypochondriacal patients are seen as excessively demanding. Anger builds on both sides, relationships deteriorate, and the hypochondriacs begin to "doctor-shop," while the physicians lose them as patients.

Although hypochondriasis is usually chronic, with periods in which it is more and less severe, temporary hypochondriacal reactions are also commonly seen. Such reactions most often occur when patients have experienced a death or serious illness of someone close to them or some other major life stressor, including their own recovery from a life-threatening illness.

When these reactions persist for less than six months, the technical diagnosis is a condition called "somatoform disorder not otherwise specified," and not hypochondriasis. When external stressors cause the reaction, the hypochondriacal symptoms usually remit when the stressors dissipate or are resolved. The important exception to this rule occurs when family, friends, or health professionals inadvertently reinforce the worry and preoccupation through inappropriate amounts of attention. In effect, they reward hypochondriacal behavior and increase the likelihood that it will persist: A mother may never have received more support and help at home than following breast cancer surgery; a father may never have felt his children's affection as much as when he recuperated from having a heart attack; an employee may have never obtained special allowances on the job or received so many calls from coworkers as when recovering from herniated disk surgery; or a student may never have gotten as special treatment or as many gifts from teammates as when treated for rheumatic fever. What began as a transient hypochondriacal reaction can become chronic, primary hypochondriasis.

The life of hypochondriacs is unhappy and unrewarding. Nervous tension, depression, hopelessness, and a general lack of interest in life mark the fabric of the hypochondriacs' daily routines. Actual clinical, depressive disorders can easily coexist with hypochondriasis, to the point that even antidepression medications will simultaneously alleviate hypochondriacal symptoms.

Hypochondriasis often accompanies physical illness in the elderly. As a group, the elderly have declining health, experience diminished physical capacities, and are at increased risk for contracting and developing disease. Sometimes, earlier tendencies toward hypochondriasis simply intensify with age. Sometimes, old age is simply when it first appears. Hypochondriasis is not, however, a typical or expected aspect of normal aging; most elderly people are not hypochondriacal. In those who are, however, hypochondriasis is most likely a symptom of depression, abandonment, or loneliness, and these are the conditions that should first be treated.

### TREATMENT AND THERAPY

The most important aspect of treating hypochondriasis is assessing whether true organic disease exists. Many diseases in their early stages are diffuse and affect multiple organ systems. Neurologic diseases (such as multiple sclerosis), hormonal abnormalities (such as Graves' disease), and autoimmune/connective tissue diseases (such as systemic lupus) can all manifest themselves early in ways that are difficult to diagnose accurately. The frantic and obsessive reporting of hypochondriacal patients can just as easily be the worried and detailed reporting of patients with early parathyroid disease; both report symptoms that are multiple, vague, and diffuse. The danger of hypochondriasis lies in its being diagnosed in place of true organic disease, which is exactly the kind of event hypochondriacs fear will happen.

Of course, there is nothing to prevent someone with true hypochondriasis from getting or having true physical illness. Worrying about illness neither protects from nor prevents illness. Moreover, barring a sudden, lethal accident or event, every hypochondriac is bound to develop organic illness sooner or later. Physical illness can coexist with hypochondriasis—and does so when attitudes, symptoms, and mental and emotional states are extreme and disproportionate to the medical problem at hand.

The goal in treating hypochondriasis is care, not cure. These patients have ongoing mental illness or chronic maladaptation and seem to need physical symptoms to justify how they feel. Neither surgical nor medical interventions will ameliorate a psychological need for symptoms. The best treatments (when hypochondriasis cannot itself be the target of treatment, which is most of the time) are long term in orientation and seek to help patients tolerate and accommodate their symptoms while health providers learn to understand and adapt to these difficult-to-treat patients.

Medications have proved useful in treating hypochondriasis only when accompanied by pharmacotherapy-sensitive conditions such as major depression or generalized anxiety. When hypochondriasis coexists with either mental or physical disease, the latter must be treated in its own right. Secondary hypochondriasis means that the primary disorder warrants primary treatment.

The course of hypochondriasis is unclear. Clinicians' anecdotal experience tends to endorse the perception that these people are impossible as patients. Outcome studies, however, belie the pessimism. The research suggests that many who are treated get better, and the more the following conditions are present, the better the outcome is likely to be: coexisting anxiety or depressive disorder, rapid onset, onset at a younger age, higher socioeconomic status, absence of organic disease, and absence of a personality disorder.

A fifty-six-year-old married male, for example, recounted his history as never having been in really good health at any time in his life. He made many physician office visits and had, over the years, seen many physicians, though without ever feeling emotionally connected to them. Over the past several months, he felt increasingly concerned that he was having headaches "all over" his head and that they were caused by an undetected tumor in the middle of his brain, "where no X ray could detect it." He had read about magnetic resonance imaging (MRI) in a health letter to which he subscribed and said that he wanted this procedure performed "to catch the tumor early." Various prescribed medications for his headache usually brought no relief.

While productive at work and promoted several times, he had been passed over for his last promotion because, he believed, his superiors did not like him. He also stated that he believed that many on the job saw him as cynical and pessimistic but that no one appreciated the "pain and mental anxiety" he endured "day in and day out."

His spouse of thirty-two years had advanced significantly at a job she had begun ten years earlier, and she seemed to him to be closer to their three children than he was. She was increasingly involved with outside voluntary activities, which kept her quite busy. She reported that she often asked him to join her in at least some of her activities but he always said no. She said that when she arrived home late, he was often in a state of physical upset, but for which she could never seem to do the "right thing to help him." In their joint interview, each admitted often feeling angry at and frustrated with the other. She could never determine why he was sick so often and why her efforts to help only seemed to make his situation worse. He could not understand how she could leave him all alone feeling as physically bad as he did. He believed that she never seemed to worry that something might happen to him while she was out being "a community do-gooder." The husband was suffering from a classic case of hypochondriasis.

### PERSPECTIVE AND PROSPECTS

Both the concept and term "hypochondriasis" have ancient origins and reflect a view that all persons are subject to their own humoral ebb and flow. Humors were once thought to be bodily fluids that maintained health, regulated physical functioning, and caused certain personality traits. In classical Greek, *hypochondria*, the plural of *hypochondrion*, referred to both a part of the anatomy and the condition known today as hypochondriasis. *Hypo* means "under," "below," or "beneath," and *chondrion* means literally "cartilage" but in this case refers specifically to the bottom tip of cartilage at the breastbone (the xiphoid or, more formally, xiphisternum). Here, below the breastbone but above the navel, two humors were thought to flow in excess in the hypochondriacal person. The liver, producing black bile, made people melancholic, depressed, and depressing; the spleen, producing yellow bile, made people bilious, cross, and cynical. This view, or a variant of it, persisted until the middle to late eighteenth century.

Sigmund Freud and other psychiatrists treated hypochondriacal symptoms with some success while approaching the disorder as a defense mechanism rather than as an excess of bodily fluids. Their treatment for the first time cast a psychological role for what had been seen as a physical problem. Mental health professionals whose theoretical orientation is psychoanalytic or psychodynamic continue to deal with hypochondriasis as they deal with other defense mechanisms.

In the 1970's, some researchers began to suggest that hypochondriasis was being incorrectly applied to describe a discrete disorder, when it was really only an adjective that described a cluster of nonspecific behaviors. They argued that hypochondriasis is not a real diagnosis. Other researchers disagreed and argued for differentiating between primary and secondary hypochondriasis. Their view has proved to have significant pragmatic utility in treating the wide range of patients who exhibit symptoms of hypochondriasis, and it remains the prevailing view.

Given the general unwillingness of patients with hypochondriasis to admit that they have a psychological problem and not some yet-to-be-found organic condition, the interpersonal difficulties that often arise between health providers and these patients, and the serious potential of concurrent organic disease, it is not surprising why hypochondriasis continues to challenge both persons afflicted with this disorder and those who treat them.   —Paul Moglia

***See also*** Anxiety; Depression; Factitious disorders; Manic-depressive disorder; Midlife crisis; Neurosis; Obsessive-compulsive disorder; Panic attacks; Phobias; Psychiatric disorders; Psychosomatic disorders; Stress.

### FOR FURTHER INFORMATION:

Barsky, Arthur J. "Somatoform Disorders." *In Comprehensive Textbook of Psychiatry*. Vol. 1, edited by Harold I. Kaplan and Benjamin J. Sadock. 5th ed. Baltimore: Williams & Wilkins, 1989. While Kaplan and Sadock's book remains the standard psychiatric reference for psychiatrists and nonpsychiatric physicians alike, Barsky's chapter includes an excellent discussion of hypochondriasis that is readily intelligible to lay readers. He includes practical recommendations for primary care physicians who deal with hypochondriacal patients as well as a careful delineation of how hypochondriasis differs from other, similar somatoform disorders.

Hill, John. *Hypochondriasis: A Practical Treatise*. New York: AMS Press, 1992. Originally published in 1766, this well-regarded and readable work presents the world of the hypochondriac in ways that challenge stereotypical and biased views of them. If the reader were to consult only one book on hypochondriasis, this should be it.

Kellner, Robert. *Somatization and Hypochondriasis*. New York: Praeger, 1986. A world authority on somatoform and somatization disorders, Kellner offers an exceptional textbook on hypochondriasis. He not only presents up-to-date information objectively but suggests approaches to the unanswered questions in clinical theory and treatment.

Kenyon, F. E. "Hypochondriacal States." *British Journal of Psychiatry* 129 (July, 1976): 1-14. In this review article, Kenyon argues strongly for discontinuing hypochondriasis as a diagnosis in its own right and using it only as a descriptive adjective when patients are preoccupied with their health. The thesis presented by this leading clinical researcher includes a discussion of how neither patient nor health practitioner benefits in trying to develop treatments for a diagnosis that, in his view, does not exist. Regardless of whether one agrees with the thesis, the review is an excellent summary of what has been happening in the field.

Pilowsky, I. "Primary and Secondary Hypochondriasis." *Acta Psychiatrica Scandinavica* 46 (1970): 273-285. This article presents the seminal opposing view to Kenyon's, noted above. Pilowsky argues persuasively that hypochondriasis is a complex diagnosis, with symptoms appearing along with several mental conditions. This view remains the prevailing one in American psychiatric and psychological circles and has given rise to several pragmatic approaches to treatment.

# HYPOGLYCEMIA

SYSTEMS AFFECTED: Endocrine, blood

SPECIALISTS: Endocrinologists, family physicians, internists

DEFINITION: The condition in which concentration of glucose in the blood is too low to meet the needs of key organs, especially in the brain; this condition limits treatments for diabetes mellitus.

KEY TERMS:

*fasting hypoglycemia:* hypoglycemia that occurs when no food is available from the intestinal tract; usually caused by failure of the neural, hormonal, and/or enzymatic mechanisms that convert stored fuels (primarily glycogen) into glucose

*glucagon:* a pancreatic hormone which signals an elevated concentration of glucose in the circulation

*gluconeogenesis:* the synthesis of molecules of glucose from smaller carbohydrates and amino acids

*glucose:* a simple sugar, readily converted to metabolic energy by most cells of the body and essential for the welfare of brain cells

*glycogen:* a storage form of carbohydrate, composed of many molecules of glucose linked together; found in many tissues of the body and serves as a major source of circulating glucose

*glycogenolysis:* the cleavage of glycogen into its constituent molecules of glucose

*hypoglycemic unawareness:* the occurrence of hypoglycemia without the warning symptoms of trembling, palpitations, hunger, or anxiety

*hypoglycemic unresponsiveness:* inadequate recovery of the circulating glucose concentration after an episode of hypoglycemia

*insulin:* a pancreatic hormone which signals a reduced concentration of glucose in the circulation

*neuroglycopenia:* abnormal function of the brain, caused by an inadequate supply of glucose from the circulation

*reactive hypoglycemia:* hypoglycemia that occurs within a few hours after ingestion of a meal

## CAUSES AND SYMPTOMS

The condition known as hypoglycemia exists when the concentration of glucose in the bloodstream is too low to meet bodily needs for fuel, particularly those of the brain. Ordinarily, physiological compensatory mechanisms are called into play when the circulating concentration of glucose falls below about 3.5 millimoles. Activation of the sympathetic nervous system and the secretion of glucagon are especially important in promoting glycogenolysis and gluconeogenesis. Symptoms of sympathetic nervous activation normally become apparent with glucose concentrations that are less than about 3 millimoles. Brain function is usually demonstrably abnormal at glucose concentrations below about 2 millimoles; sustained hypoglycemia in this range can lead to permanent brain damage.

Some of the symptoms of hypoglycemia occur as by-products of activation of the sympathetic nervous system. These symptoms include trembling, pallor, palpitations and rapid heartbeat, sweating, abdominal discomfort, and feelings of anxiety and/or hunger. These symptoms are not dangerous in themselves; in fact, they may be considered to be beneficial, as they alert the individual to obtain food. Meanwhile, the sympathetic nervous system signals compensatory mechanisms. The manifestations of abnormal brain function during hypoglycemia include blunting of higher cognitive functions, disturbed mentation, confusion, loss of normal control of behavior, headache, lethargy, impaired vision, abnormal speech, paralysis, neurologic deficits, coma, and epileptic seizures. The individual is usually unaware of the appearance of these symptoms, which can present real danger. For example, episodes of hypoglycemia have occurred while individuals were driving motor vehicles, leading to serious injury and death. After recovery from hypoglycemia, the patient may have no memory of the episode.

There are two major categories of hypoglycemia: fasting and reactive. The most serious, fasting hypoglycemia, represents impairment of the mechanisms responsible for the production of glucose when food is not available. These mechanisms include the functions of cells in the liver and brain that monitor the availability of circulating glucose. Additionally, there is a coordinated hormonal response involving the secretion of glucagon, growth hormone, and other hormones and the inhibition of the secretion of insulin. The normal consequences of these processes include the addition of glucose to the circulation, primarily from glycogenolysis, as well as a slowing of the rate of utilization of circulating glucose by many tissues of the body, especially the liver, skeletal and cardiac muscle, and fat. Even after days without food, the body normally avoids hypoglycemia through breakdown of stored proteins and activation of gluconeogenesis. There is considerable redundancy in the systems that maintain glucose concentration, so that the occurrence of hypoglycemia often reflects the presence of defects in more than one of these mechanisms.

The other category of hypoglycemia, reactive hypoglycemia, includes disorders in which there is disproportionately prolonged and/or great activity of the physiologic systems that normally cause storage of the glucose derived from ingested foods. When a normal person eats a meal, the passage of food through the stomach and intestines elicits a complex and well-orchestrated neural and hormonal response, culminating in the secretion of insulin from the beta cells of the islets of Langerhans in the pancreas. The insulin signals the cells in muscle, adipose tissue, and the liver to stop producing glucose and to derive energy from glucose obtained from the circulation. Glucose in excess of the body's immediate needs for fuel is taken up and stored as glycogen is or utilized for the manufacture of proteins. Normally, the signals for the uptake and storage of glucose reach their peak of activity simultaneously with the entry into the circulation of glucose from the food undergoing digestion. As a result, the concentration of glucose in the circulation fluctuates only slightly. In individuals with reactive hypoglycemia, however, the entry of glucose from the digestive tract and the signals for its uptake and storage are not well synchronized. When signals for the cellular uptake of glucose persist after the intestinally derived glucose has dissipated, hypoglycemia can result. Although the degree of hypoglycemia may be severe and potentially dangerous, recovery can take place without assistance if the individual's general nutritional state is adequate and the systems for activation of glycogenolysis and gluconeogenesis are intact.

### DIAGNOSIS AND TREATMENT

The diagnostic evaluation of an individual who is suspected of having hypoglycemia begins with verification of the condition. Evaluation of a patient's symptoms can be confusing. On the one hand, the symptoms arising from the sympathetic nervous system and those of neuroglycopenia may occur in a variety of nonhypoglycemic conditions. On the other hand, persons with recurrent hypoglycemia may have few or no obvious symptoms. Therefore, it is most important to document the concentration of glucose in the blood.

To establish the diagnosis of fasting hypoglycemia, the patient is kept without food for periods of time up to seventy-two hours, with frequent monitoring of the blood glucose. Should hypoglycemia occur, blood is taken for measurements of the key regulatory neurosecretions and hormones, including insulin, glucagon, growth hormone, cortisol, and epinephrine, as well as general indices of the function of the liver and kidneys. If there is suspicion of an abnormality in an enzyme involved in glucose production, the diagnosis can be confirmed by measurement of the relevant enzymatic activity in circulating blood cells or, if necessary, in a biopsy specimen of the liver.

Fasting hypoglycemia may be caused by any condition that inhibits the production of glucose or that causes an inappropriately great utilization of circulating glucose when food is not available. Insulin produces hypoglycemia through both of these mechanisms. Excessive circulating insulin ranks as one of the most important causes of fasting hypoglycemia, most cases of which result from the treatment of diabetes mellitus with insulin or with an oral drug of the sulfonylurea class. If the patient is known to be taking insulin or a sulfonylurea drug for diabetes, the cause of hypoglycemia is obvious and appropriate modification of the treatment should be made. Hypoglycemia caused by oral sulfonylureas is particularly troublesome because of the prolonged retention of these drugs in the body. The passage of several days may be required for recovery, during which time the patient needs continuous intravenous infusion of glucose.

Excessive insulin secretion may also result from increased numbers of pancreatic beta cells; the abnormal beta cells may be so numerous that they form benign or malignant tumors, called insulinomas. The preferred treatment of an insulinoma is surgery, if feasible. When the tumor can be removed surgically, the operation is often curative. Unfortunately, insulinomas are sometimes difficult for the surgeon to find. Magnetic resonance imaging (MRI), computed tomography (CT) scanning, ultrasonography, or angiography may help localize the tumor. Some insulinomas are multiple and/or malignant, rendering total removal impossible. In these circumstances, hypoglycemia can be relieved by drugs that inhibit the secretion of insulin.

Malignant tumors arising from various tissues of the body may produce hormones that act like insulin with respect to their effects on glucose metabolism. In some cases, these hormones are members of the family of insulin-like growth factors, which resemble insulin structurally. Malnutrition probably has an important role in predisposing patients with malignancy to hypoglycemia, which tends to occur when the cancer is far advanced.

Fasting hypoglycemia can be caused by disorders affecting various parts of the endocrine system. One such disorder is adrenal insufficiency; continued secretion of cortisol by the adrenal cortex is required for maintenance of normal glycogen stores and of the enzymes of glycogenolysis and gluconeogenesis. Severe hypothyroidism also may lead to hypoglycemia. Impairment in the function of the anterior pituitary gland predisposes a patient to hypoglycemia through several mechanisms, including reduced function of the thyroid gland and adrenal cortices (which depend on pituitary secretions for normal activity) and reduced secretion of growth hormone. Growth hormone plays an important physiologic role in the prevention of fasting hypoglycemia by signaling metabolic changes that allow heart and skeletal muscles to derive energy from stored fats, thereby sparing glucose for the brain. Specific replacement therapies are available for deficiencies of thyroxine, cortisol, and growth hormone.

Hypoglycemia has occasionally been reported as a side effect of treatment with medications other than those intended for treatment of diabetes. Drugs which have been implicated include sulfonamides, used for treatment of bacterial infections; quinine, used for treatment of falciparum malaria; pentamidine isethionate, given by injection for treatment of pneumocystosis; ritodrine, used for inhibition of premature labor; and propranolol or disopyramide, both of which are used for treatment of cardiac arrhythmias. Malnourished patients seem to be especially susceptible to the hypoglycemic effects of these medications, and management should consist of nutritional repletion in addition to discontinuation of the drug responsible. In children, aspirin or other medicines containing salicylates may produce hypoglycemia.

Alcohol hypoglycemia occurs in persons with low bodily stores of glycogen when there is no food in the intestine. In this circumstance, the only potential source of glucose for the brain is gluconeogenesis. When such an individual drinks alcohol, its metabolism within the liver prevents the precursors of glucose from entering the pathways of gluconeogenesis. This variety of fasting hypoglycemia can occur in persons who are not chronic alcoholics: It requires the ingestion of only a moderate amount of alcohol, on the order of three mixed drinks. Treatment involves the nutritional repletion of glycogen stores and the limitation of alcohol intake.

Severe infections, including overwhelming bacterial infection and malaria, can produce hypoglycemia by mechanisms that are not well understood. Patients with very severe liver damage can develop fasting hypoglycemia, because the pathways of glycogenolysis and gluconeogenesis in the liver are by far the major sources of circulating glucose in the fasted state. In such cases, the occurrence of hypoglycemia usually marks a near-terminal stage of liver disease. Uremia, the syndrome produced by kidney failure, can also lead to fasting hypoglycemia.

Some types of fasting hypoglycemia occur predominantly in infants and children. Babies in the first year of life may have an inappropriately high secretion of insulin. This problem occurs especially in newborn infants whose mothers had increased circulating glucose during pregnancy. Children from two to ten years of age may develop ketotic hypoglycemia, which is probably related to insufficient gluconeogenesis. These disorders tend to improve with time. Fasting hypoglycemia is also an important manifestation of a variety of inherited disorders of metabolism characterized by the abnormality or absence of one of the necessary enzymes or cofactors of glycogenolysis and gluconeogenesis or of fat metabolism (which supplies the energy for gluconeogenesis). Most of these disorders become evident in infancy or childhood. If there is a hereditary or acquired deficiency of an enzyme of glucose production, the problem can be circumvented by provision of a continuous supply of glucose to the affected individual.

There are several other rare causes of fasting hypoglycemia. A few individuals have had circulating antibodies that caused hypoglycemia by interacting with the patient's own insulin, or with receptors for insulin on the patient's cells. Although the autonomic (involuntary) nervous system has an important role in signaling recovery from hypoglycemia, diseases affecting this branch of the nervous system do not usually produce hypoglycemia; presumably, hormonal mechanisms can substitute for the missing neural signals.

Reactive hypoglycemia can occur when there is unusually rapid passage of foodstuffs through the upper intestinal tract, such as may occur after partial or total removal of the stomach. Persons predisposed to maturity-onset diabetes may also have reactive hypoglycemia, probably because of the delay in the secretion of insulin in response to a meal. Finally, reactive hypoglycemia need not indicate the presence of any identifiable disease and may occur in otherwise normal individuals.

Diagnosis of reactive hypoglycemia is made difficult by the variability of symptoms and of glucose concentrations from day to day. Adding to the diagnostic uncertainty, circulating glucose normally rises and falls after meals, especially those rich in carbohydrates. Consequently, entirely normal and asymptomatic individuals may sometimes have glucose concentrations at or below the levels found in persons with reactive hypoglycemia. Therefore, the glucose tolerance test, in which blood samples are taken at intervals for several hours after the patient drinks a solution containing 50 to 100 grams of glucose, is quite unreliable and should not be employed for the diagnosis of reactive hypoglycemia. Proper diagnosis of reactive hypoglycemia depends on careful correlation of the patient's symptoms with the circulating glucose level, preferably measured on several occasions after ingestion of ordinary meals. Some persons develop symptoms such as weakness, nausea, sweating, and tremulousness after meals, but without a significant reduction of circulating glucose. This symptom complex should not be confused with hypoglycemia.

When rapid passage of food through the stomach and upper intestine causes reactive hypoglycemia, the administration of drugs that slow intestinal transit may be helpful. When reactive hypoglycemia has no evident pathological cause, the patient is usually advised to take multiple small meals throughout the day instead of the usual three meals and to avoid concentrated sweets. These dietary modifications can help avoid hypoglycemia by reducing the stimulus to secretion of insulin.

Two rare inherited disorders of metabolism can produce reactive hypoglycemia after the ingestion of certain foods. In hereditary fructose intolerance, the offending nutrient is fructose, a sugar found in fruits as well as ordinary table sugar. In galactosemia, the sugar responsible for hypoglycemia is galactose, a major component of milk products. Management of these conditions, which usually become apparent in infancy or childhood, consists of avoidance of the foods responsible.

## PERSPECTIVE AND PROSPECTS

Fasting hypoglycemia is uncommon, except in the context of treatment of diabetes mellitus. The most serious public health problem associated with hypoglycemia is that it limits the therapeutic effectiveness of insulin and sulfonylurea drugs. Evidence suggests that elevation of the circulating glucose concentration (hyperglycemia) is responsible for much of the disability and premature death among patients with diabetes. In many of these patients, therapeutic regimens consisting of multiple daily injections of insulin or continuous infusion of insulin through a small needle placed under the skin can reduce the average circulating glucose to normal. Frequent serious hypoglycemia is the most important adverse consequence of such regimens. Persons with diabetes seem to be at especially high risk for dangerous hypoglycemia for two reasons. First, there is often a failure of the warning systems that ordinarily cause uncomfortable symptoms when the circulating glucose concentration declines, a situation termed hypoglycemic unawareness. As a consequence, when a patient with diabetes attempts to control his or her blood sugar with more frequent injections of insulin, there may occur unheralded episodes of hypoglycemia that can lead to serious alterations in mental activity or even loss of consciousness. Many patients with diabetes also have hypoglycemic unresponsiveness, an impaired ability to recover from episodes of hypoglycemia. Also, diabetes can interfere with the normal physiologic responses that cause the secretion of glucagon in response to a reduction of circulating glucose, thus eliminating one of the most important defenses against hypoglycemia. If both hypoglycemic unawareness and hypoglycemic unresponsiveness could be reversed, intensive treatment of diabetes would become safer and more widely applicable.

Reactive hypoglycemia, although seldom a clue to serious disease, has attracted public attention because of its peculiarly annoying symptoms. These symptoms, which reflect activation of the sympathetic nervous system, resemble those of fear and anxiety. The symptoms are not specific, and many patients with these complaints do not have hypoglycemia.

In summary, hypoglycemia indicates defective regulation of the supply of energy to the body. When severe or persistent, hypoglycemia can lead to serious behavioral disorder, obtunded consciousness, and even brain damage. Fasting hypoglycemia may be a clue to significant endocrine disease. Reactive hypoglycemia, while annoying, usually responds to simple dietary measures. The study of hypoglycemia has led to many important insights into the regulation of energy metabolism.   —*Victor R. Lavis*

*See also* Diabetes mellitus; Endocrine disorders; Obesity; Pancreatitis; Vitamin and mineral deficiencies.

## FOR FURTHER INFORMATION:

Bennion, Lynn J. *Hypoglycemia: Fact or Fad? What You Should Know About Low Blood Sugar*. New York: Crown, 1983. Written for lay persons by a respected clinical endocrinologist, this book presents concise information about the causes, diagnosis, prevention, and treatment of hypoglycemia. The presentation is sensible, and the medical information is accurate. The glossary is very helpful to nonspecialists.

Cryer, Philip E. "Glucose Homeostasis and Hypoglycemia." In *Williams Textbook of Endocrinology*, edited by Jean D. Wilson and Daniel W. Foster. 8th ed. Philadelphia: W. B. Saunders, 1992. A complete and definitive chapter. Delineates especially well the coordination of the nervous and hormonal systems in physiologic defense against hypoglycemia, as well as the special problems of hypoglycemia in patients with diabetes mellitus.

Davidson, Mayer B. "Hypoglycemia." In *Diabetes Mellitus: Diagnosis and Treatment*. 8th ed. New York: John Wiley & Sons, 1986. The author has made an important contribution to the study of diabetes and metabolism. The chapter offers clear explanations of the physiological abnormalities in hypoglycemia and emphasizes the importance of fasting hypoglycemia as an index of serious illness. A concise practical summary is included at the end of the chapter.

Hofeldt, Fred D. *Preventing Reactive Hypoglycemia: The Great Medical Dilemma*. St. Louis: Warren H. Green, 1983. The author, who has extensive clinical experience, points out that most individuals with symptoms of activation of the sympathetic nervous system do not have hypoglycemia. Hofeldt attempts to formulate criteria that will detect those persons who do have genuine reactive hypoglycemia, and he offers advice regarding dietary management.

Marks, Vincent, and F. Clifford Rose. *Hypoglycemia*. 2d ed. London: Blackwell Scientific Publications, 1981. This classic textbook by British authorities contains extensive clinical information as well as clear descriptions of pathologic physiology.

Smith, Robert J. "Hypoglycemia." In *Joslin's Diabetes Mellitus*, edited by Alexander Marble, Leo P. Krall, Robert F. Bradley, A. Richard Christlieb, and J. Stuart Soeldner. 12th ed. Philadelphia: Lea & Febiger, 1985. The definitive American textbook of diabetes. This chapter covers all causes of hypoglycemia, not simply those related to diabetes.

## HYPOPARATHYROIDISM. *See* HYPERPARATHYROIDISM AND HYPOPARATHYROIDISM.

## HYPOTHERMIA. *See* HYPERTHERMIA AND HYPOTHERMIA.

# IATROGENIC DISORDERS

**SYSTEMS AFFECTED:** All

**SPECIALISTS:** All

**DEFINITION:** Health problems caused by medical treatments.

## CAUSES AND SYMPTOMS

Iatrogenic disorders may be attributable to inefficient, uncaring physicians or to risks inherent in medical procedures that are necessary to prevent death or crippling disease. Such disorders are usually divided into those caused by medications, surgery, and medical misdiagnosis.

The average patient expects physicians and the medical infrastructure to deliver perfect cures for all diseases. This is not possible because some diseases have no cure and because medical treatment always involves some potential risk to persons being treated. In fact, a percentage—usually a small one—of patients treated for any disease develop unexpected health problems (adverse reactions) which can be diseases themselves.

The term "iatrogenic disorder" is a catchall used to define the many different adverse reactions that accompany the practice of modern medicine. The number of such problems has grown as medical science has become more sophisticated. They are often blamed entirely on physicians and other medical staff involved in cases producing iatrogenic disorders.

This blame is correctly directed in instances where a physician and other staff involved are uncaring, inattentive, careless, or incompletely educated. However, iatrogenic disorders often result from the nature of modern medicine. Doctors frequently attempt therapeutic methods (such as surgery) that are innovative efforts that cure serious diseases but have some inherent risk of failure. They may also use therapeutic drugs that are powerful agents for cure of specific disease processes but that have side effects causing other health problems in some people who take them. In addition, doctors often utilize complicated overall therapy having adverse consequences that patients may not acknowledge despite physicians' attempts to explain them orally and with consent forms.

## TREATMENT AND THERAPY

Despite careful efforts of most physicians—who are informed, caring, and efficient—iatrogenic disorders accompany many medical procedures. Public attention is, however, focused most on the effects of therapeutic agents, drugs and vaccines, because patients are often unaware that no therapeutic agent in use is ever perfectly safe. Even a clear physician description of the dos and don'ts associated with such therapy may be flawed by biological variation among patients, causing problems in one individual but not others.

Hence, several rules must be followed concerning therapeutic agents. First, wherever possible, these medications should be used only after other means fail and the benefits to be gained clearly outweigh the risks entailed. Second, therapy should begin with the lowest possible effective dose, and dose increase should be accompanied by frequent symptom relief and toxicity monitoring. Third, patients and responsible family members must be made aware of all possible adverse symptoms, how to best counter them, and the foods or other medications to be avoided to diminish iatrogenic potential.

Many iatrogenic disorders are caused by the presence of bacterial contamination in wounds and the fact that surgical maintenance of sterility is not absolutely perfect. For example, iatrogenesis occurs after 30 percent of surgical procedures carried out at heavily contaminated surgical sites (such as emergency surgery of abdominal wounds). In addition, the use of antibiotics can be problematic. In many cases, the large doses of these therapeutic agents required to fight primary bacterial infection will cause superinfection by other microbes, such as fungi. Furthermore, wide antibiotic use in hospitals has led to the creation of antibiotic-resistant bacteria.

For these reasons, treatment of surgical sites requires individualized attention. Clean wounds can be closed up immediately without high risk of infection, but deep wounds known to be contaminated prior to surgery are often best handled by closing up interior tissues and leaving skin and subcutaneous tissues open until it is clear that infection is under control. Many patients are frightened by such procedures and the pain involved, not understanding that it is in their best interest. Hence, they may resist treatment and accuse conscientious physicians of causing iatrogenic disorders.

Iatrogenesis resulting from misdiagnosis is too complicated an issue to be considered in depth here. In some cases, it is caused by physician inadequacy, but more often such problems are attributable to the great difficulty in diagnosing a disease absolutely.

It is essential for patients and physicians to communicate effectively. Such interaction lowers the occurrence of iatrogenic disorders because patients can decide to forgo treatment or to learn how to comply exactly with complex treatment protocols. Patients who do not receive adequate answers to questions posed to physicians should seek treatment elsewhere. Physicians should completely explain potential problems associated with therapeutic procedures by oral communication, informative consent forms, and well-educated counselors.

Because of the many iatrogenic disorders associated with medical therapy, physicians often believe that the best course of treatment—where a symptom is unclear and severe danger to patients is not imminent—is to allow nature to take its course so as to do no harm. This approach is often misunderstood by patients. To clarify the issue and to satisfy them, it should be explained—by the physician—that treatment can often be more dangerous than a perceived health problem.

It is hoped that the continued development of medical science, careful and complete therapy explanations by medical staffs, and better medical understanding and better treatment compliance by patients will decrease the incidence of iatrogenic disorders. —*Sanford S. Singer*

*See also* Nausea and vomiting.

**FOR FURTHER INFORMATION:**

Allen, Frank N., ed. *Assessing Drug Reactions: Adverse and Beneficial.* Washington, D.C.: Interdisciplinary Communication Associates, 1976.

Apfel, Roberta J., and Susan M. Fisher. *To Do No Harm: DES and the Dilemmas of Modern Medicine.* New Haven, Conn.: Yale University Press, 1984.

Carroll, Paula. *Life Wish: One Woman's Struggle Against Medical Incompetence.* Alameda, Calif.: Medical Consumers, 1986.

D'Arcy, P. F., and J. P. Griffin. *Iatrogenic Diseases.* 2d ed. New York: Oxford University Press, 1979.

Preger, Leslie, ed. *Iatrogenic Diseases.* 2 vols. Boca Raton, Fla.: CRC Press, 1986.

## IMMUNODEFICIENCY DISORDERS

**SYSTEM AFFECTED:** Immune

**SPECIALISTS:** Geneticists, immunologists

**DEFINITION:** Genetic or acquired disorders that result from disturbances in the normal functioning of the immune system.

**KEY TERMS:**

*antibody:* an immune compound secreted by B lymphocytes; the production of antibodies is induced by specific foreign invaders, and they combine with and destroy only those invaders

*B lymphocyte:* also referred to as B cells; cells of the immune system that produce antibodies and are believed to be produced within the bone marrow

*lymphocyte:* the type of immune precursor cell responsible for the production of both B and T lymphocytes

*phagocyte:* a cell of the immune system which destroys invading foreign bodies by engulfing and digesting them in a nonspecific immune response

*T lymphocyte:* a type of immune cell which kills host cells infected by bacteria or viruses or produces a chemical compound which mediates the host cells' destruction

### CAUSES AND SYMPTOMS

The defense of the body against foreign invaders is provided by the immune system. In nonspecific immunity, phagocytic cells engulf and destroy invading particles. Specific immunity consists of very specialized cell types that are synthesized in response to a particular type of foreign invader. Self-replicating stem cells within the bone marrow give rise to lymphocytes, which mediate specific immunity. Lymphocytes establish self-replacing colonies within the thymus, spleen, and lymph nodes. The various categories of T lymphocytes are derived from the thymus colonies,

and B lymphocytes are believed to develop within the bone marrow. B lymphocytes secrete highly specific antibodies that attack bacteria and some viruses. T lymphocytes do not secrete antibodies and instead either attack the body cells that have been infected with a bacterium or virus or produce chemical compounds that aid other types of T cells in destroying the infected cells. In immunodeficiency disorders, some or all of these defenses are compromised, which can have life-threatening consequences. Some immunodeficiency diseases are the result of genetic abnormalities and are present from birth; others are acquired through infection or exposure to damaging drug or radiation treatments.

The most severe immunodeficiency disorder is attributable to the absence of stem cells, which results in a total lack of B and T lymphocytes. This rare genetic condition is referred to as severe combined immunodeficiency syndrome (SCID). Affected infants show a failure to thrive from birth and can easily die from common bacterial or viral infections. One cause of SCID is a deficiency in the enzyme adenosine deaminase. This deficiency disrupts the normal deoxyribonucleic acid (DNA) synthesis in the stem cells. Another variant of SCID is Swiss-type agammaglobulinemia, in which the thymus is absent and few lymph nodes exist.

The major syndromes that involve defects in the T lymphocyte population are characterized by recurrent viral and fungal infections. Di George syndrome results from improper development of the thymus, which in turn causes the insufficient production of T lymphocytes. Deficiency of the enzyme PNP is a genetically inherited disorder in which children generally develop symptoms after infancy, including frequent viral infections, and have low T lymphocyte levels.

One genetically inherited disorder affecting B lymphocytes is hypogammaglobulinemia. This disease prevents the normal maturation of B lymphocytes, thereby blocking proper formation of antibodies. Severe bacterial infections are the most common symptom, and when the disorder is left untreated, infants generally die of severe pneumonia prior to six months of age.

Several immunodeficiency disorders are the result of partial defects in the production and/or function of B and T lymphocytes. Wiskott-Aldrich syndrome is a genetically inherited disease manifested by recurrent infections and an itchy, scaly inflammation of the skin. Certain classes of antibodies are absent or scarce. Chronic mucocutaneous candidiasis is characterized by chronic fungal infection of the skin and mucous membranes; reduced levels of T cells are responsible for this disfiguring disorder.

Numerous immunodeficiency disorders are the result of defects of the phagocytic cells, and the root cause of most of these disorders is ill-defined. In chronic granulomatosis, an inherited enzyme deficiency prevents the immune system from destroying invading bacteria. Infants affected by this disorder develop severe infections and chronic inflammations of internal organs and bones. The bacteria responsible for these symptoms are generally those which are not considered pathogens in healthy individuals.

Most of the disorders that affect the immune system are not inherited but acquired sometime during the person's life. They are either the result of an infection or a consequence of another disease or its treatment. The use of corticosteroids to treat inflammations, or the illicit use of them in muscle-building, can interfere with the proper production and function of T lymphocytes. Other immunosuppressive drugs used to diminish the possibilities of graft or transplant rejection, or in the treatment of autoimmune diseases, can severely depress antibody production. Chemotherapeutic agents used in the treatment of cancer can affect DNA replication and severely compromise the entire immune system, as can radiation treatments.

Major trauma, surgery, and burns all lead to an increased risk of infection. These experiences result in depressed function of both the nonspecific and specific immune responses. The effect is temporary, however, and generally returns to normal during the recuperative process. Advanced malignancies (cancer) are frequently associated with a depressed immune response, perhaps because of tumor proliferation and interference with the development and maturation of B and T lymphocytes.

Acquired immunodeficiency syndrome (AIDS) is believed to be caused by the human immunodeficiency virus (HIV). HIV specifically infects one type of T lymphocyte and results in severe immune depression. The virus may be harbored in an individual for years without symptoms. Initial symptoms may be quite mild, but they generally progress so that the affected individual becomes susceptible to a host of unusual bacterial and fungal infections and frequently develops a rare form of cancer called Kaposi's sarcoma. AIDS produces neurological damage in about one-third of infected individuals. HIV is transmitted primarily through unprotected sexual contact, sharing of needles for intravenous drug use, transfusion with contaminated blood products, or other contact with contaminated body fluids.

## TREATMENT AND THERAPY

Treatment of immunodeficiency disorders is targeted at the source of the deficiency. For example, in Di George syndrome, which is the congenital absence of the thymus, fetal thymus transplants can correct the problem, with improvement in lymphocyte levels seen within hours after the transplants. The use of thymus extracts has also been beneficial. Syndromes such as hypogammaglobulinemia can be managed by injection with mixtures of antibodies. Drug therapy to substitute for some absent immune components of Wiskott-Aldrich syndrome has been shown to have variable effects. The most effective treatment for chronic mucocutaneous candidiasis is aggressive antifungal medication

to eradicate the causative organism; treatment must continue for several months since fungal infections are slow to respond to therapy and frequently recur. Chronic granulomatosis is notoriously difficult to treat, and the most effective therapy has been antibiotic and antifungal agents used aggressively during an overt infection.

Because of the magnitude of the defects, many immunodeficiency disorders are difficult to treat successfully and are commonly fatal early in life. For diseases such as chronic granulomatosis, the disease is usually fatal within the first few years of life, and only about 20 percent of patients reach the age of twenty. SCID is a serious disorder in which affected infants can die before a proper diagnosis is made. For individuals with these and other serious immunodeficiency disorders, maintenance of individuals in an environment free of bacteria, viruses, and fungi, such as a sterile "bubble," has been the best means to prevent life-threatening infections. Such an approach, however, precludes the possibility of a normal life. The most effective treatment for individuals with severely compromised immune systems is bone marrow transplantation. In this procedure, bone marrow from a compatible individual is introduced into the bone marrow of the patient. If the procedure works, and the success rate is high, in approximately one to six months the transplant recipient's immune system will be reconstituted and functional. Bone marrow transplantation is a permanent cure for these disorders, since the transplanted marrow will contain stem cells that produce all the cell types of the immune system. The difficulties in transplantation include finding a compatible donor and preventing infections during the period after the transplant. Individuals are particularly susceptible to infection prior to the activation of the transplanted bone marrow. Such patients are frequently kept in sterile bubbles to limit the possibility of infection.

There is no cure for AIDS. Patients are treated with drug therapy for three different purposes: to slow down the spread of HIV; to cure or prevent bacterial, viral, and fungal infections; and to relieve unpleasant symptoms of the disease. The first drug to be approved for use to inhibit HIV was zidovudine (formerly AZT), but its success is somewhat limited and it is associated with severe side effects in some individuals. Vaccines are used to prevent influenza and certain forms of pneumonia commonly developed by AIDS patients, and a host of antibiotics are available to combat infections that may develop. Various drugs are used to ease the symptoms of AIDS, such as appetite disturbances, nausea, pain, insomnia, anxiety, depression, fever, and diarrhea. A combination of all these therapies has been shown to increase life expectancy in AIDS patients. Many patients choose to participate in clinical trials of experimental drugs not approved for general use in the hope that the new drug will be more effective at alleviating the disease. Others seek out alternative or nontraditional medical treatments that have a long history of use in non-Western cultures. These treatments include acupuncture, herbology, meditation, and homeopathy. An important aspect of therapy for AIDS patients is maintaining mental health through support groups and supportive caregivers.

Illicit use of corticosteroids can seriously compromise the immune system and may lead to permanent damage. The best therapy for this type of acquired immunodeficiency is prevention—that is, to not misuse the drugs. In their supervised use to control inflammation or other disease symptoms, normal immune function will return after treatment has been completed. A huge risk to cancer patients who are being treated with chemotherapy and/or radiation therapy is the depression of the immune system, which can lead to a host of infections being contracted and not easily fought off by the body's compromised immune system. These individuals should avoid exposure to infectious agents when possible and be attentive to lifestyle modifications that can strengthen the immune system and encourage its speedy recovery, including a nutritious diet, plenty of rest, and avoidance of stress. Close monitoring for any signs of infection facilitates rapid antibiotic therapy, which can prevent serious complications.

## PERSPECTIVE AND PROSPECTS

Prior to the gains in scientific knowledge about the mechanics of the immune system, individuals with genetic immunodeficiency disorders would die of serious infections during their first few years of life. Even when it was finally realized that these individuals suffered from defects of the immune system, little could be done for most of the disorders, except to treat infections as they developed and to avoid contact with potential disease-causing organisms—a near impossibility if one is to lead a normal life. Housing persons with SCID in sterile bubbles was uncommon because of the expense and impracticality. During the 1970's, bone marrow transplants were first developed and by the 1990's had progressed to a greater than 80 percent success rate. As a result of improved transplant-rejection drugs, transplants from donors with less-than-perfect tissue matches are now possible. Bone marrow transplantation has been a source of cure for many individuals with immune disorders.

Bone marrow transplantation is not suitable or possible in every case of immunodeficiency disorder, and scientists have long sought a means to cure the genetic defects themselves. In 1992, French Anderson of the National Institutes of Health conducted the first gene therapy trial on a young girl suffering from SCID. Some of the girl's bone marrow cells were removed from her body and exposed to a virus containing a normal gene for ADA, the defective enzyme. Some of the stem cells in the marrow incorporated the healthy gene. These engineered cells were injected into her body, and some lodged in her bone marrow. There they produced healthy immune cells.

Gene therapy is being considered for a variety of immunodeficiency conditions. In the future, bone marrow cells may be engineered to be resistant to chemotherapy and radiation therapy; therefore patients could be given more frequent dosages of cancer-fighting therapies without destroying their ability to fight infections. Bone marrow cells may also be engineered to be resistant to infection by the AIDS virus; in this way, individuals with AIDS may be given a population of cells which will provide enough immune defense so that symptoms of the disease never appear. Aging individuals develop depressed immune systems, and medical research is searching for ways to prevent this decline. These efforts toward curing immunodeficiency diseases with the tools of contemporary molecular biology are promising. —*Karen E. Kalumuck*

*See also* Acquired immunodeficiency syndrome (AIDS); Allergies; Arthritis; Asthma; Autoimmune disorders; Human immunodeficiency virus (HIV).

## FOR FURTHER INFORMATION:

Bach, Jean-Francoise, ed. *Immunology*. 2d ed. New York: John Wiley & Sons, 1982. This comprehensive guide to the field of immunology includes a detailed section on immunodeficiency disorders which the reader will find accessible and informative.

Bartlett, John G., and Ann K. Finkbeiner. *The Guide to Living with HIV Infection*. Baltimore: The Johns Hopkins University Press, 1991. This informative book developed at The Johns Hopkins University AIDS Clinic is a great resource for information about the disease and a guide for patients and caregivers in living with the disease.

Desowitz, Robert S. *The Thorn in the Starfish: How the Human Immune System Works*. New York: W. W. Norton, 1987. An accessible book written in a narrative style. Desowitz wonderfully simplifies the story of the immune system and how it functions. An excellent source for anyone interested in the mechanics of immunity, immune health maintenance, and immunodeficiency.

Dwyer, John M. *The Body at War: The Miracle of the Immune System*. New York: Penguin Books, 1988. This easy-to-read text is an excellent introduction to the functions of the immune system and such related topics as immune disorders, allergies, and immunology research.

Fox, Stuart I. *Perspectives on Human Biology*. Dubuque, Iowa: Wm. C. Brown, 1991. An understandably written and beautifully illustrated text. Includes an extensive chapter on the immune system and diseases.

Taylor, Barbara. *Everything You Need to Know About AIDS*. Rev. ed. New York: Rosen Publishing Group, 1992. This concise, large-print book pares down the complexities of the immune system and provides straightforward answers to the most common questions about the disease.

**IMPOTENCE.** *See* **SEXUAL DYSFUNCTION.**

# INCONTINENCE

**SYSTEMS AFFECTED:** Gastrointestinal, urinary

**SPECIALISTS:** Family physicians, geriatric specialists, gynecologists, internists, obstetricians, psychiatrists, urologists

**DEFINITION:** Involuntary loss of urine or feces, primarily a social and hygienic problem that particularly affects the older population.

**KEY TERMS:**

*atonic bladder:* a bladder characterized by weak muscles

*enuresis:* bed-wetting

*frequency:* urination at short intervals; a common problem accompanying incontinence

*micturition:* the act of urinating

*nocturia:* nighttime urination

*sphincter:* a ring-shaped muscle that surrounds a natural opening in the body and can open or close it by expanding or contracting

*urge incontinence:* a strong desire to urinate followed by leakage of urine

*urgency:* a strong desire to void urine immediately

## CAUSES AND SYMPTOMS

Continence is skill acquired in humans by the interaction of two processes: socialization of the infant and maturation of the central nervous system. Without society's expectation of continence, and without broadly accepted definitions of appropriate behavior, the concept of "incontinence" would be meaningless. There are many causes for urinary incontinence. Three broad (interrelated and often overlapping) categories are physiologic voiding dysfunction, factors directly influencing voiding function, and factors affecting the individual's capacity to manage voiding.

The causes of physiologic voiding dysfunction involve an abnormality in bladder or sphincter function, or both. The bladder and sphincter have only two functions: to store urine until the appropriate time for urination and then to empty it completely. Voiding dysfunction involves the failure of one or both of these mechanisms. Four basic types of voiding dysfunction can be distinguished: detrusor instability, genuine stress incontinence, outflow obstruction, and atonic bladder.

Detrusor instability is a condition characterized by involuntary bladder (detrusor muscle) contraction during filling. While all the causes of bladder instability are not fully understood, it can be associated with the following: neurologic disease (brain and spinal cord abnormalities), inflammation of the bladder wall, bladder outlet obstruction, stress urinary incontinence, and idiopathic (spontaneous or primary) dysfunction. Detrusor instability usually causes symptoms of frequency, urgency, and possibly nocturia or enuresis.

Genuine stress incontinence is caused by a failure to hold urine during bladder filling as a result of an incompetent urethral sphincter mechanism. If the closure mechanism of the bladder outlet fails to hold urine, incontinence will occur. This is usually manifested during physical exertion or abdominal stress (such as coughing or sneezing). It can occur in either sex, but it is more common in women because of their shorter urethra and the physical trauma of childbirth. Men can experience stress incontinence following traumatic or surgical damage to the sphincter.

Obstruction of the outflow of urine during voiding can produce various symptoms, including frequency, straining to void, poor urinary stream, preurination and posturination dribbling, and a feeling of urgency with resulting leakage (urge incontinence). In severe cases, the bladder is never completely emptied and a volume of residual urine persists. Overflow incontinence can result. Common causes of bladder outlet obstruction are prostatic enlargement, bladder neck narrowing, or urethral obstruction. Functional obstruction occurs when a neurologic lesion prevents the coordinated relaxation of the sphincter during voiding. This phenomenon is termed detrusor-sphincter dyssynergia.

An atonic bladder—one with weak muscle walls—does not produce a sufficient contraction to empty completely. Emptying can be enhanced by abdominal straining or manual expression, but a large residual volume persists. The sensation of retaining urine might or might not be present. If sensation is present, frequency of urination is common because only a small portion of the bladder volume is emptied each time. Sensation is often diminished, and the residual urine volume can be considerable (100 to 1,000 milliliters). Overflow incontinence often occurs.

An acute urinary tract infection can cause transient incontinence, even in a fit, healthy young person who normally has no voiding dysfunction. Acute frequency and urgency with disturbed sensation and pain can result in the inability to reach a toilet in time or to detect when incontinence is occurring. If an underlying voiding dysfunction is also present, an acute urinary tract infection is likely to cause incontinence.

Many drugs can also disturb the delicate balance of normal functioning. The most obvious category consists of diuretics, those drugs which increase urinary discharge; a large, swift production of urine will give most people frequency and urgency. If the bladder is unstable, it might not be able to handle a sudden influx of urine and urge incontinence can result. Sedation can affect voiding function directly (for example, diazepam can lower urethral resistance) or can make the individual less responsive to signals from the bladder and thus unable to maintain continence. Other commonly prescribed drugs have secondary actions on voiding function. Not all patients, however, will experience urinary side effects from these drugs.

Various endocrine disorders can upset normal voiding function. Diabetes can cause polydypsia (extreme thirst), requiring the storage of a large volume of urine. Glycosuria (sugar in the urine) might encourage urinary tract infection. Thyroid imbalances can aggravate an overactive or underactive bladder. Pituitary gland disorders can result in the production of excessive urine volumes because of an antidiuretic hormone deficiency. Estrogen deficiency in postmenopausal women causes atrophic changes in the vaginal and urethral tissues and will worsen stress incontinence and an unstable bladder.

Several bladder pathologies can also cause incontinence by disrupting normal functioning. A patient with a neoplasm (abnormal tissue growth), whether benign or malignant, or a stone in the bladder occasionally experiences incontinence as a symptom. These are infrequent causes of incontinence.

Often it takes something else in addition to the underlying problem to tip the balance and produce incontinence. This is especially true for elderly and disabled persons who are delicately balanced between continence and incontinence. For example, immobility—anything that impedes access—is likely to induce incontinence. Immobility can be the result of the gradual worsening of a chronic condition, such as arthritis, multiple sclerosis, or Parkinson's disease, until eventually the individual simply cannot reach a toilet in time. The condition may be acute—an accident or illness that suddenly renders a person immobile might be the start of failure to control the bladder.

In the case of children, most daytime wetting persists until the child reaches school age. It is less common than bed-wetting (enuresis), and the two often go together. One in ten five-year-old children, however, still wets the bed regularly. With no treatment, this figure gradually falls to 5 percent of ten-year-olds and to 2 percent of adults. It is twice as common in boys as in girls, has strong familial tendencies, and is associated with stressful events in the third or fourth year of life. A urinary tract infection is sometimes the cause.

Fecal, as opposed to urinary, incontinence is generally caused by underlying disorders of the colon, rectum, or anus; neurogenic disorders; or fecal impaction. Severe diarrhea increases the likelihood of having fecal incontinence. Some of the more common disorders that can cause diarrhea are ulcerative colitis, carcinoma, infection, radiation therapy, and the effect of drugs (for example, broad-spectrum antibiotics, laxative abuse, or iron supplements). Fecal incontinence tends to be a common, if seldom reported, accompaniment.

The pelvic floor muscles support the anal sphincter, and any weakness will cause a tendency to fecal stress incontinence. The vital flap valve formed by the anorectal angle can be lost if these muscles are weak. An increase in abdominal pressure would therefore tend to force the rectal contents down and out of the anal canal. This might be the result of congenital abnormalities or of later trauma (for example, childbirth, anal surgery, or direct trauma). A lifelong habit of straining at stool might also cause muscle weakness.

The medulla and higher cortical centers of the brain have a role in coordinating and controlling the defecation reflex. Therefore, any neurologic disorder that impairs the ability to detect or inhibit impending defecation will probably result in a tendency to incontinence, similar in causation to the uninhibited or unstable bladder. For example, the paraplegic can lose all direct sensation of and voluntary control over bowel activity. Neurologic disorders such as multiple sclerosis, cerebrovascular accident, and diffuse dementia can affect sensation or inhibition, or a combination of both. Incontinence occurs with some demented people because of a physical inability to inhibit defecation. With others, it occurs because the awareness that such behavior is inappropriate has been lost.

Severe constipation with impaction of feces is probably the most common cause of fecal incontinence, and it predominates as a cause among the elderly and those living in extended care facilities. Chronic constipation leads to impaction when the fluid content of the feces is progressively absorbed by the colon, leaving hard, rounded rocks in the bowel. This hard matter promotes mucus production and bacterial activity, which causes a foul-smelling brown fluid to accumulate. If the rectum is overdistended for any length of time, the internal and external sphincters become relaxed, allowing passage of this mucus as spurious diarrhea. The patient's symptoms usually include fairly continuous leakage of fluid stool without any awareness of control.

Most children are continent of feces by the age of four years, but 1 percent still have problems at seven years of age. More boys than girls are incontinent, suggesting that developmental factors can be relevant because boys mature more slowly. Fecal incontinence or conscious soiling in childhood (sometimes referred to as encopresis) has, like nocturnal enuresis, long been regarded as evidence of a psychiatric or psychologic disorder in the child. The evidence, however, does not support the claim that most fecally incontinent children are disturbed.

Such children usually have fastidious, overanxious parents who are intent on toilet-training. The child is punished for soiling, so defecation tends to be inhibited, both in the underwear and in the toilet. When toilet-training is attempted, the child may be repeatedly seated on the toilet in the absence of a full rectum and be unable to perform. The situation becomes fraught with anxiety, and bowel movements become associated with unpleasantness in the child's mind. The child therefore retains feces and becomes constipated. Defecation then becomes difficult and painful as well.

### TREATMENT AND THERAPY

The two primary methods of treating urinary incontinence involve medical and surgical intervention (drug therapy and surgery) and bladder training.

Many drugs can be prescribed to help those with urinary incontinence. Often the results are disappointing, although some can be useful for carefully selected and accurately diagnosed patients. Drugs are often used to control detrusor instability and urge incontinence by relaxing the detrusor muscle and inhibiting reflex contractions. This therapy is helpful in some patients. Sometimes when the drug is given in large enough doses to be effective, however, the side effects are so troublesome that the therapy must be abandoned. Drugs that reduce bladder contractions must be used cautiously in patients who have voiding difficulty, since urinary retention can be precipitated. Careful assessment must be made of residual urine. Drug therapy is also used with caution in patients with a residual volume greater than 100 milliliters. Some drugs are used in an attempt to prevent stress incontinence by increasing urethral tone. Phenylpropanolamine and ephedrine, those most often used, are thought to act on the alpha receptors in the urethra.

Drug therapy can also be used to relieve outflow obstruction. Phenoxybenzamine is most commonly used, but this drug can have dangerous side effects, such as tachycardia (an abnormally fast heartbeat) or postural hypotension. If the bladder does not contract sufficiently to ensure complete emptying, drug therapy can be attempted to increase the force of the voiding contractions. Carbachol, bethanechol, and distigmine bromide have all been used with some success. Other drugs might be useful in treating factors affecting incontinence—for example, antibiotics to treat a urinary tract infection or laxatives to treat or prevent constipation.

Many drugs can exacerbate a tendency to incontinence. For those who are prone to incontinence, medications and dosage schedules are chosen that will have a minimal effect on bladder control. For example, a slow-acting diuretic, in a divided dose, can help someone with urgency and weak sphincter tone to avoid incontinence. An analgesic might be preferable to night sedation for those who need pain relief but who wet the bed at night if they are sedated.

Turning to surgical intervention, none of the several surgical approaches that have been used in an attempt to treat an unstable bladder has gained widespread use. Cystodistention (stretching the bladder under general anesthesia) and bladder transection, for example, are presumed to act by disturbing the neurologic pathways that control uninhibited contractions. Many vaginal and suprapubic procedures are available to help correct genuine stress incontinence in women. Surgery can also be used to relieve outflow obstruction—for example, to remove an enlarged prostate gland, divide a stricture, or widen a narrow urethra.

In cases of severe intractable incontinence, major surgery is an option. For those with a damaged urethra, a neourethra can be constructed. For those with a nonfunctioning sphincter, an artificial sphincter can be implanted. In some patients, a urinary diversion with a stoma (outlet) is the only and best alternative for continence. Although a drastic solution, a urostomy might be easier to cope with than an incontinent urethra, because an effective appliance will contain the urine.

Urinary incontinence is occasionally the result of surgery, usually urologic or gynecologic but sometimes a major pelvic or spinal procedure. Such iatrogenic incontinence can be caused by neurologic or sphincter damage, leading to various dysfunctional voiding patterns.

Several different types of bladder training or retraining are distinguishable and can be used in different circumstances. The most important element for success is that the correct regimen be selected for each patient and situation. A thorough assessment identifies those patients who will benefit from bladder training and determines the most appropriate method. Other factors that contribute to the incontinence should also be treated (for example, a urinary tract infection or constipation), because ignoring them will impair the success of a program.

Bladder training is most suitable for people with the symptoms of frequency, urgency, and urge incontinence (with or without an underlying unstable bladder) and for those with nonspecific incontinence. The elderly often have these symptoms. Patients with voiding dysfunction, other than an unstable bladder, are unlikely to benefit from bladder training.

The aim of bladder training is to restore the patient with frequency, urgency, and urge incontinence to a more normal and convenient voiding pattern. Ultimately, voiding should occur at intervals of three to four hours (or even longer) without any urgency or incontinence. Drug therapy is sometimes combined with bladder training for those with detrusor instability.

Bladder training aims to restore an individual's confidence in the bladder's ability to hold urine and to reestablish a more normal pattern. Initially, a patient keeps a baseline chart for three to seven days, recording how often urine is passed and when incontinence occurs. This chart is reviewed with the program supervisor, and an individual regimen is developed. The purpose is to extend the time between voiding gradually, encouraging the patient to practice delaying the need to void, rather than giving in to the feeling of urgency. Initially, the times chosen can be at set intervals throughout the day (for example, every one or two hours) or can be variable, according to the individual's pattern as indicated by the baseline chart. When the baseline chart reveals a definite pattern to the incontinence, it might be possible to set voiding times in accordance with and in anticipation of this pattern.

A pattern of voiding is set for patients throughout the day (timed voiding). Usually no pattern is set at night, even if nocturia or nocturnal enuresis is a problem. Patients are instructed to pass urine as necessary during the night. Sometimes the provision of a suitable pad or appliance helps to increase confidence and means that, if incontinence does occur, the results will not be disastrous. If urgency is experienced, patients are taught to sit or stand still and try to suppress the sensation rather than to rush immediately to the toilet. A normal fluid intake is encouraged because the goal is to have the patient continent and able to drink fluids adequately.

As patients achieve the target intervals without having to urinate prematurely or leaking, the intervals can gradually be lengthened. The speed of progress depends on the individual and on other variables, such as the initial severity of symptoms, motivation, and the amount of professional support. Patients usually remain at one time interval for one to two weeks before it is increased by fifteen to thirty minutes for another two weeks. Once the target of three-to four-hour voiding without urgency has been achieved, it is useful to maintain the chart and set times for at least another month to prevent relapse.

Some people find that practicing pelvic muscle exercises helps to suppress urgency. Any weakness in the pelvic floor muscles will cause a tendency not only to urinary incontinence but also to fecal stress incontinence. Mild weakness can respond to pelvic muscle exercises similar to those used in alleviating the symptoms of stress incontinence, but with a concentration on the posterior rather than the anterior portion of the pelvic muscles. Rectal tone is assessed by digital examination, during which the patient is instructed to squeeze. Regular contractions on the posterior portion of the pelvic muscles are then practiced often for at least two months (usually in sets of twenty-five, three times a day).

In cases of fecal impaction, a course of disposable phosphate enemas—one or two daily for seven to ten days, or until no further return is obtained—is the treatment of choice. A single enema is seldom efficient, even if an apparently good result is obtained, because impaction is often extensive: The first enema merely clears the lowest portion of the bowel. If fecal incontinence persists once the bowel has been totally cleared (a plain abdominal X ray can be helpful in confirming this), the condition is assumed to be neurogenic in origin rather than caused by the impaction.

## PERSPECTIVE AND PROSPECTS

Historically, most health professionals have been profoundly ignorant of the causes and management of incontinence. Incontinence was often regarded as a condition over which there was no control, rather than as a symptom of an underlying physiologic disorder or as a symptom of a patient with a unique combination of problems, needs, and potentials. The unfortunate result of such limited understanding was passive acceptance of the symptom of incontinence. Incontinence, often viewed as repulsive, is often a condition that is merely tolerated. As public recognition of the implications of incontinence has increased, however, the stigma associated with it has slowly decreased. It has become common knowledge that millions of Americans suffer from incontinence, and most pharmacies and supermarkets have a section for incontinence products.

At one time, incontinence was primarily regarded as a "nursing" problem, with nurses providing custodial care—keeping the patient as clean and comfortable as possible and preventing pressure ulcers from developing. Gradually, nurses were not alone in acknowledging that incontinence was a symptom requiring investigation and intervention; those in other health professions also began to realize this need. In the 1980's, research dollars began to be allocated for the study of incontinence. In 1988, U.S. Surgeon General C. Everett Koop estimated that 8 billion dollars was being spent by the federal government on incontinence in the United States annually.

As incontinence began to be recognized by the public as a health problem rather than as an inevitable part of aging, more people admitted having the symptoms of incontinence and sought medical attention. It has been estimated that, of all cases of incontinence, more than one-third can be cured, another one-third can be dramatically improved, and most of the remainder can be significantly improved.

—*Genevieve Slomski*

*See also* Bed-wetting; Constipation; Diarrhea and dysentery; Stones; Urinary disorders.

### FOR FURTHER INFORMATION:

Azrin, Nathan H., and Richard M. Foxx. *Toilet Training in Less than a Day*. New York: Simon & Schuster, 1974. In this popular treatment of the problem of toilet-training, the authors discuss the phenomenon of bed-wetting and offer parents options for managing the process. Management problems ranging from mild to severe are discussed. A bibliography is included.

Gartley, Cheryle, ed. *Managing Incontinence*. Ottawa, Ill.: Jameson Books, 1985. An overview of the basic treatment options for urinary incontinence, including surgical and nonsurgical methods. Although somewhat technical, this work is accessible to the general reader. Includes a bibliography.

Jeter, Katherine, et al., eds. *Nursing for Continence*. Philadelphia: W. B. Saunders, 1990. This work, written by a group of nurses, addresses the diagnosis, treatment, and management of incontinence in all age groups and in special populations and circumstances in a practical, thorough, and sensitive manner. Contains illustrations, references and sources for further reading after each chapter, and appendices.

Mandelstam, Dorothy. *Incontinence*. London: William Heinemann, 1977. In this well-written volume, the author examines the etiology of incontinence, discusses its manifestations, and offers options for treatment. Also contains references.

Raz, Sholomo, ed. *Female Urology*. Philadelphia: W. B. Saunders, 1983. The book begins with fundamentals of the female genitourinary tract, then analyzes the dynamics of continence mechanisms. Female urinary incontinence is treated as a multifaceted subject. Both surgical and nonsurgical treatments are discussed. Numerous photographs and illustrations are provided.

# INDIGESTION

**SYSTEM AFFECTED:** Gastrointestinal

**SPECIALISTS:** Family physicians, gastroenterologists, internists

**DEFINITION:** Indigestion, which is also known as dyspepsia, is a digestive disorder that is often mistaken for heartburn. This burning sensation in the chest and throat is one of the symptoms of indigestion, but the patient may have other complaints as well, such as abdominal pain, belching, a bloated feeling, nausea, vomiting, and sometimes diarrhea. There is usually no organic cause for this disorder; it may be attributable to stress, the consumption of certain foods and beverages, and the excessive swallowing of air while eating. Sometimes, however, an underlying disease may be present, such as inflammation of the esophagus, a peptic ulcer, disease of the gallbladder or liver, and bacterial or viral infections. A psychological factor may also exist.

***See also*** Abdominal disorders; Alcoholism; Appendicitis; Cholecystitis; Cirrhosis; Colitis; Colon cancer; Constipation; Crohn's disease; Diarrhea and dysentery; Diverticulitis and diverticulosis; Gallbladder diseases; Gastrointestinal disorders; Heartburn; Hemorrhoids; Hernia; Intestinal disorders; Jaundice; Liver cancer; Liver disorders; Nausea and vomiting; Pancreatitis; Peritonitis; Renal failure; Stomach, intestinal, and pancreatic cancers; Ulcers.

# INFARCTION. *See* HEART ATTACK.

# INFECTION

**SYSTEMS AFFECTED:** All

**SPECIALISTS:** Family physicians, hematologists, infectious disease physicians, internists

**DEFINITION:** Invasion of the body by disease-causing organisms such as bacteria, viruses, fungi, and parasites; symptoms of infection may include pain, swelling, fever, and loss of normal function.

**KEY TERMS:**

*antibiotic:* a substance that destroys or inhibits the growth of microorganisms, such as bacteria

*antibody:* a small protein secreted from specialized white blood cells which binds to and aids in the destruction of pathogens

*antigen:* a substance found on pathogens to which the antibodies bind; also, any substance considered foreign by the body

*bacteria:* small microorganisms; some bacteria found normally in and on the body have helpful functions, while others that invade the body or disrupt the normal bacteria are harmful and often infectious

*edema:* an abnormal accumulation of fluid in the body tissues; tissue with edema is swollen in appearance

*infectious:* referring to a microorganism which is capable of causing disease, often with the ability to spread from one person to another

*inflammation:* a tissue reaction to injury which may or may not involve infection; pain, heat, redness, and edema are the usual signs of inflammation

*pathogen:* a microorganism or substance capable of producing a disease, such as a bacterium causing an infection

*phagocytosis:* the ingestion and destruction of a pathogen or abnormal tissue by specialized white blood cells known as phagocytes

*virus:* a very small organism which is dependent upon a host cell to meet its metabolic needs and to reproduce

## PROCESS AND EFFECTS

Healthy people live with potential pathogens; that is, people have on and in their bodies non-disease-causing bacteria. They live in harmony with these organisms and in fact benefit from their presence. For example, some of the bacteria found in the intestinal tract supply vitamin K, which is important in blood-clotting reactions.

The human body has several features which prevent disease-causing organisms from inducing an infection. These features include anatomical barriers, such as unbroken skin, and the mucus in the nose, mouth, and lungs, which can trap pathogens. Another defense is the acid within the stomach, and even bacteria that are normally present in certain areas of the body can force out more harmful bacteria. The immune system is specially developed to ward off intruders.

Immune cells and factors secreted from these cells provide the next line of defense against invading organisms. Antibodies are secreted from specialized white blood cells known as plasma cells. These antibodies are very specific for the recognition of pathogens. For example, one antibody will recognize a particular strain of bacteria but not another. Antibodies attach themselves to the part of the bacterium called the antigen. Once bound to the antigen, they aid in the destruction of the pathogen. In addition to plasma cells, other white blood cells help in combating infections. These include the phagocytes called macrophages and neutrophils. Both of these immune cells have the ability to eat and digest pathogens such as bacteria in a process known as phagocytosis.

Microorganisms that cause disease must, in some way, overwhelm the body's natural defenses and immune system. Bacteria capable of causing infections may even be naturally occurring organisms that have left their normal environment and overcome the elements that normally hold them at bay. For example, some normal bacteria that reside in the mouth may cause pneumonia (inflammation of the lungs) if they gain access to the lungs.

Other infections can be caused by pathogens that do not normally reside in the body. One can "catch" a cold or the flu, or even a sexually transmitted disease. These kinds of infections are called communicable or transmissible infections. Similarly, a physician treating someone who has been bitten by a bat, skunk, or dog will want to know whether the animal has rabies. Rabies is a viral infection which is transmitted via a bite which breaks the skin and contaminates the wound with infectious saliva.

No matter what the route of infection, the body must mount a response to the intruding microorganism. Often the signs and symptoms one observes are not caused by the direct action of the infecting pathogen, but rather reflect the immune system's response to the infection. The most frequent signs and symptoms include inflammation and pain at the site of infection, as well as fever.

The inflammatory response is a nonspecific defense that is triggered whenever body tissues are injured, as in the case of infection. The goal of the inflammatory response is to prevent the spread of the infectious agent to nearby tissues, destroy the pathogens, remove the damaged tissues, and begin the healing process.

The signs of inflammation include redness, edema (tissue swelling), heat, pain, and loss of normal function. At first glance, these reactions do not appear to be beneficial to the body, but they do help fight the infection and aid in the healing process. The redness is attributable to an increase in blood flow to the area of infection. This increase in blood to the site of infection helps provide nutrients to the tissue, as well as removing some of the waste products that develop as the immune system fights the infection. With this increase in blood flow comes an increase in the temperature and the amount of blood that leaks out of blood vessels into the tissue spaces, causing edema at the site of infection. Some of the blood that leaks into the site of infection contains clotting proteins that help form a clot around the infected area, thereby reducing the chances that the pathogen could escape into the bloodstream or uninfected tissue nearby. Pain is present when the damaged tissue releases waste products and the pathogen releases toxins. The swelling of the injured area and the pain associated with infections keep the patient from using that area of the body and thus aid in healing. It is interesting to note that while some painkillers such as aspirin reduce the inflammatory reaction by stopping the production of some of the chemicals released during inflammation, the aspirin-like drugs do nothing to harm the pathogen, only the body's response to the microorganism.

Some of the same chemicals that are found in inflamed tissues also cause fever. This abnormally high body temperature represents the body's response to an invading microorganism. The body's thermostat, located in a region of

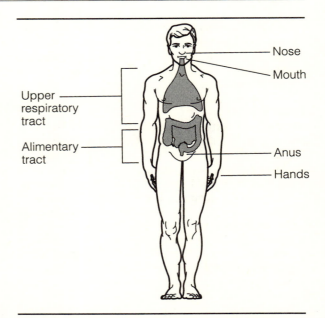

*Common sites for entry of infection into the body; in addition, a break in the skin anywhere on the body is an invitation to infection.*

the brain known as the hypothalamus, is set at 37 degrees Celsius (98.6 degrees Fahrenheit). During an infection, the thermostat is reset to a higher level. Chemicals called pyrogens are released from white blood cells called macrophages. Once again, aspirin-like drugs can be used to reduce the fever by inhibiting the action of some of these chemicals in the hypothalamus.

The body responds to viral infections in a similar way. Virally infected cells, however, secrete interferon, exerting an antiviral action which may provide protection to uninfected neighboring cells. It appears that interferon acts to inhibit the virus from replicating. Therefore, cells that are already infected must be destroyed to rid the body of the remaining virus.

In addition to being part of the inflammatory response, certain white blood cells play an important role in attempting to remove the pathogen. Soon after inflammation begins, macrophages already present at the site of infection start to destroy the microorganism. At the same time, chemicals are being released from both the damaged tissue and the macrophages, which recruit other white blood cells such as neutrophils. The neutrophils, like the macrophages, are effective at attacking and destroying bacteria but, unlike the macrophages, they often die in the battle against infection. Dead neutrophils are seen as a white exudate called pus.

Other manifestations of infection include systemic (whole-body) effects in addition to changes at the site of infection. As noted, fever is a systemic effect mediated by chemicals from the site of infection. Some of these same factors have the ability to act on the bone marrow to increase the production of white blood cells. Physicians look for fever and an increase in white blood cell number as a sign of infection. If the infection is severe, the bone marrow may not be able to keep up with the demand and an overall decrease in white blood cell number is found.

## COMPLICATIONS AND DISORDERS

Physicians and other health care workers must use patient history, signs and symptoms, and laboratory tests to determine the type of infection and the most appropriate treatment. Patient history can often tell the examiner how and when the infection started. For example, the patient may have cut himself or herself, been exposed to someone with an infectious disease, or had intimate contact with someone carrying a sexually transmitted disease. Signs of infection—edema, pain, fever—are usually rather easy to detect, but some symptoms may be rather vague, such as feeling tired and weak. These general signs and symptoms may indicate to a physician that the patient has an infection, but they will not provide information about the type of microorganism causing the infection. Nevertheless, some microorganisms do cause specific symptoms. For example, the herpes zoster virus that causes chickenpox or the paramyxovirus that causes measles leave characteristic rashes.

When the microorganism does not have a characteristic sign, physicians must use laboratory tests to determine the pathogen involved. Diagnosis of the disease relies on identifying the causative pathogen by microscopic examination of a specimen of infected tissue or body fluid, by growing the microorganism using culture techniques, or by detecting antibodies in the blood that have developed against the pathogen.

Once the physician determines what type of microorganism has caused the infection, he or she will have to determine the best treatment to eradicate the disease. Drug therapy usually consists of antibiotics and other antimicrobial agents. The selection of the appropriate drug is important, as certain pathogens are susceptible only to certain antibiotics. Unfortunately, few effective antiviral drugs are available for many infectious viruses. In these cases, drugs can be used to treat symptoms such as fever, pain, diarrhea, and vomiting rather than to destroy the virus.

Anti-infective drugs are commonly used by physicians to treat infections. Agents that kill or inhibit the growth of bacteria are known as antibiotics and can be applied directly to the site of infection (topical), given by mouth (oral), or injected. The latter two modes of administration allow the drug to be carried throughout the body by way of the blood. Some antibiotic drugs are effective against only certain strains of infectious bacteria. Antibiotics that act against several types of bacteria are referred to as broad-spectrum antibiotics. Some bacteria develop resistance to a particular antibiotic and require that the physician switch agents or use a combination of antibiotics. Antibiotic therapy for the treatment of infections should be used when the body has been invaded by harmful bacteria, when the bacteria are reproducing at a more rapid rate than the immune system can handle, or to prevent infections in individuals with an impaired immune system.

Some serious common bacterial infections include gonorrhea, which is sexually transmitted and treatable with penicillin; bacterial meningitis, which causes inflammation of the coverings around the brain and is treatable with a variety of antibiotics; pertussis (or whooping cough), which is transmitted by water droplets in air and treatable with erythromycin; pneumonia, which causes shortness of breath, is transmitted via the air, and can be treated with antibiotics; tuberculosis, which infects the lungs and is treatable with various antibiotics; and salmonella (or typhoid fever), which is transmitted in food or water contaminated with fecal material, causes fever, headaches, and digestive problems, and is treated with antibiotics. It should be noted that antibiotics are not effective in viral infections; only bacterial infections are treated with antibiotics.

Antiviral drugs such as acyclovir, amantadine, and zidovudine (formerly known as azidothymide, or AZT) are used in the treatment of infection by a virus. These drugs have been difficult to develop. Most viruses live within the cells of the patient, and the drug must in some way kill the virus without harming the host cells. In fact, antiviral agents cannot completely cure an illness, and infected patients often experience recurrent disease. Nevertheless, they do reduce the severity of these infections.

There are several common viral infections. Human immunodeficiency virus (HIV) infection, which causes acquired immunodeficiency syndrome (AIDS), is transmitted by sexual contact or contaminated needles or blood products; it is often treated with zidovudine but remains lethal. Chickenpox (herpes zoster virus), which is transmitted by airborne droplets or direct contact, is treated with acyclovir. The common cold is caused by numerous viruses that are transmitted by direct contact or air droplets and has no effective treatment other than drugs that reduce the symptoms. Hepatitis is transmitted by contaminated food, sexual contact, and blood; it causes flu-like symptoms and jaundice (a yellow tinge to the skin caused by liver problems) and may be helped with the drug interferon. Influenza viruses ("the flu") are transmitted by airborne droplets; the only treatment for the flu is of its symptoms. Measles is transmitted by virus-containing water droplets and causes fever and a rash; treatment consists of alleviating the symptoms. Mononucleosis is transmitted via saliva and causes swollen lymph nodes, fever, a sore throat, and generalized tiredness; a patient with mononucleosis can only receive treatment for the symptoms as no cure is available. Poliomyelitis (polio) is transmitted by fecally contaminated material or airborne droplets and can eventually cause paralysis; no treatment is available. Rabies is caused by a bite from an infected animal, as the virus is present in the saliva; the major symptoms include fever, tiredness, and spasms of the throat, and there is no effective treatment for rabies after these symptoms have appeared. Rubella is transmitted by virus-containing air droplets and is associated with a fever and rash; there is no treatment other than for the symptoms.

A major problem with infectious diseases is that there is almost always lag time between when the microorganism has entered the body and the onset of signs and symptoms. This gap may last from a few hours or days to several years. A patient without noticeable symptoms is likely to spread the pathogen. Thus a cycle is set up in which individuals unknowingly infect others who, in turn, pass on the disease-causing agent. Large numbers of people can quickly become infected.

One way to prevent the spread of infectious agents is to vaccinate patients. Diseases such as diphtheria, measles, mumps, rubella, poliomyelitis, and pertussis are rare in the United States because of an aggressive immunization program. When a patient is vaccinated, the vaccine usually contains a dead or inactive pathogen. After the vaccine is administered (usually by injection), the immune system responds by making antibodies against the antigens on the microorganism. Since the pathogen in the vaccine is unable to cause disease, the patient has no symptoms after immunization. The next time that the person is exposed to the infectious agent, his or her immune system is prepared to fight it before symptoms become evident.

In addition to immunization to prevent infection, individuals can largely avoid serious infectious diseases through good hygiene with respect to food and drink, frequent washing, the avoidance of contact with fecal material and urine, and the avoidance of contact with individuals who are infected and capable of transmitting the disease. When such avoidance is impractical, other protective measures can be taken.

Sexually transmitted diseases are usually preventable by using barrier contraceptives and practicing "safe sex." The most common of these diseases include chlamydial infections, trichomoniasis, genital herpes, and HIV infections. Prevention is particularly important in the viral infections of herpes and HIV, as there are no known cures.

Some infections can be acquired at birth, including gonorrhea, genital herpes, chlamydial infections, and salmonella. These microorganisms exist in the birth canal, and some infectious agents can even pass from the mother to the fetus via the placenta. The more serious infections transmitted in this manner are rubella, syphilis, toxoplasmosis, HIV virus, and the cytomegalovirus. The risk of transmitting these infections can be reduced by treating the mother before delivery or performing a cesarean section (surgical delivery from the uterus), thereby avoiding the birth canal.

## PERSPECTIVE AND PROSPECTS

The ancient Egyptians were probably the first to recognize infection and the body's response to the introduction of a disease-causing microorganism: Some hieroglyphics appear to represent the inflammatory process. Sometime in the fifth century B.C., the Greeks noted that patients who had acquired an infectious disease and survived did not usually contract the same illness a second time.

More solid scientific evidence about infections was provided in the nineteenth century by Edward Jenner, an English physician and scientist. Jenner was able to document that milkmaids seemed to be protected against smallpox because of their exposure to cowpox. With this knowledge, he vaccinated a boy with material from a smallpox pustule. The boy had a typical inflammatory response, but he showed no symptoms of the disease after being injected with smallpox a second time. His immune system protected him from the virus. Since that time, scientists have reached a much better understanding of how the body deals with infection.

Many scientists are focusing their attention on how pathogens are transmitted from the source of infection to susceptible individuals. Epidemiology is the study of the distribution and causes of diseases that are prevalent in humans. Since some infectious diseases are communicable (transmittable), epidemiologists gather data when an outbreak occurs in a population. These data include the source of infectious agents (the tissues involved), the microorganisms causing the disease, and the method by which the pathogens are transmitted from one person to another. Physicians and other health care workers help in the battle against infections by identifying susceptible individuals; developing and evaluating sources, methods, and ways to control the spread of the pathogens; and improving preventive measures, which usually includes extensive educational efforts for the general population. With this knowledge, scientists and physicians attempt to eradicate the disease.

While scientists and physicians have made great advances in the understanding of infection, many problems remain. The spread of certain diseases, such as sexually transmitted diseases, is difficult to control except by modifying human behavior. The most difficult to treat are viral illnesses in which the drugs that are used are ineffective in completely eradicating the virus and bacterial diseases in which the bacteria have developed drug resistance. Because these microorganisms evolve rapidly, new strains continually emerge. When a new infectious agent develops, it is often years before scientists can devise an effective drug or vaccine to treat the disease. In the meantime, large numbers of patients may become ill and even die. Perhaps the most effective way to combat infection is to use preventive measures whenever practical. —*Matthew Berria*

***See also*** Arthropod-borne diseases; Bacterial infections; Bites and stings; Childhood infectious diseases; Disease;

Ear infections and disorders; Fungal infections; Iatrogenic disorders; Lice, mites, and ticks; Parasitic diseases; Staphylococcal infections; Streptococcal infections; Viral infections; Zoonoses; *specific diseases.*

**FOR FURTHER INFORMATION:**

Clayman, Charles B., ed. *The American Medical Association Encyclopedia of Medicine.* New York: Random House, 1989. Covers, in alphabetical order, medical terms, diseases, and medical procedures. Lists all major infectious illnesses, their causes and treatments. Does an excellent job of explaining rather complex medical subjects for a nonprofessional audience.

*Disease Prevention/Health Promotion: The Facts.* Palo Alto, Calif.: Bull, 1988. This book was prepared by the Office of Disease Prevention and Health Promotion of the U.S. Department of Health and Human Services. It includes significant trends in disease prevention, as well as pertinent data on risk factors for infectious diseases. Readers may be particularly interested in the chapters on the surveillance and control of infectious diseases and on sexually transmitted diseases.

*Diseases.* Springhouse, Pa.: Springhouse, 1993. This text provides excellent descriptions of disease states. Chapter 2 specifically deals with infections; their causes, signs and symptoms, complications, and prevention; and the types of therapies that can eliminate the disease-causing agent.

Poole, Robert M., ed. *The Incredible Machine.* Washington, D.C.: National Geographic Society, 1986. A colorful book which describes, in layperson's terms, how the body works and how humans alter their own health. The chapter on how the immune system combats infectious agents is very well written and contains exciting pictures and drawings of inflammatory processes.

Rosenfeld, Isadore. *Modern Prevention: The New Medicine.* New York: Linden Press/Simon & Schuster, 1986. This easy-to-read book is written by a practicing physician with the ability to communicate to patients in a down-to-earth style. Rosenfeld addresses the causes and prevention of numerous common infections in both adults and children.

# INFERTILITY IN FEMALES

**SYSTEM AFFECTED:** Reproductive (female)

**SPECIALISTS:** Endocrinologists, gynecologists

**DEFINITION:** The inability to achieve a desired pregnancy as a result of dysfunction of female reproductive organs.

**KEY TERMS:**

*cervix:* the bottom portion of the uterus, protruding into the vagina; the cervical canal, an opening in the cervix, allows sperm to pass from the vagina into the uterus

*endometriosis:* a disease in which patches of the uterine lining, the endometrium, implant on or in other organs

*follicles:* spherical structures in the ovary that contain the maturing ova (eggs)

*hormone:* a chemical signal that serves to coordinate the functions of different body parts; the hormones important in female reproduction are produced by the brain, the pituitary, and the ovaries

*implantation:* the process in which the early embryo attaches to the uterine lining; a critical event in pregnancy

*ovaries:* the pair of structures in the female that produce ova (eggs) and hormones

*oviducts:* the pair of tubes leading from the top of the uterus upward toward the ovaries; also called the Fallopian tubes

*ovulation:* the process in which an ovum is released from its follicle in the ovary; ovulation must occur for conception to be possible

*pelvic inflammatory disease:* a general term that refers to a state of inflammation and infection in the pelvic organs; may be caused by a sexually transmitted disease

*uterus:* the organ in which the embryo implants and grows

*vagina:* the tube-shaped organ that serves as the site for sperm deposition during intercourse

## CAUSES AND SYMPTOMS

Infertility is defined as the failure of a couple to conceive a child despite regular sexual activity over a period of at least one year. Studies have estimated that in the United States 10 percent to 15 percent of couples are infertile. In about half of these couples, it is the woman who is affected.

The causes of female infertility are centered in the reproductive organs: the ovaries, oviducts, uterus, cervix, and vagina. The frequency of specific problems among infertile women is as follows: ovarian problems, 20 percent to 30 percent; damage to the oviducts, 30 percent to 50 percent; uterine problems, 5 percent to 10 percent; and cervical or vaginal abnormalities, 5 percent to 10 percent. Another 10 percent of women have unexplained infertility.

The ovaries have two important roles in conception: the production of ova, culminating in ovulation, and the production of hormones. Ovulation usually occurs halfway through a woman's four-week menstrual cycle. In the two weeks preceding ovulation, follicle-stimulating hormone (FSH) from the pituitary gland causes follicles in the ovaries to grow and the ova within them to mature. As the follicles grow, they produce increasing amounts of estrogen. Near the middle of the cycle, the estrogen causes the pituitary gland to release a surge of luteinizing hormone (LH), which causes ovulation of the largest follicle in the ovary.

Anovulation (lack of ovulation) can result either directly—from an inability to produce LH, FSH, or estrogen—or indirectly—because of the presence of other hormones that interfere with the signaling systems between the pituitary and ovaries. For example, the woman may have an excess production of androgen (testosterone-like) hormones, either in her ovaries or in her adrenal glands, or her pituitary may produce too much prolactin, a hormone

## Common Causes of Female Infertility

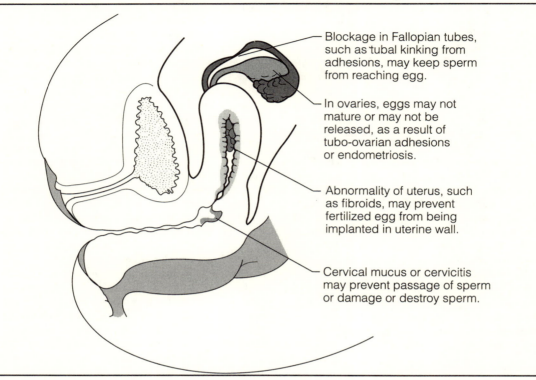

Blockage in Fallopian tubes, such as tubal kinking from adhesions, may keep sperm from reaching egg.

In ovaries, eggs may not mature or may not be released, as a result of tubo-ovarian adhesions or endometriosis.

Abnormality of uterus, such as fibroids, may prevent fertilized egg from being implanted in uterine wall.

Cervical mucus or cervicitis may prevent passage of sperm or damage or destroy sperm.

that is normally only secreted in large amounts after the birth of a child.

Besides ovulation, the ovaries have another critical role in conception since they produce hormones that act on the uterus to allow it to support an embryo. In the first two weeks of the menstrual cycle, the uterine lining is prepared for a possible pregnancy by estrogen from the ovaries. Following ovulation, the uterus is maintained in a state that can support an embryo by progesterone, which is produced in the ovary by the follicle that just ovulated, now called a corpus luteum. Because of the effects of hormones from the corpus luteum on the uterus, the corpus luteum is essential to the survival of the embryo. If conception does not occur, the corpus luteum disintegrates and stops producing progesterone. As progesterone levels decline, the uterine lining can no longer be maintained and is shed as the menstrual flow.

Failure of the pregnancy can result from improper function of the corpus luteum, such as an inability to produce enough progesterone to sustain the uterine lining. The corpus luteum may also produce progesterone initially but then disintegrate too early. These problems in corpus luteum function, referred to as luteal-phase insufficiency, may be caused by the same types of hormonal abnormalities that cause lack of ovulation.

Some cases of infertility may be associated with an abnormally shaped uterus or vagina. Such malformations of the reproductive organs are common in women whose mothers took diethylstilbestrol (DES) during pregnancy. DES was prescribed to many pregnant women from 1941 to about 1970 as a protection against miscarriage; infertility and other problems occur in the offspring of these women.

Conception depends on normal function of the oviducts (or Fallopian tubes), thin tubes with an inner diameter of only a few millimeters; they are attached to the top of the uterus and curve upward toward the ovaries. The inner end of each tube, located near one of the ovaries, waves back and forth at the time of ovulation, drawing the mature ovum into the opening of the oviduct. Once in the oviduct, the ovum is propelled along by movements of the oviduct wall. Meanwhile, if intercourse has occurred recently, the man's sperm will be moving upward in the female system, swimming through the uterus and the oviducts. Fertilization, the union of the sperm and ovum, will occur in the oviduct, and then the fertilized ovum will pass down the oviduct and reach the uterus about three days after ovulation.

Infertility can result from scar tissue formation inside the oviduct, resulting in physical blockage and inability to transport the ovum, sperm, or both. The most common cause of scar tissue formation in the reproductive organs is pelvic inflammatory disease (PID), a condition characterized by inflammation that spreads throughout the female reproductive tract. PID may be initiated by a sexually transmitted disease such as gonorrhea and chlamydia. Physicians in the United States have documented an increase in infertility attributable to tubal damage caused by sexually transmitted diseases.

Damage to the outside of the oviduct can also cause infertility, because such damage can interfere with the mobility of the oviduct, which is necessary to the capture of the ovum at the time of ovulation. External damage to the oviduct may occur as an aftermath of abdominal surgery, when adhesions induced by surgical cutting are likely to form. An adhesion is an abnormal scar tissue connection between adjacent structures.

Another possible cause of damage to the oviduct, resulting in infertility, is the presence of endometriosis. Endometriosis refers to a condition in which patches of the uterine lining implant in or on the surface of other organs. These patches are thought to arise during menstruation, when the uterine lining (endometrium) is normally shed from the body through the cervix and vagina; in a woman with endometriosis, for unknown reasons, the endometrium is carried to the interior of the pelvic cavity by passing up the oviducts. The endometrial patches can lodge in the oviduct itself, causing blockage, or can adhere to the outer surface of the oviducts, interfering with mobility.

Endometriosis can cause infertility by interfering with organs other than the oviducts. Endometrial patches on the outside of the uterus can cause distortions in the shape or placement of the uterus, interfering with embryonic implantation. Ovulation may be prevented by the presence of the endometrial tissues on the surface of the ovary. Yet the presence of endometriosis is not always associated with infertility. Thirty percent to forty percent of women with endometriosis cannot conceive, but the remainder appear to be fertile.

Another critical site in conception is the cervix. The cervix, the entryway to the uterus from the vagina, represents the first barrier through which sperm must pass on their way to the ovum. The cervix consists of a ring of strong, elastic tissue with a narrow canal. Glands in the cervix produce the mucus that fills the cervical canal and through which sperm swim en route to the ovum. The amount and quality of the cervical mucus changes throughout the menstrual cycle, under the influence of hormones from the ovary. At ovulation, the mucus is in a state that is most easily penetrated by sperm; after ovulation, the mucus becomes almost impenetrable.

Cervical problems that can lead to infertility include production of a mucus that does not allow sperm passage at the time of ovulation (hostile mucus syndrome) and interference with sperm transport caused by narrowing of the cervical canal. Such narrowing may be the result of a de-

velopmental abnormality or the presence of an infection, possibly a sexually transmitted disease.

### TREATMENT AND THERAPY

The diagnosis of the exact cause of a woman's infertility is crucial to successful treatment. A complete medical history should reveal any obvious problems of previous infection or menstrual cycle irregularity. Adequacy of ovulation and luteal-phase function can be determined from records of menstrual cycle length and changes in body temperature (body temperature is higher after ovulation). Hormone levels can be measured with tests of blood or urine samples. If damage to the oviducts or uterus is suspected, hysterosalpingography will be performed. In this procedure, the injection of a special fluid into the uterus is followed by X-ray analysis of the fluid movement; the shape of the uterine cavity and the oviducts will be revealed. Cervical functioning can be assessed with the postcoital test, in which the physician attempts to recover sperm from the woman's uterus some hours after she has had intercourse with her partner. If a uterine problem is suspected, the woman may have an endometrial biopsy, in which a small sample of the uterine lining is removed and examined for abnormalities. Sometimes, exploratory surgery is performed to pinpoint the location of scar tissue or the location of endometriosis patches.

Surgery may be used for treatment as well as diagnosis. Damage to the oviducts can sometimes be repaired surgically, and surgical removal of endometrial patches is a standard treatment for endometriosis. Often, however, surgery is a last resort, because of the likelihood of the development of postsurgical adhesions, which can further complicate the infertility. Newer forms of surgery using lasers and freezing offer better success because of a reduced risk of adhesions.

Some women with hormonal difficulties can be treated successfully with so-called fertility drugs. There are actually several different drugs and hormones that fall under this heading: Clomiphene citrate (Clomid), human menopausal gonadotropin (HMG), gonadotropin-releasing hormone (GnRH), bromocriptine mesylate (Parlodel), and menotropins (Pergonal) are commonly used, with the exact choice depending on the woman's particular problem. The pregnancy rate with fertility drug treatment varies from 20 percent to 70 percent. One problem with some of the drugs is the risk of multiple pregnancy (more than one fetus in the uterus). Hyperstimulation of the ovaries, a condition characterized by enlarged ovaries, can be fatal as a result of severe hormone imbalances. Other possible problems include nausea, dizziness, headache, and general malaise.

Artificial insemination is an old technique that is still useful in various types of infertility. A previously collected sperm sample is placed in the woman's vagina or uterus using a special tube. Artificial insemination is always performed at the time of ovulation, in order to maximize the chance of pregnancy. The ovulation date can be determined with body temperature records or by hormone measurements. In some cases, this procedure is combined with fertility drug treatment. Since the sperm can be placed directly in the uterus, it is useful in treating hostile mucus syndrome and certain types of male infertility. The sperm sample can be provided either by the woman's partner or by a donor. The pregnancy rate after artificial insemination is highly variable (14 percent to 68 percent), depending on the particular infertility problem in the couple. There is a slight risk of infection, and, if donated semen is used, there may be no guarantee that the semen is free from sexually transmitted diseases or that the donor does not carry some genetic defect.

Another infertility treatment is gamete intrafallopian transfer (GIFT), the surgical placement of ova and sperm directly into the woman's oviducts. In order to be a candidate for this procedure, the woman must have at least one partially undamaged oviduct and a functional uterus. Ova are collected surgically from the ovaries after stimulation with a fertility drug, and a semen sample is collected from the male. The ova and the sperm are introduced into the oviducts through the same abdominal incision used to collect the ova. This procedure is useful in certain types of male infertility, if the woman produces an impenetrable cervical mucus, or if the ovarian ends of the oviducts are damaged. The range of infertility problems that may be resolved with GIFT can be extended by using donated ova or sperm. The success rate is about 33 percent overall, but the rate varies with the type of infertility present.

In vitro fertilization is known colloquially as the "test-tube baby" technique. In this procedure, ova are collected surgically after stimulation with fertility drugs and then placed in a laboratory dish and combined with sperm from the man. The actual fertilization, when a sperm penetrates the ovum, will occur in the dish. The resulting embryo is allowed to remain in the dish for two days, during which time it will have acquired two to four cells. Then, the embryo is placed in the woman's uterine cavity using a flexible tube. In vitro fertilization can be used in women who are infertile because of endometriosis, damaged oviducts, impenetrable cervical mucus, or ovarian failure. As with GIFT, in vitro fertilization may utilize either donated ova or donated sperm, or extra embryos that have been produced by one couple may be implanted in a second woman. The pregnancy rate with this procedure varies from 15 percent to 25 percent.

Embryo freezing is a secondary procedure that can increase the chances of pregnancy for an infertile couple. When ova are collected for the in vitro fertilization procedure, doctors try to collect as many as possible. All these ova are then combined with sperm for fertilization. No more than three or four embryos are ever placed in the woman's uterus, however, because a pregnancy with a large number of fetuses carries significant health risks. The extra embryos can be frozen for later use, if the first ones implanted in the uterus do not survive. This spares the woman additional surgery to collect more ova if they are needed. The freezing technique does not appear to cause any defects in the embryo.

## Procedure for In Vitro Fertilization

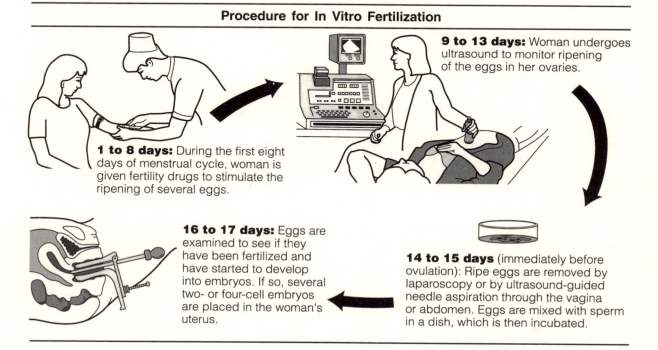

**1 to 8 days:** During the first eight days of menstrual cycle, woman is given fertility drugs to stimulate the ripening of several eggs.

**9 to 13 days:** Woman undergoes ultrasound to monitor ripening of the eggs in her ovaries.

**14 to 15 days** (immediately before ovulation): Ripe eggs are removed by laparoscopy or by ultrasound-guided needle aspiration through the vagina or abdomen. Eggs are mixed with sperm in a dish, which is then incubated.

**16 to 17 days:** Eggs are examined to see if they have been fertilized and have started to develop into embryos. If so, several two- or four-cell embryos are placed in the woman's uterus.

Some women may benefit from nonsurgical embryo transfer. In this procedure, a fertile woman is artificially inseminated at the time of her ovulation; five days later, her uterus is flushed with a sterile solution, washing out the resulting embryo before it implants in the uterus. The retrieved embryo is then transferred to the uterus of another woman, who will carry it to term. Typically, the sperm provider and the woman who receives the embryo are the infertile couple who wish to rear the child, but the technique can be used in other circumstances as well. Embryo transfer can be used if the woman has damaged oviducts or is unable to ovulate, or if she has a genetic disease that could be passed to her offspring, because in this case the baby is not genetically related to the woman who carries it.

Some infertile women who are unable to achieve a pregnancy themselves turn to the use of a surrogate, a woman who will agree to bear a child and then turn it over to the infertile woman to rear as her own. In the typical situation, the surrogate is artificially inseminated with the sperm of the infertile woman's husband. The surrogate then proceeds with pregnancy and delivery as normal, but relinquishes the child to the infertile couple after its birth.

### PERSPECTIVE AND PROSPECTS

One of the biggest problems that infertile couples face is the emotional upheaval that comes with the diagnosis of the infertility. Bearing and rearing children is an experience that most women treasure. When a woman is told that she is infertile, she may feel that her femininity and self-worth are diminished. In addition to the emotional difficulty that may come with the recognition of infertility, more stress may be in store as the couple proceeds through treatment. The various treatments can cause embarrassment and sometimes physical pain, and fertility drugs themselves are known to cause emotional swings. For these reasons, a couple with an infertility problem is often advised to seek help from a private counselor or a support group.

Along with the emotional and physical trauma of infertility treatment, there is a considerable financial burden as well. Infertility treatments, in general, are very expensive, especially the more sophisticated procedures such as in vitro fertilization and GIFT. Since the chances of a single procedure resulting in a pregnancy are often low, the couple may be faced with submitting to multiple procedures repeated many times. The cost over several years of treatment—a realistic possibility—can be staggering. Many health insurance companies in the United States refuse to cover the costs of such treatment and are required to do so in only a few states.

Some of the treatments are accompanied by unresolved legal questions. In the case of nonsurgical embryo transfer, is the legal mother of the child the ovum donor or the woman who gives birth to the child? The same question of legal parentage arises in cases of surrogacy. Does a child born using donated ovum or sperm have a legal right to any information about the donor, such as medical history? How extensive should governmental regulation of infertility clinics be? For example, should there be standards for assuring that donated sperm or ova are free from genetic defects? In the United States, some states have begun to address these issues, but no uniform policies have been set at the federal level.

The legal questions are largely unresolved because American society is still involved in religious and philosophical debates over the proprieties of various infertility treatments. Some religions hold that any interference in conception is unacceptable. To these denominations, even artificial insemination is wrong. Other groups approve of treatments confined to a husband and wife, but disapprove of a third party being involved as a donor or surrogate. Many people disapprove of any infertility treatment to help an individual who is not married. The basic problem underlying all these issues is that these technologies challenge the traditional definitions of parenthood.

—*Marcia Watson-Whitmyre*

**See also** Conception; Infertility in males; Menopause; Menstruation; Miscarriage; Ovarian cysts; Pelvic inflammatory disease (PID); Pregnancy and gestation; Sexual dysfunction; Stress.

### FOR FURTHER INFORMATION:

Andrews, Lori B. *New Conceptions: A Consumer's Guide to the Newest Infertility Treatments, Including In Vitro Fertilization, Artificial Insemination, and Surrogate Motherhood.* New York: St. Martin's Press, 1984. This outstanding book is designed to help infertile couples understand the treatments that they may be offered. The author is a lawyer known for her work in reproductive health issues. Legal aspects are well covered.

Belfort, P., J. A. Pinotti, and T. K. A. B. Eskes, eds. *Fertility, Sterility, and Contraception.* Park Ridge, N.J.: Parthenon, 1989. With chapters written by various experts in reproduction, this text offers detailed information about some of the techniques used in infertility diagnosis and treatment.

DeCherney, Alan H., Mary Lake Polan, Ronald D. Lee, and Stephen P. Boyers. *Decision Making in Infertility.* Toronto: B. C. Decker, 1988. This innovative text presents information on the diagnosis and treatment of infertility in the form of flow charts to guide decision making. The brief text provides additional details.

Fathalla, Mahmoud F., Allan Rosenfield, Cynthia Indriso, Dilup K. Sen, and Shan S. Ratnam, eds. *Reproductive Health: Global Issues.* Vol. 3 in *The FIGO Manual of Human Reproduction,* edited by Fathalla and Rosenfield. 2d ed. Park Ridge, N.J.: Parthenon, 1990. Chapter 4 in this text deals with infertility—its causes, diagnosis, and treatment—in a concise and understandable manner.

Harkness, Carla. *The Infertility Book: A Comprehensive Medical and Emotional Guide.* Berkeley, Calif.: Celestial Arts, 1992. Written as a guide for the infertile couple, this book offers emotional support as well as medical information. The text is augmented by firsthand accounts of individuals' reactions to their infertility and the treatments.

Quilligan, Edward J., and Frederick P. Zuspan, eds. *Current Therapy in Obstetrics and Gynecology*. Philadelphia: W. B. Saunders, 1990. This excellent handbook provides detailed information on procedures for various infertility causes and treatments, arranged alphabetically amid other gynecological subjects.

Speroff, Leon, Robert H. Glass, and Nathan G. Kase. *Clinical Gynecologic Endocrinology and Infertility*. 3d ed. Baltimore: Williams & Wilkins, 1983. A good basic textbook that can help the reader understand the normal functioning of the female reproductive system and the events associated with infertility.

Yeh, John, and Molly Uline Yeh. *Legal Aspects of Infertility*. Boston: Blackwell Scientific Publications, 1991. The authors, a practicing physician and a lawyer, wrote this text as a guide for doctors, but it makes fascinating reading for anyone interested in the governmental regulation of infertility treatments. Also includes medical information on the use and success of various treatments.

## INFERTILITY IN MALES

**SYSTEM AFFECTED:** Reproductive (male)

**SPECIALISTS:** Endocrinologists, urologists

**DEFINITION:** The inability to achieve a desired pregnancy as a result of dysfunction of male reproductive organs.

**KEY TERMS:**

*antibody:* a chemical produced by lymphocytes (blood cells) that enables these cells to destroy foreign materials, such as bacteria

*cryopreservation:* a special process utilizing cryoprotectants that enables living cells to survive in a frozen state

*cryoprotectant:* one of several chemicals that enables living cells to survive in a frozen state; some cryoprotectants are made by animals that survive freezing

*epididymis:* an organ attached to the testis in which newly formed sperm reach maturity (that is, become capable of fertilizing an egg)

*infertility:* the inability to produce a normal pregnancy after one year of intercourse in the absence of any contraception; it may be caused by male and/or female factors

*insemination:* the placement of semen in the female reproductive tract, which may occur naturally as a result of sexual intercourse or artificially as a result of a medical procedure

*testis:* either of two male gonads that are suspended in the scrotum and produce sperm

*varicocele:* a swollen testicular vein in the scrotum occurring as a result of improper valvular function

### CAUSES AND SYMPTOMS

To create a baby requires three things: normal sperm from a man, a normal egg from a woman, and a normal, mature uterus. Anything that blocks the availability of the sperm, egg, or uterus can cause infertility. Infertility can be thought of as an abnormal, unwanted form of contraception.

Many different factors may be responsible for infertility. In general, these factors may be infectious, chemical (from inside or outside of the body, such as illegal drugs, pharmaceuticals, or toxins), or anatomical. Genetic factors may be responsible as well, since genes control the formation of body chemicals (such as hormones and antibodies) and body structures (one's anatomy). The way that these factors work is illustrated by male infertility.

The process by which sperm are made begins in a man's testis (or testicle). Because the transformation of testis cells into sperm is controlled by genes and hormones, abnormalities can cause infertility. Sperm released from the testis become mature in the epididymis. Sperm travel from the testis to the epididymis through ducts (tubes) in the male reproductive tract. A blockage of these ducts or premature release of sperm from the epididymis can cause infertility.

A blockage of reproductive ducts can occur as a result of a bodily enlargement, such as swollen tissue, tumor, or cancer. An infection usually causes tissue swelling and can leave ducts permanently scarred, narrowed, or blocked. Infection can have a direct detrimental effect on the production of normal sperm. Cancer and the drugs or chemicals used to treat cancer can also damage a man's reproductive tract.

Another factor that may be important to male fertility is scrotal temperature. The temperature in the scrotum, the sac that holds the testis, is somewhat cooler than body tem-

## Common Causes of Male Infertility

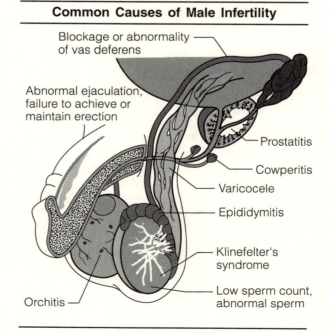

Blockage or abnormality of vas deferens

Abnormal ejaculation, failure to achieve or maintain erection

Prostatitis

Cowperitis

Varicocele

Epididymitis

Klinefelter's syndrome

Low sperm count, abnormal sperm

Orchitis

perature. The normal production of sperm seems to be dependent upon a cool testicular environment.

The leading cause of male infertility may be varicoceles, which occur when one-way valves fail in the veins that take blood away from the testicles. When these venous valves become leaky, blood flow becomes sluggish and causes the veins to swell. Many men with varicoceles are infertile, but the exact reason for this association is unknown. The reasons sometimes given are increased scrotal temperature and improper removal of materials (hormones) from the testis.

Mature sperm capable of fertilizing an egg are normally placed in the female reproductive tract by the ejaculation phase of sexual intercourse. The sperm are accompanied by fluid called seminal plasma; together, they form semen. A blockage of the ducts that transport the semen into the woman or toxic chemicals, including antibodies, in the semen can cause infertility.

For conception to take place—that is, for an egg to be fertilized after sperm enters the female tract—a normal egg must be present in the portion of the tract called the Fallopian tube and sperm must move through the female tract to that egg. If the egg is absent or is abnormal, or if normal sperm cannot reach the egg, female infertility will result. The female factors that determine whether sperm fertilize an egg are the same as the male factors: anatomy, chemicals, infection, and genes.

There are many ways to treat infertility. Female infertility may be treated, depending upon the cause, by surgery, hormone therapy, or in vitro fertilization. Treatment of male infertility may be by surgery, hormone therapy, or therapeutic (artificial) insemination. Therapeutic insemination is often performed when the couple is composed of a fertile woman and an infertile man.

The first step for therapeutic insemination is for a physician to determine when an egg is ovulated or released into the Fallopian tube of the fertile woman. At the time of ovulation, semen is placed with medical instruments in the woman's reproductive tract, either on her cervix or in her uterus.

The semen used by the physician is obtained through masturbation by either the infertile man (the patient) or a fertile man (a donor), depending on the cause of the man's infertility. The freshly produced semen from either source usually undergoes laboratory testing and processing. Tests are used to evaluate the sperm quality. An effort may be made to enhance the sperm from an infertile patient and then to use these sperm for therapeutic insemination or in vitro fertilization. Other tests evaluate semen for transmissible diseases. During testing, which may require many days, the sperm can be kept alive by cryopreservation. Freshly ejaculated sperm remains fertile for only a few hours in the laboratory if it is not cryopreserved.

There are several processes that might enhance sperm from an infertile man. If the semen is infertile because it possesses too few normal sperm, an effort can be made to

eliminate the abnormal sperm and to increase the concentration of normal sperm. Sperm may be abnormal in four basic ways: They may have abnormal structure, they may have abnormal movement, they may be incapable of fusing with an egg, or they may contain abnormal genes or chromosomes. Laboratory processes can often eliminate from semen those sperm with abnormal structure or abnormal movement. These processes usually involve replacing the seminal plasma with a culture medium. Removing the seminal plasma gets rid of substances that may be harmful to the sperm. After the plasma is removed, the normal sperm can be collected and concentrated. Pharmacologic agents can be added to the culture medium to increase sperm movement.

Testing for transmissible diseases is especially important if donor semen is used; these diseases may be genetic or infectious. There are many thousand genetic disorders. Most of these disorders are very rare and can be transmitted to offspring only if the sperm and the egg both have the same gene for the disorder. It is impossible, therefore, to test a donor for every possible genetic disorder; he is routinely tested only for a small group of troublesome disorders that are especially likely to occur in offspring. Tests for other disorders that the donor might transmit can be performed at the woman's request, usually based upon knowledge of genetic problems in her own family.

Much of the genetic information about a person is based on family history. Special laboratory procedures allow the genetic code inside individual cells to be interpreted. For this reason, it is important to store a sample of donor cells, not necessarily sperm, for many years after the procedure. These cells provide additional genetic information that might be important to the donor's offspring but not known at the time of insemination.

Semen can also be the source of infectious disease. Syphilis, gonorrhea, and acquired immunodeficiency syndrome (AIDS) are examples of venereal or sexually transmitted diseases (STDs). Tests for STDs can be done on blood and semen from a donor. These tests must be conducted in an approved manner, and the results must be negative before donor semen can be used therapeutically. In some cases, a test must be repeated in order to verify that the semen is not infectious.

Cryopreservation of sperm is important to therapeutic insemination for two major reasons. First, it gives time to complete all necessary testing. Second, it allows an inventory of sperm from many different donors to be kept constantly available for selection and use by patients. Sperm properly cryopreserved for twenty years, when thawed and inseminated, can produce normal babies.

Cryopreservation involves treating freshly ejaculated sperm with a cryoprotectant pharmaceutical that enables the sperm to survive when frozen; the cryoprotectant for sperm is usually glycerol. Survival of frozen sperm is also dependent upon the rate of cooling, the storage temperature, and the rate of warming at the time of thawing. Sperm treated with a cryoprotectant have the best chance of survival if they are cooled about 1 degree Celsius per minute and stored at a temperature of -150 degrees Celsius or colder. An environment of liquid nitrogen is often used to attain these storage temperatures. The storage temperature must be kept constant to avoid the damaging effects of recrystallization. When sperm are to be thawed, survival is enhanced if they are warmed at 10 to 100 degrees Celsius per minute.

The cryopreservation procedure involves the actual formation of ice, although the ice is confined to the extracellular medium. Intracellular ice is lethal. Ice formation during cryopreservation causes the cells to lose water and to shrink. The cryoprotectant seems to replace intracellular water and thereby maintain cell volume.

An alternative process for low temperature preservation of sperm is called vitrification. Vitrification uses temperatures as cold as cryopreservation, but it avoids ice formation altogether. Instead of using one cryoprotectant, vitrification uses a mixture of several. It employs a much slower cooling rate and a much faster warming rate. Technically, vitrification is more difficult to perform; therefore, it is seldom used by clinical sperm banks.

Human sperm can be shipped to almost any location for therapeutic insemination. Sperm is usually cryopreserved before shipment and thawed at the time of insemination.

### TREATMENT AND THERAPY

The use of therapeutic insemination to treat two kinds of male infertility will be considered here. The first example is male infertility that cannot be treated by other means. The second example is a fertile man at high risk for becoming infertile because of his lifestyle or because he is receiving treatment for a life-threatening disease.

The first example might occur when a heterosexual couple, having used no contraception for a year or longer, has been unsuccessful in conceiving a baby. In 40 percent of infertility cases, the woman has the major, but not necessarily the only, problem preventing the pregnancy. In 40 percent of the cases, the man is the major factor. In 20 percent, each person makes a substantial contribution to the problem. Therefore, both partners must deal with the infertility and be involved in the treatment.

The solution to a couple's infertility involves evaluation and therapy. The couple will be evaluated in regard to their present sexual activity and history, such as whether either one has ever contributed to a pregnancy. The medical evaluation of both partners will include a physical examination, laboratory tests, and even imaging techniques such as X rays, ultrasonography, or magnetic resonance imaging (MRI). For the man, the physical examination will include a search for the presence of varicoceles, and the laboratory tests will include a semen analysis. About 15 to 30 percent of couples entering an infertility program achieve preg-

nancy during the evaluation phase of the program, before any therapy is begun.

Varicoceles are probably the most readily detected problem that may cause male infertility. They are three times more common in infertile men than in men with proven fertility. This association does not prove that varicoceles cause infertility, however, because surgery that corrects a varicocele does not always correct infertility.

If the medical evaluation determines that the female partner has a normal reproductive tract and is ovulating on a regular basis, and if it determines that the male partner has too few normal sperm to make a pregnancy likely, the couple may be asked to consider adopting a baby or undergoing therapeutic insemination. With therapeutic insemination, the woman actually becomes pregnant and half of the baby's genes come from the mother. The other half of the genes come from the sperm donor, usually a person unknown to the couple. The physician performing therapeutic insemination may provide the couple with extensive information on several possible donors. Such information might include race, ethnic origin, blood type, physical characteristics, results of medical and genetic tests, and personal information, but the donor usually remains anonymous. The semen from each donor has undergone laboratory testing and cryopreservation. The frozen semen is thawed at the time of insemination.

Although the idea of therapeutic insemination is simple, it usually involves some very complicated emotions. Although a couple may be very happy about all other aspects of their lives together, they are usually deeply disturbed to learn of the man's infertility. It may be extremely difficult for them to discuss his infertility with anyone else. Some people ridicule infertile men as being less virile or even being impotent. (This is not the case: The majority of infertile or sterile men have normal sex lives.) These feelings will influence the couple's selection of a sperm donor. Later, they must decide whether to tell the child about the circumstances of his or her birth. Sometimes, a child who originated through therapeutic insemination will try to learn the identity of the donor.

The donor must be considered as well. In a typical sperm bank, persons are subjected to a variety of tests before they are accepted as donors. Sperm donors are typically in their second decade of life, but some are older. These men are primarily, but not solely, motivated to be sperm donors by financial compensation. Payment effectively maintains donor cooperation for a period of several years. In addition to payment, the donor usually wants an assurance that he will not be held responsible, financially or legally, for the offspring produced by his semen. As a donor grows older, however, his attitude about his donation may change: He may wonder about the children he has helped to create.

Although male-factor infertility is the situation that benefits most from insemination and semen cryopreservation procedures, these procedures might be requested by a fertile couple that is at risk for male-factor infertility. Such couples may fear that the man's lifestyle, such as working with hazardous materials (solvents, toxins, radioisotopes, or explosives), may endanger his ability to produce sperm or may harm his genetic information. The man could be facing medical therapy that will cure a malignancy, such as Hodgkin's disease or a testicular tumor, but may render him sterile. A man facing such a situation may benefit from having some of his semen cryopreserved for his own future use, in the event that he actually becomes infertile.

Therapeutic insemination with a husband's semen is usually not as effective as with donor semen, especially when cryopreservation is involved. Although cryopreservation keeps cells alive in the frozen state, not all the cells survive. Men selected to be semen donors have sperm that survive freezing much better than the sperm of most men (although the reason for this ability is unknown). If a man undergoing medical treatment is already sick at the time that the decision is made to store his sperm, his concentration of functioning sperm may be less than normal.

There are ways to compensate for decreased semen quality. The semen may be processed in ways to increase the concentration of normal sperm. The processed semen may be placed directly into the woman's uterus (intrauterine insemination) rather than on her cervix, or in vitro fertilization, a procedure in which the sperm and eggs are mixed in a laboratory and the resulting embryo implanted in the woman, may be used. All these techniques have proven helpful to infertile couples wanting children.

## PERSPECTIVE AND PROSPECTS

It has been estimated that infertility affects 8 to 15 percent of American marriages, which means that three to nine million American couples would like to, but cannot, have children without medical assistance. By the early 1990's, therapeutic insemination produced more than thirty thousand American babies yearly. This procedure advanced in the United States during the latter half of the twentieth century in large measure because of changes in attitudes, not because of new medical knowledge.

The medical knowledge to treat male infertility has been available for several centuries, even when the biological basis for pregnancy was not understood. The importance of sexual intercourse in reproduction was probably recognized by prehistoric humans. The Bible records stories of patriarchal families that knew the problem of infertility (Abraham and Sarah, Jacob and Rachel) and even indicates, in the story of Onan and Tamar (Genesis 38:9), that semen was understood to be important to reproduction. The possibility of therapeutic insemination was mentioned in the fifth century Talmud. Arabs used insemination in horse breeding as early as the fourteenth century, and Spaniards used it in human medicine during the fifteenth century.

The presence of sperm in semen was first observed by Anton van Leeuwenhoek in the seventeenth century, but their importance and function in the fertilization process was not recognized until the nineteenth century. In 1824, Jean Louis Prévost and J. A. Dumas correctly guessed the role of sperm in fertilization, and in 1876, Oskar Hertwig and Hermann Fol proved that the union of sperm and egg was necessary to create an embryo.

Therapeutic insemination became an established but clandestine procedure in the late nineteenth century in the United States and England. Compassionate physicians pioneering therapeutic insemination encouraged secrecy to protect the self-esteem of the infertile man, his spouse, the offspring, and the donor. In an uncertain legal climate, the offspring might have been viewed as the illegitimate product of an adulterous act. Even by the late twentieth century, many Americans continued to stigmatize masturbation and therapeutic insemination. Social attitudes, especially machismo, has limited the acceptability of therapeutic insemination to many infertile couples worldwide.

Cryopreservation of sperm became practical with the discovery of chemical cryoprotectants, reported in 1949 by Christopher Polge, Audrey Smith, and Alan Parkes of England. In 1953, American doctors R. G. Bunge and Jerome Sherman were the first to use this procedure to produce a human baby. Cryopreservation made possible the establishment of sperm banks; prior to this development, sperm donors had to provide the physician with semen immediately before insemination was to take place.

Therapeutic insemination and other alternative means of reproduction give rise to thorny issues of personal rights of various "parents" (social, birth, and genetic) and their offspring. In the United States, a few states have addressed these issues by enacting laws, usually to grant legitimacy to offspring of donor insemination. In the United Kingdom, Parliament established a central registry of sperm and egg donors. Offspring in the United Kingdom have access to nonidentifying donor information; these children are even able to learn whether they are genetically related to a prospective marriage partner.  —*Armand M. Karow*

**See also** Conception; Infertility in females; Pregnancy and gestation; Sexual dysfunction; Stress.

## FOR FURTHER INFORMATION:

Baran, Annette, and Reuben Pannor. *Lethal Secrets*. New York: Warner Books, 1989. The authors, medical social workers, discuss the possible consequences of secrecy in donor insemination using a series of case histories.

Karow, Armand M., and David E. Pegg, eds. *Organ Preservation for Transplantation*. 2d ed. New York: Marcel Dekker, 1981. This technical book describes in detail the theory and procedures for the cryopreservation of many human tissues. One chapter is devoted to procedures for the cryopreservation of sperm.

Noble, Elizabeth. *Having Your Baby by Donor Insemination*. Boston: Houghton Mifflin, 1987. Donor insemination is discussed from the recipient's viewpoint. Reasons for insemination, options, methods, and issues are discussed. An excellent appendix locates medical resources.

Perloe, Mark, and Linda Gail Christie. *Miracle Babies and Other Happy Endings for Couples with Fertility Problems*. New York: Rawson Associates, 1986. A physician and a psychologist talk to patients about male and female infertility. This lively, readable, and upbeat book contains a useful appendix.

Spark, Richard F. *The Infertile Male*. New York: Plenum Press, 1988. This medical book is written in a style that is easy to read by those who have taken an introductory course in biology. Discusses the factors causing infertility, diagnostic procedures, and treatment.

U.S. Congress. Office of Technology Assessment. *Infertility: Medical and Social Choices*. Washington, D.C.: Government Printing Office, 1988. This well-edited book, written by a committee, discusses the medical basis of infertility, its demographics, its monetary costs, social risks, legal status, and ethical options. Written to provide policy options to Congress.

Warnock, Mary. *A Question of Life*. New York: Basil Blackwell, 1985. This report, commissioned by the British Parliament, discusses medical procedures for alleviating infertility and social issues of family formation and inheritance. The report concludes with the recommendations that led to the Human Fertilization and Embryology Act of 1990.

# INFLAMMATION

**SYSTEMS AFFECTED:** All

**SPECIALISTS:** Burn specialists, family physicians, infectious disease physicians, internists, pathologists, rheumatologists

**DEFINITION:** The reaction of blood-filled living tissue to injury.

In inflammation, the following changes are seen locally: redness, swelling, heat, pain, and loss of function. These changes are chemically mediated. Inflammation may be caused by microbial infection; physical agents such as trauma, radiation, and burns; chemical toxins; caustic substances such as strong acids or bases; decomposing or necrotic tissue; and reactions of the immune system. Acute inflammation is of relatively short duration (from a few minutes to a day or so), while chronic inflammation lasts longer. The local changes associated with inflammation include the outflow of fluid into the spaces between cells and the inflow or migration of white blood cells (leukocytes) to the area of injury. Chronic inflammation is characterized by the presence of leukocytes and macrophages, as well as by the proliferation of new blood vessels and connective tissue.

Inflammation is a protective mechanism for the body. Redness is attributable to increased blood flow to the injured area. Swelling is caused by the flow of fluid into the spaces between cells. Heat is produced by a combination of increased blood flow and chemical reactions in the local area. Pain results from the presence of two main chemicals found in the bloodstream: prostaglandins and bradykinin. Loss of function is a result of pain (the body limits movement to reduce discomfort) and swelling (interstitial fluid limits movement).

*Acute inflammation.* Many chemicals are involved in acute inflammation. Mediators of inflammation originate from blood plasma and from both damaged and normal cells. Vasoactive amines are a class of chemicals that increase the permeability of blood vessel and cell walls. The most well studied of these are histamine and serotonin. Histamine is stored in granules in mast cells that are found in both tissue and basophils, the latter being a type of cell found in the blood. Serotonin is found in mast cells and platelets; it is another type of cell found in the bloodstream. These substances cause vasodilation (expansion of the walls of blood vessels) and increased vascular permeability (leakage through the walls of small vessels, especially veins). Histamine and serotonin can be released by trauma or exposure to cold. Other chemicals that circulate in the blood can release histamine. Two of these are part of the complement system; another is called interleukin-1. The effects of histamine diminish after approximately one hour.

Plasma proteases comprise three interrelated systems that explain much that is known about inflammation: the complement, kinin, and clotting systems. The complement system is composed of twenty different proteins involved in reactions against microbial agents that invade the body. The various chemicals act in a cascade, similar to falling dominoes: Each one sets off another in sequence. The result of these chemical actions is to increase vascular permeability, promote chemotaxis (the attraction of living cells to specific chemicals), engulf invading microorganisms, and destroy pathogens through a process called lysis.

The kinin system is responsible for releasing bradykinin, a chemical substance that causes contraction of smooth muscle tissue, dilation of blood vessels, and pain. The duration of action for bradykinin is brief because it is inactivated by the enzyme kininase. Bradykinin does not promote chemotaxis.

The clotting system is made up of a series of chemicals that result in the formation of a solid mass. The most commonly encountered example is the scab that forms at the site of a cut in the skin. Like the complement system, the clotting system is a cascade of thirteen different chemicals. In addition to producing a solid mass, the clotting system also increases vascular permeability and promotes chemotaxis for white blood cells.

Other substances are involved in acute inflammation. Among the most important of these is a class called prostaglandins. Several different prostaglandin molecules have been isolated; they are derived from the membranes of most cells. Prostaglandins cause pain, vasodilation, and fever. Aspirin counteracts the effects of prostaglandins, which explains the antipyretic (fever-reducing) and analgesic (pain-reducing) properties of the drug.

Another group of substances involved in acute inflammation are leukotrienes. The primary sources for these molecules are leukocytes, and some leukotrienes are found in mast cells. This group promotes vascular leakage but not chemotaxis. They also cause vasoconstriction (a decrease in the diameter of blood vessels) and bronchoconstriction (a decrease in the diameter of air passageways in the lungs). The effect of these leukotrienes is to slow blood flow and restrict air intake and outflow. A different type of leukotriene is found only in leukocytes. This type enhances chemotaxis but does not contribute to vascular leakage. In addition, leukotrienes cause white blood cells to stick to damaged tissues, speeding the removal of bacteria and promoting healing.

Other chemical substances are known to be involved with inflammation: platelet-activating factor, tumor necrosis factor, interleukin-1, cationic (positively charged) proteins, neutral proteases (enzymes that break down proteins), and oxygen metabolites (molecules resulting from reactions with oxygen). The sources of these are generally leukocytes, although some are derived from macrophages. They reinforce the effects of prostaglandins and leukotrienes.

There are four different outcomes for acute inflammation. There may be complete resolution in which the injured site is restored to normal; this outcome usually follows a mild injury or limited trauma where there has been only minor tissue destruction. Healing with scarring may occur, in which injured tissue is replaced with scar tissue that is rich in collagen, giving it strength but at the cost of normal function; this outcome follows more severe injury or extensive destruction of tissue. There may be the formation of an abscess, which is characterized by pus and which follows injuries that become infected with pyogenic (pus-forming) organisms. The fourth outcome is chronic inflammation.

*Chronic inflammation.* Acute inflammation may be followed by chronic inflammation. This reaction occurs when the organism, factor, or agent responsible for the acute inflammation is not removed or when the normal processes of healing fail to occur. Repeated episodes of acute inflammation may also lead to chronic inflammation, in which the stages of acute inflammation seem to remain for long periods of time. In addition, chronic inflammation may begin insidiously, such as with a low-grade infection that does not display the usual signs of acute inflammation; tuberculosis, rheumatoid arthritis, and chronic lung disease are examples of this third alternative.

Chronic inflammation typically occurs in one of the following conditions: prolonged exposure to potentially toxic substances such as asbestos, coal dust, and silica that are nondegradable; immune reactions against one's own tissue (autoimmune diseases such as lupus and rheumatoid arthritis); and persistent infection by an organism that is either resistant to drug therapy or insufficiently toxic to cause an immune reaction (such as viruses, tuberculosis, and leprosy). The characteristics of chronic inflammation are similar to those of acute inflammation but are less dramatic and more protracted.    —*L. Fleming Fallon, Jr.*

**See also** Arthritis; Bacterial infections; Burns and scalds; Bursitis; Disease; Ear infections and disorders; Food poisoning; Fungal infections; Infection; Influenza; Poisoning; Skin disorders; Staphylococcal infections; Streptococcal infections; Viral infections; *specific diseases.*

**FOR FURTHER INFORMATION:**

Cotran, Ramzi S., Vinay Kumar, and Stanley L. Robbins. *Robbins' Pathologic Basis of Disease.* 4th ed. Philadelphia: W. B. Saunders, 1989. A widely used pathology text which contains a good discussion of inflammation. Written for health professionals, but the serious nonspecialist will find a wealth of material.

Gallin, John I., Ira M. Goldstein, and Ralph Snyderman, eds. *Inflammation: Basic Principles and Clinical Correlates.* New York: Raven Press, 1988. This well-written book is for the reader who wants to know about inflammation in great detail.

Majno, Guido, Ramzi Cotran, and Nathan Kaufman, eds. *Current Topics in Inflammation and Infection.* Baltimore: Williams & Wilkins, 1982. This specialized monograph provides extensive details on the subject. It assumes that the reader is familiar with the basics of inflammation.

Ryan, G. B., and G. Majno. "Acute Inflammation: A Review." *American Journal of Pathology* 86 (January, 1977): 183-276. A comprehensive review article. Well written, but uses technical language. General readers with access to a medical dictionary should find it informative.

# INFLUENZA

**SYSTEM AFFECTED:** Respiratory

**SPECIALISTS:** Epidemiologists, family physicians, infectious disease physicians, internists, public health specialists

**DEFINITION:** Any one of a group of commonly experienced respiratory diseases caused by viruses, responsible for many major, worldwide epidemics.

**KEY TERMS:**

*antibody:* a protein substance produced by white blood cells (lymphocytes) in response to an antigen; combats bacterial, viral, chemical, or other invasive agents in the body

*antigen:* a chemical substance, often on a bacterial or viral surface, containing substances that activate the body's immune response

*pneumonia:* a respiratory tract infection that can be caused by bacteria or viruses; it is the major complication of influenza and the major cause of influenza deaths *ribonucleic acid (RNA):* the material contained in the core of many viruses that is responsible for directing the replication of the virus inside the host cell

## CAUSES AND SYMPTOMS

Epidemics of what scientists believe was influenza have been reported in Europe and Asia for at least a thousand years. Epidemics of what could have been influenza were reported by ancient Greek and Roman historians. Influenza epidemics still occur, striking isolated societies, entire nations, or, as with pandemics, the entire world. Among the great plagues that have afflicted the world over the centuries, influenza is the one that remains active today. Smallpox has been conquered, and bubonic plague (the Black Death), yellow fever, and typhus no longer erupt every few years as they once did. Cholera still breaks out, but rarely as a major epidemic. Before acquired immunodeficiency syndrome (AIDS), influenza was called "the last of the great plagues."

The term "influenza" is from the Italian and refers to the fact that some early scientists thought that the disease was caused by the malevolent influence of the planets, stars, and other heavenly bodies. To others, this "influence" was a miasma or poisonous effluvium carried in the air—a theory which is closer to the truth.

In the eighteenth and nineteenth centuries, there were about twenty major epidemics of influenza in Europe and America. They were of varying severity—some mild, some harsh. In 1918, a pandemic of influenza became one of the worst afflictions ever endured by humankind. It came in three waves, the first in the spring of 1918. This wave was relatively mild and mortality rates were low, and it spread evenly through all age groups of the population. The second wave came in the fall, and it was the most devastating outbreak of disease seen since the great plagues of the Middle Ages. Up to 20 percent of its victims died, and about half the deaths were of people in the prime of life, twenty to forty years of age. The last wave came in the winter and was not as severe. By the time that the pandemic was over, more than 20 million people worldwide had died from it, with more than 500,000 deaths in the United States alone.

In 1918, scientists understood enough about microbiology to realize that a microorganism caused influenza, but they originally thought that it was a bacterium, *Haemophilus influenzae*, because this organism was isolated from some of the victims. *H. influenzae* causes many diseases, but influenza is not among them, as researchers found when infection from it failed to produce influenza symptoms in test subjects. It soon became apparent that the organism responsible for influenza was unlike any bacterium that science had yet encountered. Bacteria were easily seen in the microscope and could be collected in filters. Whatever it was that caused influenza was invisible to the microscope, and it could not be trapped in filters. So, scientists postulated that the influenza pathogen was far smaller than bacteria. They used the term "filtrable virus" to describe it—an

interesting locution, because what they meant was that the organism could *not* be filtered by the devices that they were using. "Filter-passing virus," another term used at the time, is more accurate.

It was not until 1931, thirteen years after the great pandemic, that the first influenza virus was isolated. It was found in swine, and the methods used to discover it formed the basis for the techniques used to isolate the human influenza virus, a major event in microbiology that occurred in 1933.

It was later found that there were not one but three kinds of human influenza virus: type A, which is the major cause of severe influenza outbreaks; type B, which also causes influenza epidemics but less often and which is usually less severe than type A; and the rarest, type C, which causes a mild, coldlike illness.

Further, it was discovered that there are different strains of virus within type A and type B, subtypes that are not identical to one another but that are related. Within each subtype there are variants. As these subtypes and variants began to appear, it became clear that the virus was capable of mutation. This was a critical discovery because it meant that influenza infection of one type would not necessarily immunize the victim against influenza of another type. This ability to mutate means that new influenza virus strains are constantly being developed—and are constantly threatening new waves of disease.

For example, in 1957, a new strain of influenza virus called the Asian flu came out of China and started a pandemic. Asian flu, or variants of it, caused the flu epidemics in the years from 1957 to 1968, but immunity to it spread so that the severity of the epidemics was gradually reduced. Then the Hong Kong flu, another new strain from the Far East, appeared. People had no immunity to it, so it caused another major pandemic. Hong Kong flu and its variants caused the epidemics that occurred in the next nine years. Then, in 1977, still another pandemic arose from a newer strain, also from Eastern Asia.

In 1976, another type, swine flu, appeared in the United States. This virus infects pigs and humans and is apparently a distant descendant of the virus that caused the 1918 pandemic. It was evidently not as hardy as the 1977 virus, because that one replaced it and swine flu disappeared, although some experts predict its return.

The reason that the influenza virus can mutate readily is related to its physiological structure. The virus is usually spherical, but the shape can vary. It is extremely small, about 0.0001 millimeter in diameter. Its surface is covered with spikes of protein, hemagglutinin and neuraminidase. They are the two major antigens that trigger the body's immune system to repel the virus and provide immunity against future infection. Hemagglutinin (H) causes red blood cells to agglutinate, or clump together. Neuraminidase (N) is an enzyme.

Inside the core of the virus are two additional antigens that trigger the production of antibodies, but these antibodies do not protect against future infection. Also in the core is a feature unique to influenza virus: Instead of a single strand of ribonucleic acid (RNA), there are eight individual strands, each one a single gene. Genes are said to be "encoded" to produce specific characteristics within an organism. When the virus invades a host cell, the RNA directs a process of replication in which components of the cell are used to make new viruses. The new viruses are then released to enter other cells and continue replicating.

The H and N antigens mutate gradually over the years because of changes in the RNA genes that encode for them. This process is called antigenic drift, and it refers to slight variations that appear in the influenza virus and account for minor and localized epidemics of the disease. When a particular strain of virus has been prevalent for some time, a "herd immunity" develops in the populations exposed to it, and incidence of disease from it declines. When the H or N antigen changes radically, the process is called antigenic shift. It creates a new subtype of the virus, one that can cause a major pandemic because there is no immunity to it. There are at least thirteen variants of H (labeled H1 to H13) and at least nine variants of N (labeled N1 to N9).

Before 1968, most influenza A viruses in circulation had H2N2 antigens on its surface. This virus was the Asian flu; it had been around for some years, so the world population had become relatively immune to it. Then, in 1968, a new virus appeared in Southeast Asia, with a combination of H3N2. The H antigen had changed completely, while the N antigen remained the same, but the combination was essentially a new virus; it gave rise to the worldwide epidemic of the Hong Kong flu.

It is known that influenza viruses from animals influence the structure of the human viruses and contribute the variations that become new strains capable of causing pandemics. There is an interesting theory of how the 1957, 1968, and 1977 pandemics that came out of China developed. The Chinese people not only eat an enormous amount of duck but also keep large flocks to eat insects that attack rice crops. Ducks carry a wide variety of influenza viruses in their intestines, and they live in close proximity to humans. This theory suggests that the influenza viruses from duck droppings modified the human influenza virus and created the new strains that caused the pandemics that emanated from China. Other animals, such as pigs, which gave the world swine flu, also harbor influenza viruses that can interact with the human influenza virus.

To cause disease, the virus must be inhaled, which is why the "influence" of poisonous effluvium carried in the air is a more correct attribution of the actual cause of the disease than the influence of heavenly bodies. Inside the upper respiratory tract, there is a layer of cilia-bearing cells (cells with small, hairlike filaments) that acts as a barrier against infection. Ordinarily, the tiny cilia spread a layer of mucus over respiratory tissues. The mucus collects infectious organisms and carries them to the stomach, where they are destroyed by stomach acids. The influenza virus causes the cilia-bearing cells to disintegrate, exposing a layer of cells beneath. The virus invades these and other host cells in the respiratory tract and begins replicating. Invasion and replication by the virus destroy the host cells. Destruction of the cells starts the inflammatory process that causes the symptoms of disease.

Influenza infection grows rapidly, and symptoms can appear in only a few hours, although the incubation period in most people is two days or so. Fever, malaise, headache, muscular pain (particularly in the back and legs), coughing, nasal congestion, shivering, and a sore throat are common symptoms. The disease can spread quickly among populations because the virus is airborne. There is good reason to believe that the virus can remain infective in the air for long periods of time. It has been reported that the crew members on a ship sailing past Cuba during an epidemic there were infected with the disease, presumably from virus-laden particles carried from shore by the wind.

The major complication of influenza is pneumonia, which can be caused by the influenza virus itself (primary influenza viral pneumonia), by infection from bacteria (secondary bacterial pneumonia), or by mixed viral and bacterial infection. Pneumonia is the major cause of death from influenza. In the severe pandemic of 1918, up to 20 percent of patients developed pneumonia and, of these, about half died.

Primary influenza viral pneumonia can come on suddenly, and it often progresses relentlessly with high fever, rapidly accumulating congestion in the lungs, and difficulty in breathing. Pneumonia caused by secondary bacterial infection can be caused by a large number of pathogens. In nonhospitalized patients, both children and adults, the common causes are pneumococci, streptococci, and *Haemophilus influenzae*. In older, infirm, or hospitalized patients, the common causes are pneumococci, staphylococci, and *Klebsiella pneumoniae*.

When influenza B is the pathogen, Reye's syndrome can develop, most often in children under eighteen. This disease, which causes brain and liver damage, is fatal in about 21 percent of cases.

### TREATMENT AND THERAPY

There are two main goals of therapy for the patient with influenza: treatment and preventing the spread of the disease. The first aim of therapy is to keep the patient comfortable, address the symptoms of the disease that can be treated, and deal with any complications that may arise. Bed rest is recommended, particularly during the most severe stages of the disease. Exertion is to be avoided, in order to prevent excessive weakness that could encourage further infection. Aspirin, acetaminophen, and other drugs are given for fever, and painkillers are given to relieve aches and pains. Cough suppressants and expectorants can relieve the hacking coughs that develop. Drinking large amounts of liquids is advised to replace the fluids lost as a result of high fever and sweating.

Amantadine hydrochloride is sometimes given to patients with influenza A infection. It reduces fever and relieves respiratory symptoms. An analogue of amantadine, rimantadine, works similarly. In severe cases of influenza caused by either A or B virus, an antiviral drug called ribavirin can be administered as a mist to be breathed in by the patient. Ribavirin shortens the duration of fever and may alleviate primary influenza viral pneumonia.

Primary influenza viral pneumonia is usually treated in the intensive care unit of a hospital, where the patient is given oxygen and other procedures are used to give respiratory and hemodynamic support. Secondary bacterial pneumonia must be treated with appropriate antibiotics. Identifying the precise bacterium will help the physician decide which antibiotic to prescribe. This identification is not always feasible, however, in which case broad-spectrum antibiotics will be used. They are effective against the most common bacteria that cause these secondary infections: *Streptococcus pneumoniae*, *Staphylococcus aureus*, and *Haemophilus influenzae*.

In preventing the spread of influenza, the first line of defense is to isolate the patient from susceptible persons and to initiate a program of vaccination. Because the influenza virus is constantly mutating, vaccines are regularly reformulated to confer immunity to the current pathogens. For the most part, the differences are not great between one year's virus and the one causing the next year's disease. Current vaccines may confer immunity or may require adjustment. If a major antigenic mutation has occurred, however, immunity cannot be conferred unless a new vaccine is developed against the new strain. Because it can take months to develop a new vaccine, there is the danger that the epidemic will have run its course and infected entire populations by the time that the vaccine is ready. Fortunately, major pandemics of influenza usually start slowly, so researchers have the time to identify the new strain, create a vaccine, and disseminate it.

The usual recommendation is to vaccinate people who are at highest risk of complications from the disease. These people include those over sixty-five years of age; residents of nursing homes or other patients with chronic medical conditions; adults and children with chronic pulmonary or cardiovascular diseases, including children with asthma; adults and children who have been hospitalized during the previous year for metabolic disorders, such as diabetes mellitus, or for renal diseases, blood disorders, or immunosuppression; teenagers and children who are receiving long-term aspirin therapy (who may be at risk of developing Reye's syndrome as a result of influenza infection); and pregnant women whose third trimester occurs in winter.

When a family member brings influenza into the household, other members should be vaccinated. After vaccination, it usually takes about two weeks for immunity to develop. Amantadine may protect against influenza A in the meantime; it can be discontinued after immunity has been achieved. If, for any reason, a person cannot be vaccinated, amantadine should be given throughout the entire length of the epidemic, which may last six to eight weeks.

A history of influenza vaccine development beginning with the identification of the virus in 1933 illustrates how constant vigilance is required to combat the disease. Various influenza vaccines were developed from 1935 to 1942, but they were all unsatisfactory. Building on the work that had gone before them, Thomas Francis and Jonas Salk (who later developed the first polio vaccine) produced a vaccine in 1942 that conferred immunity against the current strains of both influenza A and influenza B. Intensive animal testing and human trials showed that the vaccine was effective for about a year.

In 1947, however, many people who had been vaccinated came down with the disease: A new strain of influenza A virus had surfaced. The old vaccine had no effect on it, and a new vaccine had to be developed. This pattern has been repeated constantly: The original vaccine of 1942 was effective until a new strain appeared and a new vaccine had to be developed. That one was satisfactory until the next new strain, the Asian flu, appeared in 1957, and the process had to be repeated to find a vaccine that would protect against it. Similarly, in 1968 and in 1977, new vaccines had to be developed, and these have had to be modified to match the changes in the virus.

The World Health Organization (WHO) maintains reference laboratories around the world to keep up with the mutations of the influenza viruses. Their vigilance discovers new varieties as they appear. The new variants are studied, and vaccines are prepared to immunize against those strains that seem likely to cause extensive epidemics. This activity blunts the force of new pandemics and saves millions of lives.

## PERSPECTIVE AND PROSPECTS

Researchers are constantly working to prevent the recurrent epidemics and pandemics of influenza, or at least to make them less severe. The fact that vaccines have to be modified periodically, and new ones developed from time to time, will probably not change.

It is theoretically possible for a pandemic of the severity of 1918 to occur. If a new subtype of the influenza virus were to arise and its initial spread were rapid, it could rage around the globe before an effective vaccine could be developed and made available. Mass devastation and death could result.

Another major concern is the enormous number of influenza virus strains that are living in animals. Hundreds of different types of influenza virus have been isolated from birds alone. These strains have the potential of causing mutations in the human influenza virus, as the Chinese ducks did in causing the Asian flu, the Hong Kong flu viruses, and the virus that caused the pandemic of 1977.

So far, medical science has been able to produce vaccines capable of protecting against the new mutant viruses as they arise. Even when a significant portion of any society is vaccinated, however, some people still become infected and there are no agents available that can kill the influenza virus. Furthermore, there are few therapeutic measures that can do any more than alleviate individual symptoms. Basically, the body's own immune system is the best therapy currently available.

Chemoprophylaxis (prevention of a disease by the use of a drug) with amantadine is effective in limiting the spread of disease caused by influenza A, but amantadine has some undesirable side effects, and the drug seems to have no effect on the virus itself. Rimantadine, a closely related compound, is equally effective as a chemoprophylactic agent and seems to be better tolerated. It is still considered an experimental drug, however, and it has not been licensed.

No chemotherapeutic agent (a drug capable of curing a disease) has yet been developed that will kill an influenza virus in the same way that an antibiotic destroys bacteria and other microorganisms. The search for antiviral agents is among the most urgent activities in medical science, and the problems are enormous. Yet the science is young. As researchers learn more about the structure, physiology, and activities of viruses, they will also develop means of controlling them.

When an agent is discovered that is safe and effective against influenza virus, it could be subject to the same limitations as the vaccines; that is, it may have to be modified periodically to remain effective against the new strains of influenza virus that are continually developing, and it may be necessary to develop new agents to deal with radically new mutants. —C. Richard Falcon

**See also** Fever; Nausea and vomiting; Pneumonia; Pulmonary diseases; Reye's syndrome; Viral infections.

## FOR FURTHER INFORMATION:

Beveridge, W. I. B. *Influenza: The Last Great Plague.* New York: PRODIST Division of Neale Watson Academic Publications, 1977. This text describes the history of influenza epidemics and pandemics. It also covers the causes of the disease and the relationship of human influenza virus to animal viruses.

Imperato, Pascal James. *What to Do About the Flu.* New York: E. P. Dutton, 1976. Imperato gives a history of influenza and relates it to the individual patient's own experiences and needs. This book contains case histories and sensible advice on how the patient should deal with a flu infection.

Kiple, Kenneth F., et al., eds. *The Cambridge World History of Human Disease.* Cambridge, England: Cambridge University Press, 1993. The section on influenza gives a useful account of the epidemics and pandemics of influenza throughout the years.

Larson, David E., ed. *Mayo Clinic Family Health Book.* New York: William Morrow, 1990. A good general medical text for the lay reader. The section on influenza is short but thorough.

Scott, Andrew. *Pirates of the Cell.* Oxford, England: Basil Blackwell, 1985. This book is admirably concise and clear in its descriptions of the influenza viruses, their physiology, structure, and activities. It is particularly useful in describing the avenues that are being explored to find effective antiviral agents against influenza and other viral diseases.

## INSECT BITES. *See* BITES AND STINGS.

## INSOMNIA AND SLEEP DISORDERS. *See* SLEEP DISORDERS.

## INTERSTITIAL PULMONARY FIBROSIS (IPF)

**SYSTEM AFFECTED:** Respiratory

**SPECIALISTS:** Occupational medicine physicians, pulmonologists

**DEFINITION:** In IPF, scarring and thickening (fibrosis) of the lung tissue occurs, causing difficulties in breathing. Its symptoms include chest pain, coughing, and shortness of breath (dyspnea). The disease is sometimes termed idiopathic or diffuse, which indicates that the cause is not known. The disease may be an autoimmune disorder, and it may be attributable to radiation therapy, lung cancer, and drug reactions. IPF has also been linked to occupational hazards, such as the repeated inhalation of organic dust (as from minerals) and chemical fumes. Such exposure may result in extrinsic allergic alveolitis (or hypersensitivy pneumonitis), which may in turn develop into IPF after several years. In IPF, the lungs may become increasingly stiff until heart failure or bronchopneumonia develops.

**See also** Pneumonia; Pulmonary diseases.

## INTESTINAL CANCER. *See* STOMACH, INTESTINAL, AND PANCREATIC CANCERS.

## INTESTINAL DISORDERS

**SYSTEM AFFECTED:** Gastrointestinal

**SPECIALISTS:** Colorectal surgeons, family physicians, gastroenterologists, general surgeons, internists

**DEFINITION:** Diseases or disorders of the small intestine, large intestine (or colon), liver, pancreas, and gallbladder.

**KEY TERMS:**

*acute:* the stage of a disease or presence of a symptom that begins abruptly, with marked intensity, and subsides after a short time *chronic:* the stage of a disease or presence of a symptom that develops slowly and usually lasts for the lifetime of the individual

*diarrhea:* the passage of approximately six loose stools within a twenty-four-hour period caused by a variety of circumstances, such as infection, malabsorption, or irritable bowel

*diverticulitis:* inflammation or swelling of one or more diverticula, caused by the penetration of fecal material through thin-walled diverticula and the collection of bacteria or other irritating agents there

*diverticulosis:* the presence of diverticula in the colon, which may lead to diverticulitis

*diverticulum:* an outpouching through the muscular wall of a tubular organ, such as the stomach, small intestine, or colon

*electrolytes:* elements or compounds found in blood, interstitial fluid, and cell fluid that are critical for normal metabolism and function

*peristalsis:* the involuntary, coordinated, rhythmic contraction of the muscles of the gastrointestinal tract that forces partially digested food along its length

*stricture:* an abnormal narrowing of an organ because of pressure or inflammation

*villi:* folds within the small intestine that are important for the absorption of nutrients into the blood

### PROCESS AND EFFECTS

Intestinal diseases and disorders are sometimes included with those of the digestive system. For the sake of clarity, this article makes the distinction between the structures of the digestive and intestinal tracts. The entire digestive tract, which includes the intestinal tract and is approximately 7.6 to 9.1 meters in length in adults, begins in the mouth and ends with the anus. It includes organs specific to digestion, such as the esophagus and stomach and their substructures. The intestinal tract, which constitutes the major part of the digestive tract, includes the small intestine, the large intestine (also known as the colon), and the organs that branch off these structures (the liver, pancreas, and gallbladder). The function of the small and large intestines is to break down food, absorb its nutrients into the bloodstream, and carry off waste products of digestion as feces.

The small intestine is approximately 6.1 meters long and 3.8 centimeters in diameter and is made up of the duodenum, the jejunum, and the ileum. It is where the process of digestion begins in full. The smaller products broken down by the stomach are received by the small intestine, where they are absorbed into the bloodstream through its lining by villi combined with bile (from the liver) and pancreatic juices.

Almost all food nutrients are absorbed in the small intestine. What passes into the large intestine is a mix of unabsorbed nutrients, water, fiber, and electrolytes. Most of the moisture from this process is removed as the mix passes

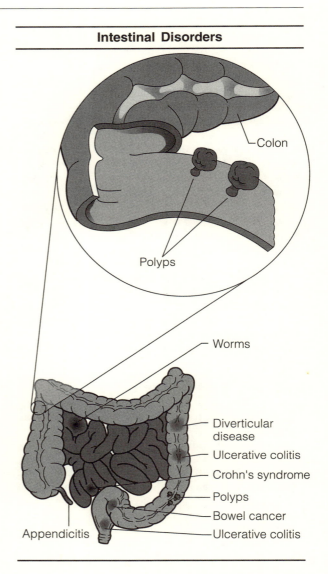

**Intestinal Disorders**

Colon

Polyps

Worms

Diverticular disease

Ulcerative colitis

Crohn's syndrome

Polyps

Bowel cancer

Ulcerative colitis

Appendicitis

through the large intestine, leaving solid waste products. Before excretion as feces, approximately 90 percent of the liquid that entered the large intestine has been reabsorbed. This reabsorption is necessary for health because it contains sodium and water.

The large intestine is approximately 1.5 meters long and connected to the small intestine at the ileocecal valve. Waste products from the digestive process pass through this valve into a large holding area of the large intestine called the cecum. The appendix is attached to this structure. The large intestine consists of the ascending colon (which begins on the right side of the abdomen and moves up toward the liver), the transverse colon (which crosses the abdomen), and the descending colon (which moves down the left side of the abdomen). The sigmoid colon is an S-shaped structure which connects to the descending colon and joins the rectum, a tube 12 to 20 centimeters long that leads to the anus. Small microorganisms in the large intestine break down waste products not broken down by the stomach and small intestines, resulting in gas (also known as flatus).

## COMPLICATIONS AND DISORDERS

Diseases and disorders of the intestinal tract constitute a major health problem affecting many individuals at one point or another in their lives. The common diseases and disorders that affect the intestinal tract are those of acute inflammatory disorders (appendicitis), diverticular disorders (diverticulosis and diverticulitis), chronic inflammatory bowel disease (Crohn's disease and ulcerative colitis), intestinal infections (intestinal parasites and bacterial infections with *Salmonella*, *Shigella dysenteriae*, and *Escherichia coli*), intestinal obstructions, cancers or tumors of the rectum and colon, and polyps.

The most common acute inflammatory disorder is appendicitis. Its symptoms usually affect individuals between the ages of ten and thirty and include abdominal pain and tenderness, nausea and vomiting, loss of appetite, rapid heart rate, fever, and an elevated white blood cell count. Normally, the appendix, whose function is not clearly understood, fills and empties with food as regularly as does the cecum, of which it is a part. It sometimes becomes inflamed because of either kinking or obstruction, producing pressure and initiating symptoms. The most common major complication associated with appendicitis is perforation, which causes severe pain and an elevation of temperature. In these cases, a physician must be notified immediately. Treatment consists of surgical removal of the appendix.

Diverticular disorders include diverticulosis and diverticulitis. Diverticulosis is the presence of diverticula without any inflammation or symptoms. Diverticulitis is the result of an inflammation or infection of the intestine produced when food or bacteria are retained in a diverticulum. Some signs of diverticulosis include cramplike pain in the left lower part of the abdomen, bowel irregularity, diarrhea, constipation, or thin stools. There may be some intermittent rectal bleeding with diverticulitis.

Inflammatory bowel disease (IBD) of unknown cause is most common in whites (usually female) between the ages of fifteen and thirty-five, occurring most frequently in the American Jewish population. The two types of IBD are Crohn's disease, which is also known as regional enteritis, and ulcerative colitis. Both disorders are considered to be separate diseases with similar characteristics.

Crohn's disease may affect any part of the intestinal tract but often affects the small intestine. The inflammation usually involves the entire thickness of the intestinal wall. Treatment for Crohn's disease depends on the presence or absence of symptoms. If there are no symptoms, treatment is not necessary. If there is evidence of inflammation, however, anti-inflammatory medication may be prescribed. Vitamin

and mineral replacement may be given because of the problems of absorption associated with this disease. Surgery may be required at some point in the disease process because of its associated complications, such as obstruction.

Ulcerative colitis is characterized by tiny ulcers and abscesses in the inner lining of the colon, where it is usually confined. There is a tendency for these ulcerations to bleed, causing bloody diarrhea. The chronic nature of inflammatory bowel disease may cause a stricture, which can result in an obstruction requiring surgical intervention. As with Crohn's disease, the treatment for ulcerative colitis depends on the type of symptoms and may consist of medication, nutrition, or surgery. Anti-inflammatory drugs are used for flare-ups of the disease. Liquid food supplements may be given to compensate for nutrients lost in diarrhea. Intravenous therapy may be prescribed if the colon is considered too diseased to tolerate food.

There are many types of infections that affect the intestinal tract. The most common bacterial infections are caused by microorganisms such as *Salmonella* and *Shigella*. *Salmonella* bacteria are commonly found in meats, fruits (through contaminated fertilizer), poultry, eggs, dairy products, and contaminated marijuana. Pet turtles are also a source of this bacteria. The source of infections for *Shigella* bacteria is feces from an infected person, with the route of transmission being oral-fecal—for example, changing the soiled diaper of an infant, or having a bowel movement, and then eating or preparing food without properly washing the hands.

Intestinal parasites may also cause infection. The most common of these parasites, *Giardia lamblia*, is present where water supplies are contaminated by raw sewage. The primary treatment for these conditions consists of replacement of lost fluids and essential electrolytes. Although not normally used because they may interfere with the elimination of the causative agent, antidiarrheal medications may be prescribed.

Intestinal obstruction occurs when the normal flow of the intestine is partially or totally impeded because of an accumulation of contents, gas, or fluid. It may also be caused by the intestine's inability to propel contents along the intestinal tract in the process called peristalsis. Peristalsis may be obstructed by scars that bind together two normally separate anatomic surfaces (adhesions), hernias, or tumors. Another cause may be a paralytic ileus, a paralysis of the peristaltic movement of the intestinal tract caused by the effect of trauma or toxins on the nerve endings that regulate intestinal movement. Conservative treatment consists of decompression of the bowel using a nasogastric tube. Surgical treatment may be indicated if the bowel is completely obstructed.

While tumors of the small intestine are rare, tumors of the colon are common. Cancer of the colon and rectum is the second most common type of cancer in the United States (with lung cancer being the most common). The majority of intestinal tumors are benign (noncancerous) and discovered between the ages of forty and sixty. There are several types of benign tumors, which do not spread. They include lipomas, leiomyomas, angiomas, and adenomas. A small percentage of tumors of the small intestine is malignant (cancerous). The most common are adenocarcinomas, leiomyosarcomas, carcinoid tumors, and lymphomas. The symptoms of these tumors include weight loss, abdominal pain, nausea and vomiting, and bleeding. Treatment is dependent upon the stage and location of the tumor. Surgical removal of the tumor may be coupled with chemotherapy and/or radiation therapy.

Polyps are benign tumors of the large intestine and are common to individuals over the age of sixty. They arise from the lining of the colon and are usually found during tests to diagnose other conditions. Polyps include several different varieties, the most common of which is a hyperplastic polyp. Hyperplastic polyps are less than one-half of a centimeter in diameter and do not pose a health risk. Juvenile polyps can occur in childhood, and inflammatory polyps are believed to result from injury or inflammation, such as after an episode of ulcerative colitis. Neither of these conditions poses a health risk. There is a major category of polyps known as adenomas, however, which have the potential for malignancy. These types of polyps are generally removed to prevent the development of cancer.

Rectal cancer and colon cancer are two types of cancer common among both men and women. Factors that predispose an individual to these types of cancer include family history or a prior history of adenomatous colon polyps, colon cancer, or ulcerative colitis. The precise cause of these cancers is unknown, but diet is believed to play a significant role, specifically low-fiber, high-animal-fat diets. One of the key symptoms of these conditions requiring immediate attention (especially for individuals over the age of forty) is rectal bleeding. Treatment consists of surgery to remove the affected part of the colon. The physician may prescribe additional treatment in the form of chemotherapy and/or radiation therapy.

## PERSPECTIVE AND PROSPECTS

Problems associated with the intestinal tract are characterized by a variety of symptoms and treatments. These problems may be temporary in nature or may be manifestations of more serious underlying conditions interfering with the normal functions of absorption, fluid and electrolyte balance, and elimination. Symptoms are signs of malfunction and should not be ignored or go untreated.

Preventing problems associated with the intestinal tract may not always be possible because the causes of some intestinal diseases and disorders are unknown. Nevertheless, there has been substantial research related to intestinal diseases and disorders to support a strong correlation between nutrition and intestinal tract health. For example, there is evidence to support the relationship between the

consumption of sugars, high amounts of animal protein and fat, and cholesterol and cancer-causing agents in the intestinal tract. Stress and its resulting influence on stomach acidity also contribute to intestinal ill health. Smoking and lack of regular exercise may also negatively influence normal peristalsis.

The prevention of these and other problems related to intestinal health are important not only to general health but also to work productivity. In the United States, for example, intestinal problems account for a large percentage of lost work time. Education about intestinal health and health issues beginning early in one's life will lower the incidence of some of the more common intestinal diseases and disorders. —*John A. Bavaro*

*See also* Abdominal disorders; Appendicitis; Arthropod-borne diseases; Cholecystitis; Cirrhosis; Colitis; Colon cancer; Constipation; Crohn's disease; Diarrhea and dysentery; Diverticulitis and diverticulosis; Gallbladder diseases; Gastrointestinal disorders; Hemorrhoids; Hernia; Jaundice; Liver cancer; Liver disorders; Obstruction; Pancreatitis; Parasitic diseases; Renal failure; Stomach, intestinal, and pancreatic cancers; Worms.

## FOR FURTHER INFORMATION:

Clayman, Charles B., ed. *The American Medical Association Encyclopedia of Medicine*. New York: Random House, 1989. Written in an encyclopedic format, this book is an authoritative guide to all aspects of medical and health topics. Contains many illustrations of various body systems and organs that are clearly presented and simple to understand. Provides useful information on staying healthy as well as contemporary medical advances in the diagnosis and treatment of various conditions.

Larson, David E., ed. *Mayo Clinic Family Health Book*. New York: William Morrow, 1990. This comprehensive medical guide was written for the general public by experts in the field of medicine. It can be used as an excellent basic source of authoritative health and medical information.

Mullen, Kathleen D., et al. *Connections for Health*. 3d ed. Madison, Wis.: Wm. C. Brown/Benchmark, 1993. A basic personal health textbook used in introductory college-level health courses. It is easily read and incorporates the concepts of wellness and disease prevention. Excellent references and recommended readings can be found at the end of each chapter.

*The New Good Housekeeping Family Health and Medical Guide*. New York: Hearst Books, 1989. A popular and useful health care reference book emphasizing the prevention of illness. Includes a color atlas of the body and an encyclopedia of medicine. The encyclopedia section of the book provides a good source for understanding basic health and medical terms.

Payne, Wayne A., and Dale B. Hahn. *Understanding Your Health*. 3d ed. St. Louis: Mosby Year Book, 1992. An introductory textbook that is easy to read. Focuses on overall health and disease prevention. Each chapter offers a list of references and recommended readings related specifically to its content.

Tapley, Donald F., et al., eds. *The Columbia University College of Physicians and Surgeons Complete Home Medical Guide.* Rev. ed. New York: Crown, 1989. An outstanding reference guide organized by each organ system and its function. Written in easily understandable terms and avoids the use of medical jargon. Includes a section containing a dictionary of medical terms and a listing of prefixes, suffixes, and roots. Part 3 of the book provides in-depth information on how the body works and includes a full-color atlas showing major organ systems.

## INTOXICATION

**SYSTEMS AFFECTED:** All

**SPECIALISTS:** Emergency physicians, psychiatrists, toxicologists

**DEFINITION:** Intoxication is the general term for poisoning of the body by toxins, such as drugs, including alcohol. It commonly refers to alcohol intoxication, or drunkenness. Of the amount of alcohol ingested, 95 percent will be absorbed directly into the wall of the stomach or small intestine and pass quickly into the bloodstream. If too much alcohol is consumed in a short period of time, the extreme slowdown of breathing and circulation can cause death; however, vomiting or coma generally precedes such an event. Intoxication decreases motor ability, reaction time, depth perception, and night vision; causes poor judgment; impairs sexual function; and may result in mood swings. If a comatose state is not reached, the intoxication will eventually resolve itself; no other method, such as coffee or cold showers, can counteract the effects of alcohol.

*See also* Alcoholism; Poisoning.

## IPF. *See* INTERSTITIAL PULMONARY FIBROSIS (IPF).

## ISCHEMIA

**SYSTEMS AFFECTED:** Blood, circulatory, all other systems

**SPECIALISTS:** Cardiologists, internists, neurologists, vascular surgeons

**DEFINITION:** Ischemia occurs when the blood supply to an organ or tissue is interrupted, usually by a narrowing of the arteries from deposits of plaque. Other causes may include blood vessel injury, an inefficient heartbeat, and spasms in the vessel wall that result in constriction. The major sites of ischemia are the eyes, kidneys, heart, brain, and legs. Insufficient blood supply to the legs or heart causes pain; ischemia in the kidneys, eyes, and brain can result in renal failure, blindness, and stroke, respectively. The circulation can be restored with vasodilator drugs or surgery, such as angioplasty or a bypass. The temporary induction of ischemia in the legs can be used to reduce bleeding in operations on the extremities.

*See also* Atherosclerotic disease; Claudication; Heart disease; Hyperlipidemia; Hypertension; Thrombosis and thrombus.

## ITCHING

**SYSTEM AFFECTED:** Skin

**SPECIALISTS:** Allergists, dermatologists, internists, toxicologists, tropical medicine physicians

**DEFINITION:** Pruritis, commonly known as itching, is an irritating skin sensation that provokes a desire to scratch the affected area. This sensation can be attributable to a wide range of environmental conditions, skin disorders, diseases, and infections; there may also be a psychological factor. Persistent and intense itching, often accompanied by a rash, is characteristic of several skin disorders, such as dermatitis, eczema, hives, chickenpox, and psoriasis. Generalized itching may also be associated with diabetes mellitus, internal cancer, jaundice, renal failure, and liver or thyroid disease. Pruritis is also common around the anal and genital area, perhaps as a result of candidiasis, worms, hemorrhoids, or chronic diarrhea. Itching can be treated with lotions, and any underlying condition must be addressed.

*See also* Chickenpox; Diabetes mellitus; Eczema; Hemorrhoids; Jaundice; Lice, mites, and ticks; Liver disorders; Psoriasis; Rashes; Renal failure; Scabies; Thyroid disorders; Worms.

## JAUNDICE

**SYSTEMS AFFECTED:** Blood, eyes, liver, skin

**SPECIALISTS:** Hematologists, internists, neonatologists

**DEFINITION:** Jaundice is a liver disorder characterized by a yellowish discoloration of the skin, the whites of the eyes, and other tissues; the urine may also darken in hue. The condition is caused by excessive amounts of bile pigments, called bilirubin, in the bloodstream. The liver excretes bilirubin in the process of breaking down red blood cells. Excess bile pigments are produced if too many red blood cells are destroyed (hemolytic jaundice), the bile ducts are blocked by a tumor or gallstones (obstructive jaundice), or the liver becomes inflamed in the condition known as hepatitis (hepatocellular jaundice). Treatment is for the underlying cause.

**See also** Cirrhosis; Hepatitis; Kwashiorkor; Liver disorders.

## JOINT DISEASES. *See* ARTHRITIS.

# KERATOSES

**SYSTEM AFFECTED:** Skin

**SPECIALISTS:** Dermatologists

**DEFINITION:** Keratoses, wartlike growths, are caused by the excessive production of the skin protein keratin; they usually occur in elderly people. Solar keratoses result from repeated exposure to the sunlight and thus appear on the face, arms, and hands. They are small and may be red or uncolored. Seborrheic keratoses, which are of unknown origin, may be small, dark brown, flat, or rough; they are generally greasy and crusted over. Seborrheic keratoses are benign, but solar keratoses may, on rare occasions, develop into a squamous cell carcinoma or other skin cancer. Both types can be removed if the patient desires, usually with cryosurgery.

*See also* Skin cancer; Warts.

# KIDNEY DISORDERS

**SYSTEM AFFECTED:** Kidneys

**SPECIALISTS:** Internists, nephrologists

**DEFINITION:** Disorders, from structural abnormalities to bacterial infections, that can affect the kidneys and may lead to renal failure.

**KEY TERMS:**

*creatinine:* the breakdown product of creatine, a nitrogenous compound found in muscle, blood, and urine

*cystinosis:* a congenital disease characterized by glucose and protein in the urine, as well as by cystine deposits in the liver and other organs, rickets, and growth retardation

*hematuria:* the abnormal presence of blood in the urine

*hydronephrosis:* the cessation of urine flow because of an obstruction of a ureter, allowing urine to build up in the pelvis of the kidney; can cause renal failure

*oliguria:* the diminished capacity to form and pass urine, so that metabolic products cannot be excreted efficiently

*reflux:* the abnormal backward flow of urine

*toxemia:* blood poisoning

*uremia:* the presence of excessive amounts of urea and other nitrogenous waste products in the blood

### CAUSES AND SYMPTOMS

Disorders of the kidney can occur for a variety of reasons. The cause may be congenital (present from birth) or may develop very quickly and at any age. Many of these problems and disorders can be easily treated. The main areas of kidney disorders are classified as malformations in development of the kidney, part of the kidney, or the ureter; glomerular disease; tubular and interstitial disease or disruption; vascular (other than glomerular) disease; and kidney dysfunction that occurs secondary to another disease.

The kidney frequently exhibits congenital anomalies, some of which occur during specific developmental stages. Agenesis occurs when the ureteric bud fails to develop normally. When the tissue does not develop, the ureter itself

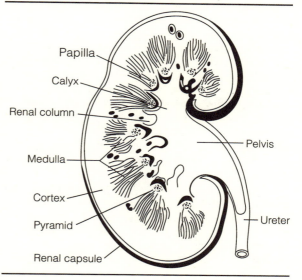

**Anatomy of the Kidney**

Papilla
Calyx
Renal column
Medulla
Cortex
Pyramid
Renal capsule
Pelvis
Ureter

fails to form. If there is an obstruction where the ureter joins the pelvis of the kidney, there may be massive hydronephrosis (dilation). One or both kidneys may be unusually small, containing too few tubules. The kidneys may be displaced, too high or offset to one side or the other. They may even be fused. All these conditions could seriously affect the manufacture of urine, its excretion, or both.

Glomerulonephritis refers to a diverse group of conditions that share a common feature—primary involvement of the glomerulus. The significance of glomerulonephritis is that it is the most common cause of end-stage renal failure. Its features include urinary casts, high protein levels (proteinuria), hematuria, hypertension, edema (swelling), and uremia. The two forms of glomerulonephritis are primary and secondary. In the primary form, only the kidneys are affected, but in the secondary form, the lesion (affected area) is only one of a series of problems.

Nephrotic syndrome is usually defined as an abnormal condition of the kidney characterized by the presence of proteinuria together with edema and high fat and cholesterol levels. It occurs in glomerular disease, in thrombosis of a renal vein, and as a complication of many systemic diseases. Nephrotic syndrome occurs in a severe, primary form characterized by anorexia, weakness, proteinuria, and edema.

Interstitial nephritis is inflammation of the interstitial tissue of the kidney, including the kidneys. Acute interstitial nephritis is an immunologic, adverse reaction to certain drugs; drugs especially associated with it are nonsteroidal anti-inflammatory drugs (NSAIDs) and some antibiotics. Acute renal failure, fever, rash, and proteinuria are indicative signs of this condition. If the medication is stopped, normal kidney function returns. Chronic interstitial nephritis is defined as inflammation and structural changes associated with such conditions as ureteral obstruction, pyelonephritis, exposure of the kidney to a toxin, transplant rejection, or certain systemic diseases.

Kidney stones (calculi) are commonly manufactured from calcium oxalate and/or phosphate, triple phosphate, uric acid (urate), or a mixture of these. Calcium stones are not necessarily the result of high serum calcium, although they can be. Struvite calculi of magnesium ammonium (triple) phosphate mixed with calcium are bigger but softer than other types; they grow irregularly, filling much of the kidney pelvis. They arise from infection with urea-splitting organisms that cause alkaline urine. Urate stones are a complication of gout.

Those who have a tendency to develop stones may experience concomitant infection known as pyonephrosis. Pyonephrosis is a result of not only blockage at the junction of the ureter and kidney pelvis but also any constricture at this location. Bacteria from the bloodstream collect and cause an abscess to form. If the tube is completely blocked, the inflammation produces enough pus to rupture a portion of the kidney, and more of the abdominal cavity becomes involved.

Pyelonephritis is inflammation of the upper urinary tract. Acute pyelonephritis may be preceded by lower tract infection. The patient complains of lethargy, fever, and back pain. The major symptoms are fever, renal pain, and body aches accompanied by nausea and toxemia. Chronic pyelonephritis often affects the renal tubules and the small spaces within the kidney. Fibrous tissue may take over these areas and cause gradual shrinking of the functional kidney. The chronic form may also result from previous bacterial infection, reflux, obstruction, overuse of analgesics, X rays, and lead poisoning.

Obstruction may be caused by inadequate development of the renal tissue itself, closing off one or both ureters. Other malformations and certain calculi can also obstruct urine flow. Reflux may occur when the contraction of the bladder forces urine backward, up toward and into the kidney. Lesser degrees of reflux do not damage the kidney, but the greater the reflux, the more likely damage will occur. Bacterial infection is often attributable to *Escherichia coli*, but other bowel bacteria may also infect the area. They generally move upward from outside the body through the urinary organs, but they may move inward from the bloodstream.

Acute renal failure is defined as a sudden decline in normal renal function that leads to an increase in blood urea and creatinine. The onset may be fast (over days) or slow (over weeks) and is often reversible. It is characterized by oliguria and rapid accumulation of nitrogenous wastes in the blood, resulting in acidosis. Acute renal failure is caused by hemorrhage, trauma, burns, toxic injury to the kidney, acute pyelonephritis or glomerulonephritis, or lower urinary tract obstruction. Occasionally, it will progress into chronic renal failure.

Chronic renal failure may result from many other diseases. Its signs are sluggishness, fatigue, and mental dullness. Patients also display other systemic problems as a result of chronic renal failure. Almost all such patients are anemic; three-fourths of them develop hypertension. The skin becomes discolored, the muddy coloration is caused by anemia and the presence of excess melanin.

Renal symptoms suggestive of renal dysfunction include increases in frequency of urination, color changes in urine, areas of edema, and hypertension. The patient may experience only one symptom but is more likely to have a series of complaints. To determine the cause of renal disease, several diagnostic tools can be used to distinguish the type of pathogenic process affecting the kidney. The degree to which other body systems are involved determines whether the disease process is systemic or confined to the kidneys. Other valuable clues may be gathered from medical history, family history, and physical examination. The key factors, however, are renal size and renal histopathology.

Examination of the urine can reveal important data relative to renal health. Stick tests may show the abnormal presence of blood, glucose, and/or protein. Assaying the kind and amount of protein may pinpoint the cause of the disease. Urine contaminated with bacteria has always been used as an indication of some form of urinary tract infection. Microscopic examination of urine sediment may help diagnose acute renal failure. Blood tests may also indicate the source of a renal disorder. A series of blood tests might reveal rising urea and creatinine levels. The urea-to-creatinine ratio may aid in determining if and which type of acute renal failure may be present. A high red cell count might suggest kidney stones, a tumor, or glomerular disease; a high white cell count would hint at inflammation and/or infection. Cells cast from the kidney tubules may indicate acute interstitial nephritis, while red cell breakdown products may mean glomerulonephritis. The diagnostician should also be diligent in tracking down possible septic causes. Repeated cultures of blood and urine should help ascertain if there is an abscess anywhere near the kidney.

X rays can provide useful information. An abdominal X ray may show urinary stones and abnormalities in the renal outline. Ultrasound will measure renal size, show scarring, and reveal dilation of the tract, perhaps as a result of an obstructive lesion. Abdominal ultrasound has become the investigation of choice because it can be performed at the patient's bedside.

Renal biopsy can give an accurate diagnosis of acute renal failure but may be more dangerous to the patient than the condition itself. The main indications for biopsy would be suspected acute glomerulonephritis and renal failure that has lasted six weeks.

### Treatment and Therapy

If glomerulonephritis is suspected or diagnosed, its treatment seeks to avoid complications of the illness. The patient is monitored daily for fluid overload; as long as the patient is retaining fluid, blood tests that measure urea, creatinine, and salt balance are also run daily. The patient should stay in bed and restrict fluid as well as potassium intake. Medications may be prescribed: diuretics, vasodilators for hypertension, and calcium antagonists. If the cause is bacterial, a course of oral antibiotics may be given. If these measures are unsuccessful, short-term dialysis may be needed. Some urinary abnormalities may last for as long as a year.

The first measure undertaken to treat acute renal failure is to rebuild depressed fluid volumes: blood if the patient has hemorrhaged, plasma for burn patients, and electrolytes for a patient who is vomiting and has diarrhea. If infection is suspected as the underlying cause, an appropriate antibiotic should be administered when blood cultures confirm the presence of bacteria. After fluid volumes have been replenished, a diuretic may be necessary to reduce swelling of tissues within the kidney.

In chronic renal failure, the major undertaking is to relieve the obstruction of the urinary tract. If the blockage is within the bladder, simple catheterization may relieve it. If a stone or some similar obstacle is blocking a ureter, however, surgery to remove it may be necessary. A tube may be inserted to allow urine drainage, and the stone will pass or be removed.

In sufferers of recurrent stones, maintaining a high urine output is important, which requires the patient to drink fluids throughout the day and even at bedtime. Those enduring intense pain may need to be hospitalized. Analgesics for pain are administered, as well as forced fluid intake to increase urine output so that the stone might be passed. If these measures do not work, surgical intervention may be necessary.

Patients suffering from progressive, incurable renal failure need medical aid managing conservation of, substitution for, and eventual replacement of nephron function. Conservation attempts to prolong kidney function for as long as possible; renal function is aided by drug treatment. Substitution means the maintenance of kidney function by dialysis, especially hemodialysis. Replacement is the restoration of renal function by a kidney transplant. By this third stage of treatment, urine formation is independent of further drug treatment, and kidney function must be achieved by other means. Patients suffering from end-stage renal failure have two options: dialysis and transplantation. A patient may go from dialysis to transplantation. In fact, if a compatible donor (preferably a sibling) is available, a transplant is advisable. For those without a suitable donor, long-term hemodialysis is the first option.

Dialysis is defined as the diffusion of dissolved molecules through a semipermeable membrane. Several types of dialysis are available. Hemodialysis filters and cleans the blood as it passes through the semipermeable membranous tube in contact with a balanced salt solution (dialysate).

Hemodialysis can be performed in a dialysis unit of a hospital or at home. It must usually be done two or three times a week, with each session lasting from three to six hours, depending on the type of membranes used and the size of the patient. Hemodialysis can lead to acute neurological changes. Lethargy, irritability, restlessness, headache, nausea, vomiting, and twitching may all occur. In some patients, neurological complications occur after dialysis is terminated. Convulsions are the most common of these consequences. In continuous abdominal peritoneal dialysis, a fresh amount of dialysate is introduced from a bag attached to a permanently implanted plastic tube. Wastes and water pass into the dialysate from the surrounding organs; then the fluid is collected four to eight hours later. Peritoneal dialysis is performed by the patient. It is continuous, so the clearance rate of wastes is higher. The most important neurological complications of peritoneal dialysis are worsening of urea-induced brain abnormalities accompanied by twitching and, rarely, psychosis and convulsions.

Transplantation of a kidney is considered for patients with primary renal diseases as well as end-stage renal failure resulting from any number of systemic and metabolic diseases. Success rates are highest for those suffering from lupus nephritis, gout, and cystinosis. If a kidney is received from a close relative, there is a 97 percent one-year survival rate. Even if the organ transplant comes from a nonrelative, the survival rate is still 90 percent.  —*Iona C. Baldridge*

***See also*** Cystitis; Edema; Glomerulonephritis; Incontinence; Male genital disorders; Nephritis; Renal failure; Stones; Urethritis; Urinary disorders.

**FOR FURTHER INFORMATION:**

Catto, Graeme R. D., and David A. Power. *Nephrology in Clinical Practice*. London: Edward Arnold, 1988. This book addresses health care professionals in particular. Its goal is to educate practitioners in methods of recognition and diagnosis and of treatment. Technically written, so some knowledge of the subject is helpful.

Dalton, John R., and Erick J. Bergquist. *Urinary Tract Infections*. London: Croom Helm, 1987. One of a series written to update clinicians' and health care workers' knowledge of urinary dysfunction. That infection anywhere in the tract can ultimately affect renal health is noted, but most attention is paid to lower tract infection.

Dische, Frederick E. *Concise Renal Pathology (Excluding Neoplasm)*. Tunbridge Wells, Kent, England: Castle House, 1987. For those in training for medical fields, this book describes renal anatomy and pathology. The terminology is somewhat simplified so that the descriptions are more understandable. A good introduction to renal pathology.

Dossetor, John B., and M. Henry Gault. *Nephron Failure*. Springfield, Mass.: Charles C Thomas, 1971. With renal disease as a premise, this book views the consequences of renal disease. Offers perspective to the three phases of treatment: conservation, substitution, and replacement. This college-level text requires some knowledge of renal morphology.

Schroeder, Steven A., Lawrence M. Tierney, Jr., Stephen J. McPhee, Maxine A. Papadakis, and Marcus A. Krupp, eds. *Current Medical Diagnosis and Treatment*. 31st ed. Norwalk, Conn.: Appleton and Lange, 1992. This reference volume covers all aspects of internal medicine. It is readable and concisely describes more than one thousand diseases and disorders, as well as their medical management.

## KWASHIORKOR

**SYSTEM AFFECTED:** Gastrointestinal
**SPECIALISTS:** Pediatricians, public health specialists

**DEFINITION:** Its name derived from a Ghanaian word, kwashiorkor is a protein-deficiency disease that usually affects young children in developing countries. When children in these countries are weaned, they may suddenly be placed on protein-poor diets that cannot provide adequate nutrients. The results of this severe malnutrition are stunted growth, weakness, and apathy. With kwashiorkor, the child suffers from edema, a swelling of the tissues, even though dehydration may be present. Serious complications of this disease include an enlarged liver, jaundice, and an ineffective immune system; a severe infection may prove fatal. Kwashiorkor can be treated with supplements to control the edema, followed by a high-protein diet; most children recover.

*See also* Bleeding; Edema; Jaundice; Malnutrition.

# LARYNGITIS

**SYSTEM AFFECTED:** Respiratory

**SPECIALISTS:** Family physicians, otolaryngologists

**DEFINITION:** An inflammation of the larynx, or voice box, laryngitis may be chronic or acute. Its most distinguishing characteristic is a hoarseness in the voice; eventually, the ability to speak may be lost. Coughing, pain, and discomfort on swallowing may also occur. Acute laryngitis is caused by an infection, either viral or bacterial. Resting the voice, drinking warm liquids, and taking antibiotics if bacteria are to blame should restore the voice. Chronic laryngitis is caused by irritation, such as that produced by alcohol, tobacco, and chemical fumes; by overuse of the voice, as sometimes found with singers; by chronic coughing; or (rarely) by a malignant tumor.

*See also* Nasopharyngeal disorders; Voice and vocal cord disorders.

# LEAD POISONING

**SYSTEMS AFFECTED:** Brain, kidneys, nervous

**SPECIALISTS:** Neurologists, occupational medicine physicians, public health specialists, toxicologists

**DEFINITION:** Poisoning as a result of an abnormally high intake of lead via the gastrointestinal tract or inhalation. Lead is the most abundant heavy metal and one of the earliest to be refined. It has been used in paint pigments and plumbing solder, providing ample opportunities for significant human exposure. Normal daily lead intake essentially passes through the body without being absorbed. An abnormally high amount of lead in the diet, however, causes an increase in body concentrations and thus lead poisoning, or plumbism. Children are more likely than adults to ingest foreign materials containing lead, a problem compounded by the fact that the effects noted in children are much greater than in adults. Lead in the respiratory tract is absorbed even more readily.

In the body, lead acts to inhibit enzymes involved in the synthesis of heme, the part of the hemoglobin that carries oxygen. In addition, lead disrupts kidney function by localizing in certain renal tissues. It also damages the nervous system, either by direct damage of nerve cells manifested in motor control problems or by the triggering of swelling in the brain. Lead has been found to affect human male fertility. The symptoms of lead poisoning include weakness and fatigue, nausea, and other nonspecific symptoms. Continued exposure results in convulsions, coma, or death. Other symptoms include wrist drop (as a result of nerve damage), anemia, and manifestations of brain damage, such as mental retardation.

Lead poisoning is quickly and effectively treated by using chelating agents, chemical substances that bind very strongly to the lead and prevent it from participating in reactions with biological materials. These chelating agents are initially administered by injection and may be followed by oral treatments. —*Craig B. Lagrone*

*See also* Poisoning.

**FOR FURTHER INFORMATION:**

Chisholm, J. Julian. "Lead Poisoning." *Scientific American* 224 (February, 1971): 15-23.

Kinder, Barry S., and Dominick Pirone. "Lead Contamination: An Important Topic for Biology Courses." *The American Biology Teacher* 56, no. 3 (1994): 152-159.

# LEARNING DISABILITIES

**SYSTEMS AFFECTED:** Brain, psychic-emotional

**SPECIALISTS:** Neurologists, pediatricians, psychologists

**DEFINITION:** A variety of disorders involving the failure to learn an academic skill despite normal levels of intelligence, maturation, and cultural and educational opportunity; estimates of the prevalence of learning disabilities in the general population range between 2 and 20 percent.

**KEY TERMS:**

*achievement test:* a measure of an individual's degree of learning in an academic subject, such as reading, mathematics, and written language

*dyslexia:* difficulty in reading, with an implied neurological cause

*intelligence test:* a psychological test designed to measure an individual's ability to think logically, act purposefully, and react successfully to the environment; yields intelligence quotient (IQ) scores

*neurological dysfunction:* problems associated with the way in which different sections and structures of the brain perform tasks, such as verbal and spatial reasoning and language production

*neurology:* the study of the central nervous system, which is composed of the brain and spinal cord

*perceptual deficits:* problems in processing information from the environment, which may involve distractibility, impulsivity, and figure-ground distortions (difficulty distinguishing foreground from background)

*standardized test:* an instrument used to assess skill development in comparison to others of the same age or grade

## CAUSES AND SYMPTOMS

An understanding of learning disabilities must begin with the knowledge that the definition, diagnosis, and treatment of these disorders have historically generated considerable disagreement and controversy. This is primarily attributable to the fact that people with learning disabilities are a highly diverse group of individuals with a wide variety of characteristics. Consequently, differences of opinion among professionals remain to such an extent that presenting a single universally accepted definition of learning disabilities is not possible. Definitional differences most frequently center on the relative emphases that alternative groups place on characteristics of these disorders. For example, experts in medical fields typically describe these disorders from a disease model and view them primarily as neurological dysfunctions. Conversely, educators usually place more emphasis on the academic problems that result from learning disabilities. Despite these differences, the most commonly accepted definitions, those developed by the United States Office of Education in 1977, the Board of the Association for Children and Adults with Learning Disabilities in 1985, and the National Joint Committee for Learning Disabilities in 1981, do include some areas of commonality.

Difficulty in academic functioning is included in the three definitions, and virtually all descriptions of learning disabilities include this characteristic. Academic deficits may be in one or more formal scholastic subjects, such as reading or mathematics. Often the deficits will involve a component skill of the academic area, such as problems with comprehension or word knowledge in reading or difficulty in calculating or applying arithmetical reasoning in mathematics. The academic difficulty may also be associated with more basic skills of learning that influence functioning across academic areas; these may involve deficits in listening, speaking, and thinking. Dyslexia, a term for reading problems, is the most common academic problem associated with learning disabilities. Because reading skills are required in most academic activities to some degree, many view dyslexia as the most serious form of learning disability.

The presumption of a neurological dysfunction as the cause of these disorders is included, either directly or indirectly, in each of the three definitions. Despite this presumption, unless an individual has a known history of brain trauma, the neurological basis for learning disabilities will not be identified in most cases because current assessment technology does not allow for such precise diagnoses. Rather, at least minimal neurological dysfunction is simply assumed to be present in anyone who exhibits characteristics of a learning disorder.

The three definitions all state that individuals with learning disabilities experience learning problems despite possessing normal intelligence. This condition is referred to as a discrepancy between achievement and ability or potential.

Finally, each of the three definitions incorporates the idea that learning disabilities cannot be attributed to another handicapping condition such as mental retardation, vision or hearing problems, emotional or psychiatric disturbance, or social, cultural, or educational disadvantage. Consequently, these conditions must be excluded as primary contributors to academic difficulties.

Reports on the prevalence of learning disabilities differ according to the definitions and identification methods employed. Consequently, statistics on prevalence range between 2 and 20 percent of the population. Many of the higher reported percentages are actually estimates of prevalence that include individuals who are presumed to have a learning disorder but who have not been formally diagnosed. Males are believed to constitute the majority of individuals with learning disabilities, and estimated sex ratios range from 6:1 to 8:1. Some experts believe that this difference in incidence may reveal one of the causes of these disorders.

A number of causes of learning disabilities have been proposed, with none being universally accepted. Some of the most plausible causal theories include neurological deficits, genetic and hereditary influences, and exposure to toxins during fetal gestation or early childhood.

Evidence to support the assumption of a link between neurological dysfunction and learning disabilities has been supported by studies using sophisticated brain imaging techniques such as positron emission tomography (PET) and computed tomography (CT) scanning and magnetic resonance imaging (MRI). Studies using these techniques have, among other findings, indicated subtle abnormalities in the structure and electrical activity in the brains of individuals with learning disabilities. The use of such techniques has typically been confined to research; however, the continuing advancement of brain imaging technology holds promise not only in contributing greater understanding of the nature and causes of learning disabilities but also in treating the disorder.

Genetic and hereditary influences also have been proposed as causes. Supportive evidence comes from research indicating that identical twins are more likely to be concordant for learning disabilities than fraternal twins and that these disorders are more common in certain families.

A genetic cause of learning disabilities may be associated with extra X or Y chromosomes in certain individuals. The type and degree of impairment associated with these conditions vary according to many genetic and environmental factors, but they can involve problems with language development, visual perception, memory, and problem solving. Despite evidence to link chromosome abnormalities to those with learning disabilities, most experts agree that such genetic conditions account for only a portion of these individuals.

Exposure to toxins or poisons during fetal gestation and early childhood can also cause learning disabilities. During pregnancy nearly all substances the mother takes in are transferred to the fetus. Research has shown that mothers who smoke, drink alcohol, or use certain drugs or medications during pregnancy are more likely to have children with developmental problems, including learning disabilities. Yet not all children exposed to toxins during gestation will have such problems, and the consequences of exposure will vary according to the period when it occurred, the amount of toxin introduced, and the general health and nutrition of the mother and fetus.

Though not precisely involving toxins, two other conditions associated with gestation and childbirth have been linked to learning disabilities. The first, anoxia or oxygen deprivation, occurring for a critical period of time during the birthing process has been tied to both mental retardation and learning disabilities. The second, and more speculative, involves exposure of the fetus to an abnormally large amount of testosterone during gestation. Differences in brain development are proposed to result from the exposure causing learning disorders, among other abnormalities. Known as the embryological theory, it may account for the large number of males with these disabilities, since they have greater amounts of testosterone than females.

The exposure of the immature brain during early childhood to insecticides, household cleaning fluids, alcohol, narcotics, and carbon monoxide, among other toxic substances, may also cause learning disabilities. Lead poisoning resulting from ingesting lead from paint, plaster, and other sources has been found in epidemic numbers in some sections of the country. Lead poisoning can damage the brain and cause learning disabilities, as well as a number of other serious problems.

The number and variety of proposed causes not only reflect differences in experts' training and consequent perspectives but also suggest the likelihood that these disorders can be caused by multiple conditions. This diversity of views also carries to methods for assessing and providing treatment and services to individuals with learning disabilities.

## TREATMENT AND THERAPY

In 1975, the U.S. Congress adopted the Education for All Handicapped Children Act, which, along with other requirements, mandated that students with disabilities, including those with learning disabilities, be identified and provided appropriate educational services. Since that time, much effort has been devoted to developing adequate assessment practices for diagnosis and effective treatment strategies.

In the school setting, assessment of students suspected of having learning disabilities is conducted by a variety of professionals, including teachers specially trained in assessing learning disabilities, school nurses, classroom teachers, school psychologists, and school administrators. Collectively, these professionals are known as a multidisciplinary team. An additional requirement of this educational legislation is that parents must be given the opportunity to participate in the assessment process. Professionals outside the school setting, such as clinical psychologists and independent educational specialists, also conduct assessments to identify learning disabilities.

Because the definition of learning disabilities in the 1975 act includes a discrepancy between achievement and ability as a characteristic of the disorder, students suspected of having learning disabilities are usually administered a variety of formal and informal tests. Standardized tests of intelligence, such as the third edition of the Wechsler Intelligence Scale for Children, are administered to determine

ability. Standardized tests of academic achievement, such as the Woodcock-Johnson Psychoeducational Battery and the Wide Range Achievement Test, also are administered to determine levels of academic skill.

Whether a discrepancy between ability and achievement exists to such a degree to warrant diagnosis of a learning disability is determined by various formulas comparing the scores derived from the intelligence and achievement tests. The precise methods and criteria used to determine a discrepancy vary according to differences among state regulations and school district practices. Consequently, a student diagnosed with a learning disability in one part of the United States may not be viewed as such in another area using different diagnostic criteria. This possibility has been raised in criticism of the use of the discrepancy criteria to identify these disorders. Other criticisms of the method include the use of intelligence quotient (IQ) scores (which are not as stable or accurate as many assume), the inconsistency of students' scores when using alternative achievement tests, and the lack of correspondence between what students are taught and what is tested on achievement tests.

In partial consequence of these and other problems with standardized tests, alternative informal assessment methods have been developed. One such method that is frequently employed is termed curriculum-based assessment (CBA). The CBA method uses materials and tasks taken directly from students' classroom curriculum. For example, in reading, CBA might involve determining the rate of words read per minute from a student's textbook. CBA has been demonstrated to be effective in distinguishing among some students with learning disabilities, those with other academic difficulties, and those without learning problems. Nevertheless, many professionals remain skeptical of CBA as a valid alternative to traditional standardized tests.

Other assessment techniques include vision and hearing tests, measures of language development, and tests examining motor coordination and sensory perception and processing. Observations and analyses of the classroom environment may also be conducted to determine how instructional practices and a student's behavior contribute to learning difficulties.

Based on the information gathered by the multidisciplinary team, a decision is made regarding the diagnosis of a learning disability. If a student is identified with one of these disorders, the team then develops an individual education plan to address identified educational needs. An important guideline in developing the plan is that students with these disorders should be educated to the greatest extent possible with their nonhandicapped peers, while still being provided with appropriate services. Considerable debate has occurred regarding how best to adhere to this guideline.

Programs for students with learning disabilities typically are implemented in self-contained classrooms, resource rooms, or regular classrooms. Self-contained classrooms usually contain ten to twenty students and one or more teachers specially trained to work with these disorders. Typically, these classrooms focus on teaching fundamental skills in basic academic subjects such as reading, writing, and mathematics. Depending on the teacher's training, efforts may also be directed toward developing perceptual, language, or social skills. Students in these programs usually spend some portion of their day with their peers in regular education meetings, but the majority of the day is spent in the self-contained classroom.

The popularity of self-contained classrooms has decreased significantly since the 1960's, when they were the primary setting in which students with learning disabilities were educated. This decrease is largely attributable to the stigmatizing effects of placing students in special settings and the lack of clear evidence to support the effectiveness of this approach.

Students receiving services in resource rooms typically spend a portion of their day in a class where they receive instruction and assistance from specially trained teachers. Students often spend one or two periods in the resource room with a small group of other students who may have similar learning problems or function at a comparable academic level. In the elementary grades, resource rooms usually focus on developing basic academic skills, whereas at the secondary level time is more typically spent in assisting students with their assignments from regular education classes.

Resource room programs are viewed as less restrictive than self-contained classrooms; however, they too have been criticized for segregating children with learning problems. Other criticisms center on scheduling difficulties inherent in the program and the potential for inconsistent instructional approaches and confusion over teaching responsibilities between the regular classroom and resource room teachers. Research on the effectiveness of resource room programs also has been mixed; nevertheless, they are found in most public schools across the United States.

Though they remain a minority, increasing numbers of students have their individual education plans implemented exclusively in a regular classroom. In most schools where such programs exist, teachers are given assistance by a consulting teacher with expertise in learning disabilities. Supporters of this approach point to the lack of stigma associated with segregating students and the absence of definitive research supporting other service models. Detractors are concerned about the potential for inadequate support for the classroom teacher, resulting in students receiving poor quality or insufficient services. The movement to provide services to educationally handicapped students in regular education settings, termed the Regular Education Initiative, has stirred much debate among professionals and parents. Resolution of the debate will greatly affect how individuals with learning disabilities are provided services.

No one specific method of teaching these students has been demonstrated to be superior to others. A variety of strategies have been developed, including perceptual training, multisensory teaching, modality matching, and direct instruction. Advocates of perceptual training believe that academic problems stem from underlying deficits in perceptual skills. They use various techniques aimed at developing perceptual abilities before trying to remedy or teach specific academic skills. Multisensory teaching involves presenting information to students through several senses. Instruction using this method may be conducted using tactile, auditory, visual, and kinesthetic exercises. Instruction involving modality matching begins with identifying the best learning style for a student, such as visual or auditory processing. Learning tasks are then presented via that mode. Direct instruction is based on the principles of behavioral psychology. The method involves developing precise educational goals, focusing on teaching the exact skill of concern, and providing frequent opportunities to perform the skill until it is mastered.

With the exception of direct instruction, research has generally failed to demonstrate that these strategies are uniquely effective with students with learning disabilities. Direct instruction, on the other hand, has been demonstrated effective but has also been criticized for focusing on isolated skills without dealing with the broader processing problems associated with these disorders. More promisingly, students with learning disabilities appear to benefit from teaching approaches that have been found effective with students without learning problems when instruction is geared to ability level and rate of learning.

## Perspective and Prospects

Interest in disorders of learning can be identified throughout the history of medicine. The specific study of learning disabilities, however, can be traced to the efforts of a number of physicians working in the first quarter of the twentieth century who studied the brain and its associated pathology. One such researcher, Kurt Goldstein, identified a number of unusual characteristics, collectively termed perceptual deficits, which were associated with head injury.

Goldstein's work influenced a number of researchers affiliated with the Wayne County Training School, including Alfred Strauss, Laura Lehtinen, Newell Kephart, and William Cruickshank. These individuals worked with children with learning problems who exhibited many of the characteristics of brain injury identified by Goldstein. Consequently, they presumed that neurological dysfunction, whether it could specifically be identified or not, caused the learning difficulties. They also developed a set of instructional practices involving reduced environmental stimuli and exercises to develop perceptual skills. The work and writings of these individuals through the 1940's, 1950's, and 1960's were highly influential, and many programs for students with learning disabilities were based on their theoretical and instructional principles.

Samuel Orton, working in the 1920's and 1930's, also was influenced by research into brain injury in his conceptualization of children with reading problems. He observed that many of these children were left-handed or ambidextrous, reversed letters or words when reading or writing, and had coordination problems. Consequently, he proposed that reading disabilities resulted from abnormal brain development and an associated mixing of brain functions. Based on the work of Orton and his students, including Anna Gilmore and Bessie Stillman, a variety of teaching strategies were developed which focused on teaching phonics and using multisensory aids. In the 1960's, Elizabeth Slingerland applied Orton's concepts in the classroom setting and they have been included in many programs for students with learning disabilities.

A number of other researchers have developed theories for the cause and treatment of learning disabilities. Some of the most influential include Helmer Mykelbust and Samuel Kirk, who emphasized gearing instruction to a student's strongest learning modality, and Norris Haring, Ogden Lindsley, and Joseph Jenkins, who applied principles of behavioral psychology to teaching.

The work of these and other researchers and educators raised professional and public awareness of learning disabilities and the special needs of individuals with the disorder. Consequently, the number of special education classrooms and programs increased dramatically in public schools across the United States in the 1960's and 1970's. Legislation on both the state and federal level, primarily resulting from litigation by parents to establish the educational rights of their children, also has had a profound impact on the availability of services for those with learning disabilities. The passage of the Education for All Handicapped Children Act in 1975 not only mandated appropriate educational services for students with learning disabilities but also generated funding, interest, and research in the field. The Regular Education Initiative has since prompted increased efforts to identify more effective assessment and treatment strategies and generated debates among professionals and the consumers of these services. Decisions resulting from these continuing debates will have a significant impact on future services for individuals with learning disabilities. —*Paul F. Bell*

*See also* Aphasia and dysphasia; Autism; Down syndrome; Dyslexia; Mental retardation; Neuralgia, neuritis, and neuropathy; Speech disorders.

## For Further Information:

Cordoni, Barbara. *Living with a Learning Disability.* Rev. ed. Carbondale: Southern Illinois University Press, 1990. Written by a professor of special education and the mother of two children with learning disabilities, this book focuses on the social skill problems associated with

these disorders. Offers suggestions to parents and professionals regarding effective counseling, teaching, and coping strategies. Included is a helpful explanation of the laws governing education for students with learning disabilities.

Lovitt, Thomas. *Introduction to Learning Disabilities.* Needham Heights, Mass.: Allyn & Bacon, 1989. This book is exceptionally well written and comprehensive in its review of topics associated with learning disabilities, including assessment and treatment issues, the history of these disorders, and recommendations for future efforts in the field. Provides balanced coverage of alternative views regarding the controversial aspects of learning disabilities.

MacCracken, Mary. *Turnabout Children: Overcoming Dyslexia and Other Learning Disabilities.* Boston: Little, Brown, 1986. Written by an educational therapist, this publication includes case histories of children with learning disabilities who have been successful in adapting to the unique difficulties that they face. Includes descriptions of assessment instruments and effective remedial techniques.

Scheiber, Barbara, and Jeanne Talpers. *Unlocking Potential.* Bethesda, Md.: Adler & Adler, 1987. This practical publication provides a step-by-step method for individuals with learning disabilities wishing to pursue postsecondary education. Advice is provided for selecting, gaining admission to, and successfully completing college, vocational, and trade school programs. Provides an excellent overview of how these disorders are diagnosed and what services are available. Includes a listing of postsecondary programs that have special accommodations for students with learning disabilities.

Snowling, M. J., and M. E. Thomson, eds. *Dyslexia: Integrating Theory and Practice.* London: Whurr, 1991. This publication includes selected papers from the second International Conference of the British Dyslexia Association, held in 1991. Chapters include detailed descriptions of theoretical and practical aspects of reading disabilities and reviews of treatment strategies for individuals from early childhood to adulthood.

## Legionnaires' disease

**System affected:** Respiratory

**Specialists:** Epidemiologists, infectious disease physicians, internists, public health specialists

**Definition:** A rapidly progressing bacterial pneumonia caused by infection with an organism of the genus *Legionella* and characterized by influenza-like illness, with high fever, chills, headache, and muscle aches.

**Key terms:**

*alveolus:* an outpouching of lung tissue in which gas exchange takes place between air in the lungs and blood capillaries

*legionellosis:* another name for any infection caused by a member of the genus *Legionella;* generally denotes Legionnaires' disease

*macrophage:* any of a variety of phagocytic cells; macrophages are found in highest numbers in tissue; alveolar macrophages are found in lungs and function to remove respiratory pathogens

*phagocytes:* white cells capable of ingesting and digesting microbes, a process referred to as phagocytosis; primarily refers to neutrophils and macrophages

*Pontiac fever:* a self-limiting, nonpneumonic disease caused by *Legionella* bacteria; clinically and epidemiologically distinct from Legionnaires' disease

*virulence factor:* a bacterial factor that enhances the pathogenic potential of the organism; includes products such as toxins and capsules

### CAUSES AND SYMPTOMS

Legionnaires' disease, or legionellosis, is an acute bacterial pneumonia that was unknown prior to 1976. In July and August of that year, an outbreak of pneumonia occurred among persons who had either attended an American Legion convention in Philadelphia or had been in the vicinity of the Bellevue-Stratford Hotel in the downtown area. The likely source of the epidemic was a contaminated air-conditioning unit in the hotel. Though speculation among the media and general public suggested all sorts of causes for the epidemic, the specific etiological agent was isolated by January, 1977. It turned out to be a somewhat common bacterium, which was subsequently given the genus and species names *Legionella pneumophila;* the genus name reflected the first known victims, while the species name meant "lung-loving."

Within several years, additional strains of *Legionella* bacteria were isolated from patients suffering from bacterial pneumonia. By 1992, thirty-two known species had been identified either as human pathogens or as microflora in environmental water sources. Most cases of Legionnaires' disease have been linked to infection by *L. pneumophila* or, to a lesser degree, *L. micdadei.*

Genetic evidence confirmed that *Legionella* was indeed a newly isolated bacterium. Several factors contributed to its previous invisibility. First, Legionnaires' disease is similar in its characteristics to other forms of nonbacterial pneumonia, such as that caused by viruses. Since no bacteria were readily isolated, there was no immediate reason to suspect a bacterium as the infectious agent. The second reason related to the initial difficulty of growing *Legionella* bacteria in the laboratory. Aspirates from pneumonia victims were inoculated onto routine laboratory media; most common bacteria grow quite readily on such media. No growth was observed, however, in the case of *Legionella.* Many nutrient supplements were tried. *Legionella* bacteria grew only on media that were supplemented with iron and the amino acid cysteine. Since the early 1980's, the medium

of choice has been agar containing buffered charcoal yeast extract. Nutrients such as amino acids, vitamins, and iron are included in the medium while the charcoal removes potentially toxic materials.

Legionellosis actually constitutes two separate clinical entities: Legionnaires' disease and Pontiac fever. Legionnaires' disease is potentially the more serious of the two. The victim is initially infected through a respiratory route. In general, the source of the infection is an aerosol generated by contaminated water supplies such as those found in the cooling units of building air-conditioning systems. Rarely, if at all, does the disease pass from person to person. Most infections are unapparent, with either mild disease or none at all. The estimate is that less than 5 percent of exposed individuals actually contract Legionnaires' disease. Certain factors seem to increase the chances that the infection will progress toward pneumonia. Often, the lungs of the victim have suffered from previous trauma, such as that caused by emphysema or smoking. The person is generally, though not always, middle-aged or older. These observations suggest that, in most instances, the person's immune system is quite capable of handling the infection.

The disease begins with a dry cough, muscle aches, and rising fever—symptoms that resemble the flu. The person may also suffer from vomiting and diarrhea. In serious cases, the disease becomes progressively more severe over the next three to six days. The alveoli, or air sacs, of the lung become necrotized, increasing the difficulty in breathing. Small abscesses may also form in the lungs, as phagocytes infiltrate the area. The mortality rate has ranged from 15 to 60 percent in various outbreaks, although with early treatment, these numbers can be significantly lowered. Patients with other underlying lung problems, or who may be immunosuppressed, are at particular risk.

Pontiac fever is a much less serious form of disease. Named for the Michigan city in which a 1968 outbreak occurred in the Public Health Department building, the disease is self-limiting, nonpneumonic, and not life-threatening. Pontiac fever also seems to follow the inhalation of the etiological agent. Though the attack rate in exposed individuals appears to approach 100 percent, there is no infiltration of lung tissue and no abscess formation. A febrile period occurs one to two days following infection, with the individual progressing to recovery after several days. The difference between the two forms of disease remains obscure. There appears to be no obvious difference between the organisms associated with the two diseases, though strains associated with Pontiac fever may not replicate as readily inside human cells.

The mechanism by which infection by *Legionella* bacteria results in pneumonia is not altogether clear. Research into this area has centered on forms of virulence factors produced by the organism and their relationships to disease. Following their infiltration into the lung, *Legionella* bacteria are phagocytized by alveolar macrophages or other leukocytes (white blood cells). Unlike other ingested microbes, however, *Legionella* bacteria often survive the process and begin a process of intracellular replication. In this intracellular state, *Legionella* bacteria are shielded from many of the host's immune defenses.

Certain questions lend themselves to understanding this approach in elucidating the mechanisms of Legionnaires' disease. First, are intracellular survival and multiplication necessary factors in the development of the disease? Second, if these factors are indeed relevant, exactly how does the organism manage to evade the killing mechanisms that exist inside the cell?

The first question has been dealt with by various animal studies. Guinea pigs were exposed to a *Legionella* aerosol, and lung aspirates were prepared after forty-eight hours. Large numbers of viable organisms were found inside alveolar macrophages. Few live *Legionella* bacteria, however, were observed outside cells. In addition, mutant *Legionella* bacteria that were incapable of intracellular growth showed reduced virulence in guinea pigs. Therefore, initial intracellular infection and multiplication does appear to be necessary to initiate the disease process.

The mechanism of intracellular survival is less clear. Macrophages are professional phagocytes that have a wide variety of means for killing ingested microorganisms. These mechanisms range from the production of reactive oxygen molecules to the synthesis of oxidizing agents such as peroxides. In addition, after a foreign microbe has been phagocytized within the membrane-bound vessel called a phagosome, a cell organelle, the lysosome, will fuse with the phagosome. Contained within the lysosome are large numbers of digestive enzymes that proceed to digest the target. Under normal circumstances, foreign microbes are ingested and digested, eliminating the threat of infection.

Somehow, *Legionella* bacteria evade these defense mechanisms. Different strains of *Legionella* bacteria appear to have evolved a variety of mechanisms for survival. In particular, there are two types of molecules, a phosphatase and a cytoxin, whose presence is correlated with intracellular survival. Both appear to act by preventing the phagocytes from producing potentially lethal oxidation molecules such as hydrogen peroxide.

Another virulence factor that appears to be important for infectivity is a surface protein known as the macrophage infectivity potentiator, or MIP. The MIP proteins are apparently unique to *Legionella* bacteria; mutants that lack the MIP gene are significantly less virulent than wild-type strains. The MIP protein appears to be necessary for the internalization of *Legionella* bacteria by the macrophage, and for survival against the array of bacteriocidal activities.

A variety of other mechanisms may also exist that allow *Legionella* bacteria to escape the killing mechanisms of the macrophage. For example, in addition to the phosphatase, which removes phosphate molecules from host proteins or lipids, *Legionella* bacteria also produce protein kinases, which can add phosphate molecules to host cell proteins. In this manner, *Legionella* bacteria can potentially regulate the metabolism of the cells in which they find themselves by adding or subtracting phosphates from various sites or metabolic pathways.

Though a precise sequence of events that leads to the development of Legionnaires' disease remains to be worked out, certain steps appear to be necessary. Following the inhalation of a *Legionella* aerosol, probably from a contaminated water source, the organism lodges in the alveoli of the lung. Resident macrophages phagocytize the microbe, resulting in its internalization. Through a variety of virulence factors, *Legionella* survives, and multiplies within the macrophage. Death of the host cells along with the concomitant infiltration of other white cells results in the inflammation and lung damage recognized as Legionnaires' disease.

## TREATMENT AND THERAPY

Despite the hysteria associated with the Philadelphia outbreak of Legionnaires' disease and the difficulty associated with the initial isolation of the etiological agent, there is nothing particularly unusual about the organism. The *Legionella* bacterium is a small, thin microbe some 2 to 10 micrometers in length, about the size of most average bacteria. Because of its characteristic staining pattern, it is classified as a gram-negative organism. This results from the molecular nature of its cell wall, which has a high lipopolysaccharide (LPS) content.

Since legionellosis can resemble other forms of pneumonia, improper diagnosis can be a problem. Though the prognosis of the disease is generally favorable with early intervention, improper or delayed treatment can prove fatal. In general, legionellosis is suspected in a patient with a progressive pneumonia for which other organisms do not appear to be a factor. *Legionella* bacteria may be observed from lung aspirates using immunofluorescent examination. In this technique, a sample of aspirate is treated with a fluorescent-labeled antibody molecule that is capable of binding to the surface of the microorganism. The microbe will then fluoresce, or glow, when observed with a microscope containing ultraviolet optics. The advantage of this method is its speed. Often, however, there are too few bacteria in the lung to be identified.

A firm diagnosis is made by culturing the bacteria on artificial media. Generally, a buffered charcoal yeast extract medium is used that contains a variety of amino acids and vitamins necessary for the organisms to grow. *Legionella* bacteria will not grow on the more conventional media used to culture other types of bacteria, which caused problems in the early attempts to isolate the organism associated with the Legionnaires' disease outbreak. Diagnosis may also be carried out by measuring the level of anti-*Legionella* antibody in the serum of the suspected patient. A rising level of antibody is indicative of active infection by the organism.

There are several aspects of the clinical significance of the gram-negative character of the organism, one of which is that this type of bacteria responds poorly to penicillin or penicillin derivatives. This serves to limit the type of antimicrobial therapy available for treatment of severe cases of legionellosis. Other antibiotics exist, of course, that exhibit antibacterial characteristics similar to those of penicillin—for example, the cephalosporins. And, indeed, penicillin derivatives have been used to treat at least some types of gram-negative infections. Legionellosis patients did not respond well, however, to treatment with any of these agents. It was subsequently found that the basis for the resistance by *Legionella* bacteria to these antibiotics lay in a type of extracellular enzyme produced by these bacteria—a beta-lactamase.

The lack of pharmacologic activity associated with the penicillins, the cephalosporins, and certain other antibiotics is thus easy to explain. The activity of these antibiotics is associated with the presence of a structure in the molecule called a beta-lactam ring. The beta-lactamase produced by the *Legionella* bacterium causes a break in the ring, rendering the antibiotic harmless to the microbe, and thus useless as a form of treatment. Such resistance has become increasingly common among bacteria, since the genes encoding the beta-lactamase are passed from organism to organism.

Fortunately, other antibiotics did prove to be useful in the treatment of legionellosis. To a certain extent, the determination of the antibiotics of choice was fortuitous. During the Philadelphia outbreak, the nature of the illness was unknown. The primary assumption was that an infectious agent was at fault, but determination of the nature of that agent lay months beyond the extent of the epidemic. Therefore, as would be true in the treatment of any illness of unknown origin, various treatments were carried out. Two antibiotics in particular proved to be useful: erythromycin and rifampin. Erythromycin, which specifically inhibits bacterial protein synthesis, has continued to be useful. Though long-term use can result in liver damage and some individuals are hypersensitive to the drug, the intravenous administration of erythromycin remains the treatment of choice for legionellosis. Rifampin is used on occasion in association with other methods of treatment, but the high frequency of bacterial resistance to the drug precludes its use as a treatment of first choice.

Since the virulent properties of the *Legionella* bacterium depend on its intracellular presence in the macrophage, those antimicrobial agents that exhibit intracellular penetration would be expected to be most effective. Erythromycin fits this requirement, as do a number of other antibiotics. Not surprisingly, these agents have proved to be most efficacious in the treatment of the disease. Thus, alternative sources of treatment exist in the event that erythromycin proves ineffective.

Other aspects of treatment center on maintaining the comfort of the individual. This may include the use of analgesics for relief of pain.

Prevention of the disease is obviously preferable to dealing with the sequelae of infection. Epidemiological studies have demonstrated that the *Legionella* bacterium is a common soil organism that is often found in bodies of water contaminated by soil. The organism has been found in lakes and pond water, and it can survive for long periods in unchlorinated tap water. In fact, contaminated water appears to have been the source of infection for most outbreaks of the illness. Problems have often been associated with cooling towers, evaporative condensers, and other water supplies found with air-conditioning units of buildings. Infectious aerosols may be generated from these units, allowing for a respiratory route of infection. Though the disease is thus spread in an airborne manner, there is no evidence that it can be passed from person to person.

The epidemiological evidence for the disease supports an airborne hypothesis. Most outbreaks have occurred in regions of soil disruption, such as that occurring during construction. Subsequent isolation of *Legionella* bacteria from the cooling towers confirmed such contamination. Though the air-conditioning unit of the Bellevue-Stratford Hotel in Philadelphia was replaced prior to isolation of the organism, the assumption is that the unit was contaminated. The outbreaks of the disease during the summer, when air-conditioning use has peaked, are consistent with the role of air-conditioning units in the spread of *Legionella* bacteria.

The method by which the *Legionella* bacterium survives in the environment has not been completely determined. The organism is somewhat resistant both to chlorine treatment and to heat as high as 65 degrees Celsius. It appears to grow best in the presence of biological factors secreted by other microflora in the environment; growth stimulation may also be enhanced by the presence of physical factors such as sediment, silicone, and rubber compounds. Its ability to survive, and indeed be transmitted, may also be related to its tendency to penetrate and multiply intracellularly within environmental protozoa or amoeba.

Prevention of disease transmission must take into account these problems. Contamination of water supplies must be minimized. The resistance of the *Legionella* bacterium to standard methods of decontamination has made the process more difficult, and methods of choice remain controversial. Chlorination at relatively high levels remains the preferred method, with subsequent treatment at lower concentrations over the long term. The disadvantages of this method include the cost of constant treatment and the eventual corrosion of the units. Continuous or intermittent heating of the water has also proved effective in decontamination.

## PERSPECTIVE AND PROSPECTS

Prior to August, 1976, Legionnaires' disease was unknown. From July 21 to 24 of that year, however, the Pennsylvania branch of the American Legion held its annual convention at the Bellevue-Stratford Hotel in Philadelphia. Some 4,000 delegates and their families attended the festivities. Following the convention, as delegates returned to their homes, a mysterious illness began to appear among the attendees. A total of 149 conventioneers and 72 others became ill. Characterized by a severe respiratory infection that progressed into pneumonia, and high fever, the illness proved fatal to 34 of the victims.

By August, it became clear to the Pennsylvania Department of Health that an epidemic was at hand. The cause of the outbreak was not clear, and rumors began to circulate. At various times, the news media explained the outbreak as a Communist plot against former military men, a Central Intelligence Agency test gone awry, and even an infectious agent arriving from space. The truth was less dramatic. By the beginning of 1977, David Fraser, Joseph McDade, and their colleagues from the Centers for Disease Control isolated the etiological agent: a bacterium subsequently named *Legionella pneumophila*.

With the isolation and identification of the organism, it became possible to explain earlier outbreaks of unusual illness. For example, during July and August of 1965, an outbreak of pneumonia at a chronic-care facility at St. Elizabeth's Hospital in Washington, D.C., resulted in 81 cases and 14 deaths. An outbreak among personnel at the Oakland County Health Department in Pontiac, Michigan, during July and August of 1968 of a disease that was subsequently called Pontiac fever was also traced to the same organism. In this case, however, though 144 persons were affected, none died. In fact, illness associated with the *Legionella* bacterium has been traced as far back as 1947. The 1976 outbreak was not new; it was merely the first time that medical personnel were able to isolate the organism that caused the disease.

The precise prevalence of the *Legionella* bacterium remains murky, but it is clearly more common than was at first realized. Despite the public's fear of the disease, in most instances it probably remains a mild respiratory infection, resembling nothing worse than a bad cold. Most cases remain undetected. Estimates have suggested that as many as 25,000 persons in the United States develop infection. Based on seroconversions—the production of anti-*Legionella* antibody in the sera of persons—it has been estimated that more than 20 percent of the population of Michigan has been exposed to the organism. There is no reason to doubt that the same situation exists in many other states.

The basis for the difference in severity between Legionnaires' disease and Pontiac fever is also unclear. There is no obvious difference between the two diseases that accounts for the differences in virulence. It also remains to be seen whether *Legionella* bacteria are associated with other illnesses.

The final lesson of Legionnaires' disease is as subtle as its initial appearance. Humans exist in an environment replete with infectious agents. Despite the battery of modern methods of treatment for illness, there always remains the potential for new outbreaks of previously unknown disease.
—*Richard Adler*

*See also* Pneumonia; Pulmonary diseases.

## FOR FURTHER INFORMATION:

Brock, Thomas D., ed. *Microorganisms: From Smallpox to Lyme Disease*. New York: W. H. Freeman, 1990. A collection of readings from *Scientific American*. The book includes a collection of accounts of the history of major infectious diseases. Divided into sections dealing with medical histories, methods of prevention, and means of transmission. Each section includes an introduction that summarizes the material.

Dowling, John N., Asish K. Saha, and Robert H. Glew. "Virulence Factors of the Family *Legionellaceae*." *Microbiological Reviews* 56 (March 1, 1992): 32. A thorough discussion of the roles played by various virulence factors related to intracellular survival of the bacterium. A review article for which basic knowledge of microbiology would be helpful. Nevertheless, the article contains a wealth of information on the subject.

Fraser, David W., et al. "Legionnaires' Disease." *New England Journal of Medicine* 297, no. 22 (1983): 1189-1197. The first detailed description of the epidemic of pneumonia determined to be Legionnaires' disease. Though requisite scientific jargon is included, the article does provide an excellent description of the epidemiological study that led to the determination of the origin of the outbreak.

Hoyle, Fred, and N. C. Wickramasinghe. *Diseases from Space*. London: J. M. Dent & Sons, 1979. As one might guess from the title, the premise of the book is not for everybody. Nevertheless, the authors discuss in a clear, concise manner the principle behind the spreading of a variety of diseases, including Legionnaires' disease. Easily read and digested by nonscientists.

Sherris, John C., ed. *Medical Microbiology*. 2d ed. New York: Elsevier, 1990. A textbook dealing with major pathogenic organisms. The section on *Legionella* is a concise outline of what is known about the disease. Some basic knowledge of science is necessary, but a detailed background in microbiology is not required.

Thomas, Gordon, and Max Morgan-Witts. *Anatomy of an Epidemic*. Garden City, N.Y.: Doubleday, 1982. A popular account of the Philadelphia outbreak. Written in the manner of a detective story, the book provides a highly readable description of the development of the epidemic and the investigation that ultimately led to its explanation. Particularly interesting are the accounts of infighting among the various state and federal agencies over jurisdiction.

## LEISHMANIASIS

SYSTEMS AFFECTED: Mucous membranes, skin

SPECIALISTS: Public health specialists, tropical medicine specialists

DEFINITION: The term "leishmaniasis" refers to several diseases associated with the single-celled parasite species *Leishmania*. Transmitted by the bite of a sandfly, the parasites cause ulcers in the skin or internal organs. There are four main types: visceral leishmaniasis, or kala-azar; and Old World cutaneous, New World cutaneous, and mucocutaneous leishmaniasis. Kala-azar is the most serious form because it affects the bone marrow and organs and may cause anemia and other disorders; it is found in Asia, Africa, and parts of South America. The cutaneous types occur either in Central and South America (New World) or in the Middle East, North Africa, and parts of the Mediterranean (Old World); a persistent skin ulcer forms and eventually heals, although disfigurement may result. Medications are available to treat all types of infection.

*See also* Protozoan diseases.

## LEPROSY

SYSTEMS AFFECTED: Nervous, skin

SPECIALISTS: Epidemiologists, immunologists, internists, public health specialists

DEFINITION: A bacterial infection that affects skin and nerves, causing symptoms ranging from mild numbness to gross disfiguration.

KEY TERMS:

*acid-fast:* the ability of a bacterium to retain a pink stain in the presence of a mixture of acid and alcohol

*antibody:* a protein found in the blood and produced by the immune system in response to bodily contact with an antigen

*antigen:* a foreign substance (such as a bacterium, toxin, or virus) to which the body makes an immune response

*bacillus Calmette-Guérin (BCG):* a vaccine for tuberculosis made from a harmless strain of *Mycobacterium bovis*

*bacterium:* microscopic single-celled organism that multiplies by simple division; bacteria are found everywhere; most are beneficial, but a few species cause disease

*cellular immune response:* the reaction of the body that produces active white blood cells that can destroy antigens associated with other body cells

*humoral immune response:* the reaction of the body that produces antibodies that can destroy antigens present in body fluids

*hypersensitivity:* an overreaction by the immune system to the presence of certain antigens; this overreaction often results in some damage to the person as well as the antigen

*immune response:* the working of the body's immune system to prevent or combat an infectious disease

### CAUSES AND SYMPTOMS

Leprosy, also known as Hansen's disease, is caused by the bacterium *Mycobacterium leprae (M. leprae)*. Humans are the only natural host for this bacterium; it can be found only in leprosy victims. Most people who are exposed to this bacterium are unaffected by it; in the remainder, the bacterium grows inside skin and nerve cells, causing a wide range of symptoms that depend upon the person's immune response to the growth of the bacteria.

*M. leprae* is an obligate intracellular parasite, which means that it can grow only inside other cells. *M. leprae* has a unique waxy coating that helps to protect it while it is growing inside human skin and nerve cells. The bacterium grows very slowly, dividing once every twelve days, whereas the average bacterium will divide every twenty to sixty minutes. *M. leprae* grows best at temperatures slightly below body temperature (37 degrees Celsius). The leprosy bacterium is the only bacterium known to destroy peripheral nerve tissue (nerves that are not a part of the central nervous system) and will also destroy skin and mucous membranes. This bacterium is closely related to the bacterium that causes tuberculosis: *Mycobacterium tuberculosis*.

Leprosy is not very contagious. Several attempts to infect human volunteers with the bacteria have been unsuccessful. It is believed that acquiring leprosy from an infected person requires prolonged intimate contact with that person, such as living in the same house for a long time. Although the precise mode of transmission of *M. leprae* bacteria is unclear, it is highly probable that the bacteria are transferred from the nasal or respiratory secretions of the victim to the nasal passages or a skin wound of the recipient.

Once inside a person, *M. leprae* will grow and reproduce inside skin and nerve cells and destroy tissue. The exact mechanism of tissue destruction is not understood, but it probably results from a combination of nerve damage, massive accumulation of bacteria, and immunological reactions. Because the bacteria grow so slowly, the length of time from infection to appearance of the symptoms (the incubation period) is quite long. The average incubation period is two to seven years, but incubation can range from three months to forty years. Since the bacteria prefer temperatures slightly lower that normal body temperature, symptoms appear first in the cooler parts of the body, such as the hands, fingers, feet, face, nose, and earlobes. In severe cases, symptoms also appear in the eyes and the respiratory tract.

The symptoms associated with leprosy can range from very mild to quite severe, and the symptoms that a person gets depend heavily on that person's ability to mount a cellular immune response against the bacteria. In a normal infection, the human body is capable of defending itself through two processes of the immune system; the humoral immune response and the cellular immune response. The humoral response produces chemicals called antibodies that can attack and destroy infectious agents that are present in body fluids such as the blood. The cellular response produces white blood cells that can destroy infectious agents that are associated with cells. Since *M. leprae* hides and grows inside human cells, a cellular response is the only type of immune response that can be of any help in fighting the infection. The ability to generate a cellular immune response against *M. leprae* is dependent upon the genetic makeup and overall health of the victim, as well as the number of infecting bacteria and their ability to invade the body and cause disease. A quick and strong cellular response by a person infected with *M. leprae* will result in no symptoms or in the mild form of the disease: tuberculoid leprosy. A slow or weak cellular response by a person exposed to leprosy may result in the more severe form of the disease: lepromatous leprosy.

Only one in two hundred people exposed to leprosy will get some form of the disease. The earliest symptom is a slightly bleached, flat lesion several centimeters in diameter that is usually found on the upper body or on the arms or legs. About three-fourths of all patients with an early solitary lesion heal spontaneously; the rest progress to tuberculoid or lepromatous leprosy or to one of the many forms that fall between these two extremes.

Tuberculoid leprosy is characterized by flat skin lesions 5 to 20 centimeters in diameter. The lesions are lighter in color than the surrounding skin and are sometimes surrounded by nodules (lumps). The lesions contain only a few bacteria, and they, along with the surrounding tissue, are numb. These lesions are caused by a hypersensitive cellular immune response to the bacteria in the nerves and skin. In an attempt to destroy the bacteria, the immune system overreacts, and some of the surrounding nerve and skin tissue is damaged while the bacteria are being killed. This causes the areas of the skin to lose pigment as well as sensation. Often, tuberculoid leprosy patients can experience more extensive physical damage if the numbness around the lesions leads to accidental loss of digits, skin, and so forth. Leprosy victims may burn and cut themselves unknowingly, since they have no feeling in certain areas of their bodies.

In lepromatous leprosy, the bacteria grow unchecked because of the weak cellular immune response. Often, there are more than 100 million bacterial cells present per square centimeter of tissue. These bacteria cause the formation of tumorlike growths called lepromas as well as tissue destruction of the skin and mucous membranes. Also, the presence of so many bacteria causes large numbers of antibacterial antibodies to be produced, but these antibodies are of no benefit in fighting off the infection. Instead, they can con-

## Lepromatous Leprosy

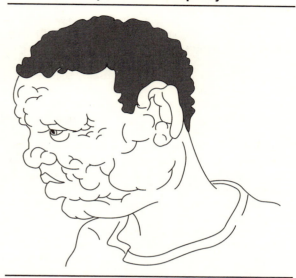

*This more severe form of leprosy occurs in the absence of a strong immune response and results in lepromas, or tumorlike growths.*

tribute to the formation of lesions and tissue damage both internally and on the skin through a process called immune complex hypersensitivity. This is a process whereby the large number of antibodies bind to the large number of bacteria in the body and form immune complexes. These complexes can be deposited in various parts of the body and trigger a chemical reaction that destroys the surrounding tissue. The large number of bacteria puts pressure on the nerves and destroys nerve tissue, which causes loss of sensation and tissue death.

The initial symptoms of lepromatous leprosy are skin lesions that can be spread out or nodular and are found on the cooler parts of the body, such as the inside of the nose, the front part of the eye, the face, the earlobes, the hands, and the feet. Often, the victim loses all facial features because the nodules enlarge the face, and the eyebrows and nose deteriorate, giving the victim a characteristic lionlike appearance. Severe lepromatous leprosy erodes bones; thus, fingers and toes become needlelike, pits form in the skull, nasal bones are destroyed, and teeth fall out. Also, the limbs become twisted and the hands become clawed. The destruction of the nerves leads to the inability to move the hands or feet, deformity of the feet, and chronic ulceration of the limbs. In addition, as is the case with tuberculoid leprosy, destruction of the small peripheral nerves leads to self-inflicted trauma and secondary infection (infection by another bacterium or virus). As the disease progresses, the growth of bacteria in the respiratory tract causes larynx problems and difficult breathing. Deterioration of the optic nerve leads to blindness. Bacteria can invade the bloodstream and spread infection throughout the whole body except the central nervous system. Death associated with leprosy usually results from respiratory obstruction, kidney failure, or secondary infection.

### Treatment and Therapy

A physician can tell whether a person has leprosy by looking for characteristic symptoms (light-colored and numb lesions, nodules, and so forth) and by determining whether the patient may have been exposed to someone with leprosy. In addition, samples of scrapings from skin lesions, nasal secretions, fluid from nodules, or other tissue secretions can be examined for the presence of *M. leprae*. Samples are treated with a procedure called the acid-fast technique. Because of *M. leprae*'s waxy coating, these bacteria retain a pink stain after being washed in an acid-alcohol mixture, whereas all other bacteria lose the pink stain. Therefore, pink, rod-shaped bacteria observed in samples treated with the acid-fast technique indicate the presence of *M. leprae*. It is easy to find the acid-fast *M. leprae* in lepromatous leprosy patients because they have so many bacteria in their lesions, but the bacteria are more difficult to find in the lesions of tuberculoid leprosy patients. The lepromin test was originally developed to be used as a diagnostic tool for leprosy, in the same way that the tuberculin test is used as a diagnostic tool for tuberculosis. Lepromin, which is heat-killed *M. leprae* taken from nodules, is injected under the skin in the lepromin test. Two reactions are possible: an early reaction that appears twenty-four to forty-eight hours later and a late reaction that appears three to four weeks later. In both reactions, a hard red lump at the injection site indicates a positive lepromin test. This test is not specific for leprosy, however, because a person who has been exposed to *M. leprae*, *M. tuberculosis*, or the tuberculosis vaccine, bacillus Calmette-Guérin (BCG), will show a positive early reaction. Even though this test is not useful as a diagnostic tool, it is useful in determining whether a patient has a strong or a weak cellular immune response to *M. leprae*. Tuberculoid leprosy patients show both the early and late reactions, while lepromatous leprosy patients show no reaction at all.

Leprosy can be treated with antibiotics. The antibiotic dapsone began to be used on a wide scale in the treatment of leprosy in 1950. Since that time, however, many dapsone-resistant strains of *M. leprae* have appeared. This means that, for some victims, this drug is no longer helpful in fighting the disease. In 1981, in response to the problem of dapsone-resistant strains, the World Health Organization recommended a multidrug regimen for leprosy victims. For lepromatous leprosy patients, dapsone, rifampin, and clofazimine are recommended, whereas tuberculoid leprosy patients need take only dapsone and rifampin. Treatment is expected to continue until skin smears are free from acid-fast bacteria, which can last from two years up to the lifetime of the patient. Since 1989, the U.S. recommendations for tuberculoid leprosy are six months of rifampin and dapsone daily, then dapsone alone for three years. For lepromatous leprosy, the recommendation is to use rifampin and dapsone daily for three years, then dapsone only for the rest of the person's life. Often, antibiotics are given to family members of leprosy patients in order to prevent them from contracting the disease. Antibiotic therapy can make a leprosy victim noncontagious, stop the progress of the disease, and in some cases cause a reversal of some of the symptoms. Until treatment is complete, however, it is recommended that patients sleep in separate bedrooms, use their own linens and utensils, and not live in a house with children. Thus, leprosy victims can lead nearly normal lives without fear of infecting others in the community.

The best ways to keep from getting leprosy are to avoid exposure to leprosy bacteria and to receive antibiotic therapy following exposure. It should be possible to control and, eventually, eliminate leprosy. If every case of leprosy were treated, the disease could not spread and the bacteria would die out with the last leprosy victim. Progress in this direction is slow, however, because of ignorance, superstition, poverty, and overpopulation in areas with many leprosy cases. The first strategy in controlling leprosy is to treat all leprosy cases with antibiotics. As of 1991, about 50 percent of all leprosy victims were not receiving drug therapy. Second, the early detection and rigid isolation of lepromatous leprosy patients are important, as is preventive antibiotic therapy for individuals in close contact with those patients. Finally, as of the early 1990's, too many countries lacked adequate basic health resources, and too many patients disabled by leprosy were not receiving adequate care. The development of a vaccine for leprosy would aid control efforts.

A global effort for the production of a vaccine for leprosy is being made under the auspices of the World Health Organization. The first problem with vaccine development is that, until recently, it was not possible to grow *M. leprae* bacteria outside of a leprosy victim; therefore, not much is known about the nature of the bacteria. Even though this bacterium was the first to be associated with a disease, it cannot be grown on an artificial laboratory medium, whereas nearly every other bacteria known can be grown artificially. It was not until 1960 that scientists at the Centers for Disease Control discovered that the bacterium could be grown in the footpads of mice. Finally, in 1969, scientists at the National Hansen's Disease Center in Carville, Louisiana, found that the bacteria would grow in the tissues of the nine-banded armadillo. Several potential vaccines for leprosy have been tested since that time. One vaccine being tested is BCG, a live bacterial vaccine of the bacteria *Mycobacterium bovis*, which is a close relative of *M. leprae*. In four major trials with BCG, a range of 20 to 80 percent protection from leprosy was obtained. It is not known why there was such a wide variation in results. As of the early 1990's, 250,000 persons in Venezuela, Malawi, and India were undergoing a preventive vaccine trial using a combination of BCG and *M. leprae* from armadillos. Because it takes so long for the disease to appear, however, five to ten years must pass before it can be determined whether this vaccine is effective in preventing leprosy. Other strategies for vaccine development include making a modified BCG that contains *M. leprae* cell wall antigens. It is more advantageous to use BCG than *M. leprae* in a vaccine because BCG is much easier to grow. In addition, scientists are trying to find a way to grow *M. leprae* artificially so that larger quantities will be available to be used for a vaccine.

## PERSPECTIVE AND PROSPECTS

Leprosy is one of the oldest known diseases. References to leprosy are contained in Indian writings that are more than three thousand years old. The Bible refers to leprosy and the isolation of lepers, although the term refers to other skin diseases as well. The examination of ancient skeletons has provided insights into how leprosy spread in past centuries. Early evidence suggests that the disease was highly contagious and that leprosy was widespread in Europe during the Middle Ages. Leprosy was so prevalent, in fact, that both governments and churches moved to deal with the problem. At that time, the cause of leprosy was unknown, and the disease was generally believed to be a punishment for some personal sin. Lepers were treated as outcasts and required to shout "unclean." They were required to wear gloves and distinctive clothes and carry a bell or clapper to warn people of their approach. They were forbidden to drink from public fountains, speak loudly, eat with healthy people, or attend church. Some lepers were even pronounced legally dead, burned at the stake, or buried alive. Later, they were isolated in asylums called leprosaria, and at one time about nineteen thousand leprosaria existed—mostly in France. There was a sharp decrease in the number of leprosy cases in the sixteenth century. Several factors may have contributed to this decline, including the isolation of lepers, a better diet, warmer clothes, the plague epidemic, and the increase in tuberculosis, which may have provided resistance to leprosy. Leprosy is no longer as deadly or contagious as it once was, yet the stigma attached to this disease has remained. In an effort to alleviate the social stigma, the Fifth International Congress on Leprosy in 1948 banned the use of the word "leper" and encouraged the use of the term "Hansen's disease" instead of leprosy. *M. leprae*, the causative agent of leprosy, was first identified in the tissues of leprosy patients by the Norwegian physician Gerhard Armauer Hansen in 1873—hence the alternate name, Hansen's disease. Today, victims of leprosy are referred to as Hansenites or Hansenotic.

From the 1960's to the 1980's, estimates of the number of cases of leprosy worldwide ranged from 10 to 12 million. In 1992, the World Health Organization revised its estimate to 5.5 million cases. Efforts to promote multidrug therapy are believed to have caused the decline in the number of cases of leprosy. Leprosy is prevalent in tropical areas such as Africa, Southeast Asia, and South America. In the United States, most cases occur in Hawaii and small parts of Texas, California, Louisiana, and Florida. In 1987, the Centers for Disease Control reported approximately thirty new cases in the United States annually—mostly in foreign-born immigrants from leprosy-prone areas. —*Vicki J. Isola*

*See also* Bacterial infections; Numbness and tingling; Parasitic diseases; Tuberculosis.

## FOR FURTHER INFORMATION:

Bloom, B. R. "Learning from Leprosy: A Perspective on Immunology and the Third World." *Journal of Immunology* 137 (July, 1986): i-x. This article discusses leprosy as a disease, the immune response to leprosy, possible leprosy vaccines, and the problems of administering vaccines in the Third World.

Brody, S. N. *The Disease of the Soul: Leprosy in Medieval Literature*. Ithaca, N.Y.: Cornell University Press, 1974. This book discusses leprosy itself, social views of the disease, church views, and the impact of leprosy on literature.

Gaylord, H., and P. J. Brennan. "Leprosy and the Leprosy Bacillus." *Annual Review of Microbiology* 41 (1987): 645-675. This article focuses on the bacterium *M. leprae*, its structure, and the human immune system's response to the bacterium.

Hastings, Robert C., ed. *Leprosy*. Edinburgh: Churchill Livingstone, 1985. This book contains a series of articles describing all aspects of leprosy, from the characteristics of the organism to the disease process to treatment.

Mandell, G. L., R. G. Douglas, and J. E. Bennett, eds. *Principles and Practice of Infectious Diseases*. 2d ed. New York: John Wiley & Sons, 1985. W. E. Bullock describes leprosy on pages 1406 to 1413. Discusses the organism, epidemiology, symptoms, complications, and diagnosis; an expanded section on therapy is included.

Marriott, H. J. L. *Medical Milestones*. Baltimore: Williams & Wilkins, 1952. This book is about the historical development of medicine. Chapter 15, "If Anyone Touches a Leper," describes social attitudes toward lepers in the United States at the turn of the century and discusses the reform that took place as knowledge of the disease increased and drugs to treat leprosy were developed.

Richards, Peter. *The Medieval Leper and His Northern Heirs*. Totowa, N.J.: Rowman & Littlefield, 1977. Discusses the history of the treatment of lepers and the spread of leprosy throughout the world. Contains translations of medieval documents written by churches and governments concerning the treatment of lepers.

Zinsser, Hans. *Zinsser Microbiology*. Edited by Wolfgang Joklik et al. 19th ed. Norwalk, Conn.: Appleton and Lange, 1988. An excellent textbook describing all infectious diseases. The information presented is thorough and logical, and it is supplemented by interesting diagrams, photographs, and charts. Chapter 33, "Mycobacteria," discusses all diseases caused by species of mycobacteria, including leprosy and tuberculosis.

## Leukemia

**System affected:** Blood

**Specialists:** Hematologists, internists, toxicologists

**Definition:** A family of cancers that affect the blood, characterized by an increase in the number of white blood cells.

**Key terms:**

*bone marrow:* the tissue within bones that produces blood cells; in children, all bones have active marrow, but in adults, blood cell production occurs only in the trunk

*bone marrow transplant:* the removal of bone marrow from an immunologically matched individual for infusion into a patient whose bone marrow has been destroyed

*chemotherapy:* the use of drugs to kill rapidly growing cancer cells; this treatment will also kill some normal cells, producing undesirable side effects

*granulocytes:* white blood cells that generally help to fight bacterial infection; they are capable of passing from the blood capillaries into damaged tissues

*hematopoiesis:* the process by which blood cells develop in the bone marrow; this maturation is regulated by specific molecules called growth factors

*immune system:* the cells and organs of the body that fight infection; destruction of these cells leaves the body vulnerable to numerous diseases

*lymphocytes:* white blood cells that specifically target a foreign organism for destruction; the two classes of lymphocytes are B cells, which produce antibodies, and T cells, which kill infected cells

*oncogenes:* genes found in every cell which are capable of causing cancer if activated or mutated

### Causes and Symptoms

The blood is essential for all the physiological processes of the body. It is composed of red cells called erythrocytes, white cells called leukocytes, and platelets, each of which has distinct functions. Erythrocytes, which contain hemoglobin, are essential for the transport of oxygen from the lungs to all the cells and organs of the body. Leukocytes are important for protecting the body against infection by bacteria, viruses, and other parasites. Platelets play a role in the formation of blood clots; therefore, these cells are critical in the process of wound healing. Blood cell development, or hematopoiesis, begins in the bone marrow with immature stem cells that can produce all three types of blood cells. Under the influence of special molecules called growth factors, these stem cells divide rapidly and form blast cells that become one of the three blood cell types. After several further divisions, these blast cells ultimately

mature into fully functional erythrocytes, leukocytes, and platelets. In a healthy individual, the number of each type of blood cell remains relatively constant. Thus, the rate of new cell production is approximately equivalent to the rate of old cell destruction and removal.

Mature leukocytes are the key players in defending the body against infection. There are three types of leukocytes: monocytes, granulocytes, and lymphocytes. In leukemia, leukocytes multiply at an increased rate, resulting in an abnormally high number of white cells. All forms of leukemia are characterized by this abnormally regulated growth; therefore, leukemia is a cancer, even though tumor masses do not form. The cancerous cells live longer than the normal leukocytes and accumulate first in the bone marrow and then in the blood. Since these abnormal cells crowd the bone marrow, normal hematopoiesis cannot be maintained in a person with leukemia. The patient will usually become weak as a result of the lack of oxygen-carrying red cells and susceptible to bleeding because of a lack of platelets. The abnormal leukocytes do not function effectively in defending the body against infection, and they prevent normal leukocytes from developing; therefore, the patient is immunologically compromised. In addition, once the abnormal cells accumulate in the blood, they may hinder the functioning of other organs, such as the liver, kidney, lungs, and spleen.

It has become clear that leukemia, which was first recognized in 1845, is actually a pathology that comprises more than one disease. Leukemia has been divided into four main types, based on the type of leukocyte that is affected and the maturity of the leukocytes observed in the blood and the bone marrow. Both lymphocytes and granulocytes can be affected. When the cells are mainly immature blasts, the leukemia is termed acute, and when the cells are mostly mature, the leukemia is termed chronic. Therefore, the four types of leukemia are acute lymphocytic (ALL), acute granulocytic (AGL), chronic lymphocytic (CLL), and chronic granulocytic (CGL). The granulocytic leukemias are also known as myologenous leukemias (AML, CML) or nonlymphoid leukemias (ANLL, CNLL). These are the main types of leukemia, although there are additional rarer forms. These four forms of leukemia account for 5 percent of the cancer cases in the United States. The incidence of acute and chronic forms is approximately equivalent, but specific forms are more common at different stages of life. The major form in children is ALL; after puberty, there is a higher incidence of AGL. The chronic forms of leukemia occur in the adult population after the fourth or fifth decade of life, and men are twice as likely to be affected as women.

The causes of leukemia are still not completely understood, but scientists have put together many pieces of the puzzle. It is known that several environmental factors increase the risk of developing leukemia. Among these are exposure to radiation, chemicals such as chloramphenicol and benzene, and possibly viruses. In addition, there is a significant genetic component to this disease. Siblings of patients with leukemia have a higher risk of developing the disease, and chromosomal changes have been found in the cells of most patients, although they disappear when the patient is in remission. These different "causes" can be linked by understanding how oncogenes function. Every person, as part of his or her genetic makeup, has several oncogenes that are capable of causing cancer. In the healthy person, these oncogenes function in a carefully regulated manner to control cell growth. After exposure to an environmental or genetic influence that causes chromosome abnormalities, however, these oncogenes may become activated or deregulated so that uncontrolled cell growth occurs, resulting in the abnormally high number of cells seen in leukemia.

Leukemia is often difficult to diagnose in the early stages because the symptoms are similar to more common or less serious diseases. Cold symptoms, sometimes accompanied by fever, may be the earliest evidence of acute leukemia, and often in children the first symptoms may be less pronounced. The symptoms quickly become more pronounced as white cells accumulate in the lymph nodes, spleen, and liver, causing these organs to become enlarged. Fatigue, paleness, weight loss, repeated infections, and an increased susceptibility to bleeding and bruising are associated with leukemia. As the disease progresses, the fatigue and bleeding increase, various skin disorders develop, and the joints become painfully swollen. If untreated, the afflicted individual will die within a few months. Chronic leukemia has a more gradual progression and may be present for years before symptoms develop. When symptoms are present, they may be vague feelings of fatigue, fever, or loss of energy. There may be enlarged lymph nodes in the neck and armpits and a feeling of fullness in the abdomen because of an increase in the size of the spleen as much as tenfold. Loss of appetite and sweating at night may be initial symptoms. Often, chronic leukemia eventually leads to a syndrome resembling acute leukemia, which is ultimately fatal.

If these symptoms are present, a doctor will diagnose the presence of leukemia in two stages. First, blood will be drawn and a blood smear will be analyzed microscopically. This may indicate that there are fewer erythrocytes, leukocytes, and platelets than normal, and abnormal cells may be visible. A blood smear, however, may show only slight abnormalities, and the number of leukemic cells in the blood may not correspond to the extent of the disease in the bone marrow. This requires that the bone marrow itself be examined by means of a bone marrow biopsy. Bone marrow tissue can be obtained by inserting a needle into a bone such as the hip and aspirating a small sample of cells. This bone marrow biopsy, which is done under local anesthetic on an outpatient basis, is the definitive test for leukemia. Visual examination of the marrow usually reveals the presence of many abnormal cells, and this finding is

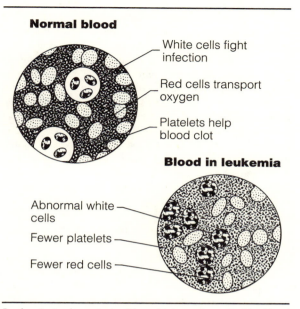

*Leukemia is characterized by a high number of white blood cells and a reduced number of red blood cells and platelets; also, abnormal cells may be visible.*

often confirmed with biochemical and immunological tests. After a positive diagnosis, a doctor will also examine the cerebrospinal fluid to see if leukemic cells have invaded the central nervous system.

### TREATMENT AND THERAPY

The treatment and life expectancy for leukemic patients varies significantly for each of the four types of leukemia. Treatment is designed to destroy all the abnormal cells and produce a complete remission, which is defined as the phase of recovery when the symptoms of the disease disappear and no abnormal cells can be observed in the blood or bone marrow. Unfortunately, a complete remission may only be temporary, since a small number of abnormal cells may still exist even though they are not observed under the microscope. These can, with time, multiply and repopulate the marrow, causing a relapse of the disease. With repeated relapses, the response to therapy becomes poorer and the durations of the remissions that follow become shorter. It is generally believed, however, that a remission that lasts five years in ALL, eight years in AGL, or twelve years in CGL may be permanent. Therefore, the goal of leukemia research is to develop ways to prolong remission.

By the time acute leukemia has been diagnosed, abnormal cells have often spread throughout the bone marrow and into several organs; therefore, surgery and radiation are usually not effective. Treatment programs include chemotherapy or bone marrow transplants or both. These treatments are aggressive and hazardous and are available only at specialized hospitals.

Chemotherapy is usually divided into several phases. In the first, or induction, phase, combinations of drugs are given to destroy all detectable abnormal cells and therefore induce a clinical remission. Vincristine, methrotrexate, 6-mercaptopurine, L-asparaginase, daunorubicin, prednisone, and cytosine arabinoside are among the drugs that are used. Combinations that selectively kill more leukemic cells than they do normal cells are available for the treatment of ALL; however, in AGL no selective agents are available, resulting in the destruction of equal numbers of diseased and healthy cells. An alternative strategy does not rely on destroying the abnormal cells, but instead seeks to induce immature leukemic cells to develop further. Once the cells are mature, they will no longer divide and will eventually die in the same way that a normal leukocyte does. Drugs such as cytarabine and retinoic acid have been tested, but the results are inconclusive.

Although the induction phase achieves clinical remission in more than 80 percent of patients, a second phase, called consolidation therapy, is essential to prevent relapse. Different combinations of anticancer drugs are used to kill any remaining cancer cells that were resistant to the drugs in the induction phase. Once the patient is in remission, higher doses of chemotherapy can be tolerated, and sometimes additional intensive treatments are given to reduce further the number of leukemic cells so that they will be unable to repopulate the tissues. During these phases of treatment, patients must be hospitalized. The destruction of their normal leukocytes along with the leukemic cells makes them very susceptible to infection. Their low numbers of surviving erythrocytes and platelets increase the probability of internal bleeding, and transfusions are often necessary. The dosages of chemotherapeutic agents must be carefully calculated to kill as many leukemic cells as possible without destroying so many normal cells that they cannot repopulate the marrow. In general, children handle intensive chemotherapy better than adults.

Following the induction and consolidation phases, maintenance therapy is sometimes used. In ALL, maintenance therapy is given for two to three years; however, its benefit in other forms of leukemia is a matter of controversy.

A second form of therapy is sometimes indicated for patients who have not responded to chemotherapy or are likely to relapse. Bone marrow transplantation has been increasingly used in leukemic patients to replace diseased marrow with normally functioning stem cells. In this procedure, the patient is treated with intensive chemotherapy and whole-body irradiation to destroy all leukemic and normal cells. Then a small amount of marrow from a normal donor is infused. The donor can be the patient himself, if the marrow was removed during a previous remission, or an immunologically matched donor, who is usually a sibling. If a sibling is not available, it may be possible to find a matched donor from the National Marrow Donor Program, which has on file approximately 350,000 people who have consented to be donors. Marrow is removed from the donor, broken up into small pieces, and given to the patient intravenously. The stem cells from the transplanted marrow circulate in the blood, enter the bones, and multiply. The first signs that the transplant is functioning normally occur in two to four weeks as the numbers of circulating granulocytes and platelets in the patient's blood increase. Eventually, in a successful transplant, the bone marrow cavity will be repopulated with normal cells.

Bone marrow transplantation is a dangerous procedure that requires highly trained caregivers. During this process, the patient is completely vulnerable to infection, since there is no functional immune system. The patient is placed in an isolation unit with special food-handling procedures. There is little chance that the patient will reject the transplanted marrow, because the immune system of the patient is suppressed. A larger problem remains, however, because it is possible for immune cells that existed in the donor's marrow to reject the tissues and organs of the patient. This graft-versus-host disease (GVHD) affects between 50 and 70 percent of bone marrow transplant patients. Even though the donor is immunologically matched, the match is not perfect, and the recently transplanted cells regard the cells in their new host as a "foreign" threat. Twenty percent of the patients who develop GVHD will die; therefore, drugs such as cyclophosphamide and cyclosporine, which suppress the immune system, are usually given to minimize this response. GVHD is not a problem if the donor is the patient. It is imperative, however, that marrow from the leukemic patient that has been removed during an earlier remission and frozen be treated to remove all leukemic cells before it is transplanted back into the patient.

Aggressive chemotherapy and bone marrow transplantation have dramatically increased the number of long-lasting remissions. For those who survive the therapy, it appears that, in ALL, approximately 60 percent of children and 35 percent of adults may be cured of the leukemia. The outlook for permanent remission is 10 to 20 percent in AGL and 65 percent for CGL patients. Statistics for chronic lymphocytic leukemia have been difficult to predict, because individual cases that have been similarly treated have had very different outcomes. The average lifespan after a diagnosis of CLL is three to four years; however, some patients live longer than fifteen years.

## PERSPECTIVE AND PROSPECTS

As the number of deaths from infectious disease has decreased, cancer has become the second most common cause of disease-related death. It is estimated that one of three people in the United States will develop a form of cancer and that the disease will kill one of five people. The search for causes and treatments of various cancers is perhaps the most active area of biological research today. Multiple lines of experimentation are being pursued, and significant advances have been made.

Leukemia is one of the cancers that scientists understand fairly well, but many unanswered questions remain. Leukemia research can be divided into two broad approaches. In the first, the researcher seeks to modify and improve the current methods for treatment: chemotherapy and bone marrow transplantation. In the second, an effort is being made to understand more about the disease itself, with the hope that completely different strategies for treatment might present themselves.

The risks involved in current therapy for leukemia have been discussed in the previous section. Treatment schedules, individually designed for each patient, will add to the understanding of how other physiological characteristics affect treatment outcome. Significant advances in reducing the risk of GVHD are likely to come quickly. In marrow transplants in which the donor is the patient, research is in progress to improve ways to screen out abnormal cells, even if they are present at very low levels, before they are infused back into the patient. In addition, for transplants in which the donor is not the patient, techniques that remove the harmful components of the bone marrow are being developed. Bone marrow cells can be partially purified, resulting in an enriched population of stem cells. Administering these to the leukemic patient should greatly reduce the risk of GVHD. Since bone marrow can be stored easily, the day may come when healthy people will store a bone marrow stem cell sample in case they contract a disease that would require a transplant.

Basic research in leukemia focuses on a simple question, "Why are leukemic cells different from normal cells?" This question is asked from a variety of perspectives in the fields of immunology, cell biology, and genetics. Immunologists are looking for markers on the surfaces of leukemic cells that would distinguish them from their normal counterparts. If such markers are found, it should be possible to target leukemic cells for destruction by using monoclonal antibodies attached to drugs. These "smart drugs" would be able to home in on the diseased cells, leaving normal cells untouched or only slightly affected. This would be a great advance for leukemia treatment, since much of the risk for the leukemic patient following chemotherapy or bone marrow transplant involves susceptibility to infection because the normal immune cells have been destroyed. Similarly, it may be possible to "teach" the patient's immune system to destroy abnormal cells that it had previously ignored.

Cell biologists are seeking to understand the normal hematopoietic process so that they can determine which steps of the process go awry in leukemia. Some of the growth factors involved in hematopoiesis have been identified, but it appears that the process is quite complex, and as yet scientists do not have a clear picture of normal hematopoiesis. When the understanding of the normal process becomes more complete, it may be possible to localize the defect in a leukemic patient and provide the missing growth factors. This might allow abnormal immature cells to complete the developmental process and relieve the symptoms of disease.

Geneticists are studying the chromosomal changes that underlie the onset of leukemia. As the oncogenes that are involved are identified, the reasons for their activation will also be determined. Once the effects of these genetic abnormalities are understood, it may be possible to intervene by genetically engineering stem cells so that they can develop normally.

These areas of research will likely converge to provide the leukemia treatments of the future. Leukemia is a cancer for which there is already a significant cure rate. It is not unreasonable to expect that this rate will approach 100 percent in the near future. —*Katherine B. Frederich*

*See also* Cancer; Malignancy and metastasis.

## FOR FURTHER INFORMATION:

Bair, Frank E., ed. *Cancer Sourcebook*. Detroit, Mich.: Omnigraphics, 1990. This extremely well-written volume provides the reader with a background against which to understand leukemia. Describes each of the four main types of leukemia in a straightforward and practical manner.

Bortin, M. M., et al. "Bone Marrow Transplantation for Acute Myelogenous Leukemia: Factors Associated with Early Mortality." *Journal of the American Medical Association* 249, no. 9 (March 4, 1983): 1166-1175. This article provides readable information on the types of risks involved in bone marrow transplantation.

Levine, A. S., ed. *Cancer in the Young*. New York: Masson, 1982. This volume contains reports by experts in the field that cover causes, symptoms, and treatments of childhood leukemia. Both lymphocytic and nonlymphocytic forms are addressed in language accessible to the layperson.

Margolies, Cynthia P., and Kenneth B. McCredie. *Understanding Leukemia*. New York: Charles Scribner's Sons, 1983. This book offers a very thorough discussion of leukemia, describing what the disease is and discussing what scientists know about its causes and treatment. In addition, a large section is devoted to helping patients and family members cope with the emotional stresses of leukemia.

# LICE, MITES, AND TICKS

**SYSTEM AFFECTED:** Skin

**SPECIALISTS:** Dermatologists, environmental medicine physicians, epidemiologists, public health specialists

**DEFINITION:** Parasites of human skin that may act as vectors of disease.

Although the term "lice" is applied to plant lice, such as psyllids and aphids in the order Homoptera, or chewing

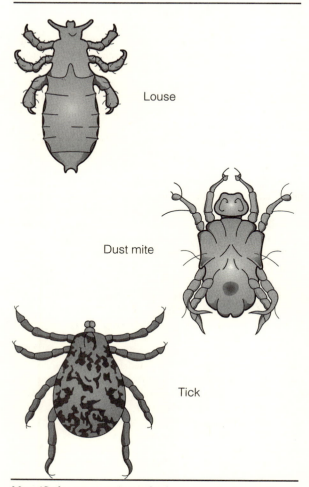

Louse

Dust mite

Tick

*Magnified representations of a louse, a mite (normally microscopic), and a tick.*

lice, as in the order Mallophaga, the medically important lice are the sucking lice in the order Anoplura. These lice are all surface parasites of mammals. Three types of lice found on humans pose serious medical problems and have changed the course of human history. Mites and ticks comprise the order Acarina, a subdivision of the class Arachnida that includes spiders, scorpions, and their relatives. There are mites or ticks that are ectoparasites of virtually all species of vertebrates above fish; several are serious vectors of human diseases.

*Lice.* The head louse *Pediculus humanus capitus* and the body louse *Pediculus humanus humanus* are considered variations of the same species, although they differ markedly in their habits. The head louse prefers the cooler region of the head and deposits its eggs on the hair shafts. The body louse prefers the warmth of the body, feeds from clothing (particularly where it wraps close to the body), and lays its

eggs in the seams of clothes. The head louse is usually spread by people sharing combs, brushes, and hats. The body louse is more often tossed aside with clothing and bedding, and the insect uses this opportunity to migrate. Both lice are relatively slender and are gray in color. The crab louse *Pthirus pubis* is shorter and crablike in appearance. Also called the pubic louse, it prefers the warmer climate of the pubic area or armpits and rarely ventures to the cooler regions of the body. The crab louse lays its eggs on the coarser hairs found in this region and migrates through physical contact or the use of infested blankets.

The occasional school outbreak of head lice may cause social concern and personal discomfort, but under conditions of poverty and wartime refugee crowding, it is the body louse that has been responsible for serious epidemics. Epidemic relapsing fever, epidemic typhus, and trench fever are all carried by this louse. The causative agents for these diseases are spirochetes and rickettsias. The spirochetes enter a louse when it feeds on an infected person, and the spiral organisms proliferate in the body of the louse. A new victim is infected when the louse is squashed and these fluids are ground into an open wound. The rickettsias are also acquired during a blood meal but are shed in the louse feces and infect a new host when the feces or squashed louse contaminates scratches. During World War I, louse-borne typhus took a terrible toll among undernourished civilian refugees and soldiers who were concentrated in unsanitary camps and trenches. In close quarters and with no bathing or change of clothes, people had no way to prevent the buildup of lice, and the fatality rate in World War I was higher from louse typhus than from armaments. World War II again brought refugees together in similar circumstances, but the use of the pesticide DDT prevented the extensive outbreaks of typhus and saved hundreds of thousands of lives.

*Mites and ticks.* The American dog tick *Dermacentor variabilis* is an example of a hard tick. A common pest of dogs, it is the principal vector of Rocky Mountain spotted fever. Larval ticks and adults of both sexes feed on blood and tissue secretions, although the female tick engorges itself when producing eggs. The lone star tick is a smaller hard tick of the southern United States and is implicated in the transmission of tularemia. Smaller still is the deer tick *Ixodes dammini*, which has spread westward in the United States and is a vector of Lyme disease. The soft-bodied ticks lack a hard, shieldlike back and infest birds or the ears of mammals. Because ticks feed on blood at all stages, and because some have developed the ability to pass disease agents across the ovary to offspring or from one larval stage to another across molting, ticks have evolved to vector many disease agents. Viruses carried by ticks cause encephalitis, hemorrhagic fever, and Colorado tick fever. In addition to Rocky Mountain spotted fever, ticks carry the rickettsias and bacteria that cause tick typhus, boutonneuse fever, relapsing fever, tularemia, and many cattle and horse diseases. Female ticks feeding near a person's neck can cause "tick paralysis," an unusual polio-like paralysis caused by a toxin in the saliva of some feeding ticks. Removal of the tick provides immediate relief.

Mites, mostly microscopic in size, are far more numerous than ticks. Some species transmit diseases, but mites can also cause dermatitis and, when they feed in large numbers, serious blood loss. The itch mite *Sarcoptes scabei* occurs worldwide and can cause rashes and lead to infection; varieties of the mite are responsible for mange in sheep, horses, dogs, and swine. Chigger mites provide an example of how microscopic female mites can cause considerable irritation by merely dissolving some surface skin. Mites are implicated as vectors of several serious diseases, including scrub typhus and Eastern hemorrhagic fever, a serious illness of troops during the Korean War. Cigar-shaped *Demodex* mites are responsible for red mange in dogs. Yet *Demodex folicularis*, the human follicle mite, is a perfectly harmless mite found in the eyelid follicles of most people, highlighting how closely related species have evolved into organisms of contrasting importance.

—*John Richard Schrock*

**See also** Arthropod-borne diseases; Bites and stings; Itching; Parasitic diseases; Typhoid fever and typhus.

**FOR FURTHER INFORMATION:**

Andrews, Michael. *The Life That Lives on Man.* New York: Taplinger, 1977. This well-illustrated book provides excellent visual images of the organisms that live on the surface of the human skin. Lice, mites, and ticks constitute a major portion of the book's content, but the structure of the skin and the role of bacterial and fungal agents are also featured.

McDaniel, Burruss. *How to Know the Mites and Ticks.* Dubuque, Iowa: Wm. C. Brown, 1979. This standard reference for identifying common mites and ticks offers ample drawings to help the beginner. Includes a brief discussion of their biology and their role as vectors for disease agents.

Zinsser, Hans. *Rats, Lice, and History.* London: G. Routledge & Sons, 1935. A classic story of how history was changed by insects.

# LIVER CANCER

**SYSTEM AFFECTED:** Liver

**SPECIALISTS:** Gastroenterologists, internists, oncologists, radiation oncologists

**DEFINITION:** Malignancies of the liver, which may be primary (arising in the organ itself) but are more likely to be secondary (metastasizing from another site).

## CAUSES AND SYMPTOMS

The liver filters the blood supply, removing and breaking down (metabolizing) toxins and delivering them through the biliary tract to the intestines for elimination with other wastes. Because of the large volume of blood flowing through the liver (about a quarter of the body's supply), blood-borne toxins or cancer cells migrating from tumors elsewhere (the process called metastasis) pose a constant threat. In fact, in the United States most liver cancers are metastatic; only about 1 percent actually originate in the liver. In Southeast Asia and sub-Saharan Africa, primary liver cancer is the most common type, accounting for as much as 30 percent of all cancers.

Two major types of cancer affect the liver: those involving liver cells (hepatocellular carcinomas) and those involving the bile ducts (cholangiocarcinomas). The first is by far the more common, although tumors may contain a mixture of both, and their development is similar. Tumors may arise in one location, forming a large mass; arise in several locations, forming nodes; or spread throughout the liver in a diffuse form. Liver cancers occur in men about four to eight times more frequently than in women and in blacks slightly more than in whites, although the proportions vary widely among different regions of the world. In the United States, most cancers arise in people fifty years old or older; in other areas, people older than forty are at risk.

Primary liver cancer has so much regional and gender variation because causative agents are more or less common in different areas and men are more often exposed. A leading risk factor in the United States and Europe is cirrhosis, a scarring of liver tissue following destruction by viruses, toxins, or interrupted blood flow. In the United States, long-term alcohol consumption is the most common cause of cirrhosis, and men have long been more likely than women to become alcoholics. Likewise, hemochromatosis, a hereditary disease leading to the toxic buildup of iron, is a cancer precursor and more common in men than in women. In Africa and Southeast Asia, the hepatitis B and C viruses are leading precancer diseases because hepatitis has long been endemic in those areas, whereas in the United States it is not widespread (although the number of infected people began to rise in the 1980's).

Diet and medical therapies have also been implicated as liver carcinogens. Food toxins, especially aflatoxin from mold growing on peanuts (which are a staple in parts of Africa and Asia); oral contraceptives; anabolic steroids; and the high levels of sex hormones used in some treatments are thought to increase the likelihood of hepatobiliary tumors. Genetic factors, radiation, and occupational exposure to volatile chemicals may also play a minor role.

Although researchers generally agree about which agents are liver cancer precursors, the exact mechanism leading to tumor development is not thoroughly understood. Nevertheless, one factor may be universal. Viruses and toxins injure or destroy liver and bile duct cells; the body reacts to repair the damage with inflammation and an increased rate of new cell growth, a condition called regenerative hyperplasia. If the toxin damage continues, triggering ever

## Liver Cancer

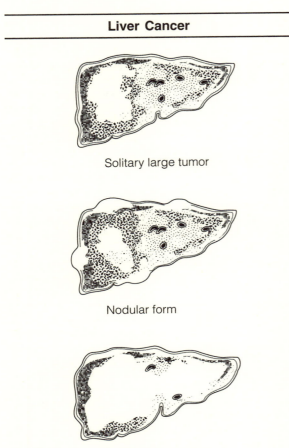

Solitary large tumor

Nodular form

Diffuse growth

*The liver is a frequent site of cancer, most commonly from malignancies that have spread from their original site. The particular form the cancer takes depends on several factors, notably the primary source and its possible cause.*

more hyperplasia, as is the case with hepatitis and alcoholic cirrhosis, formation of a tumor becomes almost inevitable.

Like lymph nodes, the liver collects migrating cancer cells, so the cancers that physicians detect there often are metastases from cancers arising elsewhere in the body. In fact, liver involvement may be found before the primary cancer has been recognized. Colorectal cancer is especially given to metastasizing to the liver, since the digestive tract's blood supply is directly linked to the liver through the portal vein; similarly, lung and breast cancer may spread to the liver. Such metastases indicate advanced cancers that do not bode well for the patient's survival.

Symptoms may be ambiguous. Two common symptoms are jaundice and enlargement of the liver, with accompanying tenderness. Jaundice, a yellowing of the skin and eyes, is caused by an accumulation of bilirubin. Bilirubin builds up because a tumor has blocked the bile duct that normally empties it into the small intestine. (Both symptoms may also occur as a result of either gallstones or cirrhosis.) Patients with liver cancer may also have a fever and retain fluid in the abdominal cavities.

### TREATMENT AND THERAPY

Doctors suspecting liver cancer conduct tests designed to distinguish this disease from other disorders. Palpation of the liver may reveal that the organ is enlarged or contains an unusual tissue mass, which is likely to be a tumor. A rubbing sound heard through the stethoscope may also come from a tumor. Hepatocellular carcinoma often elevates the alpha-fetoprotein level in blood. Abdominal ultrasound or computed tomography (CT) scans can provide good evidence of a tumor in the liver, and a biopsy will supply a tissue sample capable of proving the presence of cancer, especially if the biopsy is done with CT scan or ultrasound guidance. A tumor can also disrupt normal biochemical action in the body, which doctors may detect in blood tests. Liver function blood tests may be abnormal with both primary and secondary liver cancer.

Under even the most favorable circumstances, the outlook for patients with liver cancer is still not good. If a primary cancer is found while still fairly small, surgical removal is the surest and fastest treatment, although it is a difficult, risky procedure because of the liver's complex, delicate structure. Radiation and chemotherapy have not succeeded in shrinking tumors effectively. Because symptoms usually appear late in the development of primary liver cancer, it seldom is found early enough for surgical cure; patients usually live only one to two months after detection. Those found with small, removable cancers live an average of twenty-nine months. Most liver cancers are metastases, however, and removal of the liver tumor will not rid the patient of cancer. In general, hepatobiliary cancer patients have a 5 percent chance of living five years after diagnosis.

Liver cancer screening tests can locate tumors while they are still treatable, although routine physical examinations in Western nations seldom include such tests. Usually only patients with cirrhosis or chronic hepatitis are screened. The best ways to ward off liver cancer are to avoid viral infection and to abstain from alcohol. For those at risk for infection, such as health care workers, the most effective primary prevention is vaccination for hepatitis B.

—*Roger Smith*

***See also*** Alcoholism; Cancer; Cirrhosis; Hepatitis; Jaundice; Liver disorders; Malignancy and metastasis.

### FOR FURTHER INFORMATION:

Renneker, Mark, ed. *Understanding Cancer*. 3d ed. Palo Alto, Calif.: Bull, 1988.

Sachar, David B., Jerome D. Waye, and Blair S. Lewis. *Pocket Guide to Gastroenterology*. Rev. ed. Baltimore: Williams & Wilkins, 1991.

Steen, R. Grant. *A Conspiracy of Cells: The Basic Science of Cancer*. New York: Plenum Press, 1993.

# LIVER DISORDERS

**SYSTEM AFFECTED:** Liver

**SPECIALISTS:** Gastroenterologists, internists

**DEFINITION:** As one of the most complex organs in the body, the liver is the target of a wide variety of toxins, infectious agents, and cancers that lead to hepatitis, cirrhosis, abscesses, and liver failure.

**KEY TERMS:**

*abscess:* a localized collection of pus and infectious microorganisms

*ascites:* the presence of free fluid in the abdominal cavity

*bilirubin:* a major component of bile, derived from the breakdown products of red blood cells

*cirrhosis:* the fibrous scar tissue that replaces the normally soft liver after repeated damage by viruses, chemicals, and/or alcohol

*hepatitis:* inflammation of the liver, such as that caused by viruses or toxins

*jaundice:* a yellow discoloration of the skin, eyes, and membranes caused by excess bilirubin in the blood

*portal hypertension:* elevated pressures in the portal veins caused by resistance to blood flow through a diseased liver; produces many regional problems, including ascites

*portal system:* a system of veins, unique to the liver, that carry nutrient-rich blood from the digestive organs to the liver

## CAUSES AND SYMPTOMS

The liver is the largest internal organ, lying in the upper-right abdominal cavity. Intricately attached to it by a system of ducts on its lower surface is the pear-shaped gallbladder. Unique to the liver is its blood supply that derives from two separate sources: the hepatic artery, carrying freshly oxygenated blood from the heart, and the portal vein, carrying blood rich in the products of digestion from the digestive organs. The liver cells, or hepatocytes, are arranged in thin sheets that are separated by large pores, blood vessels, and ducts. The result is a very soft, spongy organ filled with a large volume of blood.

The liver performs a wide variety of complex and diverse functions, more so than any other organ. Most commonly known is the production of bile, which is formed from the breakdown of red blood cells, cholesterol, and salts; stored in the gallbladder; and used in the small intestine to digest fats. The liver also serves that all-important purpose of detoxification by chemically altering harmful substances such as alcohol, drugs, and ammonia from protein digestion. Additionally, the liver is involved in the formation of such essential materials as blood proteins, blood-clotting factors, and sugar and fat storage compounds.

Because of the liver's many responsibilities and unique position as an intermediary between the digestive process and the blood (via the portal vein), it easily falls prey to many disease-causing agents. Chemicals, illegal drugs, al-

cohol, viruses, parasites, hormones, and even medical drugs can damage the liver and have widespread effects on the rest of the body. The liver is also the most frequent target of cancer cells that have spread beyond their primary site. In the United States and other industrialized countries, liver disease is usually related to alcoholism and cancer, while in Third World countries it is often the result of infectious contamination by viruses and parasites.

There are two simplified methods of classifying liver disorders: The first is based on cause: infections (viruses and parasites), injury (alcohol and other toxins), inheritance (inability to perform certain functions), infiltration (iron and copper deposits), and tumors (both benign and malignant). The second method of classification is based on the result: hepatitis (infections), cirrhosis (injury from alcohol or other toxins), and cancer, for example.

Each of these liver diseases produces a particular set of signs and symptoms depending on the length of time and the specific disruption of structure and function. Pain and swelling rarely occur alone and are usually associated with one or more of the following: nausea and vomiting, jaundice, ascites, blood-clotting defects, and encephalopathy. Indeed, in some cases liver failure ensues, leading to coma and death.

Jaundice, a yellow discoloration of the skin and whites (sclera) of the eyes, is caused by the secretion of bile precursors (bilirubin) from the damaged liver cells directly into the blood rather than into the ducts leading to the gallblad-

## Liver Disorders

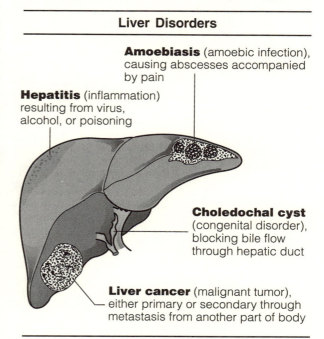

**Amoebiasis** (amoebic infection), causing abscesses accompanied by pain

**Hepatitis** (inflammation) resulting from virus, alcohol, or poisoning

**Choledochal cyst** (congenital disorder), blocking bile flow through hepatic duct

**Liver cancer** (malignant tumor), either primary or secondary through metastasis from another part of body

*The liver's unique structure and functions leave it vulnerable to a wide range of diseases.*

der. Consequently, bilirubin accumulates in the body's tissues, including the skin and eyes. Ascites, the collection of fluid beneath the liver in the abdomen, is an important sign of liver disease. This fluid comes primarily from the portal vein system, which lies between the liver and the digestive organs. As the liver becomes congested and enlarged in response to injury or infection, blood flow becomes difficult and pressure begins to build, causing liquid to leak from the blood vessels into the abdominal cavity. Easy bruising, excessive bleeding, and other problems with blood clotting are important signs that reflect the failure of the liver to produce essential blood proteins. Neuropsychiatric symptoms such as a flapping hand tremor and encephalopathy (a state of mental confusion and disorientation that can quickly progress to coma) are not well understood, but it is likely that they result from an accumulation of toxic substances that would normally be cleared from the blood by the liver. Several other problems, such as the enlargement of male breasts, atrophy of the testicles, and other sexual changes, derive from the inability of the liver to clear the blood of hormones.

Hepatitis, an inflammation of the liver generally caused by viruses, is one of the most common diseases in the world. Hepatitis A and B, Epstein-Barr virus (the causative agent of mononucleosis), and herpes are a few of the organisms that can infect the liver. Hepatitis A, transmitted through contaminated food, water, and shellfish, is usually a self-limited disease that resolves itself. Hepatitis B, transmitted through contact with infected blood and body secretions, is much more serious, with a carrier state, progressive organ damage, cancer, and death as possible sequelae. Noninfectious causes of hepatitis in susceptible people include

## Signs and Symptoms of Liver Disease

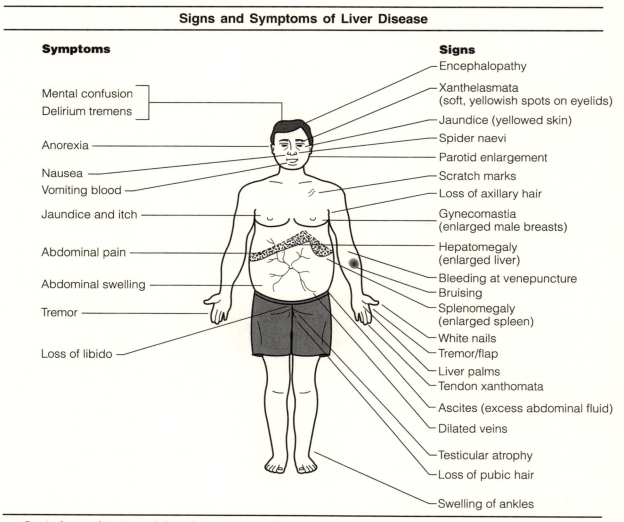

**Symptoms**

Mental confusion
Delirium tremens
Anorexia
Nausea
Vomiting blood
Jaundice and itch
Abdominal pain
Abdominal swelling
Tremor
Loss of libido

**Signs**

Encephalopathy
Xanthelasmata
(soft, yellowish spots on eyelids)
Jaundice (yellowed skin)
Spider naevi
Parotid enlargement
Scratch marks
Loss of axillary hair
Gynecomastia
(enlarged male breasts)
Hepatomegaly
(enlarged liver)
Bleeding at venepuncture
Bruising
Splenomegaly
(enlarged spleen)
White nails
Tremor/flap
Liver palms
Tendon xanthomata
Ascites (excess abdominal fluid)
Dilated veins
Testicular atrophy
Loss of pubic hair
Swelling of ankles

*Particular combinations of these factors can provide clues to both the diagnosis and the extent of liver damage.*

such frequently used substances as acetaminophen (Tylenol), halothane (general anesthesia), and oral contraceptives.

Cirrhosis is the result of continuous toxic exposure that injures the liver beyond repair. Fibrous scar tissue replaces the normally soft, spongy organ, making it small and firm, with few hepatocytes capable of functioning normally. Chronic alcohol abuse is by far the most frequent factor in the development of cirrhosis. Severe ascites, bleeding disorders, encephalopathy, and sex organ changes often herald imminent liver failure and death from this disease.

Liver cancer is most often secondary to malignancies that have spread from other sites. In Asia and Africa, primary tumors of the liver itself are much more common, in part because of several factors: a high incidence of hepatitis B infection, food toxins, and parasite infestation. Chronic injury appears to play the critical role in liver cancer; hence the risk factors that have been established are cirrhosis, hepatitis B, and long-term exposure to a variety of chemicals, hormones, and drugs. Benign tumors may occur in young women who use oral contraceptives, but they are relatively infrequent.

Several other hepatic diseases warrant mention. Liver abscesses, encapsulated areas filled with infectious material, can be caused by bacteria, fungi, and parasites. These organisms enter the bloodstream through ingestion, skin puncture, or even intestinal rupture (as occurs in appendicitis and diverticulitis), and travel to the liver. Two unusual but notable disorders of iron and copper metabolism—hemochromatosis and Wilson's disease, respectively—have prominent liver involvement. While the disease mechanisms are not well understood, these essential metals are retained in excess and deposited in body tissues in toxic levels, causing damage. Finally, several genetic disorders of bile production run the gamut from mere nuisances to death in infancy. Disruption in bilirubin metabolism, the handling of red blood cell waste products by incorporation into bile, is affected to varying degrees. Severe jaundice reflects the accumulation of toxic levels of bilirubin in all body tissues, including the brain.

### TREATMENT AND THERAPY

The diagnosis of a patient with suspected liver disease occurs in an orderly process that begins with a thorough history and physical examination, supported by a number of valuable blood tests and imaging techniques. Liver biopsy, the obtaining of a tissue sample for microscopic analysis, is often a final and definitive procedure if the disorder remains ambiguous. Both the cause and the chronology or state of the disease (whether of recent onset or advanced) determine treatment and outcome. While many signs and symptoms are nonspecific—nausea, vomiting, pain, hepatic enlargement, and jaundice—others such as ascites, encephalopathy, blood-clotting defects, and sex organ changes reflect significant organ damage and an advanced

stage of disease. Careful questioning of the recent and past history of a patient can elicit facts that point to a diagnosis: exposure to known liver toxins such as alcohol, anesthetics, certain medications, and occupational chemicals; travel to countries with known contaminated water supplies (hepatitis A); blood transfusions, kidney dialysis, sexual promiscuity, or intravenous drug abuse (hepatitis B); weight loss that is unexplained (cancer); or even a history of gallstones (blocked bile ducts between the liver and gallbladder). Armed with suspicions from the history, the physician uses the physical examination to note signs that confirm or reject the possibilities. A small and firm liver with ascites, tremor, enlarged male breasts, and small, shrunken testicles all point to an advanced stage of cirrhosis, for example. An enlarged painful liver, with vomiting, jaundice, fever, and recent raw shellfish ingestion, would likely suggest hepatitis A.

Blood tests play the second critical role in evaluating liver disease. An elevated bilirubin level would correlate with the severity of jaundice. Blood protein levels (albumin) and blood-clotting factors (prothrombin) may be dangerously low, revealing a near inability of the hepatocytes to synthesize these vital substances. Special chemicals that exist primarily in liver cells (hepatic enzymes and the aminotransferases) may be quite high, as the cells die and release their contents into the blood. Finally, elevated white blood cell counts and special tests for individual infections (viruses, bacteria, fungi, and parasites) can positively establish the diagnosis.

Depending on the suspected disease, confirmation may be needed from various imaging techniques, chosen specifically for a particular diagnosis. Plain X rays do little to visualize the liver, although they can reveal air in the abdomen, a consequence of a perforated intestine, appendix, or ulcer. A much more advanced method, the computed tomography (CT) scan, combines computer-generated views of multiple cross-sectional X rays, providing a highly detailed examination of the liver and thereby establishing a diagnosis in the majority of cases. Two other techniques that have more specific uses are ultrasound, which uses sound wave transmission, and magnetic resonance imaging (MRI), which uses magnetic fields to create an image. Ultrasound can readily distinguish solid masses from those that are fluid-filled (tumors versus abscesses) and can view the bile ducts. MRI is quite helpful in determining blood flow problems such as portal hypertension.

Finally, if a precise diagnosis remains ambiguous, a biopsy is performed. A sample of liver tissue is obtained using a large needle inserted through the skin, under the guidance of an ultrasound image. The sample is then viewed microscopically, and both the cause and the extent of liver damage are readily apparent.

Treatment options for the majority of liver diseases are few, and often little can be done beyond symptomatic relief and supportive care. For example, if drug toxicity is suspected, especially from alcohol, immediate withdrawal of the agent can prevent further damage, as has been shown in cirrhosis. Obstructing gallstones can be surgically removed to relieve pressure in the bile ducts. Combinations of surgery, radiation, and chemotherapy are used in liver cancer, but the prognosis is poor. Little can be done for the inherited diseases of bilirubin metabolism, while some success has been achieved in treating the iron and copper storage diseases. Infections of viral origin have no effective antibiotic treatment, but the prevention of hepatitis A and B is possible if pooled serum immunoglobulin is given immediately after exposure. This substance is a concentrated form of antibodies obtained from infected individuals whose diseases have completely resolved; essentially, it is a method of giving passive immunity. One area in which effective treatment does exist is in bacterial, fungal, and parasitic infections and abscesses. Appropriate antibiotics and surgical drainage yield dramatic improvement in most cases.

In the majority of cases of liver disease, symptom relief and nutritional support, often carried out in the hospital, are the only options. Pain relief and the administration of intravenous fluid and nutrients to counteract vomiting and dehydration are the first steps. Ascites is relieved through bed rest, salt restriction, and paracentesis, a procedure that uses ultrasound to guide a needle into the abdomen and withdraw fluid. Attempts to correct encephalopathy by removing toxins such as ammonia from the blood are generally ineffective, and mental changes, along with other intractable symptoms, often herald complete liver failure and imminent death.

Clearly, preventive measures are the most important factor in liver disease. One effective measure that is widely available is the hepatitis B vaccine, which is recommended for anyone at high risk of contracting the virus. A three-injection series is suggested for health care personnel, kidney dialysis patients, sexually promiscuous people, and anyone else who is frequently in contact with blood and body secretions.

## PERSPECTIVE AND PROSPECTS

Little in the field of hepatology is as exciting or hopeful as liver transplantation, the replacement of the diseased organ by a normal, donated one. Begun experimentally in the early 1960's after decades of low success rates (less than 20 percent), it has finally been accepted as a life-saving operation, with survival rates exceeding 60 percent at five years. Technical improvements, especially intraoperative blood circulation and cadaver organ preservation, have been combined with advances in immunosuppressive therapy that counteracts rejection and refined patient selection and timing. The result is that liver transplantation has become the method of choice for patients whose liver disease is life-threatening, progressive, and unresponsive to other treatments.

Specific guidelines exist for both children and adults to be considered candidates for the procedure. It is imperative that the person is otherwise healthy and that the heart, lungs, kidneys, and brain are functioning well. Malignancy, human immunodeficiency virus (HIV) infection, incorrectable congenital defects, and continuing drug or alcohol abuse are obvious contraindications. On the other hand, infants with inherited, inevitably fatal liver disorders are good candidates, as are adults with end-stage liver failure from chronic hepatitis, for example. Controversial indications, requiring case-by-case evaluation, include advanced viral hepatitis (as recurrent infection in the donated organ often occurs) and alcohol-induced cirrhosis (because of the likelihood of damage to other organs and the high relapse rate after surgery). Relapse is also very common if the transplantation is done for a primary liver cancer.

Careful donor selection is equally important. The principal source of cadaver organs is victims of head trauma who are declared brain-dead. Organs are accepted from those sixty years of age or younger who had no viral, bacterial, or fungal infections and who were otherwise healthy up to the time of death. In the United States, recipient-donor matches are made through a nationwide organ transplantation registry, with highest priority going to those most critically ill. Only twelve to eighteen hours can elapse between organ retrieval and implantation—beyond that, liver tissue begins to degenerate.

The use of immunosuppressive therapy, drugs that keep the recipient's immune system in check, has contributed significantly to success and survival. Rejection of the transplanted organ remains one of the most feared postoperative complications, along with hemorrhaging. Because the body recognizes the organ as foreign tissue, the immune system's white blood cells attack and damage the implanted donor liver. The use of drugs to counteract this process allows the new liver to heal and the body to adapt to the presence of foreign tissue. Despite the use of these potent drugs, which themselves have serious side effects, rejection continues to be a problem. Nevertheless, one-year survival rates approach 85 percent, and at five years, nearly 60 percent of transplant patients are alive. —*Connie Rizzo*

*See also* Alcoholism; Cirrhosis; Hepatitis; Jaundice; Liver cancer.

## FOR FURTHER INFORMATION:

Fishman, Mark, et al. *Medicine*. 3d ed. Philadelphia: J. B. Lippincott, 1991. This excellent soft cover text is the perfect place to start. Used by medical students and other health professionals, it is clear and understandable, exploring normal biology and the process of disease. The section on gastroenterology has several chapters devoted to liver disorders.

Wyngaarden, James, Lloyd H. Smith, Jr., and J. Claude Bennett. *Cecil's Textbook of Medicine*. 19th ed. Philadelphia: W. B. Saunders, 1992. This bible of internal medicine has a superb section on liver diseases that is somewhat difficult but so well written and thorough that it is worth the effort. The text is well supplemented with diagrams and photographs.

Yamada, Todataka, et al. *Textbook of Gastroenterology.* Philadelphia: J. B. Lippincott, 1991. The reference text used by specialists in the field, covering all aspects of the digestive system. A large section is devoted to the liver and gallbladder.

Zakim, David, and Thomas D. Boyer. *Hepatology: A Textbook of Liver Disease.* 2d ed. Philadelphia: W. B. Saunders, 1990. This extraordinary book is devoted entirely to the liver, with wonderful photographic atlases accompanying each disease. The text is difficult, as it is highly detailed, and should only be read after other, more comprehensive books have been used. The section on liver transplantation is first-rate.

# Lockjaw. *See* Tetanus.

# Lou Gehrig's disease. *See* Motor neuron disorders.

# Lumps, breast. *See* Breast cancer; Breast disorders.

# Lung cancer

**System affected:** Respiratory
**Specialists:** Internists, occupational medicine physicians, oncologists, pulmonologists, radiation oncologists
**Definition:** The appearance of malignant tumors in the lungs, which is usually associated with cigarette smoking.

### Causes and Symptoms

Most forms of lung cancer fall within one of four categories: squamous cell (or epidermoid) carcinomas and adenocarcinomas (each of which accounts for approximately 30 percent of all pulmonary cancers), small or oat cell carcinomas (accounting for about 25 percent of lung cancers), and large cell carcinomas (which represent about 15 percent of lung cancers). Each of these forms can be further categorized on the basis of cell differentiation within the tumor: either well differentiated (resembling the original cell type) or moderately or poorly differentiated. Upon biopsy, stage groupings are also determined on the basis of size, invasiveness, and possible extent of metastasis.

Oat or small cell carcinomas usually consist of small, tightly-packed, spindle-shaped cells, with a high nucleus-to-cytoplasm ratio within the cell. Oat cell carcinomas tend to metastasize early and widely, often to the bone marrow or brain. As a result, by the time that symptoms become apparent, the disease is generally widely disseminated within the body. Coupled with a resistance to most common forms of radiation and chemotherapy, oat cell carcinomas present a particularly poor prognosis. In general, patients diagnosed with this form of cancer have a survival period measured, at most, in months.

Adenocarcinomas are tumors of glandlike structure, presenting as nodules within peripheral tissue such as the bronchioles. Often these forms of tumors may arise from previously damaged or scarred tissue, such as has occurred among smokers. The development of adenocarcinoma of the lung is not as dependent upon smoke inhalation, however, as are other forms of lung cancer.

Squamous cell, also called epidermoid, carcinomas tend to be slower-growing malignancies which form among the flat epithelial cells on the surface of a variety of tissues, including the bladder, cervix, or skin, in addition to the lung. The cells are often polygonal in shape, with keratin nodes on the surface of lesions. Squamous cell carcinomas tend to metastasize less frequently than other forms of lung cancer, allowing for a more optimistic prognosis as compared to other forms.

Large cell carcinomas are actually a more general form of cancer in which the cells are relatively large in size, with the cell nucleus being particularly enlarged. Often these carcinomas have arisen as either squamous cell carcinomas or adenocarcinomas. Metastasis, when it occurs, is frequently within the gastrointestinal tract.

There is no question that the single leading cause or factor resulting in lung cancer is smoking. Persons who do not smoke, and indeed even smokers who smoke fewer than five cigarettes per day, are at relatively low risk of developing any form of lung cancer. Those who smoke more than five cigarettes per day run an increased risk of developing lung cancer at rates approaching two hundred times that of the nonsmoker. This risk is greatest for oat cell carcinomas and least for adenocarcinomas (but still approximately a tenfold risk over that for nonsmokers). The relative risk is related to the number of cigarettes smoked: The more cigarettes, the greater the risk. In addition, though other environmental hazards can be related to the development of lung cancers, the risk associated with those hazards is without exception amplified by cigarette smoke.

Exposure to other specific environmental factors has also been associated with the formation of certain forms of pulmonary cancers. Individuals chronically exposed to materials such as asbestos, hydrocarbon products (coal tars or roofing materials), nickel, vinyl chloride, or radiochemicals (uranium and pitchblende) are at increased risk. Chronically damaged lungs, for whatever reason, are at significantly increased risk for development of cancer.

The symptoms of lung cancer may represent the damage caused by the primary tumor or may be the result of metastasis to other organs. The most common symptom is a persistent cough, sometimes accompanied by blood in the sputum or difficulty breathing. Chest pain may be present, especially upon inhalation. There may also be repeated attacks of bronchitis or pneumonia that tend to persist for abnormal periods of time.

## TREATMENT AND THERAPY

Diagnosis of a tumor in the lung generally includes a chest X ray, along with use of a variety of diagnostic tests: bronchography (X-ray observation of the bronchioles following application of an opaque material), tomography (cross-sectional observation of tissue), and cytologic examination of sputum or bronchiole washings. Confirmation of the diagnosis, in addition to determination of the specific type of tumor and its clinical stage, generally requires a needle biopsy of material from the lung.

The treatment of the tumor is dependent on the form of the disease and on the extent of its spread. Surgery remains the preferred method of treatment, but because of the nature of the disease, less than half the cases are operable at the time of diagnosis. Of these, a large proportion are beyond the point at which the surgical removal of the cancer and resection of remaining tissue are possible. A variety of chemotherapeutic measures are available and along with the use of radiation therapy can be used to produce a small number of cures or at least temporary alleviation of symptoms. Nevertheless, only a small proportion of lung cancers, perhaps 10 percent, respond with a permanent remission or cure.

Lung cancer represents the leading cause of cancer deaths among American men and the second leading cause of cancer deaths among American women. By the 1990's, however, lung cancer was gaining among women and was poised to surpass breast cancer as the major cause of cancer deaths for this group. Each year, between 150,000 and 175,000 new cases of lung cancer are diagnosed in the United States, with about 50,000 deaths. The prognosis for most forms of lung cancer remains poor.    —*Richard Adler*

*See also* Addiction; Cancer; Malignancy and metastasis; Tumors.

### FOR FURTHER INFORMATION:

Patterson, James T. *The Dread Disease: Cancer and Modern American Culture*. Cambridge, Mass.: Harvard University Press, 1987. A general text dealing with all major forms of cancer.

Steen, R. Grant. *A Conspiracy of Cells: The Basic Science of Cancer*. New York: Plenum Press, 1993. Provides a fine discussion on a variety of factors which cause cancers to develop.

Williams, C. J. *Lung Cancer: The Facts*. 2d ed. Oxford, England: Oxford University Press, 1992. A work that deals specifically with pulmonary cancer.

# LUNG DISEASES. *See* PULMONARY DISEASES.

# LUPUS ERYTHEMATOSUS

**SYSTEMS AFFECTED:** Connective tissue, skin

**SPECIALISTS:** Dermatologists, immunologists, internists, nephrologists

**DEFINITION:** A chronic inflammation of connective tissue that may prove fatal if it becomes systemic and spreads to the kidneys. Known popularly as lupus, but not to be confused with a variety of unrelated diseases with this name—especially lupus vulgaris, a form of tuberculosis; these diseases share only the symptoms of red or purple lesions appearing on the face.

**KEY TERMS:**

*antigen:* a protein in the blood serum which represents foreign material detrimental to the body; the presence of antigens results in the manufacture of other serum proteins (antibodies) that attack the foreign material in an attempt to protect the system

*autoimmunity:* sensitivity to one's own body in which antibodies may attack some of the body's cells

*edema:* the collection of serous fluid in the spaces between cell structures or body cavities

*etiology:* the physical basis of a disease, especially its medical study

*L.E. cell:* a white blood cell that has destroyed the nucleus of another white blood cell and shows particular staining characteristics

*leukocyte:* a white blood cell; these cells are vital in the body's defenses against disease

*nucleic acids:* very large molecules that control the synthesis of proteins and carry basic information determining heredity

*phagocytosis:* the process in which white blood cells destroy bacteria and other unwanted components of body fluids

*tuberculosis:* a large family of diseases which may affect virtually any of the tissues of the body

## CAUSES AND SYMPTOMS

It is essential that a careful distinction be made among several diseases known by the same popular name of lupus. For example, lupus erythematosus and lupus vulgaris are radically different from each other yet share one highly visible symptom—a red rash often limited to the face. In the nineteenth century, it was observed that the rash leads to extensive, ragged deterioration of structures beneath the skin of the face in the vulgaris form. This early diagnostic confusion and the similarity of its manifestation on the face to an attack by a hungry animal produced the alarming designation of "lupus" (meaning "wolf").

The most striking difference between these two most common forms of lupus is their relationship to sunlight. This subject is of significance in a discussion of their treatment and management. A second important distinction is the frequency of occurrence. Lupus vulgaris is essentially of historical interest because it is actually a well-described form of tuberculosis that can now be cured. Lupus erythematosus, however, has no known etiology and remains a significant area of research.

A fascinating, and maddening, aspect of lupus erythematosus lies in its huge array of manifestations. Typically, the physician sees a patient who complains of aches and pains in the joints. Often this symptom is accompanied by swollen and inflamed joints. The joints of the hands are the usual site, but sometimes the elbows, wrists, hips, knees, or ankles are affected; other joints are not. Bones too are rarely involved in cases eventually diagnosed as lupus. Along with fatigue and low-grade fever, these symptoms are found in approximately 90 percent of lupus patients. Sensitivity to sunlight is often reported.

Efforts to understand the disease, and especially to facilitate correct and early diagnosis, have produced well documented lists of typical symptoms together with their frequency of occurrence. The characteristic "butterfly rash" that led to the earliest description of lupus erythematosus is found in less than half of the cases studied. In the 1970's and 1980's, the American Rheumatism Association compiled a list of common symptoms as a result of a massive survey of experts in the diagnosis of lupus. The original list of about sixty signs was studied for specificity in differentiating this condition from others with similar symptoms. The number of criteria was reduced to fourteen, and it was concluded by the committee of physicians that a patient must show at least four to establish lupus as the condition under treatment.

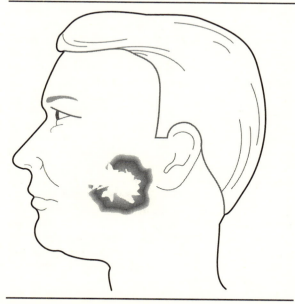

*Lupus erythematosus and lupus vulgaris are radically different from each other yet often share the symptom of a red rash on the face; however, this rash does not occur in all cases. In lupus erythematosus, the rash may be a circular, thickened, reddened area with white scar tissue in the center. More typically, those suffering from lupus erythematosus complain of aches and pains in the joints, fatigue, and low-grade fever.*

While such studies are of immense importance in diagnosis and in directing further study of the disease, they also point out how inadequate understanding remains. For example, it is not known why women are afflicted more than ten times as often as men; why, among women, African Americans are three or perhaps more times as frequently diagnosed, or why several studies have shown higher incidence or mortality rates among Asians. These unsolved pieces of the puzzle remain intriguing clues, but they lack solid ties to the root causes of lupus erythematosus.

In 1948, Malcolm M. Hargraves and his colleagues at the Mayo Clinic made an important discovery related to lupus. Microscopic study of properly stained bone marrow material revealed a particular type of white blood cell called a polymorphonuclear leukocyte. This imposing name denotes one of the most important advances in lupus research. In plain language, Hargraves found cells with more than one collection of nuclear substance because one cell has, in essence, destroyed the nucleus of another. They designated this process with the elegant term "aberrant phagocytosis."

From this key observation came a blood test which, while not foolproof, is of significance in diagnosing lupus. The new direction suggested was even more important, proven by the fact that present research continues to progress along the same lines. It is well established that the body protects itself against disease-causing organisms through a system of antigen-antibody reactions. An example can be seen in the immunity of the body after a case of measles or vaccination against that virus.

In the late 1950's, a class of antibodies that act against the nuclear material of cells in general, rather than specific disease-causing antigens, was found in essentially all lupus patients. A condition in which antibodies act against the body's own cells is called autoimmunity. These antinuclear antibodies do not enter living cells, but react with the nucleic acids that control protein synthesis and transmit heredity information. It is quite possible that these antibodies are activated by liberated proteins and lead to the formation of L.E. cells, which subsequently destroy the nuclei of other cells.

Although these studies and many others reveal much about the causes of lupus, there is still much to be explained. One especially fortunate finding was that a particular strain of mice native to New Zealand spontaneously develop an autoimmune hemolytic anemia. The breeding of hybrids produced a mouse which developed an ailment bearing a striking resemblance to lupus. Much of the research accomplished since 1960 is directly related to the development of these laboratory animals.

A most promising line of research into the cause of lupus erythematosus lies among the viruses. Several types of known viral organisms have been discounted. Among these are the arboviruses, which are transmitted by ticks or mosquitoes, and the myxoviruses or influenza viruses. On the other hand, large quantities of antibodies that fight the paramyxoviruses (including measles, mumps, and perhaps rubella) are reported in all lupus studies. While the actual virus has not been located, these data show an important future direction.

The other major condition known as lupus, lupus vulgaris, is rare to the point of extinction. It is a form of tuberculosis, and the tireless efforts of Niels Ryberg Finsen, the third Nobel laureate in physiology or medicine (1903), account for its disappearance. Finsen was so ill that he was unable to write or deliver the traditional Nobel lecture, but his book *La Photothérapie* (1899) provides a full discussion of his thoughts and the technical progress that he achieved. The following remarks are based on *Phototherapy*, the English translation of that work published in 1901.

Finsen begins his treatise with a review of earlier applications of light to medical problems. In evaluating these studies, he accepts the hypothesis that light is bactericidal. He attributes the absence of positive clinical results in his predecessors' work to their use of weak sources and short treatment times. He concludes that a systematic scientific study is needed. Experimenting with pure bacterial cultures and a variety of filtering apparatuses on the ear, Finsen was able to offer convincing evidence that concentrated rays were more effective. In the course of these studies, he also discovered that the radiant energy was even more effective when the ear was partially deprived of blood. From these carefully considered experiments, Finsen was prepared to make the intellectual leap to the treatment of lupus vulgaris.

### TREATMENT AND THERAPY

Few medical conditions have been more fully described in terms of patient-physician relationships than has lupus erythematosus. Because of the terrifying nature of the name itself—coupled with its unknown cause, its difficulty of diagnosis, and its uncertain prognosis—the sufferer will probably need careful counseling and reassurance. The physician too is faced with a substantial emotional investment in trying to deal with a condition which is so unpredictable.

The most important fact for the patient to understand is that lupus is a manageable malady. In fact, the great majority of people afflicted with lupus have only some of its symptoms, and the most serious and fatal forms involving kidney failure are rare indeed. Sir William Osler, who at the beginning of the twentieth century described the involvement of the kidneys in lupus, made the most penetrating observation concerning medical conditions such as lupus: "If you want to live a long life, get a chronic disease and learn how to take care of it."

The lupus sufferer, as well as the physician, must be content with treating symptoms; no cause or cure has yet been discovered. In spite of this sobering reality, much has been learned that makes such treatment useful. As Osler's comment suggests, a basic premise lies in the recognition of the importance of adequate rest and the avoidance of tension. These two ingredients of a balanced life are crucial to the well-being of the lupus patient.

One of the most common complaints of the patient is fatigue. Many find that doing their normal, daily chores demands most or all of their strength. Some physicians treating lupus cases believe that reduced work schedules, greater-than-average time for sleep, and strict rest periods are essential for good control. Others advocate a more active program during the characteristic periods of remission.

Closely related to the need for rest is another truism of good living—the demand to avoid stress. A number of chronic ills respond to either physical or emotional stress; among the most widely known of these conditions are peptic ulcers, migraine headaches, and heart disease. Lupus too has such a connection, and in relation to other factors specific to this disease, it is of even greater concern.

There are several erratic aspects of lupus, all of which contribute directly to feelings of stress. Most important are the variable periods of remission and activity and the shifting symptoms within an individual. There is evidence that infections, injuries, cold, sunlight, or ultraviolet radiation all may set in motion active phases of lupus. Avoiding such situations is important to all who desire a healthy life; for the lupus patient, such a sensible lifestyle becomes a necessity.

There is clear evidence of the patient's vital role in the successful management of lupus. Several excellent books and articles have described in detail the nature of the team effort of patients and doctors and the benefits to be obtained from it. A specific example is found in the need to seek the advice of one's physician before using any over-the-counter drugs. Even the most innocent of these materials might cause allergic reactions, which seem to be much more common in lupus sufferers. There is also the distinct possibility that such medications might interfere with the utility of a drug that has been prescribed.

Perhaps the most common of all materials on the medical scene, aspirin, continues to be the treatment of choice for the very common painful inflammation of arthritis that comes with lupus. This utility is obviously related to aspirin's cost and effectiveness. Of greater significance is the ability of many patients to take large quantities of the drug over long periods of time with very limited side effects. A number of other drugs are available to combat pain and inflammation, and in specific cases they may be used to great benefit.

Many lupus patients require more aggressive treatment for inflammation than the nonsteroidal drugs described above. Traditionally, the alternative has been cortisone and an array of related steroid hormones. So much has been written concerning the adverse effects associated with the misuse of steroids, especially by athletes, that it is easy to lose sight of their benefits. While careful supervision of their use, by both patient and physician, is essential, these materials can relieve much suffering.

While some kidney malfunction occurs in 50 percent of lupus patients, most of these cases are mild and produce no symptoms. In the much rarer circumstance, when kidney functions drop to less than 25 percent of normal, symptoms of nausea, fatigue, or edema are found. In all cases, careful attention must be paid to blood and urine tests, and any observed abnormalities must be treated to prevent further damage. The only treatments for life-threatening kidney dysfunction currently available are dialysis or transplant surgery. Both of these alternatives make clear how far medical science is from a cure for lupus.

The treatment of lupus vulgaris differs greatly from that of lupus erythematosus. Finsen's life work in the study of radiant energy and its bactericidal properties was focused largely on this condition. The sensitivity to sunlight in lupus erythematosus offers a marked contrast to the cure he achieved using high-powered radiation.

In introducing Finsen as the winner of the 1903 Nobel Prize in Physiology or Medicine, Count K. A. H. Mörner, the rector of the Royal Caroline Institute, proclaimed that Finsen's work would never be forgotten in the history of medicine. His contribution to the treatment of skin diseases through the advancement of knowledge of phototherapy was such an "immense step forward" that he "deserves the eternal gratitude of suffering humanity." The great success of these treatments with light (or "photothérapie") caused Mörner to concur with Finsen in proclaiming that the disease would soon be permanently eradicated.

From Finsen's first treatments in November, 1895, until the summary report of November, 1901, eight hundred cases of lupus vulgaris were treated. A complete cure was achieved in 50 percent of these, and marked improvement resulted in an additional 45 percent of cases, even among those patients who had been afflicted for as long as fifty years. That early diagnosis and treatment enhanced the likelihood of a complete cure was shown with the treatment of three hundred additional cases during the period following this report up to the time of the Nobel Prize presentation. The symptoms in the majority of these cases were in the early stages, and Finsen stated that here the cure was almost certain. Finsen had crossed a major hurdle, for Denmark could henceforth consider this disease conquered.

X rays have also been studied as a treatment for lupus vulgaris, and some reports of cure have been published. Like phototherapy, these more powerful energies ultimately were replaced by the use of drugs. Today, sulfa drugs are used to some extent, but isoniazid provides the most effective treatment by inhibiting certain key enzymes.

## PERSPECTIVE AND PROSPECTS

The family of conditions known as lupus has an ancient pedigree. Hippocrates may have been referring to it when he wrote (c. 300 B.C.) of "an erosive, disfiguring malady, eating away at the skin and flesh of the face." In the sixteenth century, the great iatrochemist Paracelsus, along with several of his contemporaries and successors, recognized similar maladies. It was in the mid-nineteenth century that the term "lupus" was first used, and shortly afterward, the distinction between the two rather different conditions of lupus erythematosus and lupus vulgaris was made. These two forms of lupus present a vivid contrast in terms of their importance to medical science as a whole, their present significance, and probable future development.

Lupus erythematosus represents a significant field of research and has for many years. There is an extensive literature of original author research, textbook chapters, and reports of international conferences all dealing with the study of the causes and treatment of this disease. As more sensitive diagnostic methods become available, researchers come to understand that what was once thought to be a rare and certainly fatal condition is neither. Of greater importance is the appreciation gained of the suffering of its victims. Much of this suffering is the direct result of ignorance and misunderstanding on the part of the patient, the physician, and the general public.

In a general way, the study of this complicated disease is likely to contribute significantly to the development of methodology useful in the study of other important conditions. For example, since there is significant evidence of viral involvement in lupus, its study seems virtually certain to enhance medical science's ability to deal effectively with a range of totally unrelated viral conditions. In a similar fashion, the need to produce and assess new drugs in the treatment of lupus makes it likely that an increase in medical knowledge will follow.

While lupus vulgaris might now be considered of mere historical interest, one ought to be careful of something being "merely historical." Examples of "extinct" diseases that return to catch the scientific community unawares are not unknown. One of the most pressing problems of modern pharmaceutical research and productivity is the emergence of strains of organisms resistant to the available drugs. —*K. Thomas Finley*

**See also** Arthritis; Kidney disorders; Rashes; Stress; Tuberculosis.

## FOR FURTHER INFORMATION:

Aladjem, Henrietta. *Understanding Lupus*. Rev. ed. New York: Charles Scribner's Sons, 1985. Written by a patient with lupus, working with a team of physicians experienced in treating the disease. Offers extensive background concerning the problem. Also contains supplementary materials, such as a glossary and a bibliography.

Aladjem, Henrietta, and Peter H. Schur. *In Search of the Sun*. Rev. ed. New York: Charles Scribner's Sons, 1988. A collaboration between a patient and physician, with alternating chapters describing their complementary views of their joint problems with lupus. Contains an extensive glossary, a bibliography, and support group data.

Blau, Paul Sheldon, and Dodi Schultz. *Lupus: The Body Against Itself*. Garden City, N.Y.: Doubleday, 1977. A brief, and somewhat dated, account of the disease, its treatment, and future research possibilities. Nevertheless, it is extremely well written. Valuable reading for an appreciation and understanding of lupus.

De Kruif, Paul. *Men Against Death*. New York: Harcourt, Brace, 1932. De Kruif is justly famous for his writing of scientific biography, and while the intellectual purists might scoff at his "popular" stories, he has the gift for interesting the lay reader in scientific questions. While remaining accurate, he presents in vivid detail what other scientists write in dry, pedantic prose. Contains a chapter that is obligatory for anyone wishing to appreciate Niels Finsen and his work.

Finsen, Niels R. *Phototherapy*. Translated by James H. Sequeira. London: Edward Arnold, 1901. From the German edition, with an appendix by the translator. A reprint of several of Finsen's original publications. This work constitutes a first-person source in readable English.

Fyfe, Herbert C. "The Finsen Light-Cure in England." *Scientific American* 89 (November 28, 1903): 389-390. This article does far more than describe the English scene at the beginning of the twentieth century. With its excellent photographs, the article is a well-documented essay on the nature of Niels Finsen's work and its application at the time of the Nobel Prize.

Stehlin, Dori. "Living with Lupus." *FDA Consumer* 23 (December, 1989): 8-12. An excellent example of the literature of personal stories of the courage of lupus sufferers. Especially strong on the problems of pregnancy for those with lupus.

# LYME DISEASE

**SYSTEMS AFFECTED:** Skin, joints, nervous, heart
**SPECIALISTS:** Environmental medicine physicians, internists, public health specialists, rheumatologists
**DEFINITION:** Named for the town of Lyme, Connecticut, where it was first discovered in 1975, Lyme disease is a multisymptom disorder transmitted by the bite of a tick, *Borrelia burgdorferi*. The infection often begins with flulike symptoms and a rash surrounding the bite area. If the disease is diagnosed at this stage, antibiotic treatment is usually effective, with no permanent damage. If unnoticed or untreated, however, Lyme disease can cause complications, including neurological problems (such as meningitis) and heart problems (such as myocarditis). The joints may swell as arthritis develops. At this stage, nonsteroidal anti-inflammatory drugs (NSAIDs) or corticosteroid drugs may be used; patients will recover, but some suffer recurrent bouts of fatigue and joint pain.
*See also* Arthritis; Lice, mites, and ticks.

# LYMPHADENOPATHY AND LYMPHOMA

**SYSTEM AFFECTED:** Lymphatic
**SPECIALISTS:** Hematologists, internists, oncologists
**DEFINITION:** Lymphadenopathy, or enlarged lymph nodes, refers to any disorder related to the lymphatic vessels of lymph nodes; lymphoma is a group of cancers consisting of unchecked multiplication of lymphatic tissue cells.

**KEY TERMS:**

*B lymphocyte:* a blood and lymphatic cell that plays a role in the secretion of antibodies

*Hodgkin's disease:* a malignant disorder of lymphoid tissue, generally first appearing in cervical lymph nodes, which is characterized by the presence of the Reed-Sternberg cell

*lymphoma staging:* a classification of lymphomas based upon the stage of the disease; used in the determination of treatment

*non-Hodgkin's lymphoma:* any malignant lymphoproliferative disorder other than Hodgkin's disease

*Reed-Sternberg cell:* a large atypical macrophage with multiple nuclei; found in patients with Hodgkin's disease

*T lymphocyte:* a blood and lymphatic cell that functions in cell-mediated immunity, which involves the direct attack of diseased tissues; subclasses of T cells aid B lymphocytes in the production of antibodies

### CAUSES AND SYMPTOMS

The lymphatic system consists of a large complex of lymph vessels and groups of lymph nodes ("lymph glands"). The lymph vessels include a vast number of capillaries that collect fluid and dissolved proteins, carbohydrates, and fats from tissue fluids. The lacteals of the intestinal villi are lymph vessels that serve to absorb fats from the intestine and transport them to the bloodstream.

Lymph nodes are found throughout the body but are concentrated most heavily in regions of the head, neck, armpits, abdomen, and groin. Nodes function to filter out foreign materials, such as bacteria or viruses, which make their way into lymphatic vessels.

The sizes of lymph nodes vary: some are as small as a pinhead, some as large as a bean. In general, they are shaped much like kidney beans, with an outer covering. Internally, they consist of a compartmentalized mass of tissue that contains large numbers of B and T lymphocytes as well as antigen-presenting cells (APC). The lymphatic circulation into the lymph nodes consists of a series of entering, or afferent, vessels, which empty into internal spaces, or sinuses. A network of connective tissue, the reticulum, regulates the lymph flow and serves as a site of attachment for lymphocytes and macrophages. The lymphatic circulation leaves the node through efferent, or exiting, vessels in the lower portion of the organ, the hilum.

Among the functions of lymph nodes are those of the immune response. B and T lymphocytes tend to congregate in specialized areas of the lymph nodes: B cells in the outer region, or cortex, and T cells in the underlying paracortex. When antigen is presented by an APC, T- and B-cell interaction triggers B-cell maturation and proliferation within the germinal centers of the cortex. The result may be a significant enlargement of the germinal centers, and subsequently of the lymph node itself.

Lymphadenopathy, or enlarged lymph nodes, may signify a lymphoma, or cancer of the lymphatic system. More commonly, however, the enlarged node is secondary to other phenomena, usually local infections. For example, an ear infection may result in the entrance of bacteria into local lymphatic vessels. These vessels drain into regional nodes of the neck. The result is an enlargement of the nodes in this area, as an immune response is carried out.

Enlarged nodes caused by infections can, in general, be easily differentiated from those caused by malignancies. Infectious nodes are generally smaller than 2 centimeters in diameter, soft, and tender. They usually occur in areas where common infections occur, such as the ears or the throat. Malignant lymph nodes are often large and occur in groups. They are generally firm and hard, and they often appear in unusual areas of the body (for example, along the diaphragm). In order to confirm a malignancy, a biopsy of material may be necessary.

Infectious nodes can also be caused by diseases such as infectious mononucleosis, tuberculosis, and acquired immunodeficiency syndrome (AIDS). Lymphadenopathy syndrome (LAS), a generalized enlargement of the lymph nodes, is a common feature of the prodromal AIDS-related complex (ARC).

Since lymphadenopathy can be caused by any immune proliferation in the germinal centers, allergy-related illnesses may also cause enlargement of the lymph nodes. Consequently, immune disorders such as rheumatoid arthritis, systemic lupus erythematosus, and even hay fever allergies may show enlarged nodes as part of their syndromes.

As is the case for any cell in the body, cells constituting the lymphatic system may undergo a malignant transformation. The broadest definition of these lymphoproliferative diseases, or lymphomas, can include both Hodgkin's disease and non-Hodgkin's lymphomas, in addition to acute and chronic lymphocytic leukemias (ALL and CLL). With the understanding of, and ability to detect, specific cell markers, it is possible to classify many of these lymphomas on the basis of their cellular origin. Such is the case for ALL, CLL, Burkitt's lymphoma, and many other forms of non-Hodgkin's lymphomas. The cell type that ultimately forms the basis for Hodgkin's disease remains uncertain.

Hodgkin's disease is a malignant lymphoma that first presents itself as a painless enlargement of lymphoid tissue. Often, this is initially observed in the form of swollen lymph nodes in the neck or cervical region. Occasionally, the victim may exhibit a mild fever, night sweats, and weight loss. Untreated, the disease spreads from one lymphatic region to another, resulting in diffuse adenopathy. An enlarged spleen (splenomegaly) is a common result. As the disease spreads, other organs such as the liver, lungs, and bone marrow may be involved.

The disease is characterized by the presence of a characteristic cell type—the Reed-Sternberg cell. Reed-Sternberg cells appear to be of macrophage origin, with multilobed nuclei or multiple nuclei. They may also be present in other lymphatic disorders, but their presence is considered to be indicative of all cases of Hodgkin's disease. The precise relationship of the cell to the lymphoma is unclear, but some researchers in the field believe that the Reed-Sternberg cell is the actual malignant cell of the disease. The other infiltrative cells present in the node, including many B and T lymphocytes, may simply represent the reaction to the neoplasm. This interpretation, however, has been disputed.

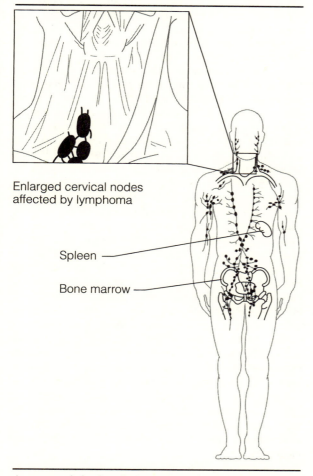

Enlarged cervical nodes affected by lymphoma

Spleen

Bone marrow

*Anatomy of the lymphatic system, showing major lymph nodes; enlarged lymph nodes may occur for a wide variety of reasons, including but not limited to lymphoma (cancer).*

Lymphoma staging is a system of classifying lymphomas according to the stage of development of the disease. Staging is important in that the prognosis and basis for treatment are in part determined by the stage of disease. Characterizing the form of Hodgkin's disease, therefore, involves two forms of classification. The first is a four-part classification based on the histology or cell type (Rye Conference classification). This scheme is based upon the proportion of Reed-Sternberg cells, ranging from their being "hard to find" to their being the predominant type. The prognosis becomes less favorable as the proportion of these cells increases.

Clinical staging, like that based on histology, is a four-part classification scheme (it is actually six parts, since stage III can be divided into subclasses). In this system, classification is based upon the extent of spread or extralymphatic involvement. For example, stage I features the involvement of a single lymph node region or a single extralymphatic site. Stage IV involves multiple disseminated foci. Early-stage disease is more easily treated and has a better prognosis than late-stage disease.

Non-Hodgkin's lymphomas (NHLs) represent a multitude of malignant disorders. Unlike Hodgkin's disease, they frequently arise in lymphatic tissue that is not easily observed; for example, in the gastrointestinal tract, tonsils, bone, and central nervous system. They have a tendency to spread rapidly, with malignant cells being released into the bloodstream early in the disease. Consequently, by the time diagnosis of NHL is made, the disease has often spread and the prognosis may be poor.

Though the etiology of most forms of NHL remains unknown, certain characteristics are evident in some forms of these diseases. For example, a portion of chromosome 14 is elongated in about 60 percent of NHL patients. Nearly one-third of patients with NHLs of B-cell origin demonstrate a chromosomal translocation, often involving a piece of chromosome 14 being translocated to chromosome 18. Though the relationship of these changes to disease is unclear, one can surmise that chromosomal defects play at least some role in the development of some forms of these disorders.

At least two forms of NHL are either caused by viruses or related to their presence: Burkitt's lymphoma and adult T-cell lymphoma/leukemia. Burkitt's lymphoma, which was first described by Denis Burkitt in central Africa, is a B-cell tumor that occurs primarily in children. It is generally presented as a large tumor of the jaw. This type of lymphoma is associated with early infection by the Epstein-Barr virus, or EBV (also the etiological agent of infectious mononucleosis). The relationship of the disorder to the virus remains unclear, and EBV may be either a specific cause or a necessary cofactor.

Specific chromosomal abnormalities are also associated with Burkitt's lymphoma. In 75 percent of cases, a translocation from chromosome 8 to chromosome 14 is evident, while in most other cases, a portion of chromosome 8 is translocated to either chromosome 2 or chromosome 22. Each of these translocations involves the transfer of the same gene from chromosome 8, the c-myc gene. The site to which the c-myc is translocated is in each instance a region that encodes protein chains for antibody production, proteins that are produced in large quantities. The c-myc gene product normally plays a role in committing a cell to divide. By being translocated into these specific regions, the c-myc gene product is overproduced, and the B cell undergoes continual replication.

Approximately 80 percent of NHL tumors are of B-cell origin; the remainder are primarily of T-cell origin. Those lymphomas that arise within the thymus, the organ of T-cell maturation, are called lymphoblastic lymphomas. Those that originate as more differentiated and mature T cells outside the thymus include a heterogeneous group of diseases (for example, peripheral T-cell lymphomas and Sézary syndrome). Often, by the time of diagnosis, these disorders have spread beyond the early stage of classification and have become difficult to treat.

## TREATMENT AND THERAPY

Treatment and other means of dealing with lymphadenopathy depend on the specific cause. In the case of lymph node enlargement that is secondary to infections, treatment of the primary cause is sufficient to restore the normal appearance of the node. For example, in a situation in which nodes in the neck region are enlarged as the result of a throat infection, antibiotic treatment of the primary cause— that is, the bacterial infection—is sufficient. The nodes will resume their normal size after a short time.

Dealing with lymph node enlargement caused by lymphoma requires a much more aggressive form of treatment. There are many kinds of lymphomas, which differ in type of cell involvement and stage of differentiation of the involved cells. The manifestations of most lymphomas, however, are similar. In general, these disorders first present themselves as painless, enlarged nodes. Often, this occurs in the neck region, but in many forms of NHL, the lymphadenopathy may manifest itself elsewhere in the lymphatic system. As the disease progresses, splenomegaly (enlarged spleen) and hepatomegaly (enlarged liver) may manifest themselves. Frequently, the bone marrow becomes involved. If the enlarged node compresses a vital organ or vessel in the body, immediate surgery may be necessary. For example, if one of the veins of the heart is compressed, the patient may be in immediate, life-threatening danger. Treatment generally includes radiation therapy and/or chemotherapy.

As is true for lymphomas in general, Hodgkin's disease is found more commonly in males than in females. In the United States, it occurs at a rate of 2 per 100,000 population per year, resulting in more than 6,000 cases being diagnosed each year. Approximately 1,500 persons die of the disease each year. The cause of the disease is unknown, though attempts have been made to assign the Epstein-Barr virus to this role.

Hodgkin's disease has an unusual age incidence. The age-specific incidence exhibits a bimodal curve. The disease shows an initial peak among young adults between 15 and 30 years of age. The incidence drops after age 30, only to show an additional increase in frequency after age 50. This is in contrast to NHL, which shows a sharp increase in incidence only after age 45. The reasons for this are unknown.

As noted earlier, the staging of Hodgkin's disease is important in determining methods of treatment; the earlier the stage, the better the prognosis. Patients in stage I (single node or site of involvement) or stage II (two or more nodes on the same side of the diaphragm involved, or limited extralymphatic involvement) have a much better prognosis than patients in stages III and IV (splenic or disseminated disease). Prior to the mid-1960's, a diagnosis of Hodgkin's disease was almost a death sentence. The development of radiation therapy and chemotherapy has dramatically increased the chances for survival; long-term remission can be achieved in nearly 70 percent of patients, and the "cure" rate may be higher than 90 percent with early detection. In part, this has been the result of understanding the progression of the disease (reflected in the process of staging) and utilizing a therapeutic approach to eradicate the disease both at its current site and at likely sites of spreading.

Radiation therapy is the treatment of choice for patients in stages I and II; spreading beyond local nodes is still unlikely in these stages. The body is divided into three regions to which radiation may be delivered: the mantle field covers the upper chest and armpits, the para-aortic field is the region of the diaphragm and spleen, and the third field is the pelvic area. For example, a patient presenting lymphadenopathy in a single node in the neck region may undergo only "mantle" irradiation. As noted above, with early detection, such treatment is effective 90 percent of the time (based on five-year disease-free survival).

Beyond stage II, a combination of radiation therapy and chemotherapy treatment is warranted. A variety of chemotherapy programs have been developed, the most common of which is known by the acronym MOPP (nitrogen mustard/Oncovin/procarbazine/prednisone). With combined radiation therapy and chemotherapy, even stage-III disease may go into remission 60 to 70 percent of the time, while 40 to 50 percent of stage-IV patients may enter remission. In general, therapy takes six to twelve months.

Non-Hodgkin's lymphomas represent a heterogeneous group of malignancies. Eighty percent are of B-lymphocyte origin. The wide variety of types has made classification difficult. The most useful method of classification for clinical purposes is based on the relative aggressiveness of the disease, low-grade being the slowest growing, followed by intermediate-grade and high-grade, which is the most aggressive.

NHLs often arise in lymphoid areas outside the mainstream. For example, the first sign of disease may be an abdominal mass or pain. Fever and night sweats are uncommon, at least in the early stages. Consequently, once the disease is presented, it is often deep and widespread. Because the disorder is no longer localized by this stage, radiation therapy by itself is of limited use. For comparison, nearly half of Hodgkin's disease patients are in stage I at presentation; not quite 15 percent of NHL patients are in stages I and II. Consequently, treatment almost always involves extensive chemotherapy.

A variety of aggressive forms of chemotherapy may be applied. These may include either single drugs such as alkaloids (vincristine sulfate) and alkylating agents (chlorambucil) or combination programs such as that of MOPP. Low-grade types of NHL are frequently slow growing and respond well to less aggressive forms of therapy. Low-grade NHL patients often enter remission for years. Unfortunately, the disorder often recurs with time and may become resistant to treatment; remission may occur in 50 percent of the patients, but only about 10 percent survive disease-free after ten years. High-grade lymphomas are rapidly growing, and the prognosis for most patients in the short term is not good. Those patients who do achieve remission with aggressive therapy, however, often show no recurrence of disease. As many as 50 percent of these persons may be "cured." The difference in prognosis between low-grade and high-grade disease may relate to the characteristics of the malignant cell. A rapidly growing cancer cell may be more susceptible to aggressive therapy than a slow-growing cancer, and more likely to die as a result. Thus, if a patient enters remission following therapy, there is greater likelihood that the cancer has been eradicated.

## PERSPECTIVE AND PROSPECTS

What was likely Hodgkin's disease was first described in 1666 as an illness in which lymphoid tissues and the spleen had the appearance of a "cluster of grapes." The disorder was invariably fatal. In 1832, Thomas Hodgkin published a thorough description of the disease, including its progression from the cervical region of the body to other lymphatic regions and organs. The unusual histological appearance of the cellular mixture characteristic of Hodgkin's disease was noted during the nineteenth century. It was early in the twentieth century, however, that Dorothy Reed and Karl Sternberg described the cell that is characteristic of the disorder: the Reed-Sternberg cell. As noted earlier, the number and proportion of such cells are the bases for the classification of the disease.

Two forms of non-Hodgkin's lymphoma are known to be associated with specific viruses: Burkitt's lymphoma (BL) and adult T-cell leukemia (ATL). BL was described by Denis Burkitt, who studied the pattern of certain forms of lymphomas among Ugandan children during the late 1950's. He noted that nearly all cases were found in children between the ages of 2 and 14, and noted that most cases in Africa were found in the malarial belt. Burkitt suspected that a mosquito might be involved in the transmissions of BL. Though no link has been found with arthropod transmission, the idea that BL might be associated with a viral agent bore fruit. In 1964, Michael Epstein and Yvonne Barr reported the presence of a particle in BL tissue that resembled the herpes virus. The Epstein-Barr virus was eventually linked to BL, though the specific role played by the virus remains elusive.

Adult T-cell leukemia was first noted in Japan during the 1970's. Japanese scientists observed that the majority of NHLs there were of T-cell origin and exhibited a similar clinical spectrum. The disease was later observed in the Caribbean basin, the southeastern United States, South America, and central Africa. In 1980, Robert Gallo isolated the etiological agent, the human T-cell lymphophic type I virus (HTLV-I).

The treatment of Hodgkin's disease represents one of the few success stories in dealing with cancers. In addition, some forms of NHL—notably, Burkitt's lymphoma—respond well to treatment. The prognosis for most patients with NHL, however, is less than optimal. In addition, the specific causes of most NHL syndromes are not known. Those with which a virus is linked may, in theory, be prevented by means of vaccination. The etiological agents or factors associated with the development of other forms of lymphomas remain elusive.   —*Richard Adler*

*See also* Cancer; Hodgkin's disease; Infection; Malignancy and metastasis.

**FOR FURTHER INFORMATION:**

Beck, William S., ed. *Hematology*. 5th ed. Cambridge, Mass.: MIT Press, 1991. A series of lectures dealing with hematology. Though the text was written for medical students, the material is not excessively detailed. The book is appropriate for anybody with a basic knowledge of biology, and the section on lymphomas is easy to follow. Numerous tables and photographs.

Bruning, Nancy. *Coping with Chemotherapy*. Rev. ed. New York: Ballantine Books, 1993. Written by a woman who survived breast cancer and its aftermath, this book provides a vivid description of chemotherapy. The author discusses methods of treatment and her own experiences.

Franks, L. M., and N. M. Teich, eds. *Introduction to the Cellular and Molecular Biology of Cancer*. 2d ed. New York: Oxford University Press, 1991. A general description of cancer and areas of research. The text discusses features of cancer and its possible origins. The possible role of oncogenes in the disease is also included. Though not intended for the layperson, the book does present a good overview of the subject.

Jandl, James H. *Blood*. Boston: Little, Brown, 1987. A textbook on hematology. The book is quite detailed but is recommended for anyone who is seriously interested in the subject. Though the lymphatic system is not specifically covered, blood and lymphatic cells are extensively covered. The nature of hematological disorders is the subject of nearly half the book.

Levine, Arnold. *Viruses*. New York: W. H. Freeman, 1992. A discussion of viruses and the diseases with which they are associated. Included are sections that deal with viruses and human cancers. The book is vividly illustrated and is intended for a general audience with some basic knowledge of biology. From the *Scientific American* library.

Roitt, Ivan. *Essential Immunology*. 7th ed. Boston: Blackwell Scientific, 1991. An outstanding textbook on immunology written by a leading researcher in the field. The early chapters on the lymphatic system, lymph nodes, and the immune response provide an excellent background for the subject. The diagrams are clear, as are the numerous photographs. Written at a level appropriate for those with a limited background in the subject.

Varmus, Harold, and Robert Weinberg. *Genes and the Biology of Cancer*. New York: Scientific American Library, 1993. The authors provide an excellent discussion of the role played by genetic factors in development of cancers. Several chapters deal with chromosome translocation as a possible cause of certain cancers, including Burkitt's lymphoma. Vividly illustrated with diagrams and photographs. Recommended for those with a basic knowledge of genetics.

**LYMPHATIC DISORDERS.** *See* **LYMPHADENOPATHY AND LYMPHOMA.**

**LYMPHOMA.** *See* **LYMPHADENOPATHY AND LYMPHOMA.**

# MACULAR DEGENERATION

**SYSTEM AFFECTED:** Visual

**SPECIALISTS:** Ophthalmologists

**DEFINITION:** Macular degeneration is a disease of the retinas; the macula is the part of the eye that allows for detailed sight in the center of the field of vision, with a dense concentration of rods and cones. The progressive breakdown of tissues in this area in one or both eyes forms scars, blocking vision until all sight in this field is gone, causing legal blindness. The surrounding vision may be unaffected or merely blurred, however, allowing many patients to function with the aid of special magnifying glasses. Macular degeneration may be an inherited condition, but it usually strikes the elderly as part of the aging process. Laser treatments to seal leaks during the degeneration process may halt the disease.

*See also* Aging; Blindness; Visual disorders.

# MALARIA

**SYSTEMS AFFECTED:** Brain, blood, kidneys, liver

**SPECIALISTS:** Epidemiologists, hematologists, public health specialists, tropical medicine specialists

**DEFINITION:** A serious parasitic infection borne by mosquitoes in tropical and subtropical regions and characterized by recurrent bouts of severe fever, chills, sweating, vomiting, and damage to kidneys, blood, brain, and liver.

**KEY TERMS:**

*Anopheles:* the genus of mosquito that transmits malaria parasites to human hosts

*falciparum, ovale, malariae, vivax:* the species or kinds of *Plasmodium* parasites that cause malaria in humans

*merozoite:* the stage of the malaria parasite's residence in the human host at which the red blood cells are infected

*oocyst:* the encysted or encapsulated ookinete in the wall of an infected mosquito's stomach

*ookinete:* the fertilized form of the malaria parasite in the mosquito's body

*Plasmodium:* the genus of the protozoan parasite that contains the different species of malaria parasites that infect humans

*pulmonary edema:* accumulation of fluid on the lungs, which may lead to death

*schizogony:* the process in which sporozoites develop into merozoites within the liver of a human host

*schizont:* a multinucleate parasite that reproduces by schizogony

*vector:* an organism (such as a mosquito) that transmits a pathogen (such as the malaria parasite), especially from one human to another

## CAUSES AND SYMPTOMS

Malaria in humans is caused by one of four species of protozoan parasites of the genus *Plasmodium*: *P. falciparum*, *P. vivax*, *P. ovale*, and *P. malariae*. The most severe form of malaria is caused by *P. falciparum*; the symptoms of this type include fever and chills occurring at irregular intervals. *P. vivax* is the most widespread parasite, causing most of the malaria infections in the world; this type of malaria results in recurrent periods of fever known as relapses. *P. malariae* is also widespread but has a patchier distribution than *P. falciparum* or *P. vivax*. *P. malariae* is common in many parts of Central Africa. It also occurs in India, Malaya, the East Indies, New Guinea, North Africa, and South America. *P. ovale* is found primarily in tropical Africa. These parasites belong to the subphylum Sporoza and the family Plasmodiidae. Malaria parasites also infect birds, lizards, and monkeys; the *Culex* mosquito carries parasites that infect birds. These other forms of malaria do not infect humans.

People may carry the malaria parasite but not develop the disease. Many variables determine whether the disease develops from *Plasmodium* infection. A person's age and genetic makeup, the species of the parasite, the density of the infection, and duration of exposure to mosquitoes carrying the parasites may influence the severity of the disease.

The clinical aspects of malaria are varied. Often a person with malaria has shaking chills to drenching sweats to intense fevers. Severe, complicated malaria is most often caused by *P. falciparum*; about 80 percent of the deaths from this parasite are caused by cerebral malaria, which is characterized by altered consciousness and often coma. Renal failure, hypoglycemia, severe anemia, pulmonary edema, and shock may also play a role in fatal malaria cases. Pregnant women that contract malaria may miscarry. They may also suffer severe anemia. If they survive childhood, people in areas of endemic malaria may have a moderate level of resistance to the disease. They often suffer recurrent but nonfatal fevers.

A definitive diagnosis of malaria is made by microscopic examination of stained blood smears for the presence of parasites. Because the parasite may disappear from the blood during the process of schizogony or not be visible in its early stages, blood smears must be taken at frequent intervals to diagnose the disease properly.

Of the twenty-five hundred known species of mosquitoes worldwide, only fifty to sixty species of the genus *Anopheles* transmit malarial parasites to humans by their bite. *Anopheles* mosquitoes are both a host and a vector of the malaria parasite. The females need blood meals to reproduce; it is during this biting and sucking of blood that the malaria parasite is passed to the human or the protozoan parasite is introduced into the mosquito's own system. During feeding, the mosquito injects a small amount of saliva into the host to increase blood flow to the area. Sporozoites are transmitted to the human host by this salivary fluid.

*Anopheles* mosquitoes can be identified from other genera of mosquitoes by their characteristic stance; they appear to be standing on their heads. (Other mosquitoes hold their bodies parallel to the surface on which they are resting.) The mosquito has four stages of growth: egg, larva, pupa, and adult. It is the bite of the adult *Anopheles* mosquito that transmits the malaria parasite to the human host. An adult mosquito will emerge from an egg in seven to twenty days. Females live at least a month.

The life cycle of the malaria parasite is complex. It has three phases in the mosquito and two in the human host; twelve different life history stages exist. The parasite is transmitted to humans as the sporozoite forms in the saliva of infected female *Anopheles* mosquitoes.

After entering the human host, the sporozoites invade liver cells, where during the next five to fifteen days, they develop into schizonts. Each schizont contains between ten thousand and thirty thousand daughter parasites called merozoites. The merozoites are released from the liver cells and invade the red blood cells. Once inside a red blood cell, the merozoite matures into a schizont containing eight to thirty-two new merozoites. The red blood cell ruptures and releases these merozoites so that they can invade additional red blood cells. The rupturing of the red blood cells is associated with fever and signals the clinical onset of malaria. Some merozoites differentiate into sexual forms, gametocytes, which are ingested by a mosquito during its next blood meal. Once in the mosquito, the sexual forms leave the blood cells, and male and female gametes fuse to form a zygote. In twelve to forty-eight hours, the zygote elongates to form an ookinete, which penetrates the wall of the mosquito's stomach and becomes an oocyst. During the next seven days or more, depending on the species of *Plasmodium* and the temperature in the gut of the mosquito, the oocyst enlarges, forming more than ten thousand sporozoites. The oocyst ruptures, and its sporozoites immigrate to the mosquito's salivary glands. The sporozoites are then injected into the next human host that the female mosquito bites.

Mosquitoes seek their hosts in response to a combination of chemical and physical stimuli, including carbon dioxide plumes, body odors, color, warmth, and movement of the host. Anopheline mosquitoes feed most frequently at night or in heavily shaded or dark areas during the early morning hours.

## Cycle of Malaria Infection

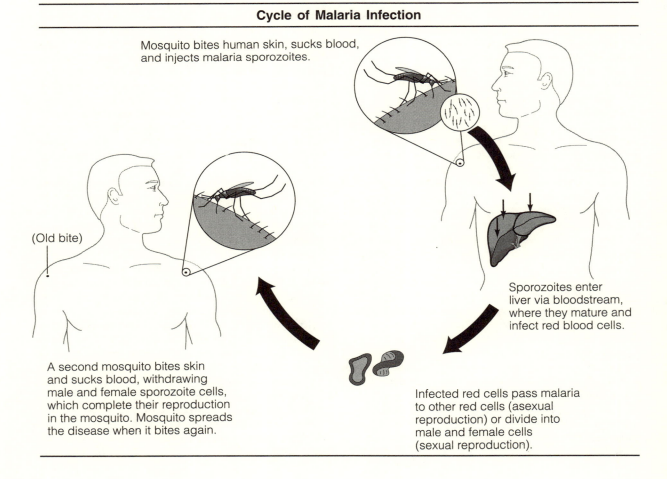

Mosquito bites human skin, sucks blood, and injects malaria sporozoites.

(Old bite)

A second mosquito bites skin and sucks blood, withdrawing male and female sporozoite cells, which complete their reproduction in the mosquito. Mosquito spreads the disease when it bites again.

Sporozoites enter liver via bloodstream, where they mature and infect red blood cells.

Infected red cells pass malaria to other red cells (asexual reproduction) or divide into male and female cells (sexual reproduction).

## TREATMENT AND THERAPY

It is still not understood why some people develop the disease malaria after being infected by the *Plasmodium* parasite from an *Anopheles* mosquito's bite while others do not. *P. falciparum* causes almost all the cases of severe and complicated malaria. Cerebral malaria, hypoglycemia, and malarial anemia are all serious diseases caused by this parasite. Fluid concentration in the lungs, kidney failure, and enlargement of the spleen also may occur with this disease.

Even without complications, malaria has a variety of symptoms: fever, headache, malaise, cough, nausea, vomiting, and diarrhea. Visitors to areas where malaria is found benefit from preventive drug therapy. Chloroquine is effective and safe, but chloroquine-resistant *P. falciparum* and *P. vivax* require alternative drugs for malaria prevention, such as mefloquine. While residents in malaria zones have no optimal treatment alternatives, the drugs dapsone and pyrimethamine, used to protect pregnant women from malaria, have been effective in Gambia.

Microscopic examination of blood smears provides definitive proof of infection by malaria parasites. Two drops of blood, usually from the tip of a finger pricked by a lancet, are placed on a glass microscope slide. One is smeared to a thin film, and both are air-dried. Chemicals are then added that fix and stain the parasites so that they are visible through a microscope. The quantitative buffy coat (QBC) technique, based on fluorescence microscopy, is also used to detect the presence of the malaria parasite; however, it is more expensive than usual microscopic screening and requires more technical equipment. Immunoassays are also possible diagnostic tools for malaria detection.

Controlling malaria is focused on destroying the *Anopheles* mosquito. If the females bearing the malarial parasite do not bite a human host, the vector chain is broken and the disease will be prevented. Once a female mosquito is infected, however, it remains so for life. Spraying of insecticides to kill adult mosquitoes is the best antivector method in malaria control. Long-lasting or residual insecticides are preferred. The use of chemicals to kill the larvae of *Anopheles* mosquitoes in aquatic habitats has only limited application. Other ways to destroy mosquito larvae include intermittent flushing of ponds with fresh water; aquatic plant control; use of larvae-eating fishes, such as mosquito fish (*Gambusia affinis*); and covering or draining hatching sites such as wells, small ponds, or water barrels.

There are many simple ways that individuals may protect themselves from mosquitoes bearing the malaria parasite. Repellents, such as skin lotions or those applied or built into clothing, may work well. Mosquito coils, material that releases insecticide when burned, may be used. Insecticide-impregnated netting around beds and screens on the windows and doors of homes will often prevent mosquitoes from entering and biting human hosts.

The economic cost of malaria is high, but precise estimates of its exact economic impact are difficult to make. Premature death, loss of productivity as a result of illness, and the failure to grow certain crops or to use new lands productively occur because of the presence of malaria. The costs of medical treatment for the disease may also be high, especially for those in poor countries. Migration to find work or to avoid malaria often spreads the disease to other areas.

About 40 percent of the world's population lives where malaria may occur. This is primarily in the tropics, but malaria can also be found in temperate regions, including the Middle East and Asia. Malaria is present in 102 countries and causes millions of clinical cases and several million deaths each year. Control of this disease was partially successful in the 1950's and 1960's, but by the 1970's and 1980's, cases of malaria were increasing worldwide.

Drug-resistant strains of *P. falciparum* and *P. vivax* reduce the effectiveness of drugs used to treat the disease. The mosquitoes that carry malaria to humans are now resistant to some chemicals that were once able to kill them. Some of the vector mosquitoes avoid insecticide-treated surfaces, making control of *Anopheles* mosquitoes less effective.

People who travel to many different parts of the world may expose themselves to the threat of malaria. The lack of adequate health care facilities and the often-critical economic conditions in malaria-infected areas of the world prevent effective malaria control and its eradication. In fact, although considered a single disease, malaria is more correctly viewed as many diseases, each different because of biological, ecological, sociological, and economic conditions that interact to determine its final morbidity (rate of incidence) and mortality (fatality rate) within a population. While malariologists do not agree on how best to treat and control this disease, it is agreed that malaria must be attacked on the local, regional, and global levels for any control to be effective.

Effective treatment of malaria requires trained personnel and the efforts and resources of health care organizations. More funds are needed for research on the development of a malaria vaccine. Long-term, guaranteed support for malaria research must be provided by funding agencies. Malaria surveillance should monitor high-risk groups and detect potential malaria epidemics early in their development. Drug discovery and development must also continue so that drug-resistant strains of malaria can be treated with new medicines. Better vector-control methods should be developed.

The most basic priority in malaria control is to prevent infected individuals from becoming severely ill and dying. Effective clinical treatment involves diagnostic and referral actions that provide treatment for infected patients in the early stages of the disease. Personal protection measures, such as insecticide-treated netting, screens, and mosquito coils, reduce the risk of infection for individuals living in endemic areas. Draining or filling small bodies of water where mosquito larvae develop and widespread use of residue insecticides are needed to reduce vector mosquito populations. Malaria control is in crisis in many areas of the world; it represents one of the greatest challenges for health professionals.

## PERSPECTIVE AND PROSPECTS

European colonization of the New World probably spread malaria to the Americas; it is unclear if the disease existed there before that time. Malaria became one of the most widespread and dehabilitating diseases of early North America. *P. vivax* and *P. malariae* were introduced by the English in 1607 when they settled Jamestown, Virginia. The importation of African slaves in 1620 brought the virulent *P. falciparum* to North America. Boston was hard hit by malaria-related illness and death in the seventeenth century, and in the eighteenth and nineteenth centuries, malaria was endemic in the southern and western portions of the Colonies. During the Civil War, eight thousand soldiers died from malaria and 1.2 million cases of the disease were recorded. As recently as the early 1900's, 500,000 cases of malaria were reported each year in the United States, most occurring in the South.

European explorers found South Americans using cinchona tree bark to combat fevers. In 1639, Jesuit missionaries brought some of the bark to Europe, where it became a popular treatment. It was not until 1820, however, that French chemists Pierre-Joseph Pelletier and Joseph-Bienaimé Caventou identified quinine as the active ingredient in cinchona bark that effectively fought these fevers.

In 1846, the Italian physician Giovanni Rasori theorized that a parasite caused malaria. In 1880, Charles-Louis-Alphonse Laveran, a French army medical officer, observed live parasites in blood taken from a feverish soldier in Algeria. In 1898, Giovanni Battista Grassi, Amico Bignami, and Guiseppe Bastianelli documented the transmission of human malaria parasites by *Anopheles* mosquito bites. Sir Ronald Ross, a British military doctor, did research on malaria transmission at the same time as the Italian team. Sir Patrick Manson was the first scientist to speculate that mosquitoes spread malaria, but Ross was the first to demonstrate the complete cycle of malaria in mosquitoes. Ross was awarded the Nobel Prize in Physiology or Medicine in 1902 for his work on malaria.

The first efforts to control malaria were made by the Greeks and Romans in the sixth century B.C. when they drained many marshy areas. Malaria control by drainage had minimal success, however, until the twentieth century. General William C. Gorgas directed a complex malaria control program during the construction of the Panama Canal from 1904 to 1914. This program included drainage, application of chemicals to kill the larval stage of the mosquitoes, and treatment of workers in the malaria zone of the Panama Canal with quinine. Malaria was eliminated from the Canal Zone by 1910.

From the mid-1940's through the mid-1950's, public health officials tried to eradicate malaria throughout the world. The development of the powerful insecticide DDT during World War II made this eradication seem possible. DDT was sprayed widely to kill *Anopheles* mosquitoes. The World Health Organization (WHO) directed this effort, and by the mid-1960's malaria was essentially controlled in North America and Europe. It had become evident, however, that eradication was not technically or economically feasible in many areas of the world. In 1969, WHO malaria-control efforts shifted from eradication to control. Because of the environmental problems that it caused, DDT was banned from use in the United States in 1972 and its production in the United States stopped in 1982. More toxic and expensive insecticides, such as dieldrin and malathion, were used to replace DDT in mosquito-control actions.

Beginning in the early 1970's, resistance by the *Plasmodium* parasite to antimalarial drugs became prevalent. In many areas of the world, no effective drugs exist to control malaria. Cholorquine, once the treatment of choice for *P. falciparum*, is of limited effectiveness. Research using irradiated sporozoites, however, indicates that development of a vaccine for malaria may be possible. In addition, the antimalarial drugs mefloquine and halofantrine are useful in fighting the disease. Yet political and social instability has increased the incidence of this disease by limiting or preventing its eradication and treatment. A shortage of malariologists also complicates fighting this disease. In 1986, 2.3 million deaths and 489 million clinical cases of malaria were reported.

Many governmental and private organizations around the world support malaria prevention, research, and control efforts. The World Bank, the European Commission, and WHO contribute extensively to solving this disease problem. In the United States, the U.S. Agency for International Development (USAID), the Centers for Disease Control (CDC), the Department of Defense (DOD), and the National Institute of Allergy and Infectious Diseases (NIAD) of the National Institutes of Health (NIH) all work to reduce the effects of malaria.  —*David L. Chesemore*

*See also* Arthropod-borne diseases; Bites and stings; Parasitic diseases.

## FOR FURTHER INFORMATION:

Brown, A. W. A., J. Haworth, and A. R. Zahar. "Malaria Eradication and Control from a Global Standpoint." *Journal of Medical Entomology* 13, no. 1 (1976): 1-25. This journal article provides a good overview of malaria-control activities through 1976. Can be understood by the nonscientist and provides some excellent statistical information about malaria control.

Harrison, Gordon. *Mosquitoes, Malaria, and Man: A History of the Hostilities Since 1880*. New York: E. P. Dutton, 1978. Written by a historian, this book is rich in detail about the people trying to solve the malaria puzzle. Provides an extensive listing of references and historical sources dealing with malaria. A good place to start.

Oaks, Stanley C., Jr., Violaine S. Mitchell, Greg W. Pearson, and Charles C. J. Carpenter, eds. *Malaria: Obstacles and Opportunities*. Washington, D.C.: National Academy Press, 1991. One of the best books available, with up-to-date information about malaria all over the world. Extremely easy to read for the nonspecialist. Provides a thorough discussion of the problems associated with malaria and the possible solutions to controlling and eradicating the disease.

Thompson, Paul E., and Leslie M. Werbel. *Antimalarial Agents: Chemistry and Pharmacology*. New York: Academic Press, 1972. A technical book for those with a good background in chemistry. Deals with the chemicals used to treat the various malarial infections. Extensive detail is offered, but it is sometimes difficult to ferret out the facts from the chemical formulas.

Williams, Greer. *The Plague Killers*. New York: Charles Scribner's Sons, 1969. A good review of the search for the cause and cures for both malaria and yellow fever. Written for a general audience, so it is easily read by the layperson seeking insights into the way in which scientists try to solve complex problems.

## MALE GENITAL DISORDERS

**SYSTEM AFFECTED:** Reproductive (male)

**SPECIALISTS:** Family physicians, oncologists, psychologists, urologists

**DEFINITION:** Disorders and diseases of the male reproductive system, including sexual dysfunction, infertility, genital cancer, and sexually transmitted diseases.

**KEY TERMS:**

*autonomic nervous system:* the part of the vertebrate nervous system that controls involuntary actions

*dysfunction:* the disordered or impaired function of a body system or organ

*endocrine:* relating to the production or action of a hormone

*hormone:* a substance which creates a specific effect in an organ distant from its site of production

*impotence:* the inability to have or maintain an erection satisfactory for sexual intercourse

*organic:* pertaining to, arising from, or affecting a body organ

*parasympathetic nervous system:* the part of the autonomic nervous system that stimulates digestion, slows the heart, and dilates blood vessels, acting in opposition to sympathetic nerves

*psychogenic:* originating in the mind or in mental conditions and activities

*spermatogonia:* cells of the testes that become sperm during spermatogenesis

*sphincter:* a ringlike muscle which constricts or relaxes to close or open a body orifice or passage, as required by normal body function

*sympathetic nervous system:* the part of the autonomic nervous system that represses digestion, speeds up the heart, and constricts blood vessels, acting in opposition to parasympathetic nerves

### PROCESS AND EFFECTS

Before discussion of male genital disorders and diseases, it is useful to describe the male genital system, which is composed of the scrotum, testes, epididymis, vas deferens, prostate and bulbourethral glands, seminal vesicles, penis, and urethra. The scrotum, composed of skin and underlying muscle, encloses the two testes and protects these sperm-making organs.

Each human testis is an ovoid structure about 5.0 centimeters long and 3.3 centimeters in width. A testis is composed of seminiferous tubules, a structure which surrounds the sperm-producing tubules, and accessory cells (the Leydig cells). The production of sperm, spermatogenesis, is controlled by hormones from the brain's hypothalamus and pituitary glands. It begins with the secretion of testosterone, the main male hormone, by Leydig cells. Brain hormone

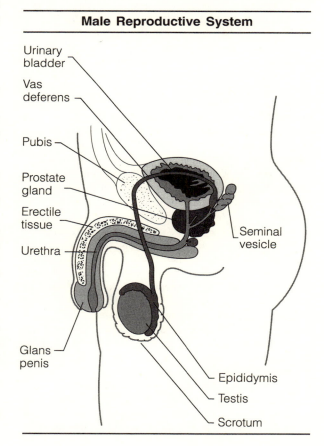

**Male Reproductive System**

Urinary bladder

Vas deferens

Pubis

Prostate gland

Erectile tissue

Urethra

Glans penis

Seminal vesicle

Epididymis

Testis

Scrotum

and testosterone actions cause the metamorphosis of cells called spermatogonia into sperm during a two-month passage through the seminiferous tubules.

The highly coiled seminiferous tubules, tiny in diameter and more than 200 meters long, coalesce into the efferent tubules, which release sperm into the epididymis. In a twelve-day trip through the highly coiled, 4.5-meter-long epididymis, sperm attain the ability to move (motility) and to fertilize a human egg cell, or ovum. Next, they enter the vas deferens, paired structures that connect the epididymis of each testis to its ejaculatory duct and the urethra. The only known vas function is to transport sperm, as a result of the action of nearby nerves and muscles, into the latter structures. The vas are cut in bilateral vasectomy surgery, which is often used for male sterilization.

The prostate, seminal vesicles, and bulbourethral glands produce the secretions that constitute most sperm-containing semen, which is ejaculated during intercourse. The prostate gland is situated immediately below the urinary bladder and surrounds the portion of the urethra closest to the bladder. It is a fibromuscular gland which empties into the male urethra on ejaculation. Prostate secretions contain important enzymes and make up a quarter of the seminal fluid.

The seminal vesicles are 7.5 centimeters long and empty into the ejaculatory ducts. They produce more than half of the liquid portion of semen, contributing fluid rich in fructose, the main nutrition source of sperm. The tiny, paired bulbourethral (or Cowper's) glands are located below the prostate. They secrete lubricants into the male urethra that ease semen passage.

The male urethra passes from the urinary bladder, through the prostate, and then through the penis. At the end of the penis, it reaches the outside of the body, to pass semen and urine. The penis, a cylindrical erectile organ, surrounds most of the male urethra and contains three cavernous regions. One, the corpus spongiosum, is found around the urethra. The others, the paired corpora cavernosa, are erectile tissues that fill with blood to produce an erection upon male sexual arousal. Erection is a complex reflex which involves both the sympathetic and parasympathetic portions of the human nervous system.

At the time of erection, nerve impulses dilate blood vessels that communicate with the corpora cavernosa and allow them to fill with blood. Sphincters then close off the portion of the urethra closest to the urinary bladder. At the same time, sperm, prostate secretions, bulbourethral gland secretions, and seminal vesicle secretions enter the urethra. Next, muscle contractions propel the ejaculate out of the urethra. The blood then leaves the corpora cavernosa, and the penis resumes its unexcited state.

### COMPLICATIONS AND DISORDERS

Proper male sexual function involves several closely coordinated hormone, nervous, and chemical processes. After a discussion of the male genital system, it thus becomes clear that many factors can cause male genital problems and diseases. Male infertility, for example, can be attributable to inadequate sperm production; undersecretion by the seminal vesicles, Cowper's glands, and/or prostate; malfunction of other endocrine glands or of the nervous system; and dysfunction or lack of the epididymis. Impotence, the inability to have or maintain a satisfactory erection for intercourse, is another frequent male genital problem. It may be psychogenic or caused by anatomic dysfunction, disease, or medications used to treat health problems.

The male sexual response cycle is mediated by the complex interplay of parasympathetic and sympathetic nerves. For example, penis erection is mostly parasympathetic, while ejaculation is largely attributable to sympathetic enervation. Dysfunction disorders include low sexual desire, impotence (erectile dysfunction), and lost orgiastic control (premature ejaculation). Impotence is the most frequent of these problems.

Erectile dysfunction is said to occur when the failure to complete successful intercourse occurs at least 25 to 30 percent of the time. Most often, it is short term (secondary impotence) and related to individual partners or to temporary damage to male self-esteem. Secondary impotence may also be caused by diseases such as diabetes mellitus, medications such as tranquilizers and amphetamines, alcoholism and other psychoactive drug addictions, and minor genital abnormalities. Aging is not necessarily a cause of impotence, even in octogenarians.

Long-lasting (or primary) impotence that occurs despite corrective medical treatment is generally attributable to severe psychopathology and must be treated by psychotherapy and counseling. Psychogenic impotence is implicated when an erection can be achieved by masturbation. The treatment of impotence caused by organic problems may include testosterone administration, the discontinuation of drug therapy or addictive drugs, or corrective surgery, which may include inflatable penis implants.

Male infertility is a problem found in about a third of all cases in which American couples are unable to have children. The problem is thus estimated to occur in 4 to 5 percent of American men. There are a wide number of causes for male infertility, which is always caused by the failure to deliver adequate numbers of mature sperm into the female reproductive tract as a result of organic problems. Impaired spermatogenesis, a frequent cause of male infertility, may have numerous causes. Examples include severe childhood mumps, brain and/or testicular hormone imbalances, drug abuse, obstruction or anatomic malformation of the seminal tract (especially the seminiferous tubules and epididymis), and a defective prostate gland.

Diagnosis includes careful physical examination by a urologist and evaluation of ejaculated semen to identify the number, activity, and potential for fertilization of its sperm. Blood tests will identify hormone imbalances and other possible causative agents. Many treatments are possible for male infertility, ranging from medications, to corrective surgery, to artificial insemination with sperm collected and frozen until enough are on hand to effect fertilization.

Cancer of the male genital organs may occur in the prostate, urethra, penis, or testis. The most important of these is prostate cancer. Urethral cancer is rare. More common is carcinoma of the penis, which occurs most often in uncircumcised men who practice poor genital hygiene. It is very often located beneath the foreskin and does not spread quickly. Total or partial removal of the penis is often required in advanced cases that have been ignored for long periods. Testicular cancers account for most solid genital malignancies in young men. These cancers appear as painful scrotal masses which increase rapidly in size. Any large, firm mass arising from a testis is suspicious and should be examined immediately by X ray, computed tomography (CT) scan, and tests for various tumor markers seen in the blood. Treatment of these tumors includes surgery, radiation, and chemotherapy. Survival rates vary greatly and depend upon the cancer type. Cancer of the prostate and other male genital organs is not clearly understood and may have hormonal and chemical bases. It is believed that periodic self-examination is the most valuable preventive methodology.

Common disorders of the male genital organs include priapism, hydrocele and spermatocele, testicular torsion, and varicocele. Priapism is persistent, painful erection not accompanied by sexual arousal. It is caused by a poorly understood mechanism and is characterized by both pain and much-thickened blood in the corpora cavernosa. Priapism often occurs after prolonged sexual activity and may accompany prostate problems, genital infections such as syphilis, and addictive drug use. Treatment of priapism includes spinal anesthesia, anticoagulants, and surgery. In the absence of prompt, effective treatment, priapism may end male sexual function permanently.

Hydrocele is a common, noncancerous scrotum lesion most common in men over forty. The problem is caused by fluid accumulation resulting from testis inflammation. Hydrocele is not painful and is removed surgically only if excessive in size. Closely related in appearance is a spermatocele, which contains sperm and occurs adjacent to an epididymis. Both hydroceles and spermatoceles are said to transilluminate: They are both so transparent that a flashlight beam will pass through them. Testicular torsion is a twisting of the vas deferens, which causes pain and swelling; surgery is required to return blood flow to the testis. Varicocele describes varicose veins of the testis, which is common and usually harmless.

Sexually transmitted diseases can also affect the male genitals. These diseases include herpes, gonorrhea, syphilis, chlamydia, and genital warts. For the prevention of sexually transmitted diseases, abstention, the careful choice of sexual partners, and the use of male or female condoms are useful.

## PERSPECTIVE AND PROSPECTS

Treatment of the various types of male genital disorders and diseases has evolved greatly. Particularly valuable are the strides made in the treatment of impotence. It has been realized that such sexual dysfunction is often a consequence of organic problems that may be remedied by the cessation of causative medication use or by minor surgery. In addition, the utilization of inflatable penis implants in the cases where insoluble psychogenic or organic problems occur has been a milestone in the treatment of this emotionally devastating male genital problem.

Wide examination of the entire spectrum of male genital problems has led to numerous advantageous treatments and to an understanding that withholding unneeded medical treatments can be beneficial. For example, information regarding spermatoceles, hydroceles, and many related nonacute male genital problems has decreased the incidence of unnecessary male genital surgery, and its related risks, for patients.

Another important concept is that of frequent self-examination of the male genitals. This practice has led to a shortening of the time lag between the appearance of a suspicious mass in the scrotum, testes, or other male sex organ and medical attention from professionals (such as urologists) trained both to evaluate their seriousness and to treat them. Early detection has diminished the severity of many genital cancers and facilitated their treatment. Moreover, several clinical tests for such lesions have become more available and more widely used by the public.

It is hoped that these avenues and others, as well as further advances in both diagnostic techniques and treatment possibilities, will eventually eradicate male genital diseases and disorders. Two areas in need of advancements are priapism and prostate cancer, which is an effective killer.

—*Sanford S. Singer*

**See also** Acquired immunodeficiency syndrome (AIDS); Gonorrhea; Herpes; Infertility in males; Prostate cancer; Sexual dysfunction; Sexually transmitted diseases; Stones; Syphilis.

## FOR FURTHER INFORMATION:

American Psychiatric Association. *Diagnostic and Statistical Manual of Mental Disorders*. Rev. 3d ed. Washington, D.C.: Author, 1980. This compilation includes diagnostic criteria and other useful facts about mental problems associated with male genital diseases. It thus provides insight into the psychogenic aspects of these afflictions.

Berkow, Robert, and Andrew J. Fletcher. *The Merck Manual of Diagnosis and Therapy*. 15th ed. Rahway, N.J.: Merck Sharp & Dohme Research Laboratories, 1987. This book abounds with useful data on the characteristics, etiology, diagnosis, and treatment of male genital disorders and diseases. Written for physicians, it is also quite useful to general readers.

Montague, Drogo K. *Disorders of Male Sexual Function*. Chicago: Year Book Medical Publishers, 1988. This medical text is useful to all readers wishing detailed information on aspects of men's health, including male reproductive anatomy and physiology, terminology, clinical evaluation, pharmacology, and the treatment of male sexual diseases.

Rajfer, Jacob. *Urologic Endocrinology*. Philadelphia: W. B. Saunders, 1986. This technical text is useful for those who wish detailed information. Offers sections on urogenital tract development, sex differentiation disorders, prostate disease, normal and abnormal aspects of penis and testis development or function, male infertility, and male genital cancer.

Sherwood, Lauralee. *Human Physiology: From Cells to Systems*. St. Paul, Minn.: West, 1989. This college text contains useful information on the male genital system, background endocrinology, spermatogenesis, aspects of sexual dysfunction, and sexually transmitted diseases in men. Also a source of many explanatory illustrations.

Swanson, Janice M., and Katherine A. Forrest. *Men's Reproductive Health*. New York, N.Y.: Springer, 1984. This book contains useful information on many aspects of men's health. Included are sections on male reproductive system anatomy and physiology, sexually transmitted disease, diseases of the male reproductive system, male infertility, and problems associated with medicinal drugs.

Tseng, C. Howard, T. Guilas Villaneuva, and Alvin Powell. *Sexually Transmitted Diseases: A Handbook of Protection, Prevention, and Treatment*. Saratoga, Calif.: R and E, 1987. This popular book contains useful information on acquired immunodeficiency syndrome (AIDS), herpes, gonorrhea, syphilis, chlamydia, genital warts, and other sexually transmitted diseases. Descriptive material on symptoms, ideas for prevention, and treatment modes are included.

# MALIGNANCY AND METASTASIS

**SYSTEMS AFFECTED:** All

**SPECIALISTS:** Colorectal surgeons, dermatologists, general surgeons, internists, oncologists, pathologists, plastic and reconstructive surgeons

**DEFINITION:** "Malignancy" is the uncontrolled growth of tumor cells that invade and compress surrounding tissues and break through the skin or barriers within the body; "metastasis" describes the tendency of malignant cells to break loose from their tumor or origin to travel to other locations within the body.

**KEY TERMS:**

*benign tumors:* tumors that grow relatively slowly, do not interfere with normal body functions, and do not metastasize

*carcinogen:* a natural or artificial substance inducing the transformation of cells toward the malignant state

*chemotherapy:* the use of chemicals to kill or inhibit the growth of cancer cells

*multistep progression:* the typical pathway of induction of cancer, beginning with an initial alteration to a gene and progressing to the fully malignant state

*oncogene:* a gene directly or indirectly inducing the transformation of cells from the normal to the malignant state; most oncogenes have normal counterparts in body cells

*retrovirus:* a virus infecting mammalian and other cells that sometimes carries and introduces oncogenes into host cells

*transfection:* a technique used to introduce genes into cells by exposing the cells to fragmented deoxyribonucleic acid (DNA) under conditions that promote the uptake and incorporation of DNA

*tumor suppressor gene:* a gene that, in its normal form, inhibits cell division

## CAUSES AND SYMPTOMS

Cancer cells are characterized by two primary features. One of these is uncontrolled cell division: Cells enter an unregulated, rapid growth phase by losing the controls that normally limit division rates to the amount required for normal growth and maintenance of body tissues. The second feature is metastasis, in which tumor cells lose the connections that normally hold them in place in body tissues, break loose, and spread from their original sites to lodge and grow in other body locations. Tumor cells with these characteristics are described as malignant.

The detrimental effects of solid malignant tumors result from the interference of rapidly growing masses of cancer cells with the activities of normal tissues and organs, or from the loss of vital functions because of the conversion of cells with essential functions to nonfunctional forms. Some malignant tumors of glandular tissue upset bodily functions by producing and secreting excessive quantities of hormones.

Solid malignant tumors, as they grow, compress surrounding normal tissues; they destroy normal structures by cutting off blood supplies and interrupting nerve function. They may also break through barriers that separate major body regions, such as internal membranes and epithelia or the gut wall. They may also break through the skin. Such breakthroughs cause internal or external bleeding and infection, and they destroy the organization and separation of body regions necessary for normal function. Both compression and breakthroughs can cause pain that, in advanced cases, may become extreme.

Malignant tumors of blood tissues involve cell lines that normally divide to supply the body's requirements for red and white blood cells. Cancer in these cell lines crowds the bloodstream with immature, nonfunctional cells that are unable to accomplish required activities, such as the delivery of oxygen to tissues or the activation of the immune response.

When the total mass of actively growing and dividing malignant cells becomes large, their demands for nutrients may deprive normal cells, tissues, and organs of their needed supplies, leading to generally impaired functions, fatigue, weakness, and weight loss.

Not all unregulated tissue growths are malignant. Some tumors, such as common skin warts, are benign—they do not usually interfere with normal body functions. They grow relatively slowly and do not metastasize. Often, benign tumors are surrounded by a closed capsule of connective tissue that prevents or retards expansion and breakup. Some initially benign tumors, however, including even common skin warts, may change to malignant forms.

Individual cells of a malignant tumor exhibit differences from normal cells in activity, biochemistry, physiology, and structure. First and foremost is the characteristic of uncontrolled division. Cancer cells typically move through the division cycle much more rapidly than normal cells. The rapid division is accompanied by biochemical changes characteristic of dividing cells such as high metabolic rates; increases in the rate of transport of substances across the plasma membrane; increases in protein phosphorylation; raised cytoplasmic concentrations of sodium, potassium, and calcium ions; and an elevated pH. Often chromosomal abnormalities are present, including extra or missing chromosomes, exchanges of segments between chromosomes, and breakage.

Cancer cells also typically fail to develop all the characteristics and structures of fully mature cells of their type. They may also lose mature characteristics if these were attained before conversion to the malignant state. Frequently, loss of mature characteristics involves disorganization or disappearance of the cytoskeleton. Alterations are also noted in the structure and density of surface carbohydrate groups. Cancer cells lose tight attachments to their neighbors or to supportive extracellular materials such as collagen; some cancer cells secrete enzymes that break cell connections and destroy elements of the extracellular material, aiding their movement into and through surrounding tissues. If removed from the body and placed in test-tube cultures, most cancer cells have the capacity to divide indefinitely. In contrast, most normal body cells placed in a culture medium eventually stop dividing.

The conversion of normal cells to malignant types usually involves multiple causes inducing a series of changes that occur in stages over a considerable length of time. This characteristic is known as the multistep progression of cancer. In most cases, the complete sequence of steps leading from an initiating alteration to full malignancy is unknown.

The initial event in a multistep progression usually involves the alteration of a gene from a normal to an aberrant form known as an oncogene. The gene involved is typically one that regulates cell growth and division or that takes part in biochemical sequences with this effect. The alteration may involve substitutions or the loss of DNA sequences, the movement of the gene to a new location in the chromosomes, or the movement of another gene or its controlling elements to the vicinity of the gene. In some cases, the alteration involves a gene that in normal form suppresses cell division in cells in which it is active. Loss or alteration of function of such genes, known as tumor suppressor genes, can directly or indirectly increase growth and division rates.

An initiating genetic alteration may be induced by a long list of factors, including exposure to radiation or certain chemicals, the insertion of viral DNA into the chromosomes, or the generation of random mutations during the duplication of genetic material. In a few cancers, the initiating event involves the insertion of an oncogene into the DNA by an infecting virus that carries the oncogene as a part of its genetic makeup.

In some cases, about 5 percent in humans, an initiating oncogene or faulty tumor suppressor gene is inherited, producing a strong predisposition to the development of malignancy. Among these strongly predisposed cancers are familial retinoblastoma, familial adenomatous polyps of the colon, and multiple endocrine neoplasia, in which tumors develop in the thyroid, adrenal medulla, and parathyroid glands. In addition to the strongly predisposed cancers, some, including breast, ovarian, and colon cancers other than familial adenomatous polyps, show some degree of disposition in family lines—members of these families show a greater tendency to develop the cancer than individuals in other families.

Subsequent steps from the initiating change to the fully malignant state usually include the conversion of additional genes to oncogenic form or the loss of function of tumor suppressor genes. Also important during intermediate stages are further alterations to the initial and succeeding oncogenes that increase their activation. The initial conversion of a normal gene to oncogenic form by its movement to a new location in the chromosomes may be compounded at successive steps, for example, by sequence changes or the multiplication of the oncogene into extra copies. The subsequent steps in progression to the malignant state are driven by many of the sources of change responsible for the initiating step. Because genetic alterations often occur during the duplication and division of the genetic material, an increase in the cell division rate by the initiating change may increase the chance that further alterations leading to full malignancy will occur.

A change advancing the progression toward full malignancy may take place soon after a previous change or only after a long delay. Moreover, further changes may not occur, leaving the progression at an intermediate stage, without the development of full malignancy, for the lifetime of the individual. The avoidance of environmental factors inducing genetic alterations—such as overexposure to radiation sources such as sunlight, X rays, and radon gas and chemicals such as those in cigarette smoke—increases the chance that progressions toward malignancy will remain incomplete.

The last stage in progression to full malignancy is often metastasis. After the loss of normal adhesions to neighboring cells or to elements of the extracellular matrix, the separation and movement of cancer cells from a primary tumor to secondary locations may occur through the development of active motility or from breakage into elements of the circulatory system.

Relatively few of the cells breaking loose from a tumor survive the rigors of passage through the body. Most are destroyed by various factors, including deformation by passage through narrow capillaries and destruction by blood turbulence around the heart valves and vessel junctions. Furthermore, tumor cells often develop changes in their surface groups that permit detection and elimination by the immune system as they move through the body. Unfortunately, the rigors of travel through the body may act as a sort of natural selection for the cells that are most malignant—that is, those most able to resist destruction—and that can grow uncontrollably and spread by metastasis.

Many natural and artificial agents trigger the initial step in the progression to the malignant state or push cells through intermediate stages. Most of these agents, collectively called carcinogens, are chemicals or forms of radiation capable of inducing chemical changes in DNA. Some, however, may initiate or further this progression by modifying ribonucleic acids (RNAs) or proteins, or they may act by increasing the rate of DNA replication and cell division.

## TREATMENT AND THERAPY

Cancer is treated most frequently by one or a combination of three primary techniques: surgical removal of tumors, radiation therapy, and chemotherapy. Surgical removal is most effective if the growth has remained localized so that the entire tumor can be detected and removed. Often, surgery is combined with radiation or chemotherapy in an attempt to eliminate malignant cells that have broken loose from a primary tumor and lodged in other parts of the body. Surgical removal followed by chemotherapy is presently the most effective treatment for most forms of cancer, especially if the tumor is detected and removed before extensive metastasis has taken place. Most responsive to surgical treatments have been skin cancers, many of which are easily detected and remain localized and accessible.

Radiation therapy may be directed toward the destruction of a tumor in a specific body location. Alternatively, it may be used in whole-body exposure to kill cancer cells that have metastasized and lodged in many body regions. In either case, the method takes advantage of the destructive effects of radiation on DNA, particularly during periods when the DNA is under duplication. Because cancer cells undergo replication at higher rates than most other body cells, the technique is more selective for tumors than for normal tissues. The selection is only partial, however, so that body cells that divide rapidly, such as those of the blood, hair follicles, and intestinal lining, are also affected. As a consequence, radiation therapy often has side effects ranging from unpleasant to serious, including hair loss, nausea and vomiting, anemia, and suppression of the immune system. Because radiation is mutagenic, radiation therapy carries the additional disadvantage of being carcinogenic—the treatment, while effective in the destruction or inhibition of a malignant growth, may also initiate new cancers or push cells through intermediate stages in progression toward malignancy.

When possible, radiation is directed only toward the body regions containing a tumor in order to minimize the destruction of normal tissues. This may be accomplished by focusing a radiation source on the tumor or by shielding body regions outside the tumor with a radiation barrier such as a lead sheet.

Chemotherapy involves the use of chemicals that retard cell division or kill tumor cells more readily than normal body cells. Most of the chemicals used in chemotherapy have been discovered by routine screening of substances for their effects on cancer cells in cultures and test animals. Several hundred thousand chemicals were tested in the screening effort that produced the thirty or so chemotherapeutic agents available for cancer treatment.

Many of the chemicals most effective in cancer chemotherapy alter the chemical structure of DNA, produce breaks in DNA molecules, slow or stop DNA duplication, or interfere with the natural systems repairing chemical lesions in DNA. The effects inhibit cell division or interfere with cell functions sufficiently to kill the cancer cells. Because DNA is most susceptible to chemical alteration during duplication and cancer cells duplicate their DNA and divide more rapidly than most normal tissue cells, the effects of these chemicals are most pronounced in malignant types. Normal cells, however, are also affected to some extent, particularly those in tissues that divide more rapidly. As a result, chemotherapeutic chemicals can produce essentially the same detrimental side effects as radiation therapy. The side effects of chemotherapy are serious enough to be fatal in 2 to 5 percent of persons treated. Because they alter DNA, many chemotherapeutic agents are carcinogens and carry the additional risk, as with radiation, of inducing the formation of new cancers.

Not all chemicals used in chemotherapy alter DNA. Some act by interfering with cell division or other cell processes rather than directly modifying DNA. Two chemotherapeutic agents often used in cancer treatment, vinblastine and taxol, for example, slow or stop cell division through their ability to interfere with the spindle structure that divides chromosomes. The drugs can slow or stop tumor growth as well as the division of normal cells.

Tumors frequently develop resistance to some of the chemicals used in chemotherapy, so that the treatment gradually becomes less effective. Development of resistance is often associated with random duplication of DNA segments, commonly noted in tumor cells. In some, the random duplication happens to include genes that provide resistance to the chemicals employed in chemotherapy. The genes providing resistance usually encode enzymes that break down the applied chemical or its metabolic derivatives, or transport proteins of the plasma membrane capable of rapidly excreting the chemical from the cell. One gene in particular, the multidrug resistance gene (MDR), is frequently found to be duplicated or highly activated in resistant cells. This gene, which is normally active in cells of the liver, kidney, adrenal glands, and parts of the digestive system, encodes a transport pump that can expel a large number of substances from cells, including many of those used in chemotherapy. Overactivity of the MDR pump can effectively keep chemotherapy drugs below toxic levels in cancer cells. Cells developing resistance are more likely to survive chemotherapy and give rise to malignant cell lines with resistance. The chemotherapeutic agents involved may thus have the unfortunate effect of selecting cells with resistance, thereby ensuring that they will become the dominant types in the tumor.

Success rates with chemotherapy vary from negligible to about 80 percent, depending on the cancer type. For most, success rates do not range above 50 to 60 percent. Some cancer types, including lung, breast, ovarian, and colorectal tumors, respond poorly or not at all to chemotherapy. The overall cure rate for surgery, radiation, and chemotherapy combined, as judged by no recurrence of the cancer for a period of five years, is about 50 percent.

Full success in the treatment of cancer hopefully will come from the continued study of the genes controlling cell division and the regulatory mechanisms that modify the activity of these genes in the cell cycle. An understanding of the molecular activities of these genes and their modifying controls may bring with it a molecular means to reach specifically into cancer cells and halt their growth and metastasis.

## PERSPECTIVE AND PROSPECTS

Indications that malignancy and metastasis might have a basis in altered gene activity began to appear in the nineteenth century. In 1820, a British physician, Sir William Norris, noted that melanoma, a cancer involving pigmented skin cells, was especially prevalent in one family under study. More than forty kinds of cancer, including common types such as cancer of the breast and colon, have since been noticed to occur more frequently in some families than in others. Another indication that cancer has a basis in altered gene activity was the fact that the chromosomes of many tumor cells show abnormalities in the chromosomes, such as extra chromosomes, broken chromosomes, or rearrangements of one kind or another. These abnormalities suggested that cancer might be induced by altered genes with activities related to cell division.

These indications were put on a firm basis by research with tumors caused by viruses infecting animal cells, most notably those caused by a group of viruses infecting mammals and other animals, the retroviruses. Many retroviral infections cause little or no damage to their hosts. Some, however, are associated with induction of cancer. (Another type of pathogenic retrovirus is responsible for acquired immunodeficiency syndrome, or AIDS.) The cancer-inducing types among the retroviruses were found to carry genes capable of transforming normal cells to the malignant state. The transforming genes were at first thought to be purely viral in origin, but DNA sequencing and other molecular approaches revealed that the viral oncogenes had normal counterparts among the genes directly or indirectly regulating cell division in cells of the infected host. Among the most productive of the investigators using this approach were J. Michael Bishop and Harold E. Varmus, who received the 1989 Nobel Prize in Medicine for their research establishing the relationship between retroviral oncogenes and their normal cellular counterparts.

The discovery of altered host genes in cancer-inducing retroviruses prompted a search for similar genes in nonviral cancers. Much of this work was accomplished by transfection experiments, in which the DNA of cancer cells is extracted and introduced into cultured mouse cells. Frequently, the mouse cells are transformed into types that grow much more rapidly than normal cells. The human oncogene responsible for the transformation is then identified in the altered cells. Many of the oncogenes identified by transfection turned out to be among those already carried by retroviruses, confirming by a different route that these genes are capable of contributing to the transformation of cells to a cancerous state. The transfection experiments also identified some additional oncogenes not previously found in retroviruses.

In spite of impressive advances in treatment, cancer remains among the most dreaded of human diseases. Recognized as a major threat to health since the earliest days of recorded history, cancer still counts as one of the most frequent causes of human fatality. In technically advanced countries, it accounts for about 15 to 20 percent of deaths each year. In a typical year, more persons die from cancer in the United States than the total number of Americans killed in World War II and the Vietnam War combined. Smoking, the most frequent single cause of cancer, is estimated to be responsible for about one-third of these deaths.

*—Stephen L. Wolfe*

*See also* Cancer; Carcinoma; Lymphadenopathy and lymphoma; Tumors.

**FOR FURTHER INFORMATION:**

Alberts, Bruce, et al. *Molecular Biology of the Cell.* 2d ed. New York: Garland, 1989. Chapter 21 describes the development and characteristics of malignance and metastasis. The text is clearly written at the college level and is illustrated by numerous diagrams and photographs. An extensive bibliography of technical and scientific articles appears at the end of each chapter.

Cairns, John. *Cancer: Science and Society.* San Francisco: Freeman, 1978. A clearly written evaluation of the characteristics of cancer and its impact on human society. Although written at an advanced level, the work is accessible to the general reader.

Darnell, James, Harvey Lodish, and David Baltimore. *Molecular Cell Biology.* 2d ed. New York: Scientific American Books, 1990. An excellent textbook written at the college level. Chapter 24 provides an unusually complete discussion of the characteristics and causes of malignancy and metastasis. Many highly illustrative diagrams and photographs are included. A very extensive bibliography of technical articles and books is provided at the end of each chapter.

Weinberg, Robert A. "Finding the Anti-oncogene." *Scientific American* 259 (September, 1988): 44-51. A lucidly written description of tumor suppressor genes and their possible use as a means to inhibit tumor growth. Many innovative and informative illustrations are included with the article.

Wolfe, Stephen L. *Molecular and Cellular Biology.* Belmont, Calif.: Wadsworth, 1993. Chapter 22, "The Cell Cycle, Cell Cycle Regulation, and Cancer," describes the cellular factors and processes regulating the growth and division of both normal and malignant cells. The book, written at the college level, is readable and illustrated with many useful and informative diagrams and photographs.

# MALNUTRITION

**SYSTEMS AFFECTED:** All

**SPECIALISTS:** Registered dietitians, public health specialists

**DEFINITION:** Impaired health caused by an imbalance, either through deficiency or excess, in nutrients.

**KEY TERMS:**

*anemia:* a condition in which there is a lower-than-normal concentration of the iron-containing protein in red blood cells, which carry oxygen

*famine:* a lack of access to food, the cause of which can be a natural disaster, such as a drought, or a situation created by humans, such as a civil war

*kwashiorkor:* the condition that results from consuming a diet that is sufficient in energy (kilocalories) but inadequate in protein content

*marasmus:* the condition that results from consuming a diet that is deficient in both energy and protein

*osteoporosis:* a bone disorder in which the bone's mineral content is decreased over time, resulting in a weakening of the skeleton and susceptibility to bone fractures

*protein-energy malnutrition (PEM):* a deficient intake of energy (kilocalories) and/or protein, the most common type of undernutrition in developing countries; the two major types of PEM are kwashiorkor and marasmus

*undernutrition:* continued ill health caused by a long-standing dietary deficiency of the energy (kilocalories) and the nutrients that are required to maintain health and provide protection from disease

## CAUSES AND SYMPTOMS

Malnutrition literally means "bad nutrition." It can be used broadly to mean an excess or deficiency of the nutrients that are necessary for good health. In industrialized societies, malnutrition typically represents the excess consumption characterized by a diet containing too much energy (kilocalories), fat, and sodium. Malnutrition is most commonly thought, however, to be undernutrition or deficient intake, the consumption of inadequate amounts of nutrients to promote health or to support growth in children. The most severe form of undernutrition is called protein-energy malnutrition, or PEM. It commonly affects children, who require nutrients not only to help maintain the body but also to grow. Two types of PEM occur: kwashiorkor and marasmus.

Kwashiorkor is a condition in which a person consumes adequate energy but not enough protein. It usually is seen in children between one and four who are weaned so that the next baby can be breast-fed. The weaning diet consists of gruels made from starchy foods that do not contain an adequate supply of amino acids, the building blocks of protein. These diets do, however, provide enough energy.

Diets in many developing countries are high in bulk, making it nearly impossible for a child to consume a sufficient volume of foods such as rice and grain to obtain an adequate amount of protein for growth. The outward signs of kwashiorkor are a potbelly, dry unpigmented skin, coarse reddish hair, and edema in the legs. Edema results from a lack of certain proteins in the blood that help to maintain a normal fluid balance in the body. The potbelly and swollen limbs often are misinterpreted as signs of being "fat" among the developing world cultures. Other signs requiring further medical testing include fat deposits in the liver and decreased production of digestive enzymes. The mental and physical growth of the child are impaired. Children with kwashiorkor are apathetic, listless, and withdrawn. Ironically, these children lose their appetites. They become very susceptible to upper-respiratory infection and diarrhea. Children with kwashiorkor also are deficient in vitamins and minerals that are found in protein-rich foods. There are symptoms caused by these specific nutrient deficiencies as well.

Marasmus literally means "to waste away." It is caused by a deficiency of both Calories (kilocalories) and protein in the diet. This is the most severe form of childhood malnutrition. Body fat stores are used up to provide energy, and eventually muscle tissue is broken down for body fuel. Victims appear as skin and bones, gazing with large eyes from a bald head with an aged, gaunt appearance. Once severe muscle wasting occurs, death is imminent. Body temperature is below normal. The immune system does not operate normally, making these children extremely susceptible to respiratory and gastrointestinal infections.

A vicious cycle develops once the child succumbs to infection. Infection increases the body's need for protein, yet the PEM child is so protein deficient that recovery from even minor respiratory infections is prolonged. Pneumonia and measles become fatal diseases for PEM victims. Severe diarrhea compounds the problem. The child is often dehydrated, and any nourishment that might be consumed will not be adequately absorbed.

The long-term prognosis for these PEM children is poor. If the child survives infections and is refed, PEM returns once the child goes home to the same environment that caused it. Children with repeated episodes of kwashiorkor have high mortality rates.

Children with PEM are most likely victims of famine. Typically, these children either were not breast-fed or were breast-fed for only a few months. If a weaning formula is used, it has not been prepared properly; in many cases, it is mixed with unsanitary water or watered down because the parents cannot afford to buy enough to use it at full strength.

It is difficult to distinguish between the cause of kwashiorkor and that of marasmus. One child ingesting the same diet as another may develop kwashiorkor, while the other may develop marasmus. Some scientists think this may be a result of the different ways in which individuals adapt to nutritional deprivation. Others propose that kwashiorkor is caused by eating moldy grains, since it appears only in rainy, tropical areas.

Another type of malnutrition involves a deficiency of vitamins or minerals. Vitamin A is necessary for the maintenance of healthy skin, and even a mild deficiency causes susceptibility to diarrhea and upper respiratory infection. Diarrhea reinforces the vicious cycle of malnutrition, since it prevents nutrients from being absorbed. With a more severe vitamin A deficiency, changes in the eye and, eventually, blindness result. Night blindness is usually the first detectable symptom of vitamin A deficiency. The blood that bathes the eye cannot regenerate the visual pigments needed to see in the dark. Eventually, the tissues of the eye become infected and total blindness results. Vitamin A deficiency, the primary cause of childhood blindness, can result from the lack of either vitamin A or the protein that transports it in the blood. If the deficiency of vitamin A occurs during pregnancy or at birth, the skull does not develop normally and the brain is crowded. An older child deficient in vitamin A will suffer growth impairment.

Diseases resulting from B-vitamin deficiencies are rare. Strict vegetarians called vegans, who consume no animal products, are at risk for vitamin $B_{12}$ deficiency resulting in an anemia in which the red blood cells are large and immature. Too little folate (folic acid) in the diet can cause this same anemia. Beriberi is the deficiency disease of thiamine (vitamin $B_1$) in which the heart and nervous systems are damaged and muscle wasting occurs. Ariboflavinosis (lack of riboflavin) describes a collection of symptoms such as cracks and redness of the eyes and lips; inflamed, sensitive eyelids; and a purple-red tongue. Pellagra is the deficiency disease of niacin (vitamin $B_3$). It is characterized by "the Four Ds of pellagra": dermatitis, diarrhea, dementia, and death. Isolated deficiency of a B vitamin is rare, since many B vitamins work in concert. Therefore, a lack of one hinders the function of the rest.

Scurvy is the deficiency disease of vitamin C. Early signs of scurvy are bleeding gums and pinpoint hemorrhages under the skin. As the deficiency becomes more severe, the skin becomes rough, brown, and scaly, eventually resulting in impaired wound healing, soft bones, painful joints, and loose teeth. Finally, hardening of the arteries or massive bleeding results in death.

Rickets is the childhood deficiency disease of vitamin D. Bone formation is impaired, which is reflected in a bow-legged or knock-kneed appearance. In adults, a brittle bone condition called osteomalacia results from vitamin D deficiency.

Malnutrition of minerals is more prevalent in the world, since deficiencies are observed in both industrialized and developing countries. Calcium malnutrition in young children results in stunted growth. Osteoporosis occurs when calcium reserves are drawn upon to supply the other body parts with calcium. This occurs in later adulthood, leaving bones weak and fragile. General loss of stature and fractures of the hip, pelvis, and wrist are common, and a humpback appears. Caucasian and Asian women of small stature are at greatest risk for osteoporosis.

Iron-deficiency anemia is the most common form of malnutrition in developing societies. Lack of consumption of iron-rich foods is common among the poor, especially in women who menstruate. This deficiency, which is characterized by small, pale red blood cells, causes weakness, fatigue, and sensitivity to cold temperatures. Anemia in children can cause reduced ability to learn and impaired ability to think and to concentrate.

Deficiencies of other minerals are less common. Although these deficiencies are usually seen among people in developing nations, they may occur among the poor, pregnant women, children, and the elderly in industrialized societies. Severe growth retardation and arrested sexual maturation are characteristics of zinc deficiency. With iodine deficiency, the cells in the thyroid gland enlarge to try to trap as much iodine as possible. This enlargement of the thyroid gland is called simple or endemic goiter. A more severe iodine deficiency results from a lack of iodine that leads to a deficiency of thyroid hormone during pregnancy. The child of a mother with such a deficiency is born with severe mental and/or physical retardation, a condition known as cretinism.

The causes of malnutrition, therefore, can be difficult to isolate, because nutrients work together in the body. In addition, the underlying causes of malnutrition (poverty, famine, and war) often are untreatable.

### TREATMENT AND THERAPY

Treatment for PEM involves refeeding with a diet adequate in protein, Calories, and other essential nutrients. Response to treatment is influenced by many factors, such as the person's age, the stage of development in which the deprivation began, the severity of the deficiency, the duration of the deficiency, and the presence of other illnesses, particularly infections. Total recovery is possible only if the underlying cause that led to PEM can be eliminated.

PEM can result from illnesses such as cancer and acquired immunodeficiency syndrome (AIDS). Victims of these diseases cannot consume diets with enough energy and protein to meet their body needs, which are higher than normal because of the illness. Infections also increase the need for many nutrients. The first step in treatment must be to cure the underlying infection. People from cultures in which PEM is prevalent believe that food should not be given to an ill person.

Prevention of PEM is the preferred therapy. In areas with unsafe water supplies and high rates of poverty, women should be encouraged to breast-feed. Education about proper weaning foods provides further defense against PEM. Other preventive efforts involve combining plant proteins into a mixture of high-quality protein, adding nutrients to cereal products, and using genetic engineering to produce grains with a better protein mix. The prevention of underlying causes such as famine and drought may not be feasible.

Prekwashiorkor can be identified by regular plotting of the child's growth. If treatment begins at this stage, patient response is rapid and the prognosis is good. Treatment must begin by correcting the body's fluid imbalance. Low potassium levels must be corrected. Restoration of fluid is followed by adequate provision of Calories, with gradual additions of protein that the patient can use to repair damaged immune and digestive systems. Treatment must happen rapidly yet allow the digestive system to recover—thus the term "hurry slowly." Once edema is corrected and blood potassium levels are restored, a diluted milk with added sugar can be given. Gradually, vegetable oil is added to increase the intake of Calories. Vitamin and mineral supplements are given. Final diet therapy includes a diet of skim milk and other animal protein sources, coupled with the addition of vegetables and fat.

The residual effects of PEM may be great if malnutrition has come at a critical period in development or has been of long duration. In prolonged cases, damage to growth and the digestive system may be irreversible. Mortality is very high in such cases. Normally, the digestive tract undergoes rapid cell replacement; therefore, this system is one of the first to suffer in PEM. Absorptive surfaces shrink, and digestive enzymes and protein carriers that transport nutrients are lacking.

Another critical factor in the treatment of PEM is the stage of development in which the deprivation occurs. Most PEM victims are children. If nutritional deprivation occurs during pregnancy, the consequence is increased risk of infant death. If the child is carried to term, it is of low birth weight, placing it at high risk for death. Malnutrition during lactation decreases the quantity, but not always the nutritional quality, of milk. Thus, fewer Calories are consumed by the baby. Growth of the child is slowed. These babies are short for their age and continue to be shorter later in life, even if their diet improves.

During the first two years of life, the brain continues to grow. Nutritional deprivation can impair mental development and cognitive function. For only minimal damage to occur, malnutrition must be treated in early stages. Adults experiencing malnutrition are more adaptive to it, since their protein-energy needs are not as great. Weight loss, muscle wasting, and impaired immune function occur, and malnourished women stop menstruating.

Successful treatment of a specific nutrient deficiency depends on the duration of the deficiency and the stage in a person's development at which it occurs. Vitamin A is a fat-soluble vitamin that is stored in the body. Thus, oral supplements or injections of vitamin A can provide long-term protection from this deficiency. If vitamin A is given early enough, the deficiency can be rapidly reversed. By the time the child is blind, sight cannot be restored, and frequently the child dies because of other illnesses. Treatment also is dependent upon adequate protein to provide carriers in the blood to transport these vitamins. Treatment of the B-vitamin deficiencies involves oral and intramuscular injections. The crucial step in treatment is to initiate therapy before irreversible damage has occurred. Scurvy (vitamin C deficiency) can be eliminated in five days by administering the amount of vitamin C found in approximately three cups of orange juice. Treatment of vitamin D deficiency in children and adults involves an oral dose of two to twelve times the recommended daily allowance of the vitamin. Halibut and cod liver oils are frequently given as vitamin D supplements.

Successful treatment of a mineral deficiency depends on the timing and duration of the deficiency. Once the bones are fully grown, restoring calcium to optimal levels will not correct short stature. To prevent osteoporosis, bones must have been filled to the maximum with calcium during early adulthood. Estrogen replacement therapy and weight-bearing exercise retard calcium loss in later years and do more than calcium supplements can.

Iron supplementation is necessary to correct iron-deficiency anemia. Iron supplements are routinely prescribed for pregnant women to prevent anemia during pregnancy. Treatment also includes a diet with adequate meat, fish, and poultry to provide not only iron but also a factor that enhances absorption. Iron absorption is also enhanced by vitamin C. Anemias caused by lack of folate and vitamin $B_{12}$ will not respond to iron therapy. These anemias must be treated by adding the appropriate vitamin to the diet.

Zinc supplementation can correct arrested sexual maturation and impaired growth if it is begun in time. In areas where the soil does not contain iodine, iodine is added to salt or injections of iodized oil are given to prevent goiter. Cretinism cannot be cured—only prevented.

In general, malnutrition is caused by a diet of limited variety and quantity. The underlying causes of malnutrition—poverty, famine, and war—are often untreatable. Overall treatment lies in prevention by providing all people with a diet that is adequate in all nutrients, including vitamins, minerals, and Calories. Sharing the world's wealth and ending political strife and greed are essential elements of the struggle to end malnutrition.

## PERSPECTIVE AND PROSPECTS

Over the years, the study of malnutrition has shifted to include the excessive intake of nutrients. In developing countries, the primary causes of death are infectious diseases, and undernutrition is a risk factor. In industrialized societies, however, the primary causes of death are chronic diseases, and overnutrition is a risk factor. The excessive consumption of sugar is linked to tooth decay. Also, overnutrition in terms of too much fat and Calories in the diet leads to obesity, high blood pressure, stroke, heart disease, some cancers, liver disease, and one type of diabetes.

Historically, the focus of malnutrition studies was deficiencies in the diet. In the 1930's, classic kwashiorkor was described by Cicely Williams. Not until after World War II was it known that kwashiorkor was caused by a lack of protein in the diet. In 1959, Derrick B. Jelliffe introduced the term "protein-calorie malnutrition" to describe the nutritional disorders of marasmus, marasmic kwashiorkor, and kwashiorkor.

PEM remains the most important public health problem in developing countries. Few cases are seen in Western societies. Historically, the root causes have been urbanization, periods of famine, and the failure to breast-feed or early cessation of breast-feeding. Marasmus is prevalent in urban areas among infants under one year old, while kwashiorkor is prevalent in rural areas during the second year of life.

Deficiencies of specific nutrients have been documented throughout history. Vitamin A deficiency and its cure were documented by Egyptians and Chinese around 1500 B.C. In occupied Denmark during World War I, vitamin A deficiency, caused by dairy product deprivation, was common in Danish children. Beriberi, first documented in the Far East, was caused by diets of polished rice that were deficient in thiamine. Pellagra was seen in epidemic proportions in the southern United States, where corn was the staple grain, during World War I.

Zinc deficiency was first reported in the 1960's. The growth and maturation of boys in the Middle East were studied. Their diets were low in zinc and high in substances that prevented zinc absorption. Consequently, the World Health Organization recommended increased zinc intake for populations whose staple is unleavened whole grain bread. Goiter was documented during Julius Caesar's reign. Simply adding iodine to salt has virtually eliminated goiter in the United States.

If classic malnutrition is observed in industrialized societies, it usually is secondary to other diseases, such as AIDS and cancer. Hunger and poverty are problems that contribute to malnutrition; however, the malnutrition that results is less severe than that found in developing countries.

Specific nutrients may be lacking in the diets of the poor. Iron-deficiency anemia is prevalent among the poor, and this anemia may impair learning ability. Other deficiencies may be subclinical, which means that no detectable signs are observed, yet normal nutrient pools in the body are depleted. Homelessness, poverty, and drug or alcohol abuse are the major contributing factors to these conditions. In addition, malnutrition as a result of poverty is exacerbated by lack of nutritional knowledge and/or poor food choices.
—*Wendy L. Stuhldreher*

**See also** Anorexia nervosa; Beriberi; Botulism; Bulimia; Cholesterol; Eating disorders; Food poisoning; Hyperlipidemia; Kwashiorkor; Lead poisoning; Obesity; Osteoporosis; Poisoning; Scurvy; Vitamin and mineral deficiencies; Weight loss and gain.

## FOR FURTHER INFORMATION:

Bender, Arnold E., and David A. Bender. *Nutrition for Medical Students*. New York: Vail-Ballou Press, 1982. Two major sections of this book are devoted to the problem of nutrition in industrialized nations (overnutrition) and the problem in developing countries (undernutrition). Some of the information is quite technical, yet the average reader can obtain further information on nutrition and disease and avoid the technical descriptions.

Christian, Janet L., and Janet L. Greger. *Nutrition for Living*. 3d ed. Redwood City, Calif.: Benjamin/Cummings, 1991. This introductory textbook of nutrition is easy to understand. It provides brief explanations of various vitamin and mineral deficiencies, as well as of PEM. Photographs showing symptoms are included.

Davidson, L. Stanley Patrick, Reginald Passmore, and Martin A. Eastwood. *Davidson and Passmore Human Nutrition and Dietetics*. 8th ed. New York: Churchill Livingstone, 1986. Several chapters in this book provide information on malnutrition, from PEM to specific nutrient deficiencies. History, causes, symptoms, and treatments of the disorders are covered. An excellent list of references is provided. Photographs of victims of deficiency diseases are included.

Kreutler, Patricia A., and Dorice M. Czajka-Narins. *Nutrition in Perspective*. 2d ed. Englewood Cliffs, N.J.: Prentice-Hall, 1987. This textbook provides a chapter on the food supply, including issues for meeting the problem of undernutrition. It also describes the deficiency diseases for vitamins and minerals and PEM in various chapters.

Physician Task Force on Hunger in America. *Hunger in America*. Scranton, Pa.: Harper & Row, 1985. This document provides a synopsis of the findings by the Task Force on the extent of hunger, regional variations, the assessment of health effects, and recommendations for remedying the problem in America.

Wardlaw, Gordon M., Paul M. Insel, and Marcia F. Seyler. *Contemporary Nutrition*. St. Louis: Mosby Year Book, 1991. Chapter 18 of this text covers undernutrition. This chapter emphasizes the types of undernutrition and hunger found in America.

Whitney, Eleanor Noss, and Sharon Rady Rolfes. *Understanding Nutrition*. 6th ed. St. Paul, Minn.: West, 1993. This is an introductory nutrition textbook. Various chapters have information about the different nutrient deficiencies and malnutrition.

Winick, Myron, Brian L. G. Morgan, Jaime Rozovski, and Robin Marks-Kaufman, eds. *The Columbia Encyclopedia of Nutrition*. New York: G. P. Putnam's Sons, 1988. Brief synopses of marasmus and kwashiorkor are provided. Descriptions of isolated nutrient deficiencies also can be found in the sections on specific nutrients.

# Manic-depressive disorder

**System affected:** Psychic-emotional
**Specialists:** Psychiatrists, psychologists
**Definition:** A recurrent affective (mood) illness characterized either by alternating periods of extreme depression and extreme elation or, less often, by only one of these moods.

**Key terms:**

*affective disorders:* a group of disorders characterized by a disturbance of mood accompanied by a full or partial manic or depressive syndrome that is not caused by any other physical or mental disorder

*bipolar:* a manic-depressive course with both manias and depressions

*lithium:* a drug used in the treatment of manic-depression

*psychosis:* any mental disorder in which the personality is seriously disorganized

*unipolar:* a manic-depressive course with recurrent depression and no mania

## Causes and Symptoms

Although the causes of manic-depressive illness (often called manic-depression) are not known, research indicates that some persons may be genetically predisposed to respond readily with mania or depression to internal and external influences. It is believed that insufficient resolution of deep personality problems may also play a role. While changes in the metabolism of the brain are thought to be significant in the development of manic-depressive episodes, both psychological and nonpsychological stresses are able to precipitate such episodes. It is often not possible, however, to find one precipitating factor, since there is presumably a complex interaction between the effects of internal and external influences in persons suffering from this disease.

Manic-depression is an illness that occurs in attacks, or episodes. These may be attacks of mania (periods of extreme elation and increased activity) or attacks of depression (periods of abnormal sadness and melancholy). A patient may have both manias and depressions (a bipolar course). Some patients have only depressions, and a few have only manias. Occasionally, the disease presents a mixture of manic and depressive features; this condition is referred to as a "mixed state." The degree, type, and chronicity of cognitive, perceptual, and behavioral disorganization determine the subclassifications, or stages, of mania. In increasing order of severity, these stages are hypomania, acute mania, and delirious mania (severe mania with psychotic overtones).

Manic-depression is a fairly common disease. About one to two persons out of every hundred develop, at some time in life, symptoms of such severity that hospitalization is required. More women than men suffer from the disease. The onset of the disease frequently occurs between the ages of thirty and fifty, but it may appear for the first time at fifteen to twenty years of age and as late as sixty to seventy years. Manic and depressive episodes present themselves differently in different persons; they can even vary within a particular patient from one time to another. Although mania has characteristic features, not all features are present during each manic episode.

Prominent features of manic episodes are elation, easily aroused anger, and increased mental activity. The elation varies from unusual vigor to uninhibited enthusiasm. The anger most often takes the form of irritability. Manic patients become annoyed if other people are unable to keep up with their racing thoughts. Intellectual activity takes place with lightning speed, ideas race through the mind, speech flows with great rapidity and almost uninterruptedly, and puns alternate with caustic commentary.

During a manic episode, patients are often excessively self-confident and lacking in self-criticism. This produces a previously unknown energy, and when that energy is combined with racing thoughts, indefatigability, and lack of inhibition, the consequences are often disastrous. During manic episodes, patients may destroy their relationships, ruin their reputations, or create financial disasters.

Manic patients usually sleep very little. They rarely feel tired and are usually kept awake by the rapid flow of ideas. Sexual activity may also be increased. Manic patients often neglect to eat and may lose weight. The combination of violent activity, decreased food intake, and an inadequate amount of sleep may lead to physical exhaustion.

Depressions are in many respects the opposite of manias. They are characterized by sadness, a lack of self-confidence, and decreased mental activity. The sadness may vary from a slight feeling of being "down" to the bleakest despair. Ideas are few, thoughts move slowly, and memory function is impaired. Frequently, depressed patients feel tired and emotionally drained; they feel the need to cry but are unable to do so. Weighed down by feelings of guilt and self-reproach, they may contemplate or even commit suicide.

The depressed patient's courage and self-confidence are eroded, and as a result the patient is resigned, lacks initiative and energy, feels that obstacles are insurmountable, and has difficulty making even trivial decisions. Because of their low self-esteem and feelings of inadequacy, patients suffering from depression often fear social interaction and become anxious, agitated, and restless in a crowd. Sleep disturbances are also frequent. Occasionally, there is an increased need for sleep, but more often patients have difficulty sleeping. Some patients find it difficult to fall asleep, others wake up frequently during the night, and others wake up early with feelings of anxiety. Depressed patients often experience variations in mood over the course of a day. They are, typically, depressed late at night and in the early morning. The desire to stay in bed is overwhelming, and the first hours of the day are difficult to get through.

Depressions are often accompanied by physical transformations. The muscles give the impression of being slack, the facial expression is static, and movement is slow. There may be constipation, menstruation may stop, and sexual interest and activity usually decrease. Appetite is reduced, and there is a resulting loss of weight. The cessation of depression is sometimes followed by a light and transient mania, which may be seen as a reaction to the depression or as a sign of relief that it is over.

In addition to manias and depressions, manic-depressive disease may present mixed states during which signs of mania and depression are present concurrently. Patients who experience mixed states may be sad and without energy but also irritable, or they may be manic and restless yet feel an underlying melancholy. Mixed states may occur as independent episodes, but they are seen more often during transitions from mania to depression or from depression to mania. During these periods of transition, the condition may alternate between mania and depression several times within the course of a day. During the intervals between episodes, the patients often enjoy mental health and stability.

## TREATMENT AND THERAPY

Until the 1950's, manic-depressive illness had remained intractable, frustrating the best efforts of clinical practitioners and their predecessors. This long history ended abruptly with the discovery of lithium's therapeutic benefits. In an ironic turn of events, the pharmacologic revolution then initiated a renaissance in the psychotherapy of manic-depressive patients. Substantially freed from the severe disruptions of mania and the profound withdrawal of depression, patients, with the help of their therapists, could focus on the many psychological issues related to the illness and also confront basic developmental tasks. Even a combination of drugs and psychotherapy, however, cannot yield a completely satisfactory outcome for every patient. Yet the treatment approaches that are available do allow most manic-depressive patients to lead relatively normal lives.

Electroconvulsive therapy (ECT) is one alternative to medications in treating acute manic-depressive disorder. Although ECT may be used to treat severely manic patients, those who have proven unresponsive to drugs, and those in mixed states with a high risk of suicide, it is used primarily for severe depressions. In ECT, following narcosis (an unconscious state induced by narcotics), certain parts of the patient's brain are stimulated electrically through electrodes placed on the skin. This stimulation elicits a seizure, but since the drug relaxes the muscles, the seizure manifests as muscle twitching only. The patients do not feel the treatment, but during the hours following the treatment, they may have headaches and feel tenderness of the muscles. Transitory memory impairment may also occur. Treatment, which occurs two to four times a week for three to four weeks, leads to amelioration of symptoms in most patients. ECT may be given at a hospital or on an outpatient basis.

For treatment of manic agitation, the so-called neuroleptics are often used. These are sedative drugs such as chlorpromazine (Largactil, Thorazine) and haloperidol (Haldol). Neuroleptics exert a powerful tranquilizing effect on anxiety, restlessness, and tension. They also attenuate or relieve hallucinations and delusions. Neuroleptics are not specific for any single disease. They may be used, possibly in conjunction with lithium, in the treatment of mania, and they may be used in depressions that are accompanied by delusions. Neuroleptics may, however, produce side effects involving the muscles and the nervous system.

Antidepressants act, as the name indicates, on depression, but only on abnormal depression; they do not affect ordinary sadness or grief. They are drugs such as imipramine (Tofranil) and amitriptyline (Elavil, Tryptizol). The side effects of antidepressants may include tiredness, mouth dryness, tremor, constipation, difficulty in urinating, and a tendency to faint. Changes in heart rate and rhythm may also occur, and careful evaluation is necessary in patients with cardiac disease.

Treatment with antidepressants is most often continued for some time after disappearance of the symptoms; for example, three to four months. Occasionally, antidepressant therapy precipitates episodes of mania, and patients with previous attacks of mania may have to discontinue antidepressants earlier than other patients. In patients with a bipolar course who require prophylactic (preventive) treatment, lithium is indicated. Patients with a unipolar course may be treated prophylactically with either lithium or antidepressants.

Lithium, a metallic element discovered by a Swedish chemist in 1818, is produced from lithium-containing minerals such as spodumene, amblygonite, lepidolite, and petalite. As a drug, lithium is always used in the form of one of its salts; for example, lithium carbonate or lithium citrate. It is the lithium portion of these salts that is effective medically.

Lithium was introduced into medicine in 1850 for the treatment of gout, and during the following century many medical uses of the element were proposed. It was used, for example, as a stimulant, as a sedative, for the treatment of diabetes, for the treatment of infectious diseases, as an additive to toothpaste, and for the treatment of malignant growths. The efficacy of lithium in these conditions was not proved, however, and lithium treatment never became widespread.

In 1949, an Australian psychiatrist, John Cade, published an article that forms the basis of all later lithium treatment. The prophylactic action of lithium in manic-depressive illness was debated in the psychiatric literature for some years, but extensive trials in many countries have fully documented the efficacy of the drug. Its prophylactic action is exerted against both manic and depressive relapses, and it can be seen in unipolar as well as bipolar patients.

One of the characteristic features of lithium is that it removes manic symptoms without producing sedation, unlike treatment with neuroleptics, which are also effective in the treatment of mania but which exert sedative action. Lithium may occasionally produce side effects, such as nausea, stomachache, tremor of the hands, and muscle weakness, but these symptoms are usually neither severe nor incapacitating. The greatest drawback of the treatment is that the full antimanic effect is usually not seen until after six to eight days of treatment, and sometimes it is necessary to supplement lithium with a neuroleptic drug.

In addition to being used in the treatment of manic episodes, lithium is also used in the prevention of manic-depressive illness; moreover, the drug's prophylactic effect is almost as beneficial in the treatment of depression as it is in the treatment of mania. While lithium may also be used to treat depressive episodes, this use is less widespread because treatment with antidepressants and electric convulsive therapy appear to be more effective in cases of depression.

Although prophylaxis denotes prevention, lithium is unable to prevent the development of manic-depressive illness. Lithium prophylaxis merely prevents relapse so that manic and depressive recurrences become less frequent or disappear during treatment. Thus, prophylactic lithium keeps the illness under control but does not cure it. If the patient's lithium therapy ceases, the disease is likely to reappear, exhibiting episodes as frequent and severe as those that occurred before therapy. Therefore, it is necessary that patients continue taking lithium during periods in which no signs of illness are present.

Manic-depressive illness is treated most effectively with a combination of lithium or other medications and adjunctive psychotherapy. Drug treatment, which is primary, relieves most patients of the severe disruptions of manic and depressive episodes. Psychotherapy can assist them in coming to terms with the repercussions of past episodes and in comprehending the practical implications of living with manic-depressive illness.

Although not all patients require psychotherapy, most can benefit from individual, group, and/or family therapy. Moreover, participation in a self-help group is often useful in supplementing or supplanting formal psychotherapy. Psychotherapeutic issues are dictated by the nature of the illness: Manifested by profound changes in perception, attitudes, personality, mood, and cognition, manic-depressive illness can lead to suicide, violence, alcoholism, drug abuse, and hospitalization. Although reactions vary widely, patients typically feel angry and ambivalent about both the illness and its treatment. They may deny its existence, its severity, or its consequences, and they are often concerned about issues such as relationships and the possibility of genetically transmitting the illness to their children.

No one technique has been shown to be superior in the psychotherapy of manic-depressive patients. The therapist is guided by knowledge of both the illness itself and its manifestation in the individual patient. In style and technique, the therapist must remain flexible in order to adjust to the patient's fluctuating levels of dependency and mood change, cognition and behavior. The therapist must be especially alert to the countertransference issues that commonly occur when working with manic-depressive patients. In addition, educating patients and their families is essential because it helps them to recognize new episodes.

### PERSPECTIVE AND PROSPECTS

Manic-depressive illness is among the most consistently identifiable of all mental disorders, and it is also one of the oldest; it is discernible in descriptions in the Old Testament, and it was recognized in clinical medicine almost two thousand years ago. The medical writers of ancient Greece (the

Hippocratic school) conceived of mental disorders in terms that sound remarkably modern. They believed that melancholia was a psychological manifestation of an underlying biological disturbance—specifically, a perturbation in brain function. Early conceptions of "melancholia" and "mania" were, however, broader than those of modern times. These two terms, together with "phrenitis," which roughly corresponds to an acute organic delirium, comprised all mental illnesses throughout most of the ancient period.

As they did with other illnesses, the Hippocratic writers argued forcefully that mental disorders were not caused by supernatural or magical forces, as primitive societies had believed. Their essentially biological explanation for the cause of melancholia, which survived until the Renaissance, was part of the prevailing understanding of all health as an equilibrium of the four humors—blood, yellow bile, black bile, and phlegm—and all illness as a disturbance of this equilibrium. First fully developed in the Hippocratic work *Nature of Man* (c. 400 B.C.), the humoral theory linked the humors with the seasons and with relative moistness. An excess of black bile was seen as the cause of melancholia, a term that literally means "black bile." Mania, by contrast, was usually attributed to an excess of yellow bile.

Reflections on the relationship between melancholia and mania date back at least to the first century B.C. and Soranus of Ephesus. Artaeus of Cappadocia, who lived in the second century A.D., appears to have been the first to suggest that mania was an end-stage of melancholia, a view that was to prevail for centuries to come. He isolated "cyclothymia" (an obsolete term for mild fluctuations of the manic-depressive type) as a form of mental disease presenting phases of depression alternating with phases of mania. Although Artaeus included syndromes that in the twentieth century would be classified as schizophrenia, his clear descriptions of the spectrum of manic conditions are impressive even in modern times.

The next significant medical writer, Galen of Pergamon (A.D. 131-201), firmly established melancholia as a chronic condition. His few comments on mania included the observation that it can be either a primary disease of the brain or secondary to other diseases. His primary contribution was his all-encompassing elaboration of the humoral theory, a system so compelling that it dominated medical thought for more than a millennium.

Medical observations in succeeding centuries continued to subscribe to the conceptions of depression and mania laid down in classical Greece and Rome. Most authors wrote of the two conditions as separate illnesses yet suggested a close connection between them. Yet where mania and depression are considered in the historical medical literature, they are almost always linked.

The explicit conception of manic-depressive illness as a single disease entity dates from the mid-nineteenth century. Jean Pierre Falret and Jules Baillarger, French "alienists,"

independently and almost simultaneously formulated the idea that mania and depression could represent different manifestations of a single illness. In 1854, Falret described a circular disorder that he expressly defined as an illness in which the succession of mania and melancholia manifested itself with continuity and in an almost regular manner. That same year, Baillarger described essentially the same thing, emphasizing that the manic and depressive episodes were not two different attacks, but two different stages of the same attack. Despite the contributions of Falret, Jeanne-Étienne-Dominique Esquirol, and other observers, however, most clinical investigators continued to regard mania and melancholia as separate chronic entities that followed a deteriorating course.

It was left to the German psychiatrist Emil Kraepelin (1856-1926) to distinguish psychotic illnesses from one another and to draw the perimeter clearly around manic-depressive illness. He emphasized careful diagnosis based on both longitudinal history and the pattern of current symptoms. By 1913, in the eighth edition of Kraepelin's textbook of psychiatry, virtually all of melancholia had been subsumed into manic-depressive illness.

Wide acceptance of Kraepelin's broad divisions led to further explorations of the boundaries between the two basic categories of manic-depressive illness and dementia praecox, the delineation of their similarities, and the possibility that subgroups could be identified within two basic categories. Kraepelin's synthesis was a major accomplishment because it formed a solid and empirically anchored base for future developments.

During the first half of the twentieth century, the views of Adolf Meyer (1866-1950) gradually assumed a dominant position in American psychiatry, a position that they maintained for several decades. Meyer believed that psychopathology emerged from interactions between an individual's biological and psychological characteristics and his or her social environment. This perspective was evident in the label "manic-depressive reaction" in the first official American Psychiatric Association diagnostic manual, which was published in 1952. When the Meyerian focus, considerably influenced by psychoanalysis, turned to manic-depressive illness, the individual in the environment became the natural center of study, and clinical descriptions of symptoms and the longitudinal course of the illness were given less emphasis.

Eugen Bleuler (1857-1939), in his classic contributions to descriptive psychiatry, departed from Kraepelin by conceptualizing the relationship between manic-depressive (affective) illness and dementia praecox (schizophrenia) as a continuum without a sharp line of demarcation. Bleuler also broadened Kraepelin's concept of manic-depressive illness by designating several subcategories and using the term "affective illness." His subcategories of affective illness anticipated the principal contemporary division of the classic manic-depressive diagnostic group—the bipolar-unipolar distinction. The bipolar-unipolar distinction represents a major advance in the classification of affective disorders primarily because it provides a basis for evaluating genetic, pharmacological, clinical, and biological differences rather than representing a purely descriptive subgrouping.

—*Genevieve Slomski*

*See also* Anxiety; Depression; Psychiatric disorders.

**FOR FURTHER INFORMATION:**

Goodwin, Frederick K., and K. R. Jamison. *Manic Depressive Illness*. New York: Oxford University Press, 1990. Drawing on their extensive clinical and research experience, the authors have analyzed and interpreted the literature on manic-depressive illness and presented a unique synthesis of information for the acute and chronic management of manic-depressive patients. This 938-page work contains more than 100 pages of references.

Mondimore, Francis M. *Depression: The Mood Disease*. Rev. ed. Baltimore: The Johns Hopkins University Press, 1993. In this excellent scholarly work, the author discusses the biological basis of and medical treatment for depression, mood swings, and other affective disorders. Contains a bibliography.

Rosenthal, Norman E. *Seasons of the Mind*. New York: Bantam Books, 1989. An insightful popular account of depression. The author discusses the etiology of the "winter blues" and what can be done about it. Charting moods to obtain an objective pattern of moods and treatment responses is one useful technique suggested by Rosenthal. Contains a useful reading list.

Winokur, George, et al. *Manic Depressive Illness*. St. Louis: C. V. Mosby, 1969. This book discusses manic-depressive illness in terms of data collected over the course of many years. In reviewing previous studies and presenting their own data, the authors have attempted to offer a set of clinical and genetic findings that are fundamental to the understanding of the illness. Both etiologies and treatment are discussed. Appendices and glossary included.

Wolpert, Edward A., ed. *Manic Depressive Illness: History of a Syndrome*. New York: International Universities Press, 1977. This lengthy and scholarly work presents a collection of papers that are historically significant in the development of understanding of manic-depressive illness. The aim of demonstrating the developmental history of the idea embodied in the syndrome allows the reader to transcend an enumeration of symptoms and arrive at an understanding of the syndrome itself.

# MASTITIS

**SYSTEM AFFECTED:** Breasts

**SPECIALISTS:** Gynecologists

**DEFINITION:** Mastitis is an infection of the female breast resulting in inflammation, tenderness, swelling, and pain.

The condition often occurs with breast-feeding, when bacteria enter through the nipple. The infection does not spread rapidly, generally remaining localized, because the breast is composed of much fatty tissue and has a widely dispersed system of blood vessels. An abscess may form, in which the infected tissue hardens and becomes walled off from healthy tissue. Antibiotics usually destroy the bacteria; if not, a needle biopsy, mammogram, or surgical biopsy may be indicated to rule out cancer. Mastitis can also be caused by changes in sex hormones in newborns and at puberty, and chronic mastitis, which is characterized by lumps in the breasts, may be attributable to hormone changes as well.

*See also* Abscesses; Breast disorders; Breast-feeding.

# MEASLES, RED

**SYSTEMS AFFECTED:** Immune, respiratory, skin

**SPECIALISTS:** Epidemiologists, family physicians, infectious disease physicians, pediatricians, public health specialists

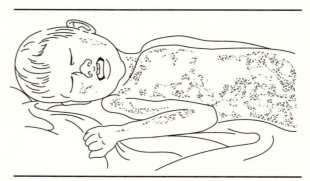

*Red measles most often affects children; its calling card is the rash that appears on the face and spreads downward.*

**DEFINITION:** Also known as rubeola, red measles was once a major childhood infectious disease but is now controlled through immunization. Measles is a viral illness; one attack gives the patient lifetime immunity. Measles is highly contagious and causes a wide range of symptoms: a low-grade fever, coughing, a runny nose, and sore eyes or conjunctivitis. Between two and four days after these first symptoms, a rash appears on the face and may spread downward. The fever may rise, perhaps dramatically. The illness usually begins to subside from one to three days later; if not, then complications can develop, such as a relapse of rash and fever, gastrointestinal disorders, pneumonia, or ear infections. In rare cases, encephalitis, seizures, and coma may occur.

*See also* Childhood infectious diseases; Rubella; Rubeola; Roseola.

# MELANOMA. *See* SKIN CANCER.

## MEMORY LOSS. *See* AMNESIA AND MEMORY LOSS.

## MÉNIÈRE'S DISEASE

**SYSTEM AFFECTED:** Auditory

**SPECIALISTS:** Audiologists, neurologists, otolaryngologists

**DEFINITION:** Ménière's disease is a dysfunction of the inner ear, or labyrinth; it is thought to result from a buildup of fluid in the labyrinth, which creates pressure. Consequently, hearing and balance are affected, with severe vertigo, tinnitus (ringing or buzzing in the ears), and progressive hearing loss. In addition, acute attacks of vertigo can occur, lasting from ten minutes to several hours. These attacks may cause nausea, vomiting, and sweating. Periods of remission may increase along with hearing loss, and attacks may stop completely with total loss of hearing. At this point, in order to restore balance, surgery may be used to destroy the inner ear, since hearing can no longer be affected.

*See also* Ear infections and disorders; Hearing loss.

## MENINGITIS

**SYSTEMS AFFECTED:** Brain, nervous

**SPECIALISTS:** Emergency physicians, infectious disease physicians, neurologists, public health specialists

**DEFINITION:** An inflammation of the meninges of the brain and spinal cord.

### CAUSES AND SYMPTOMS

The meninges is the three-layered covering of the spinal cord and brain. The layers are the outer dura mater, inner pia mater, and middle arachnoid. Meningitis is the inflammation or infection of the arachnoid and pia mater. It is characterized by severe headaches, vomiting, and pain and stiffness in the neck. These symptoms may be preceded by an upper-respiratory infection. The age of the patient may affect which signs and symptoms are displayed. Newborns may exhibit either fever or hypothermia, along with lethargy or irritability, disinterest in feeding, and abdominal distension. In infants, examination may find bulging of the fontanelles (the soft areas between the bones of the skull found in newborns). The elderly may show lethargy, confusion, or disorientation. As pressure in the skull increases, nausea and vomiting may occur. With meningococcal meningitis, a rash of pinpoint-sized or larger dots appears.

Most cases of meningitis are the result of bacterial infection. These cases are sometimes referred to as septic meningitis. The bacteria invade the subarachnoid space and may have traveled from another site of infection, having caused pneumonia, cellulitis, or an ear infection. It is unclear if the bacteria make their way from the original area

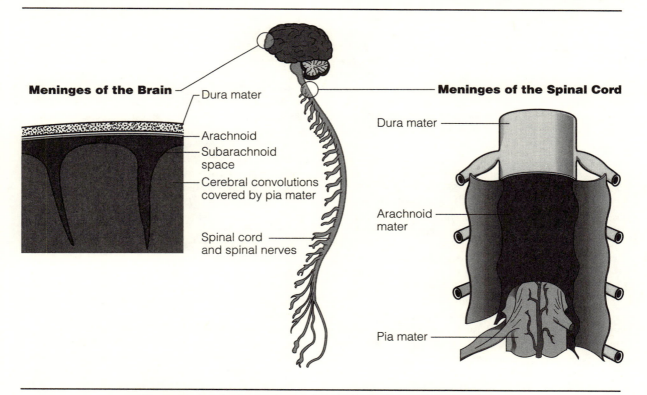

Meninges of the Brain

- Dura mater
- Arachnoid
- Subarachnoid space
- Cerebral convolutions covered by pia mater
- Spinal cord and spinal nerves

Meninges of the Spinal Cord

- Dura mater
- Arachnoid mater
- Pia mater

*Meningitis attacks the meninges of the brain or the spinal cord or both.*

of infection to the meninges by the bloodstream or the lymphatic system. Once they have entered the subarachnoid space, they divide without inhibition since there is no impediment posed by defensive cells. In other words, the cerebrospinal fluid (CSF) contains very few white blood cells to inactivate the bacteria. More rarely, some bacteria may be introduced into the area by neurological damage or surgical invasion.

The most common cause of bacterial meningitis in adults and older children is meningococcus (*Neisseria meningitidus*). It is a diplococcus that typically does its damage inside the cell. The incidence of meningococcal meningitis is 2 to 3 cases per 100,000 people per year, and it most often affects schoolchildren and military recruits. *Haemophilus influenzae* is the most common culprit infecting babies between two months and one year of age. Complications or residual effects often follow bacterial meningitis. These may include deafness, delayed-onset epilepsy, hydrocephalus, cerebritis, and brain abscess. In addition, for several weeks after resolution of the disease the patient may experience headaches, dizziness, and lethargy.

Aseptic meningitis is meningitis attributable to causes other than bacteria. These causes include neurotropic viruses, such as those that cause poliomyelitis or encephalitis; other viruses such as those that cause mumps, herpes, mononucleosis, hepatitis, chickenpox, and measles; spirochetes; bacterial products from brain abscesses or previous cases of bacterial meningitis; and foreign bodies, such as those found in the air or chemicals, in the CSF. Most cases of aseptic meningitis are viral in origin. The signs and symptoms are similar to those of bacterial meningitis. Onset is usually gradual, with symptoms starting mildly. The slight headache becomes worse over the course of several days, the neck becomes characteristically stiff, and photophobia (dislike of bright light) occurs.

Tuberculous meningitis is different from most other forms of meningitis because it lasts longer, has a higher mortality rate, and affects the CSF less. It mostly strikes children and is usually the result of a bacillus infection from the respiratory tract or the lymphatic system that has relocated to the meninges. When the bacilli are translocated to the central nervous system, they form tubercles that release an exudate. If tuberculous meningitis is left untreated, death may occur within three weeks. Even with treatment, it may result in neurologic abnormalities.

### TREATMENT AND THERAPY

If meningitis is suspected, the first testing procedure is an examination of the CSF. To obtain CSF, a lumbar puncture, sometimes called a spinal tap, is made. Opening pressure, protein and glucose concentrations, total cell count, and cultures of microbes are determined. In cases of meningitis, the CSF is almost always cloudy and generally comes out under higher-than-normal pressure. An elevated white blood cell count in the CSF would be one indication that the patient has bacterial meningitis; another would be lowered serum glucose but slightly raised protein concentration, especially albumin. About 90 percent of bacterial meningitis cases show gram-positive staining. The examination of this slightly atypical fluid, along with presenting symptoms and signs, gives the diagnostician some confidence in diagnosing meningitis accurately. Further cultures and a repeat puncture are necessary to pinpoint the kind of meningitis and to check the effect of the treatment.

Bacterial meningitis should be promptly treated with antibiotics specific for the causative bacteria. The success of treatment is contingent on the magnitude of the bacterial count and the quickness with which the bacteria can be controlled. Virtually all bacterial cases are treated with ampicillin or penicillin. Cases aggressively treated with very large doses of antibiotics are the most successful. If antibiotics do not destroy the areas of infection, surgery should be considered. Surgery is especially effective if meningitis is recurrent or persistent. Viral meningitis may be treated with adenine arabinoside if the cause is herpes simplex. No medication will kill other viruses causing the infection. The condition usually resolves itself in a few days, even without treatment. When necessary, supportive therapy should be employed, including blood transfusions. Young children with open fontanelles often undergo subdural taps to relieve pressure caused by CSF buildup.

Mortality rates in meningitis vary with age and the pathogen responsible. Those suffering from meningococcal meningitis (without overwhelming bacterial numbers) have a fatality rate of only 3 percent. Newborns suffering from gram-negative meningitis, however, have a 70 percent mortality rate. In addition, the younger the patient, the more likely the incidence of lasting neurological damage.

There are two basic ways to prevent meningitis: chemoprophylaxis for likely candidates of the disease and active immunization. Those exposed to a known case are usually treated with rifampin for four days; rifampin is especially useful in inactivating *H. influenzae*. Active immunization is suggested for toddlers eighteen to twenty-four months of age, especially for those in situations where there is a high risk of exposure (such as day care centers).

—*Iona C. Baldridge*

## MENOPAUSE

**SYSTEMS AFFECTED:** Reproductive (female), psychic-emotional

**SPECIALISTS:** Endocrinologists, gynecologists

**DEFINITION:** The time during a woman's life when her ability to conceive and bear children ends, marked by irregular, and eventually complete cessation of, menstruation, accompanied by hormonal changes such as the dramatic reduction in the body's production of estrogen.

## KEY TERMS:

*climacteric:* that phase in the aging process of women marking the transition from the reproductive stage of life to the nonreproductive stage

*estrogen:* the female hormones estradiol and estrone, produced by the ovary and responsible for the development of secondary sex characteristics

*exogenous:* originating outside an organ or part

*osteoporosis:* a condition characterized by a loss of bone density and an increased susceptibility to fractures

*progesterone:* a hormone, released by the corpus luteum and placenta, responsible for changes in the uterine endometrium

### PROCESS AND EFFECTS

The word "menopause" comes from two Greek words meaning "month" and "cessation." It is used medically to mean a cessation of, not a "pause" in, menstrual periods. Technically, the menopause begins the moment a woman has had her final menstrual period; until then, her menstrual periods may have shown a wide variety of irregularities, including missed periods.

Medical experts refer to the time when the body is noticeably preparing for the menopause as the perimenopause, which can begin anywhere from a few months to a few years before the menopause. During that time, a woman still experiences menstrual periods, but they are erratic. Some women stop menstruating suddenly, without irregularities; however, they are in the minority. For some women, signs of the menopause, such as hot flashes, may begin during the perimenopause. For even more women, such signs begin, or at least increase in intensity, at the menopause.

The term "climacteric" covers a longer span and includes all the years of diminishing estrogen production, both before and after a woman's last menstrual period. Some experts believe that women may undergo declines in their levels of estrogen even when they are in their late twenties; almost all experts believe that estrogen levels drop at least by a woman's mid-thirties, and the process accelerates in the late forties.

The average age at which the menopause occurs in women from the United States is 51.4 years, with the usual range between ages forty-five and fifty-five. For some it occurs much earlier, for others much later. Only 8 percent of women reach the menopause before age forty, and only 5 percent continue to menstruate after age fifty-three. A very few have menstrual periods until they are sixty.

Even after the menopause, the climacteric continues. Declining hormonal levels bring more changes, until the situation stabilizes. A decade or more of noticeable changes can take place before the climacteric is completed. Unlike the climacteric, the menopause itself is usually considered completed after one full year without a period. After two years, a woman can be reasonably certain that her periods

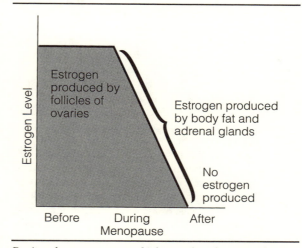

*During the menopause, which may last for several years, estrogen production diminishes; after the menopause, estrogen is no longer produced by the body.*

have ceased permanently. The signs and symptoms of the menopause, however, can linger for years longer.

Starting in her mid-forties, a woman's ovaries gradually lose their ability to respond to the follicle-stimulating hormone (FSH), which is released by the pituitary into the blood, triggering the release of estrogen from the ovaries. A few eggs do remain even after menstrual flows have ceased, and the production of estrogen does not stop completely after the menopause; in much smaller amounts, it continues to be released by the adrenal glands, in fatty tissue, and in the brain. At the menopause, however, the blood levels of estrogen are drastically reduced—by about 75 percent. Many experts believe that the presence of some estrogen is important for a woman's total well-being, bone health, and skin suppleness and for the prevention of heart disease.

About two to four years before the menopause, many women stop ovulating or ovulate irregularly or only occasionally. Although almost all the follicles enclosing the eggs are depleted by this time, the ovaries continue to produce estrogen. Estrogen continues to build up the endometrium (the lining of the uterus), but without ovulation no progesterone is produced to shed the extra lining. Therefore, instead of regular periods, a woman may bleed at unexpected times as the extra lining is shed sporadically.

During the perimenopause, menstrual periods may be late or early, longer than usual or shorter, and lighter than before or heavier. They may disappear for several months, then reappear for several more. It has been noted that in 15 to 20 percent of women the typical menopausal symptoms, sometimes accompanied by noticeable mood swings similar to premenstrual tension, begin during the perimenopausal period.

According to the National Institutes of Health, about 80 percent of women experience mild or no signs of the menopause. The rest have symptoms troublesome enough to seek medical attention. The two most important factors in determining how a woman will fare are probably the rate of decline of her female hormones and the final degree of hormone depletion. A woman's genes, general health, lifetime quality of diet, level of activity, and psychological acceptance of aging are also major influences. The most severe symptoms occur in women who lose their ovaries through surgery or radiation when they are perimenopausal.

When only the uterus is removed (hysterectomy) and the ovaries remain intact, menstrual periods stop but all other aspects of the menopause occur in the same way and at the same age. When only one ovary is removed, the menopause occurs normally. If both ovaries are removed, a complete menopause takes place abruptly, sometimes with intense effects. Women who have had a tubal ligation to prevent pregnancy will experience a normal menopause because tubal ligation does not affect ovaries, the uterus, or hormonal secretions.

Although experts disagree about the causes of a variety of symptoms that may appear at the menopause, there is no disagreement about the fact that the majority of women experience hot flashes, or flushes. For two out of three women, hot flashes can start well before the last menstruation. Generally, however, hot flashes increase dramatically at menopause and continue to occur, with intermittent breaks (sometimes lasting several months), for five years or so.

While hot flashes are not dangerous, they are uncomfortable. Many women have only three or four episodes a day—or even a week—and hardly notice them. Others have as many as fifty severe flashes a day. The intense waves of heat generally last several minutes, but some unusual flashes have been reported to last as long as an hour. Usually there is some perspiration; with a severe flash, there is heavy perspiration. Because the blood vessels dilate (expand) and then contract, the hot flash is often followed by chills, even intense shivering. Since the flashes are usually worse at night, they can cause insomnia.

Other vasomotor symptoms can also appear with the menopause. Experts believe that they are the result of disruptions of the same mechanisms—vasomotor instability—that are manifested as hot flashes. Palpitations, which are distinct and rapid heartbeats, may also occur. A woman may experience dizziness or may feel faint or nauseated at times. She may have peculiar sensations in her arms and hands, especially her fingers. Some feel these sensations as tingling, or pins and needles, while others say that their fingers occasionally feel numb. One of the oddest, most frightening sensations associated with the menopause is formication, a feeling of insects crawling over the skin.

Headaches, depression, mood swings, insomnia, and weight gain often affect women at the menopause and may be related to the body's hormonal readjustments. Insomnia is second only to hot flashes as the symptom that causes women to seek out their doctors' help at the menopause. The hypothalamus controls sleep as well as temperature and hormone production; insomnia is caused by changes in sleep patterns and brain waves from the same hypothalamic disturbances that result in the hot flashes and an overstimulated central nervous system.

## COMPLICATIONS AND DISORDERS

One of the problems that women encounter with the menopause is calcium deficiency. Many experts believe that before the menopause a woman requires a minimum of 1,000 milligrams of calcium a day in food or supplements. At the menopause, however, a woman who is not taking estrogen needs 1,500 milligrams of calcium a day. Since it is very difficult to obtain these daily allotments from food without consuming considerable amounts of milk or milk products, calcium supplements are often recommended for menopausal and postmenopausal women.

If the calcium deficiency is allowed to persist, osteoporosis, a loss of bone density that can lead to dangerous fractures, can result. Osteoporosis is known to have less of a damaging effect on women who are somewhat overweight because estrogen continues to be produced in fatty tissues after the menopause. Cigarettes, alcohol, and caffeine increase bone loss because they interfere with the body's ability to absorb calcium. A well-balanced diet, calcium supplements, and regular exercise—especially weightbearing exercise—are effective ways of controlling osteoporosis. Hormone-replacement therapy is another means of coping with osteoporosis brought on by the menopause. Since nearly half of all women do not develop osteoporosis, however, many physicians do not believe that administering estrogen therapy to combat this disease is worth the risks except in women at high risk for osteoporosis.

Although estrogen was isolated as a substance in the 1920's, the modern study of hormones—how they work, where they are produced, what their benefits are—began in the 1940's. Originally, estrogen was administered cautiously to women who had lost their ovaries through surgery and to those with severe distress after the menopause. It was not until the 1960's that estrogen replacement therapy became widespread, however, when books such as Robert A. Wilson's *Feminine Forever* (1966) promoted its use as the newfound fountain of youth for women. The replacement of estrogen was suddenly fashionable, with the hormone being viewed as a miracle drug that could keep women looking and feeling youthful well into their later years. Physicians began prescribing it for women well before the menopause, and it was recommended for use throughout life. Often, large doses were prescribed.

By the mid-1970's, twenty million American women were taking estrogen. A decade later, however, the number had fallen to four or five million. Beginning in 1975, research studies began documenting dramatic increases—sometimes as high as 500 percent—in cases of cancer of the lining of the endometrium among women taking estrogen, compared with those not taking it. Other studies at that time found higher rates of breast cancer as well as other problems, such as gallbladder conditions, among women taking estrogen.

Some studies found the overall risk of contracting uterine cancer increased 350 percent for women who took estrogen for a year or more. Some women who were on the therapy for long periods were judged to be as much as 100 percent more likely to contract uterine cancer. Furthermore, contrary to expectations, some studies claimed that the risk persisted even ten years after the estrogen use was discontinued. Other studies also found that the risk of cancer persisted, though for a shorter period.

All those studies were based on replacement therapy using estrogen only. Estrogen stimulates the growth of cells in the endometrium, which is one of the aspects of the development of cancer. Yet the researchers also reported that a newer treatment in which estrogen was combined with a form of progesterone appeared to reduce the risk of uterine cancer. Further studies have shown lower rates of both endometrial and breast cancer, as well as lower rates of heart disease among women using the two hormones, compared with nonusers.

The most widely recommended regimen in the early 1990's called for using estrogen in the lowest effective dose three weeks each month. During the last week to thirteen days of this therapy, a form of progesterone is added. Then both hormones are stopped. Uterine bleeding, similar to that of a menstrual period, may occur. This bleeding allows the progesterone to break down any excess buildup of cells in the endometrium.

During the menopause, the walls of the vagina become smooth and dry and produce less lubrication, producing a condition called atrophic vaginitis. It has been assumed that this condition is attributable to a lack of estrogen. Despite doubts concerning the relationship between circulating estrogen and objective measures of vaginal atrophy, estrogen (often topical) is frequently prescribed and effectively used in the alleviation or elimination of symptoms.

To help alleviate menopausal symptoms, many women require only short-term therapy; other women, such as those at risk for developing osteoporosis, may need the therapy for years or even for the rest of their lives. Some physicians believe that estrogen should not be taken during the perimenopause, when there may still be high levels of estrogen in the patient's system. Other physicians believe that the levels of estrogen should be checked using a vaginal smear test during the perimenopause and estrogen prescribed if necessary.

Some physicians prescribe estrogen therapy for women with severe symptoms after a surgical menopause. The therapy is usually continued for at least five years or until the time that the natural menopause would have occurred, unless the woman has an estrogen-dependent malignancy.

The most popular method for administering hormone-replacement therapy is oral, but this method is relatively ineffective because of poor gastrointestinal absorption. One way of increasing the effectiveness of oral medication is to provide it in micronized form; micronization increases the total surface area of the medication by reducing the size of the particles and increasing their numbers, thereby facilitating dissolution and absorption. Estrone increases at a faster rate than does estradiol when hormone-replacement therapy is administered orally because the intestines and the liver convert estradiol, the more active form of estrogen, to estrone. Other routes of administration, such as a transdermal patch, have been studied in order to discover a method that might bypass the gut and liver and avoid the rapid conversion of estradiol to estrone.

Another method of administering hormone-replacement therapy is intravaginally, which also bypasses the gut and liver. When intravaginal administration was compared to oral administration at a variety of doses, it was found that at each dosage level, the vaginal route resulted in significantly lower blood estrogen values than did the oral route. Relief from vaginal symptoms was achieved in all cases, however, where the hormone was administered vaginally. Routes that bypass the liver and gut produce a more natural ratio of estrone to estradiol.

There is considerable evidence that exogenous estrogen treatment in menopausal women is associated with an increase in the probability of developing uterine cancer; it has also been linked to cancer of the breast. Initially, hormone replacement therapy consisted of estrogen administered on a continual basis. Since the increased risk of uterine cancer was thought to be the result of the hyperplastic effects of unopposed estrogen on the endometrium, other forms of medication have been advocated. For example, estrogen is sometimes given on a cyclic basis, with twenty-five days of medication and five days off. The rationale for this form of treatment is that it more precisely conforms to premenopausal hormone levels and, more important, that it prevents hyperplasia (enlargement of the uterus).

Anecdotal evidence suggests that stress reduction, a regular exercise program, and/or vitamin E therapy are useful in reducing the frequency and severity of hot flashes, although none of these approaches has been tested empirically to determine its effectiveness.

## PERSPECTIVE AND PROSPECTS

The menopause, in various guises, was referred to in many early cultures and texts. Initially, an association was made between age and the loss of fertility. By the sixth century, written records on the cessation of menstruation were well documented. At that time, it was believed that menstruation did not cease before the age of thirty-five, nor did it usually continue after the age of fifty. It was thought that obese women ceased menstruation very early and that the periods remained normal or abnormal and increased in flow or became diminished depending on age, the season of the year, the habits and peculiar traits of women, the types of food eaten, and complicating diseases. Similar descriptions of menstrual cessation and its age of onset continued for another thousand years. It was not until the late eighteenth and early nineteenth centuries, however, that much advancement in the knowledge of the topic took place.

John Leake, influenced by William Harvey's historic description of the circulatory system, made one of the first reasonable attempts to explain the etiology of the menopause in his 1777 book *Medical Instructions Towards the Prevention and Cure of Chronic or Slow Diseases Peculiar to Women*. He believed that as long as the "prime of life" continued, along with the circulating force of the blood being more than equal to the resistance of the uterine vessels, the menses would continue to flow. When these vessels became firm from the effect of age, however, the diminished current of blood would be insufficient to force the uterine vessels open, and then periodic discharge would cease.

A later development in the history of menstruation studies was to link menstruation with all sorts of other problems, both emotional and organic. Leake commented that at the time of cessation of menses, women were often afflicted by various chronic diseases. He added that some women were prone to pain and lightheadedness, others were plagued by an intolerable itching at the neck of the bladder, and some were affected by low spirits and melancholy. Leake thought, because it seemed extraordinary that so many disorders should result from such a natural occurrence in a woman's life, that these symptoms could be explained away by indulgence in excesses, luxury, and an "irregularity" in the passions. Laying the blame for complications with the menopause on societal (in particular, female) excesses continued for some time.

Specific disease associations were also made; in 1814, John Burns announced that the cessation of menses seemed to cause cancer of the breast in some women. Edward John Tilt, a British physician, wrote one of the first full-length books on *The Change of Life in Health and Disease* (1857). Some of his views were that women should adhere to a strict code of hygiene during menstruation because they are often afflicted with cancer, gout, rheumatism, and nervous disorders.

These beliefs reflect a tendency from the mid-nineteenth century onward for medical literature to associate the menopause with many negative sociological features. For example, Colombat de l'Isère, in his book *Traité des maladies des femmes et de l'hygiène spéciale de leur sexe* (1838; *A Treatise on the Diseases and Special Hygiene of Females*, 1845), believed that during the menopause women ceased

to live for the species and lived only for themselves. He thought that it was prudent for men to avoid having erotic thoughts about women in whom these feelings ought to have become extinct; he believed that after the menopause sexual enjoyment for women was ended forever.

Not all physicians, however, took such a negative attitude. Some believed that examining this phase in a woman's life presented a challenge. They believed that the boundaries between the physiological and the pathological in this field of study were ill-defined and that it was in the interest of the male gender that more research into this stage of a woman's life be done. The narrow boundary between normal physiology and pathology was not fully defined nearly a hundred years later, nor did the many negative and unsubstantiated theories cease. Well into the 1960's, the menopause was still considered "abnormal" and a "negative" state by some physicians.

Three major milestones exist in the history of menopause research in the twentieth century. The first event was the achievement of Adolf Butenandt, a Nobel Prize winner in chemistry. He succeeded in 1929 in isolating and obtaining, in pure form, a hormone from the urine of pregnant women which was eventually called estrone. The second development was the publication of the book *Feminine Forever*, by Robert A. Wilson, in 1966. The book, which became an instant best-seller, popularized a theory called "estrogen-replacement treatment" or "hormone-replacement therapy." As a result of the book's publication, physicians were prompted to take sides in a heated and continuing debate. The third landmark was the publication of an editorial and two original articles in *The New England Journal of Medicine* of December 4, 1975, claiming an association between exogenous estrogens and endometrial cancer. This claim brought about legal action by initiating, at least in the United States, a series of health administration inquiries.

—*Genevieve Slomski*

**See also** Aging; Atherosclerotic disease; Breast cancer; Cervical, ovarian, and uterine cancers; Endometrial cancer; Heart disease; Infertility in females; Menstruation; Obesity; Osteoporosis; Ovarian cysts.

**FOR FURTHER INFORMATION:**

Cutler, Winnifred B., and Celso-Ramon Garcia. *The Medical Management of Menopause and Premenopause*. Philadelphia: J. B. Lippincott, 1984. This combined effort by a biologist and a gynecologist represents an attempt to clarify the facts about this subject and their potential interpretations. Focuses on the endocrine system's relation to symptomatology. Contains charts, graphs, and a bibliography.

Gannon, Linda R. *Menstrual Disorders and Menopause*. New York: Praeger, 1985. Presents an integration and synthesis of scholarly research on the biological, psychological, and cultural aspects of menstruation, menstrual disorders, and the menopause to help the reader better understand the variables that influence the predisposition, development, and treatment of menstrual and menopausal symptoms. Extensive references are included.

Hammond, Charles B., et al., eds. *Menopause*. New York: Liss, 1989. A series of essays on the evaluation and treatment of and the health concerns surrounding the menopause, stressing hormone replacement therapy in particular. Contains numerous charts and graphs.

Sheehy, Gail. *The Silent Passage: Menopause*. New York: Random House, 1992. Expanding on an article that she published in the October, 1991, issue of *Vanity Fair*, Sheehy draws from more than one hundred interviews conducted with women experiencing various stages of the menopause, as well as interviews with dozens of experts in many disciplines. A good popular account for the general reader.

Swartz, Donald P. *Hormone Replacement Therapy*. Baltimore: Williams & Wilkins, 1992. Discusses the physiological role of the sex hormones and the growing evidence for the pathology that results from a long-term deficiency in these hormones. Raises such questions as "Which patients can benefit the most from hormone replacement therapy on a long-term basis?" "Which patients should be excluded from therapy?" and "How long should hormone replacement therapy be continued?"

Utian, Wulf H. *Menopause in Modern Perspective*. New York: Appleton-Century-Crofts, 1980. The purpose of this book is to define clearly the climacteric and its related effects, to evaluate the status of hormone replacement therapy (including risks and benefits), and to provide guidelines in the care of the perimenopausal patient.

# MENORRHAGIA

**SYSTEM AFFECTED:** Reproductive (female)

**SPECIALISTS:** Gynecologists

**DEFINITION:** Menorrhagia is excessive or prolonged bleeding during menstruation. Large amounts of blood (up to three times the normal amount) may be lost during the menstrual cycle each month, and iron-deficiency anemia may result. There are several possible causes of such abnormal bleeding, such as uterine tumors or polyps and endometriosis, in which uterine tissue grows in other locations in the body. Changes in the production and release of hormones may also be suspected. Hormone therapy may be used, and hysterectomy is required in some cases. *See also* Endometriosis; Menstruation.

# MENSTRUATION

**SYSTEM AFFECTED:** Reproductive (female)

**SPECIALISTS:** Endocrinologists, gynecologists, obstetricians, pediatricians

**DEFINITION:** The monthly discharge of blood and tissue (menses) by women of childbearing age, caused by changes in hormonal levels.

**KEY TERMS:**

*endometrium:* the layer of cells lining the inner cavity of the uterus; the source of menstrual discharge

*feedback:* a system in which two parts of the body communicate and control each other, often through hormones; can be either negative (inhibitory) or positive (stimulatory)

*follicle:* a spherical structure within the ovary that contains a developing ovum and that produces hormones; each ovary contains thousands of follicles

*hormone:* a chemical signal produced in some part of the body that is carried in the blood to another body part, where it has some observable effect

*menstrual cycle:* the cycle of hormone production, ovulation, menstruation, and other changes that occurs on an approximately monthly schedule in women

*ovary:* the organ that produces ova and hormones; the two ovaries lie on either side of the uterus, within the abdominal cavity

*ovulation:* the process by which an ovum is released from its follicle in the ovary; occurs in the middle of each menstrual cycle

*ovum* (pl. *ova*): the egg or reproductive cell produced by the female, which when fertilized by a sperm from the male will develop into an embryo

*prostaglandins:* chemical signals that have local effects on the organ that produces them

*uterus:* the organ that nourishes and supports the developing embryo; also called the womb

## PROCESS AND EFFECTS

Menstruation is the monthly discharge of bloody fluid from the uterus. It occurs in humans and in other primates (apes and monkeys), but not in all mammals; for example, horses, cats, and dogs do not menstruate. The menstrual fluid consists of blood, cells and debris from the endometrial lining of the uterus, and mucus and other fluids. The color of the discharge varies from dark brown to bright red during the period of flow. The menstrual discharge does not normally clot after leaving the uterus, but it may contain endometrial debris that resembles blood clots. The flow lasts from four to five days in most women, with spotting (the discharge of scant fluid) possibly continuing another day or two. The volume of fluid lost ranges from 10 to 80 milliliters, with a median of about 40 milliliters. The blood in the menstrual discharge amounts to only a small fraction of the body's total blood volume of about 5,000 milliliters, and so normal physiological functioning is not usually impaired by the blood loss that occurs during menstruation.

The first menstruation (menarche) begins when a girl goes through puberty at the age of twelve or thirteen; the last episodes of menstruation occur some forty years later at the time of menopause. Menstruation does not occur during the months of pregnancy or for the first few months after a woman has given birth.

## Menstrual Cycle

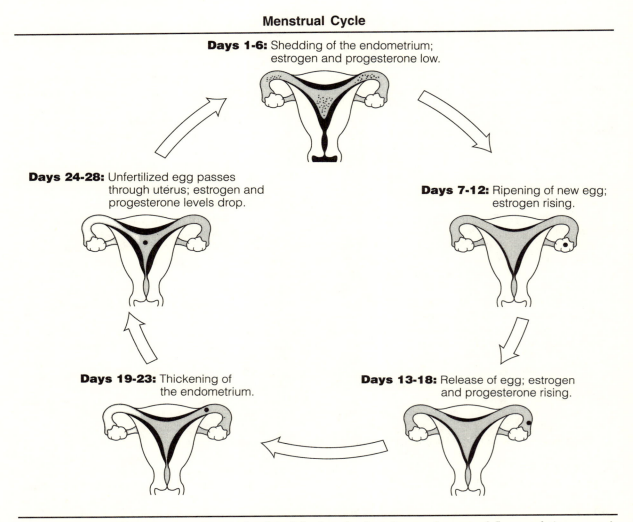

**Days 1-6:** Shedding of the endometrium; estrogen and progesterone low.

**Days 24-28:** Unfertilized egg passes through uterus; estrogen and progesterone levels drop.

**Days 7-12:** Ripening of new egg; estrogen rising.

**Days 19-23:** Thickening of the endometrium.

**Days 13-18:** Release of egg; estrogen and progesterone rising.

*Exact timing varies from woman to woman; day 1 is defined as the day of onset of menstrual flow; ovulation occurs in mid-cycle (around day 14). Hormonal levels are rising and falling throughout the cycle.*

Menstruation is the most visible event of the woman's monthly menstrual cycle. The average length of the menstrual cycle in the population is about 29.1 days, but it may vary from 16 to 35 days, with variation occurring between different individuals and in one individual from month to month. Girls who have just gone through puberty and women who are approaching the menopause tend to have more variation in their cycles than do women in the middle of their reproductive years. There is also an age-related change in cycle length: Cycles tend to be relatively long in teenagers, then decrease in length until a woman is about forty years old, after which cycles tend to lengthen and become irregular.

Hormones cause menstruation to be coordinated with other events in the menstrual cycle. Uterine function is regulated by two hormones, estrogen and progesterone, that are produced in the ovaries. In turn, the production of estrogen and progesterone is controlled by follicle-stimulating hormone (FSH) and luteinizing hormone (LH), both of which are produced in the pituitary gland. The hormones from the ovaries and from the pituitary have mutual control over each other: They participate in a feedback relationship. The fact that females produce ova only once a month, in a cycle, rather than continuously, is the result of a change in the feedback relationships between the ovarian and pituitary hormones as the menstrual cycle proceeds.

In the first half of the cycle, the follicular phase, a predominant negative feedback effect keeps pituitary hormone levels low while allowing estrogen to increase. Day 1 of the menstrual cycle is defined as the day of the onset of the menstrual flow. During the days of menstrual bleeding, levels of estrogen and progesterone are low, but FSH levels are high enough to cause the growth of follicles in the ovary. As the follicles start to grow, they secrete estrogen, and increasing amounts are secreted as the follicles continue to enlarge over the next five to ten days. The estrogen exerts negative feedback control over the pituitary: FSH and LH production is inhibited by estrogen, so levels of these hormones remain low during the follicular phase. Besides producing estrogen, the growing follicles contain ova that are maturing and preparing for ovulation. Meanwhile, estrogen acts on the uterus to cause the growth of the endometrial lining. The lining becomes thicker and its blood supply increases; glands located in the lining also grow and mature. These uterine changes are known as endometrial proliferation.

As the woman nears the middle of her cycle, a dramatic change in hormonal feedback occurs. The increasing secretion of estrogen shifts the hormonal system into a positive feedback mode, whereby an increase in estrogen stimulates the release of LH and FSH from the pituitary instead of inhibiting it. Thus, at the middle of the cycle (around day 14), simultaneous peaks in levels of estrogen, LH, and FSH occur. The peak in LH triggers ovulation by causing changes in the wall of the follicle, allowing it to break open to release its ovum. Although a group of follicles had matured up to this point, usually only the largest one ovulates, and the remainder in the group die and cease hormone production.

Following ovulation, negative feedback is reestablished. The follicle that just ovulated remains as a functional part of the ovary; it becomes transformed into the corpus luteum, a structure which produces estrogen and progesterone throughout most of the second half of the cycle, the luteal phase. During this phase, the combined presence of estrogen and progesterone reestablishes negative feedback over the pituitary, and LH and FSH levels decline. A second ovulation is prevented because an LH peak is not possible at this time. The combined action of estrogen and progesterone causes the uterus to enter its secretory phase during the second half of the cycle: The glands in the thickened endometrium secrete nutrients that will support an embryo if the woman becomes pregnant, and the ample blood supply to the endometrium can supply the embryo with other nutrients and oxygen. If the woman does in fact become pregnant, the embryo will secrete a hormone that will ensure the continued production of estrogen and progesterone, and because of these hormones, the uterus will remain in the secretory condition throughout pregnancy. Menstruation does not occur during pregnancy because of the high levels of estrogen and progesterone, which continually support the uterus.

If the woman does not become pregnant, the corpus luteum automatically degenerates, starting at about the twenty-fourth day of the menstrual cycle. As the corpus luteum dies, it fails to produce estrogen and progesterone, so levels of these hormones decrease. As the amounts of estrogen and progesterone drop, the uterus begins to produce prostaglandins, chemicals that act as local signals within the uterus. The prostaglandins cause a number of changes in uterine function: Blood flow to the endometrium is temporarily cut off, causing the endometrial tissue to die, and the uterine muscle begins to contract, causing further changes in blood flow. The decreased blood flow and the muscle contractions contribute to the cramping pain that many women feel just before and at the time of menstrual bleeding. Menstrual bleeding starts when the blood flow to the endometrium is reestablished and the dead tissue is sloughed off and washed out of the uterus. This event signals the start of a new menstrual cycle.

## COMPLICATIONS AND DISORDERS

Many disorders involving menstruation exist. Toxic shock syndrome is a disease that, while not caused directly by menstruation, sometimes occurs during menstruation in women who use tampons to absorb the menstrual flow. The symptoms of toxic shock syndrome—fever, rash, a drop in blood pressure, diarrhea, vomiting, and fainting—are caused by toxins produced by the bacterium *Staphylococcus aureus*. This bacterium is normally present in limited numbers within the vagina, but the use of high-absorbency tampons is associated with a higher-than-normal bacterial growth and toxin production. Toxic shock syndrome requires immediate medical attention, since it may be fatal if left untreated. Women can reduce the risk of toxic shock syndrome by changing tampons often, using lower-absorbency types, and by alternating the use of tampons and sanitary napkins.

Amenorrhea is defined as the absence of menstruation. It is usually, but not always, coincident with lack of ovulation. Amenorrhea may be primary (the woman has never menstruated) or secondary (menstrual cycles that were once normal have stopped). The condition is usually associated with abnormal patterns of hormone secretion, but the problem in hormone secretion may itself be merely the symptom of some other underlying disorder. One of the most common situations leading to both primary and secondary amenorrhea is low body weight, caused by malnutrition, eating disorders, or sustained exercise. Body fat has two roles in reproduction: It provides energy needed for tissue growth and cell functions, and it contributes to circulating estrogen levels. Loss of body fat may create a situation in which the reproductive system ceases to function because of low estrogen levels and because of lack of needed energy. The result is seen as amenorrhea. Emotional or physical stress may also cause amenorrhea, because stress results in the release of hormones that interfere with the reproductive hormones. Ideally, amenorrhea is treated by removing its cause; for example, a special diet or a change in an exercise program can bring about an increase in body fat stores, or stress level can be reduced through changes in lifestyle or with counseling. Ironically, sometimes birth control pills are prescribed for women with amenorrhea. The pills do not cure the amenorrhea, but they counteract some of the long-term problems associated with it, such as changes in the endometrial lining and loss of bone density.

Dysmenorrhea refers to abnormally intense uterine pain associated with menstruation. It is estimated that 5 to 10 percent of women experience pain intense enough to interfere with their school or work schedules. Dysmenorrhea may be primary (occurring in women with no known disease) or secondary (caused by a disease condition such as a tumor or infection). Studies have shown uterine prostaglandin levels to be correlated with the degree of pain perceived in primary dysmenorrhea, and drugs that interfere with prostaglandins offer an effective treatment for this condition. These drugs include aspirin, acetaminophen, ibuprofen, and naproxen; some formulas are available without a doctor's prescription, but the stronger drugs require one. Secondary dysmenorrhea is best managed by removing the underlying cause; if this is not possible, the antiprostaglandin drugs may be useful in controlling the pain.

Menorrhagia is excessive menstrual blood loss, usually defined as more than 80 milliliters of fluid lost per cycle. This condition can have serious health consequences because of the loss of red blood cells, which are essential for carrying oxygen to tissues. Women who have given birth to several children are more likely to suffer from menorrhagia, possibly because of enlargement of the uterine cavity and interference with the mechanisms that limit menstrual blood flow. Women who have diseases that interfere with blood clotting may also have menorrhagia. Although the menstrual discharge itself does not usually form clots after it leaves the uterus, clots do form within the uterine endometrium; these clots normally prevent excessive blood loss. Treatment for menorrhagia may begin with iron and vitamin supplements to induce increased red blood cell production, or transfusions may be used to replace the lost red blood cells. If this is unsuccessful, treatment with birth control pills, destruction of the endometrium by laser surgery, or a hysterectomy (surgical removal of the uterus) may be necessary.

Endometriosis is a condition in which endometrial cells from the uterus become misplaced within the abdominal cavity, adhering to and growing on the surface of some organ. The outside of the uterus, the oviducts (Fallopian tubes), the surface of the ovaries, and the outer surface of the intestines can all support the growth of endometrial tissue. Endometriosis is thought to arise during menstruation, when endometrial tissue enters the oviducts instead of being carried outward through the cervix and vagina. Through the oviducts, the endometrial tissue has access to the abdominal cavity. Since the misplaced endometrial tissue responds to hormones in the same way that the normal endometrium does, it undergoes cyclic changes in thickness and attempts to shed at the time of menstruation. Endometriosis results in intense pain during menstruation and can cause infertility because of interference with ovulation, ovum or sperm transport, or uterine function. Endometriosis is treated with birth control pills or with drugs that suppress menstrual cycles, or the endometrial tissue may be removed surgically.

Premenstrual syndrome (PMS) is a set of symptoms that occurs in some women in the week before the start of menstruation, with the symptoms disappearing once menstruation begins. Researchers and physicians who study PMS have struggled to devise a standard definition for the disorder, but the list of possible symptoms is lengthy and varies from woman to woman and even within one woman from month to month. The possible symptoms include both psychological and physical changes: irritability, nervous tension, anxiety, moodiness, depression, lethargy, insomnia, confusion, crying, food cravings, fatigue, weight gain, swelling and bloating, breast tenderness, backache, headache, dizziness, muscle stiffness, and abdominal cramps. A diagnosis of PMS requires that the symptoms show a clear relation to the timing of menstruation and that they recur during most menstrual cycles. Researchers estimate that 3 to 5 percent of women have PMS symptoms that are so severe that they are incapacitating, but that milder symptoms occur in about 50 percent of all women. Because of the variability in symptoms between women, some researchers believe that there are several subtypes of PMS, each with its own cluster of symptoms. It is possible that each subtype has a unique cause. Suggested causes of PMS include an imbalance in the ratio of estrogen to progesterone following ovulation, changes in the hormones that control salt and water balance (the renin-angiotensin-aldosterone system), increased levels of prolactin (a hormone that acts on the breast), changes in amounts of brain chemicals, altered functioning of the biological clock that determines daily rhythms, poor diet or sensitivity to certain foods, and psychological factors such as attitude toward menstruation, stresses of family or professional life, and underlying personality disorders. Studies evaluating these theories have yielded contradictory results, so that no one cause of PMS has yet been found. Current treatments for PMS include dietary therapy, hormone administration, and psychological counseling, but no treatment has been found effective in all PMS patients.

An interesting phenomenon associated with menstruation is menstrual synchrony, also known as the "dormitory effect." Among women who live together, menstrual cycles gradually become synchronized, so that the women begin to menstruate within a few days of one another. Researchers have found that this phenomenon probably occurs because of pheromones, chemical signals that are produced by an individual and that have an effect on another individual. Pheromones act on the brain through the sense of smell, even though there may not be an odor that is consciously perceived.

## PERSPECTIVE AND PROSPECTS

Early beliefs about menstruation were based on folk magic and superstition rather than on scientific evidence. Even today, some cultures persist in believing that menstruating women possess deleterious powers: that the presence of a menstruating woman can cause crops to fail, farm animals to die, or beer, bread, jam, and other foods to be spoiled. Some people believe that these incidents will occur even if the menstruating woman has no evil intention. Because of the possibility of these events, some cultures prohibit menstruating women from interacting with others. In the most rigorous example of such a taboo, some societies require that menstruating women live in special huts for the duration of the bleeding period.

Folk beliefs about menstruating women have been bolstered by religious views of menstruating women as "unclean" and in need of purification. In Orthodox Judaism, there are detailed proscriptions to be observed by a menstruating woman, including the avoidance of sexual intercourse. Seven days after her menstrual flow has stopped, the Orthodox Jewish woman undergoes a ritual purification, after which she may resume sexual relations with her husband. Early Christians absorbed the Jewish belief in the uncleanliness of a menstruating woman and prohibited her from entering church or receiving the sacraments. These injunctions were lifted by the seventh century, but the view of women as spiritually and bodily impure persists in some Christian groups to this day.

In the United States, most couples abstain from intercourse during the woman's menstrual period. There is no medical justification for this behavior; in fact, research has demonstrated that intercourse can alleviate menstrual cramping, at least temporarily. Still, surveys have shown that a majority of both men and women think that it is wrong for a woman to have intercourse while menstruating.

There are also persistent beliefs that women's physical and mental abilities suffer during menstruation. In fact, this was the predominant medical opinion up through the nineteenth and early twentieth centuries. Medical writings from this time are filled with injunctions for women to rest and refrain from exercise and intellectual strain while menstruating. It was a common belief that education could actually cause physical harm to women. Some men used this advice as justification for excluding women from equal opportunities in education and employment. Starting in the late 1800's, however, scientific studies clearly demonstrated that education has no harmful effects and that there is no diminution of intellectual or physical performance during menstruation. Nevertheless, the latter finding has been one that the general population finds difficult to accept.

The latest view of menstruation is that, far from being harmful, menstrual bleeding is directly beneficial to a woman's health. Margie Profet, an evolutionary biologist at the University of California, theorizes that menstruation evolved as a means of periodically removing disease-causing bacteria and viruses from the woman's uterus. These organisms might enter the uterus along with sperm after sexual activity. In Profet's view, the energetic cost of replacing the blood and tissue lost through menstruation is more than outweighed by the protective benefits of menstruation. Her theory implies that treatments which suppress menstruation, as birth control drugs sometimes do, are not always advantageous. —*Marcia Watson-Whitmyre*

*See also* Amenorrhea; Cervical, ovarian, and uterine cancers; Childbirth; Conception; Dysmenorrhea; Endometriosis; Female genital disorders; Infertility in females; Menopause; Menorrhagia; Ovarian cysts; Pregnancy and gestation; Premenstrual syndrome (PMS).

## FOR FURTHER INFORMATION:

Asso, Doreen. *The Real Menstrual Cycle*. Chichester, England: John Wiley & Sons, 1983. This book presents a complete description of physiological and psychological changes during the menstrual cycle. Contains especially good coverage of the various factors that can affect the cycle. Menopause is also well addressed.

Covington, Timothy R., and J. Frank McClendon. *Sex Care: The Complete Guide to Safe and Healthy Sex*. New York: Pocket Books, 1987. Parts 1 and 2 deal with contraception and sexually transmitted diseases, but part 3 covers some topics directly related to menstruation: premenstrual syndrome, toxic shock syndrome, feminine hygiene, and various myths.

Golub, Sharon. *Periods: From Menarche to Menopause*. Newbury Park, Calif.: Sage Publications, 1992. An exceptionally complete book that presents information on all aspects of the menstrual cycle. The chapters dealing with scientific studies are accurate and easy to read. The author includes her thoughts on how society could make menstruation easier for women and on further research that needs to be done.

Laws, Sophie. *Issues of Blood: The Politics of Menstruation*. Basingstoke, England: Macmillan, 1990. Written by a sociologist, the text explores the results of the author's interviews with men about their attitudes toward menstruation. It is the premise of the author that the dominant group in a society determines the beliefs of the oppressed; thus, women's feelings about menstruation can be understood by referring to what men think. Highly recommended.

Quilligan, Edward J., and Frederick P. Zuspan, eds. *Current Therapy in Obstetrics and Gynecology*. Philadelphia: W. B. Saunders, 1990. A standard medical reference on treatment for women's disorders, arranged in an encyclopedia format, with short articles on each topic. There is a particularly good description of premenstrual syndrome, written by Guy E. Abraham and Richard J. Taylor. This article describes the authors' classification of PMS into four different subtypes and presents detailed information on a dietary treatment program that they have devised.

Riddick, Daniel H., ed. *Reproductive Physiology in Clinical Practice*. New York: Thieme Medical Publishers, 1987. This text is noteworthy for its scientific yet understandable approach to human reproduction, including a complete description of the menstrual cycle and the functioning of the endometrium.

# MENTAL RETARDATION

**SYSTEM AFFECTED:** Brain

**SPECIALISTS:** Geneticists, psychiatrists, psychologists

**DEFINITION:** Significant subaverage intellectual development and deficient adaptive behavior accompanied by physical abnormalities.

**KEY TERMS:**

*educable mentally retarded (EMR):* individuals with mild-to-moderate retardation; they can be educated with some modifications of the regular education program and can achieve a minimal level of success

*idiot:* an expression which was formerly used to describe a person with profound mental retardation; such an individual requires custodial care

*inborn metabolic disorder:* an abnormality caused by a gene mutation which interferes with normal metabolism and often results in mental retardation

*mental handicap:* the condition of an individual classified as "educable mentally retarded"

*mental impairment:* the condition of an individual classified as "trainable mentally retarded"

*neural tube defects:* birth defects resulting from the failure of the embryonic neural tube to close; usually results in some degree of mental retardation

*trainable mentally retarded (TMR):* individuals with moderate-to-severe retardation; only low levels of achievement may be reached by such persons

## CAUSES AND SYMPTOMS

Mental retardation is a condition in which a person demonstrates significant subaverage development of intellectual function, along with poor adaptive behavior. Diagnosis can be made fairly easily at birth if physical abnormalities also accompany mental retardation. An infant with mild mental retardation, however, may not be diagnosed until problems arise in school. Estimates of the prevalence of mental retardation vary from 1 to 3 percent of the world's total population.

Diagnosis of mental retardation takes into consideration three factors: subaverage intellectual function, deficiency in adaptive behavior, and early-age onset (before the age of eighteen). Intellectual function is a measure of one's intelligence quotient (IQ). Four levels of retardation based on IQ are described by the American Psychiatric Association. An individual with an IQ between 50 and 70 is considered mildly retarded, one with an IQ between 35 and 49 is moderately retarded, one with an IQ between 21 and 34 is severely retarded, and an individual with an IQ of less than 20 is termed profoundly retarded.

A person's level of adaptive behavior is not as easily determined as an IQ, but it is generally defined as the ability to meet social expectations in the individual's own environment. Assessment is based on development of certain skills: sensory-motor, speech and language, self-help, and socialization skills. Tests have been developed to aid in these measurements.

To identify possible mental retardation in infants, the use of language milestones is a helpful tool. For example, parents and pediatricians will observe whether children begin to smile, coo, babble, and use words during the appropriate age ranges. Once children reach school age, poor school achievement may identify those who are mentally impaired. Psychometric tests appropriate to the age of the children will help with diagnosis.

Classification of the degree of mental retardation is never absolutely clear, and dividing lines are often arbitrary. There has been debate about the value of classifying or labeling persons in categories of mental deficiency. On the one hand, it is important for professionals to understand the amount of deficiency and to determine what kind of education and treatment would be appropriate and helpful to each individual. On the other hand, such classification can lead to low self-esteem, rejection by peers, and low expectations from teachers and parents.

There has been a marked change in the terminology used in classifying mental retardation from the early days of its study. In the early twentieth century, the terms used for moderate, severe, and profound retardation were "moron," "imbecile," and "idiot." In Great Britain, the term "feebleminded" was used to indicate moderate retardation. These terms are no longer used by professionals working with the mentally retarded. "Idiot" was the classification given to the most profoundly retarded until the middle of the twentieth century. Historically, the word has changed in meaning, from William Shakespeare's day when the court jester was called an idiot, to an indication of psychosis, and later to define the lowest grade of mental deficiency. The term "idiocy" has been replaced with the expression "profound mental retardation."

Determining the cause of mental retardation is much more difficult than might be expected. More than a thousand different disorders that can cause mental retardation have been reported. Some cases seem to be entirely hereditary, others to be caused by environmental stress, and others the result of a combination of the two. In a large number of cases, however, the cause cannot be established. The mildly retarded make up the largest proportion of the mentally retarded population, and their condition seems to be a recessive genetic trait with no accompanying physical abnormalities. From a medical standpoint, mental retardation is considered to be a result of disease or biological defect and is classified according to its cause. Some of these causes are infections, poisons, environmental trauma, metabolic and nutritional abnormalities, and brain malformation.

Infections are especially harmful to brain development if they occur in the first trimester of pregnancy. Rubella is a viral infection that often results in mental retardation. Syphilis is a sexually transmitted disease which affects adults and infants born to them, resulting in progressive mental degeneration.

Poisons such as lead, mercury, and alcohol have a very damaging effect on the developing brain. Lead-based paints linger in old houses and cause poisoning in children. Children tend to eat paint and plaster chips or put them in their mouths, causing possible mental retardation, cerebral palsy, and convulsive and behavioral disorders.

Traumatic environmental effects that can cause mental retardation include prenatal exposure to X rays, lack of oxygen to the brain, or a mother's fall during pregnancy. During birth itself, the use of forceps can cause brain damage, and labor that is too brief or too long can cause mental impairment. After the birth process, head trauma or high temperature can affect brain function.

Poor nutrition and inborn metabolic disorders may cause defective mental development because vital body processes are hindered. One of these conditions, for which every newborn is tested, is phenylketonuria (PKU), in which the body cannot process the amino acid phenylalanine. If PKU is detected in infancy, subsequent mental retardation can be avoided by placing the child on a carefully controlled diet, thus preventing buildup of toxic compounds that would be harmful to the brain.

The failure of the neural tube to close in the early development of an embryo may result in anencephaly (an incomplete brain or none at all), hydrocephalus (an excessive amount of cerebrospinal fluid), or spina bifida (an incomplete vertebra, which leaves the spinal cord exposed). Anencephalic infants will live only a few hours. About half of those with other neural tube disorders will survive, usually with some degree of mental retardation. Research has shown that if a mother's diet has sufficient quantities of folic acid, neural tube closure disorders will be rare or nonexistent.

Microcephaly is another physical defect associated with mental retardation. In this condition, the head is abnormally small and does not allow for normal brain growth. Microcephaly may be inherited or caused by maternal infection, drugs, irradiation, or lack of oxygen at birth.

Abnormal chromosome numbers are not uncommon in developing embryos and will cause spontaneous abortions in most cases. Those babies that survive usually demonstrate varying degrees of mental retardation, and incidence increases with maternal age. A well-known example of a chromosome disorder is Down syndrome (formerly called mongolism), in which there is an extra copy of the twenty-first chromosome. Gene products caused by the extra chromosome cause mental retardation and other physical problems. Other well-studied chromosomal abnormalities involve the sex chromosomes. Both males and females may be born with too many or too few sex chromosomes, which often results in mental retardation.

Mild retardation with no other noticeable problems has been found to run in certain families. It occurs more often in the lower economic strata of society and probably reflects only the lower end of the normal distribution of intelligence in a population. The condition is probably a result of genetic factors interacting with environmental ones. It has been found that culturally deprived children have a lower level of intellectual function because of decreased stimuli as the infant brain develops.

## TREATMENT AND THERAPY

Diagnosis of the level of mental retardation is important in meeting the needs of the intellectually handicapped. It can open the way for effective measures to be taken to help these persons achieve the highest quality of life possible for them.

Individuals with an IQ of 50 to 70 have mild-to-moderate retardation and are classified as "educable mentally retarded" (EMR). They can profit from the regular education program when it is somewhat modified. The general purpose of all education is to allow for the development of knowledge, to provide a basis for vocational competence, and to allow opportunity for self-realization. The EMR can achieve some success in academic subjects, make satisfactory social adjustment, and achieve minimal occupational adequacy if given proper training. In Great Britain, these individuals are referred to as "educationally subnormal" (ESN).

Persons with moderate-to-severe retardation generally have IQs between 21 and 49 and are classified as "trainable mentally retarded" (TMR). These individuals are not educable in the traditional sense, but many can be trained in self-help skills, socialization into the family, and some degree of economic independence with supervision. They need a developmental curriculum which promotes personal development, independence, and social skills.

The profoundly retarded (formerly called idiots) are classified as "totally dependent" and have IQs of 20 or less. They cannot be trained to care for themselves, to socialize, or to be independent to any degree. They will need almost complete care and supervision throughout life. They may learn to understand a few simple commands, but they will only be able to speak a few words. Meaningful speech is not characteristic of this group.

EMR individuals need a modified curriculum, along with appropriately qualified and experienced teachers. Activities should include some within their special class and some in which they interact with students of other classes. The amount of time spent in regular classes and in special classes should be determined by individual needs in order to achieve the goals and objectives planned for each. Individual development must be the primary concern.

For TMR individuals, the differences will be in the areas of emphasis, level of attainment projected, and methods used. The programs should consist of small classes that may be held within the public schools or outside with the help of parents and other concerned groups. Persons trained in special education are needed to guide the physical, social, and emotional development experiences effectively.

A systematic approach in special education has proven to be the best teaching method to make clear to students what behaviors will result in the successful completion of goals. This approach has been designed so that children work with only one concept at a time. There are appropriate remedies planned for misconceptions along the way. Progress is charted for academic skills, home-living skills, and prevocational training. Decisions on the type of academic training appropriate for a TMR individual is not based on classification or labels, but on demonstrated ability.

One of the most important features of successful special education is the involvement of parents. Parents faced with rearing a retarded child may find the task overwhelming and have a great need of caring support and information about their child and the implications for their future. Parental involvement gives the parents the opportunity to learn by observing how the professionals facilitate effective learning experiences for their children at school.

Counselors help parents identify problems and implement plans of action. They can also help them determine whether goals are being reached. Counselors must know about the community resources that are available to families. They can help parents find emotional reconciliation with the problems presented by their special children. It is important for parents to be able to accept the child's limitations. They should not lavish special or different treatment on the retarded child, but rather treat this child like the other children.

Placing a child outside the home is indicated only when educational, behavioral, or medical controls are needed which cannot be provided in the home. Physicians and social workers should be able to do some counseling to supplement that of the trained counselors. Those who offer counseling should have basic counseling skills and relevant knowledge about the mentally retarded individual and the family.

EMR individuals will usually marry, have children, and often become self-supporting. The TMR will live in an institution or at home or in foster homes for their entire lives. They will probably never become self-sufficient. The presence of a TMR child has a great impact on families and

may weaken family closeness. It creates additional expenses and limits family activities. Counseling for these families is very important.

Sheltered employment provides highly controlled working conditions, helping the mentally retarded to become contributing members of society. This arrangement benefits the individual, the family, and society as the individual experiences the satisfaction and dignity of work. The mildly retarded may need only a short period of time in the sheltered workshop. The greater the degree of mental retardation, the more likely shelter will be required on a permanent basis. For the workshop to be successful, those in charge of it must consider both the personal development of the handicapped worker and the business production and profit of the workshop. Failure to consider the business success of these ventures has led to failures of the programs.

There has been a trend toward deinstitutionalizing the mentally retarded, to relocate as many residents as possible into appropriate community homes. Success will depend on a suitable match between the individual and the type of home provided. This approach is most effective for the mentally retarded if the staff of a facility is well trained and there is a fair amount of satisfactory interaction between staff and residents. It is important that residents not be ignored, and they must be monitored for proper evaluation at each step along the way. Top priority must be given to preparation of the staff to work closely with the mentally impaired and handicapped.

In the past, there was no way to know before a child's birth if there would be abnormalities. With advances in technology, however, a variety of prenatal tests can be done and many fetal abnormalities can be detected. Genetic counseling is important for persons who have these tests conducted. Some may have previously had a retarded child, or have retarded family members. Others may have something in their backgrounds that would indicate a higher-than-average risk for physical and/or mental abnormalities. Some come for testing before a child is conceived, others do not come until afterward. Tests can be done on the fetal blood and tissues that will reveal chromosomal abnormalities or inborn metabolic errors.

Many parents do not seek testing or genetic counseling because of the stress and anxiety that may result. Though most prenatal tests result in normal findings, if problems are indicated the parents are faced with what may be a difficult decision: whether to continue the pregnancy. It is often impossible to predict the extent of an abnormality, and weighing the sanctity of life in relation to the quality of life may present an ethical and religious dilemma. Others prefer to know what problems lie ahead and what their options are.

### PERSPECTIVE AND PROSPECTS

Down through history, the mentally retarded were first ignored, and then subjected to ridicule. The first attempts to educate the mentally retarded were initiated in France in the mid-nineteenth century. Shortly afterward, institutions for them began to spring up in Europe and the United States. These were often in remote rural areas, separated from the communities nearby, and were usually ill-equipped and understaffed. The institutions were quite regimented and harsh discipline was kept. Meaningful interactions usually did not occur between the patients and the staff.

The medical approach of the institutions was to treat the outward condition of the mentally retarded and ignore them as people. No concern for their social and emotional needs was shown. There were no provisions for children to play, nor was there concern for the needs of the family of those with mental handicaps.

Not until the end of the nineteenth century were the first classes set up in some U.S. public schools for education of the mentally retarded. The first half of the twentieth century brought about the expansion of the public school programs for individuals with both mild and moderate mental retardation. After World War II, perhaps in response to the slaughter of mentally handicapped persons in Nazi Germany, strong efforts were made to provide educational, medical, and recreational services for the mentally retarded.

Groundbreaking research in the 1950's led to the normalization of society's attitude about the mentally retarded in the United States. Plans to help these individuals live as normal a life as possible were made. The National Association for Retarded Citizens was founded in 1950 and had a very strong influence on public opinion. In 1961, President John F. Kennedy appointed the Panel on Mental Retardation and instructed it to prepare a plan for the nation, to help meet the complex problems of the mentally retarded. The panel presented ninety recommendations in the areas of research, prevention, medical services, education, law, and local and national organization. Further presidential commissions on the topic were appointed and have had far-reaching effects for the well-being of the mentally retarded.

A "Declaration of the Rights of Mentally Retarded Persons" was adopted by the General Assembly of the United Nations in 1971, and the Education for All Handicapped Children Act was passed in the United States in 1975, providing for the development of educational programs appropriate for all handicapped children and youth. These pieces of legislation were milestones in the struggle to improve learning opportunities for the mentally retarded.

Changes continue to take place in attitudes toward greater integration of the retarded into schools and the community, leading to significant improvements. The role of the family has increased in emphasis, for it has often been the families themselves that have worked to change old, outdated policies. The cooperation of the family is very important in improving the social and intellectual development of the mentally retarded child. Because so many new and innovative techniques have been used, it is very im-

portant that programs be evaluated and compared to one another to determine which methods provide the best training and education for the mentally retarded.
—*Katherine H. Houp*

**See also** Birth defects; Down syndrome; Fetal alcohol syndrome; Genetic diseases; Phenylketonuria; Pregnancy and gestation.

**FOR FURTHER INFORMATION:**

Carter, Charles H., ed. *Medical Aspects of Mental Retardation*. Springfield, Ill.: Charles C Thomas, 1965. Each chapter is written by a medical researcher of a particular aspect of mental retardation. The book covers many medical abnormalities that may accompany mental retardation. Frequency, causation, pathology, symptoms, and treatment are discussed for each of the conditions. Photographs are included.

Clarke, Ann M., Alan D. B. Clarke, and Joseph M. Berg. *Mental Deficiency: The Changing Outlook*. 4th ed. New York: Free Press, 1985. A classic text in the field of mental retardation which summarizes the tremendous amount of knowledge that has been amassed on the subject. Covers the genetic and environmental causes of mental retardation, prevention, help, intervention, and training.

Gearheart, Bill R., and Freddie W. Litton. *The Trainable Retarded*. 2d ed. St. Louis: C. V. Mosby, 1979. An excellent text for students training to work with moderately to severely retarded individuals. Provides a history of work in the field, and emphasizes the great strides taken in the mid-twentieth century. The topics covered include assessment, education and training, parental training, and alternatives in residential services.

Hurley, Rodger. *Poverty and Mental Retardation*. New York: Random House, 1969. This text summarizes a study of the high prevalence of mental retardation among the poor and the effects of cultural deprivation on mental development.

Jakab, Irene, ed. *Mental Retardation*. New York: Karger, 1982. A clearly written text for training health professionals who work with the mentally retarded. Contains useful, practical information and emphasizes those things which can be done to improve the quality of life for the mentally retarded.

Koch, Richard, and Kathryn J. Koch. *Understanding the Mentally Retarded Child*. New York: Random House, 1975. A helpful book written to inform and encourage parents of mentally retarded children. Discussion includes causes of mental retardation, common abnormalities that may accompany retardation, and ways by which the mentally retarded may progress toward a normal life.

Matson, Johnny L., and Rowland P. Barrett, eds. *Psychopathology in the Mentally Retarded*. New York: Grune & Stratton, 1982. This book addresses an often-neglected topic: the psychological problems that may be found in mentally retarded individuals. Discusses special emotional problems of various types of mentally retarded persons based on the causation of their deficiency. Descriptions of major disorders and their treatments are given.

## METASTASIS. *See* CANCER; MALIGNANCY AND METASTASIS.

## MIDLIFE CRISIS

**SYSTEM AFFECTED:** Psychic-emotional

**SPECIALISTS:** Psychiatrists, psychologists

**DEFINITION:** The emotional, psychological, physical, spiritual, and relationship crises that arise during the transition from early to later adulthood.

**KEY TERMS:**

*development:* a generally predictable process of physical, emotional, cognitive, and/or spiritual growth or differentiation

*developmental stressors:* the events or other characteristics associated with the developmental process, which may be experienced as causing subjective or objectively measurable discomfort

*midlife crisis:* a crisis resulting from stressors related to the transition from early adulthood to later adulthood

*situational stressors:* the events or characteristics that may be experienced unpredictably during life and that may cause subjective or objectively measurable discomfort

### CAUSES AND SYMPTOMS

Before the nature of the midlife crisis can be explored, it is first helpful to identify what is meant by "midlife." As the average life expectancy has changed throughout history, so has the period termed midlife. For example, by the 1990's, the human life expectancy in the United States had risen to approximately seventy-four years for men and seventy-eight years for women. These figures are more than twice as long as the average life expectancy during the time of the Massachusetts Bay Colony, and more than three and a half times as long as someone in ancient Greece could have expected to live.

Life expectancy changes as it is influenced by any number of factors, including nutrition, health care and prevention, stress and lifestyle issues, historical period, culture, race, individual variability, gender, and social context. Consequently, there is no precise age at which midlife can be said to commence. It is also difficult to state unequivocally when the possibility for a midlife crisis ends. Nevertheless, some developmental theorists, such as D. J. Levinson, suggest the period from forty to forty-five is the time of the midlife transition or "crisis." Others have indicated that this time period may last until the age of fifty-three. Yet the results of these studies, collected primarily from Caucasian males in the United States, may not be applicable to the general population.

Other researchers, Carol Gilligan among them, have engaged in a critique of the assumptions underlying previous comments on midlife crises and theories of how human beings develop, pointing out how this research may be based on outdated and/or incomplete studies of human development and experience. Gilligan's book *In a Different Voice* (1982) demonstrates, for example, how it may be that women have an experience of the aging process which is different from the one commonly experienced by men. As a result, the process of normal adult development and the nature of this crisis remain less than crystal clear.

Midlife crisis experiences seem to arise in response to a variety of precipitating factors, including both normal developmental changes and severe or numerous stressors. This variability raises another interesting challenge to the notion of a midlife crisis. Is experience of a midlife crisis a predictable event or an aberration? Some experts claim that the belief in a "midlife crisis" is one of the many myths about the aging process.

Richard Schulz and Robert B. Ewen, in their book *Adult Development and Aging* (1988), insist that many adults do not experience an unusually severe crisis at midlife. It is the perspective of these authors that those who do experience a significant midlife crisis tend to have suffered similar crises throughout their adulthood. The stresses involved in the transitions in midlife may be similar to, and not necessarily occurring more frequently than, those experienced by the same individual in any stage of life. If so, the adjective "midlife," as indicative of a qualitatively different kind of crisis, may be misleading.

On the other hand, Lois Tamir states that clinical studies reveal the male population in midlife to have a significant increase in mental health problems, including depression, alcoholism, and suicide. In *Men in Their Forties* (1982), Tamir insists that most studies of adulthood display something atypical among middle-aged men, whether dramatic or subtle.

Caution is necessary when making general statements about a phenomenon such as midlife crisis, but for the sake of this discussion, a more general perspective is taken. It is assumed that midlife crises, however varied in form, intensity, or duration, do commonly occur. In addition, they are best understood from a holistic and contextual perspective on the individual's life.

A developmental framework which describes the cycle that an individual experiences in life further clarifies an understanding of midlife crises. The life changes of an individual may be seen as summative and consecutive. During this life cycle, one stage, with its tasks and crises, is lived and resolved before another is reached. In *Adulthood* (1978), Erik Erikson developed one framework for understanding the individual life cycle and its tasks, crises, and stages. Life crises are attributable in large part to the stress of transitioning from one part of life to another. The stage relevant to a discussion of midlife crises is termed generativity versus stagnation; in other words, midlife is the period of time during which individuals strive to come to terms with whether they are and may continue to be productive, or whether they will stagnate.

Development is also a physical experience. Therefore, an individual's psychological and emotional responses are influenced by changing physiology and health. One common midlife example in women is menopause and its attendant hormonal changes. At few other times in a woman's life is there such a complex interaction between physical and psychological factors. Along with the physical stresses brought about by hormonal changes, the psychological and emotional reactions of each woman to this normal transition vary depending on her lifestyle, attitudes, self-image, and network of supportive relationships. This type of experience may contribute to crises in midlife.

In addition to the impact of changing physiology, the experience of midlife is emotional, cognitive, and spiritual. Midlife crises may be precipitated by an individual's reflection on or reevaluation of the meaning of life. Similarly, midlife may be a time during which people begin or intensify the process of spiritual evaluation and reckoning. It is a time during which people take stock of their lives and come to grips with their mortality.

A decline or change in physical functioning may trigger thoughts about mortality and death. A frequent phenomenon is evident in the change of one's perspective on time, from a focus on "time since birth" to one on "time left to live." Self-assessment may lead to greater emphasis on long-neglected aspects of the self or relationships with others.

All these issues are known as developmental issues or stressors, which are more or less predictable in life according to the person's stage of development. Situational stressors also contribute to the development of life crises. Situational stressors include such things as unexpected illness or injury, unemployment, and war—all those things which are not necessarily related to the person's chronological age or development through time. Consequently, it is reasonable to conclude that these factors may be potent in midlife as well.

Typically, individuals live not in isolation from one another but within the context of relationships. The most common network of relationships is the family. A discussion of issues that have biological, emotional, psychological, and social components, therefore, must include an examination of what is happening with other family members and the family as a group. These factors, including what is termed the family life cycle, may influence the development or severity of the subjective experience of midlife crisis. In fact, the crises of midlife often arise from the interaction between individual and family factors.

Those experiencing midlife crisis are usually members of what has become known as the "sandwich generation": a generation sandwiched between, and with the responsibility for taking care of, those in two others. For example, a middle-aged woman may have responsibilities with aging parents on the one hand and with an adolescent son on the other. Any crisis experience that she might have then becomes much more than the psychological or emotional process of an individual. The coincidence of adolescence, with her son's focus on the development of an identity and his constant evaluation of his own and his parents' values, beliefs, and behaviors, may only exacerbate her similar search for meaning. She also may be reevaluating her accomplishments and striving to do more of what she believes has been meaningful so far in life. In contrast, the elder generation may be struggling to find some sense of integrity about a life which is coming to an end. Each individual in the family becomes a point of contact, contrast, or conflict with the other.

The various manifestations of a midlife crisis are much like the symptoms exhibited by people in response to stress. The symptoms include an anxious or depressed mood, loss of interest in normal activities, an intensified reevaluation of life (both past and future), sudden changes in relationships, difficulty with organic processes (such as sleeping, eating, and concentration), and a subjective feeling of the need for a change. Extreme reactions may be a function of the psychology and emotional makeup of a particular individual in the context of his or her life. In addition, people who have less social support or who are living a lifestyle which they have long been aware was unfulfilling are more likely to experience a more significant crisis.

Not only do people and family groups vary in their reactions to midlife stress, but different ethnic and cultural groups do as well. The meaning associated with life events is generated within the context of these various social groups. Each social group develops its own culture with its own rules and regulations regarding how to respond or behave. In other words, individuals understand and respond to stressors as they do because of their experience within larger social groups. For example, within the Caucasian culture in the United States, a certain mythology has developed around the midlife crisis. Midlife is sometimes seen as a time when a man will buy a red sports car and leave his middle-aged wife for a young blonde. Someone else might give up her booming career and begin working with the underprivileged. As a result, within the context of this particular culture, dramatic lifestyle changes are predicted, explained, and possibly even supported.

In summary, midlife crisis are those crises that may arise during the developmental stage associated with midlife. Like crises or other stress reactions, midlife crises vary in timing, intensity, duration, and character from one person, family, and social group to another. Crises in midlife seem to be no more frequent than crises at other stages of development.

### TREATMENT AND THERAPY

Medical science has contributed to the understanding of the concept of midlife crisis through research, theory building, and the development and testing of treatment strategies, including the use of medication and psychotherapeutic techniques. Yet there are no specific treatments for a midlife or any other kind of crisis because the needs of the individual and the family group vary considerably. The range of possible treatments or clinical applications of medical science to this area are largely in the form of supporting the preexisting resources and coping skills of the individual and his or her family and other social support systems.

As with other life skills, an individual's ability to cope with and manage crises depends on the nature of one's character and personality, past experiences in managing crises, and degree of social support. The more well developed the person's character and coping mechanisms, the more numerous his or her experiences in successfully resolving past crises, and the greater amount of perceived support from family and friends, the more likely he or she will be able to resolve conflicts and crises in the present and future successfully.

Since midlife crises can differ from those in other stages, because of the particular tasks to be negotiated at this stage, resolution may involve the need to address certain tasks constructively. An individual may be called on to reevaluate or reassess his or her life, putting into perspective what is hoped for relative to what has transpired. An individual struggling with crises associated with midlife should be encouraged to explore the contributing situational and developmental issues openly. This process may involve cognitive reevaluation, working through feelings, or spiritual and existential reassessment.

Tamir suggests several tasks that must be addressed in order to facilitate the successful resolution of a midlife crisis. The individual must reckon with his or her own mortality, go through a process of self-assessment, examine sex-role obligations and expectations, and gain perspective on his or her generativity. Self-assessment involves taking stock and putting life into perspective. Life's polarities and contradictions must be examined and resolved in some manner.

One central polarity involves sex roles. The traditional differences between men and women often break down during the period of midlife. This process is facilitated by the life review accompanying a midlife crisis. For example, a woman may decide that she has devoted much of her life to the care and nurture of others while putting her own needs second. As a result, she may attempt to remedy the situation by developing the more stereotypical male characteristics of being assertive and goal-directed. Similarly, a male may turn away from his career as the primary source of self-esteem and gratification to developing richer interpersonal relationships.

Clinical and research evidence as reported by Richard Rahe and Thomas Holmes in *Life Change, Life Events, and Illness* (1989) demonstrates a solid link between life crisis

and disease onset. Consequently, medical health professionals may be called on to assist individuals struggling with the effects of a midlife crisis. These professionals, as well as other concerned individuals, may intervene in a variety of ways.

In a preventive fashion, helpers may offer what is termed anticipatory guidance to the individual approaching midlife transitions. In other words, conversations can include predictive or educative content orienting the person toward what may be expected as he or she approaches or anticipates these changes. An individual in the midst of midlife review and crisis may also need assistance, support, and/or direction in resolving generativity issues. The individual needs to resolve how he or she will make a significant contribution to others rather than stagnate and become increasingly self-absorbed. Accomplishment of these tasks may involve repercussions in work, family, and social relationships.

Physicians occasionally are called on to treat an individual exhibiting physical and/or psychological symptoms. While the prescription of medication for symptoms of depression and anxiety is recommended only in relatively extreme circumstances, antidepressant and antianxiety medications are very effective with some conditions, normally those in which the symptoms are impairing the person's ability to function over an extended period of time.

These various forms of assistance may be offered in an office visit for brief counseling, within the process of psychotherapy for a longer term approach, or during an informal conversation. Regardless of the context, however, being able to anticipate or coming to grips with the issues involved helps an individual to feel less out of control and to believe that the problems are being dealt with constructively.

Family and social support are very helpful in times of crisis. The degree to which these relationship contexts are flexible and supportive can either exacerbate problems or ameliorate struggles. A balance between permission and validation, with encouragement for the individual to continue managing daily functioning and obligations, is important. In the absence of an individual's ability to negotiate and resolve successfully the conflicts associated with the crisis, and perhaps without the presence of a supportive network of family and friends, individual and/or family therapy or a support group may be of help. These modes of therapy and support provide helpful perspective, normalization of the experience, and training or advice regarding constructive problem-solving and conflict resolution techniques.

## PERSPECTIVE AND PROSPECTS

In many areas of medical science pertaining to human behavior and emotional experience, important ideas from different theories are often integrated to yield a more comprehensive understanding. Congruently, several theoretical frameworks shape approaches to and perspectives on the understanding of midlife crises. Rudolf H. Moos explains in *Coping with Life Crises* (1986) that these include evolutionary theory, human growth and development, theories about the life cycle, behavior theory, family systems theory, learning theory, and theories of stress and coping.

The theory of evolution proposed by Charles Darwin provides the understanding of human beings as living interdependently, as well as adapting to their changing environment. The development of effective coping strategies ensures survival and promotes human community. Midlife crises present the individual and his or her social context with an opportunity for testing the effectiveness of these strategies.

The work of psychologist Abraham Maslow emphasized the tendency of human beings to strive toward the maintenance of life and the promotion of growth. An individual negotiating transitions in life taps into this growth motivation in order to maximize and enrich personal experience. In the midst of crisis, basic necessities of life are the first priority. Once the fundamental needs for food, shelter, and physical survival are satisfied, an individual will strive toward fulfilling what Maslow termed higher-level goals, such as emotional security and spiritual enlightenment.

According to Moos, crisis theory deals with the impact of disruptions on established patterns of personal and social identity. This framework suggests that, in addition to seeking to maximize human growth and potential, each individual first struggles to maintain a state of social and psychological equilibrium. In crisis, the midlife adult will seek homeostasis or balance prior to exploring opportunities for productive change. Thus, the similarity between crisis theory and theories of human growth and development may be apparent. The crises involved in midlife are more often related to the higher-level goals defined within each of these frameworks.

The stage or developmental theories described previously provide a framework within which to understand some of these transitions and the emotional, psychological, and physical changes that are involved. In addition, the perspective of the individual as developing, growing, evolving, and coping within the context of a family system enriches the view of midlife crisis.

The resulting context for an understanding of midlife crisis, then, is one of an integration of ideas and theories. This integration supports an understanding of midlife crisis as a product of the normative development and transitions in life. An individual's reaction to the required transitions depends on his or her personal characteristics, coping skills, family and social relationships, aspects of the transition or crisis itself, and other features of the physical and social environments. *—Layne A. Prest*

*See also* Aging; Anxiety; Death and dying; Depression; Factitious disorders; Hypochondriasis; Menopause; Neurosis; Panic attacks; Psychiatric disorders; Psychosomatic disorders; Sexual dysfunction; Sexuality; Stress.

**FOR FURTHER INFORMATION:**

Erikson, Erik H., et al. *Adulthood: Essays.* New York: Norton, 1978. A classic work in the field of adult development. May be understood by the general reader.

Gilligan, Carol. "New Maps of Development: New Visions of Maturity." *American Journal of Orthopsychiatry* 52 (April, 1982): 199-212. In this article, Gilligan begins to map out her alternatives to previously accepted theories of adult development. These alternatives are based on comparative research that contrasts male and female experiences. The author suggests that a woman's development cannot be measured according to the same yardstick as a man's. The female experience of development is colored by the network or web of relationships within which women live.

Holmes, Thomas H., and E. M. David, eds. *Life Change, Life Events, and Illness.* New York: Praeger, 1989. The editors of this book have compiled an important collection of research and clinical applications of stress and coping theories to practical and everyday experience. The authors of the various papers clarify the connection between life stressors and both psychological and physical illness.

Levinson, D. J. "A Conception of Adult Development." *American Psychologist* 41 (January, 1986): 3-13. Levinson's article includes an explanation of his framework for understanding adult development, including the phenomena related to midlife crisis.

Moos, Rudolf H., ed. *Coping with Life Crises.* New York: Plenum Press, 1986. Moos is a pioneer in the field of stress, families, and development. The book and its authors provide a view of midlife crises within the larger context of life development and transitions, as well as of crises in general. The authors emphasize the perspective that many crises are normal and/or normative. In addition, they point out that, given adequate support and effective skills, people often cope effectively without the help of professionals or the interventions of medical science.

Schulz, Richard, and Robert B. Ewen. *Adult Development and Aging.* New York: Macmillan, 1988. This textbook can be easily understood by the general reader and includes a comprehensive view of the development and aging processes. The areas covered include physiology, sensory experiences, learning, creativity, personality, relationships, work and retirement, stress and coping, and death and dying.

Tamir, Lois M. *Men in Their Forties: The Transition to Middle Age.* New York: Springer, 1982. This book is based on the author's research with men in midlife and represents the classic and commonly accepted notions about the midlife transition and its crises.

## MIGRAINE HEADACHES

**SYSTEM AFFECTED:** Brain

**SPECIALISTS:** Neurologists

**DEFINITION:** The cause of migraine headaches, which are characterized by intense, throbbing pain that may incapacitate the sufferer, is not known. Studies have shown, however, that they are linked to the constriction and dilation of arteries in the brain and scalp and that abnormalities in the body's biochemistry may occur during a migraine. The two main types of migraine headaches are common migraine and classic migraine. Common migraines are preceded by fatigue, nausea, vomiting, and fluid imbalance; during an attack, extreme sensitivity to noise and light occurs. With classic migraines, visual, sensory, and motor disturbances may foretell an attack, such as diagonal lines and bright spots in the field of vision, tingling in the face and hands, and a tendency to stagger. Certain drugs, when taken at the onset of an attack, can stop the migraine from proceeding.

*See also* Cluster headaches; Headaches.

## MISCARRIAGE

**SYSTEM AFFECTED:** Reproductive (female)

**SPECIALISTS:** Obstetricians

**DEFINITION:** Miscarriage, sometimes called spontaneous abortion, is the expulsion of the embryo or fetus before it is viable outside the uterus. About 20 percent of all pregnancies end in miscarriage, but because such a high percentage of these happen in the first trimester, the miscarriage may occur before the woman even knows that she is pregnant. Among the causes of miscarriage are abnormalities and structural defects in the fetus (as a result of genetic defects, syphilis, or drug use) and hormone imbalance in the mother (perhaps as a result of severe stress); contributing factors may include the excessive ingestion of alcohol or caffeine, heavy smoking, and poor nutrition. Most women who suffer a miscarriage will have no future problems in carrying a baby to term, but some women show a pattern of failed pregnancies.

*See also* Alcoholism; Ectopic pregnancy; Stillbirth; Syphilis.

## MITES. *See* BITES AND STINGS; LICE, MITES, AND TICKS; PARASITES.

## MITRAL INSUFFICIENCY

**SYSTEM AFFECTED:** Heart

**SPECIALISTS:** Cardiologists, family physicians, internists

**DEFINITION:** The inability of the mitral valve in the heart to close properly.

### CAUSES AND SYMPTOMS

The mitral valve connects the heart's left ventricle and left atrium. The oxygenated blood, having already passed through the right heart chambers and the lungs, arrives in the left atrium through the pulmonary veins and then passes through the mitral valve into the left ventricle. Compression of the left ventricle pumps the blood into the aorta and on to the rest of the body. A properly functioning mitral valve closes and prevents regurgitation or backflow into the left atrium. Mitral insufficiency occurs when the three leaves of the mitral valve close imperfectly, allowing leakage. This condition, known also as mitral valve prolapse, is the most common cardiac syndrome. Found in all segments of society, it is most common in young adult women.

Mitral valve prolapse has several possible causes including rheumatic fever, inflammation of the heart lining (endocarditis), cardiac tumors, or most often, genetic error. Its symptoms are undue fatigue after exercise, shortness of breath, and chest pain. Other common complaints are anxiety, depression, and panic, all related to stress. The number of diagnosed cases in Western countries is rising markedly and may be the result of more sophisticated diagnostic techniques or the increasing stress in modern society.

### PERSPECTIVE AND PROSPECTS

Until the 1960's, the detection of mitral insufficiency was through a characteristic "click" heard by the physician when the mitral leaves attempted to close. Now the use of echocardiograms, allowing ultrasound images of the beating heart and blood flow, are standard practice.

People with mitral valve prolapse lead a normal life, and many are unaware that they have the condition. Repeated irregularity in breathing or an inexplicable shortness of breath is a sign to see one's physician. Regular exercise and good eating habits are recommended for this mild con-

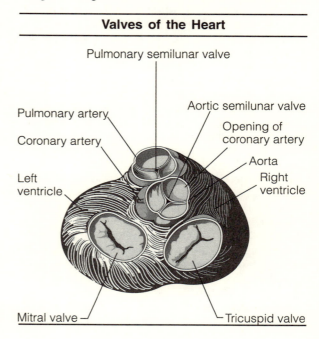

### Valves of the Heart

Pulmonary semilunar valve

Aortic semilunar valve

Pulmonary artery

Opening of coronary artery

Coronary artery

Aorta

Left ventricle

Right ventricle

Mitral valve

Tricuspid valve

dition. Fear and anxiety, however, can cause a disastrous situation: People should know that only in severe cases is mitral valve prolapse treated surgically or considered life-threatening. —*K. Thomas Finley*

*See also* Congenital heart disease; Endocarditis; Heart disease.

**FOR FURTHER INFORMATION:**

Boudoulas, Harisios, and Charles F. Wooley. *Mitral Valve Prolapse and the Mitral Valve Prolapse Syndrome.* Mount Kisco, N.Y.: Futura, 1988.

Frederickson, Lyn. *Confronting Mitral Valve Prolapse Syndrome: The Mysterious Heart Condition of the Young and Healthy.* San Marcos, Calif.: Slawson Communications, 1988.

## MONONUCLEOSIS

**SYSTEM AFFECTED:** Respiratory

**SPECIALISTS:** Family physicians, infectious disease physicians, internists

**DEFINITION:** An infectious respiratory illness caused by the Epstein-Barr virus.

Mononucleosis is commonly spread by oral transmission, such as kissing or eating and drinking with the same utensils used by an infected person. An infection in a child may be without symptoms or may resemble other common upper-respiratory infections. In adolescents and young adults, the disease is more likely to cause the characteristic symptoms of fatigue, fever, sore throat, and swollen, painful lymph nodes.

The virus invades B lymphocytes, a type of white blood cell important to the function of the immune system. Microscopic examination of a blood sample reveals that these cells have increased in number and are abnormal in appearance. An antibody test called the heterophil agglutination test confirms the diagnosis.

Treatment primarily consists of bed rest and good nutrition. Nonaspirin pain relievers, such as acetaminophen, are usually recommended. Care should be taken to wash eating utensils and dishes thoroughly to prevent the spread of the infection to family members. The patient is usually able to resume near normal activities in two to three weeks. Fatigue will persist for several months, however, and strenuous activity should be avoided during that time.

*The Epstein-Barr virus.* The virus responsible for mononucleosis is in the herpesvirus family. It is also associated with disorders other than mononucleosis. Researchers have discovered that the Epstein-Barr virus is present in cases of Burkitt's lymphoma, a cancer of the lymph nodes primarily found in Africa. Certain throat cancers in China and Hodgkin's disease are also associated with the Epstein-Barr virus. Researchers believe that the study of these diseases may aid in understanding of the roles that viruses, inheritance, age, and environmental influences play in the development of cancer.

The Epstein-Barr virus has also been implicated in chronic fatigue syndrome. Symptoms of this disorder, such as fatigue and reduction in mental abilities, are very similar to those experienced by mononucleosis patients. Although infection with Epstein-Barr virus has not been confirmed as the definitive cause, it does appear to play a role in some cases of chronic fatigue syndrome. —*Edith K. Wallace*

*See also* Chronic fatigue syndrome; Fatigue; Viral infections.

**FOR FURTHER INFORMATION:**

Berkow, Robert, ed. "Infectious Mononucleosis." In *The Merck Manual of Diagnosis and Therapy.* 16th ed. Rahway, N.J.: Merck Sharp & Dohme Research Laboratories, 1992.

Fettner, Ann Giudici. *The Science of Viruses: What They Are, Why They Make Us Sick, How They Will Change the Future.* New York: Quill/William Morrow, 1990.

Rosenbaum, Michael, and Murray Susser. *Solving the Puzzle of Chronic Fatigue Syndrome.* Tacoma, Wash.: Life Sciences Press, 1992.

## MOSQUITO BITES. *See* ARTHROPOD-BORNE DISEASES; BITES AND STINGS.

## MOTION SICKNESS

**SYSTEMS AFFECTED:** Gastrointestinal, auditory

**SPECIALISTS:** Aerospace physicians, family physicians, internists, otolaryngologists

**DEFINITION:** A feeling of nausea brought on by motion.

### CAUSES AND SYMPTOMS

Motion sickness results from exposure to unusual motion such as that experienced in a boat, airplane, or automobile. It is often accompanied by pallor and, if severe, vomiting. It probably has the same cause as space sickness, which is suffered by more than half of cosmonauts and astronauts. Humans are differentially susceptible to motion sickness: Some are affected by a short ride on an amusement park carousel; others are unaffected by the wildest rides available. Dogs, cats, horses, rats, and other animals are also susceptible to motion sickness.

According to one theory, motion sickness is the result of a mechanism which normally defends an organism against ingested toxins. The theory holds that the first bit of toxin absorbed into the blood upsets the balance among a delicate array of equilibrium mechanisms involving feedback to the cerebellum (the part of the brain responsible for balance and coordination) from the eye, the equilibrium receptors in the inner ear, and stretch receptors in the joints and muscles. This upset triggers vomiting, purging the stomach of the remainder of the toxin. According to the theory, unusual motion upsets the same balance when conflicting information is fed to the cerebellum from the inner ear, eyes, or other receptors.

Motion sickness has been treated with acupuncture at a point two inches above the wrist, wrist bands worn to put pressure on that point, autogenic-feedback training (learning to control physiological responses that are normally automatic), adaptation (repeated exposure to motion that causes motion sickness), and drugs taken orally or from a patch applied to the skin. Each method has its supporters, but none always works. Research indicates that the most effective drugs are scopolamine combined with d-amphetamine (Dexedrine), followed closely by promethazine (Phenergan) combined with d-amphetamine and by dimenhydrinate (Dramamine), which can also be combined with d-amphetamine. All have side effects (drowsiness, dizziness, and dry mouth), some of which are lessened or increased when used in the combinations listed.

—*Carl W. Hoagstrom*

*See also* Nausea and vomiting.

**FOR FURTHER INFORMATION:**

Crampton, George H., ed. *Motion and Space Sickness*. Boca Raton, Fla.: CRC Press, 1990.

Daunton, N. G., W. R. Mehler, and K. R. Brizzee. *Mechanisms of Motion-Induced Vomiting*. New York: Karger, 1983.

Young, L. R. "Space and the Vestibular System: What Has Been Learned?" *Journal of Vestibular Research* 3, no. 3 (Fall, 1993): 203-206.

# MOTOR NEURON DISEASES

**SYSTEMS AFFECTED:** Muscular, nervous

**SPECIALISTS:** Neurologists

**DEFINITION:** Progressive, debilitating, and eventually fatal diseases affecting nerve cells in muscles.

**KEY TERMS:**

*Babinski's sign:* an abnormal response to a neurological test involving a brisk stroke with a sharp object on the bottom of the foot; the normal response is for the toes to bunch together and curve downward, while the abnormal response is for the big toe to pull upward and not in unison with the other toes

*corticospinal tracts:* neurological pathways descending from the brain to the spinal cord that control and allow voluntary movement

*fasciculations:* spontaneous electrical impulses from neurons that result in irregular, involuntary muscular contractions; in motor neuron disease, these contractions indicate nerve death

*lower motor neuron:* a nerve cell whose cell body resides either in the brain stem (to form a cranial nerve) or in the spinal cord (to form a spinal motor neuron)

*motor neuron:* a nerve that functions either directly or indirectly to control a target organ

*muscular atrophy:* a wasting of muscle mass; a greatly reduced size of muscle cells caused by the lost innervation (neuron death) or disuse of muscles

*spasticity:* an abnormal condition in which the limbs demonstrate resistance to passive movement as a result of damage to the corticospinal tracts; the reflexes are hyperactive

*tropic factors:* chemicals released from nerve cells that have a vital influence on muscle health; in the absence of tropic factors, muscles atrophy

*upper motor neuron:* a nerve whose cell body resides within the brain but whose axon descends the brain stem and spinal cord to form a corticospinal tract

**CAUSES AND SYMPTOMS**

In motor neuron diseases, certain nerves die, specifically those that allow any and all body movement. The actual cause of spontaneous motor neuron death is unknown, but genetic defects, neurotoxins, viruses, autoimmune disruptions, and metabolic disorders are contributing factors.

The predominant features of motor neuron disorders are muscular weakness, muscular wasting, and the presence of fasciculations. As a nerve dies, it can no longer effectively innervate its target muscle, but neighboring nerves may sprout to keep the muscle active. A consequence of nerve sprouting is the onset of brief, spontaneous contractions, or twitches. These visible twitches are called fasciculations. Eventually, as increasing numbers of nerves die, fewer healthy nerves are left to sprout until, finally, all muscles are denervated. Dead nerves cannot prompt muscle movement, nor can they release tropic factors as they do in health. This loss of tropic input from the neuron causes muscular atrophy and renders the muscle useless.

Motor neuron diseases are usually first noticed in the hands or upper limbs, where muscle weakness and decreased ability to use arms or hands causes problems. Unlike some disorders, motor neuron diseases fail to show stages of exacerbation or remission. Rather they progress—either rapidly or slowly, but unrelentingly—until death, usually as a result of respiratory complications.

Although there are childhood forms of motor neuron diseases, they are more likely to strike between the ages of fifty and fifty-five, and they are seen in males more than females by a ratio of 1.5 to 1. Motor neuron diseases seem to occur rarely in the obese person and tend to afflict otherwise healthy, thin, and perhaps athletic persons. A famed person afflicted by the debilitating motor neuron disease amyotrophic lateral sclerosis (ALS) was baseball player Lou Gehrig, in whose honor it is often called Lou Gehrig's disease.

Motor neuron diseases are often subgrouped into three categories: ALS, progressive spinal muscular atrophy, and progressive bulbar (brain-stem) palsy. In the plural form, motor neuron diseases refer to all forms of the affliction, whereas the singular form, motor neuron disease, is synonymous with ALS.

Amyotrophic lateral sclerosis is the most familiar of the motor neuron diseases primarily because it accounts for a full 60 percent of all such disorders. The name has clinical meaning: "Amyotrophy" refers to the loss of muscle bulk as a result of missing tropic factors from dying or dead neurons; "lateral" refers to the locations within the spinal cord that are affected; and "sclerosis" refers to the hardened quality of the lateral regions of the diseased spinal cord, which otherwise would be soft tissue. The brain stem may also be sclerotic (hardened). ALS has an incidence of 1 or 2 persons per 100,000, although some Pacific islands, such as Guam, seem to have a higher incidence attributable to undetermined genetic factors. In addition, some populations show an autosomal dominant genetic component. ALS is fatal, and death generally occurs as a result of respiratory failure within three to five years after the onset of symptoms.

ALS is characterized by upper and lower motor neuron signs of neural death; thus the presence of both fasciculations and spasticity is required for a diagnosis. Spasticity is a medical term that describes a certain kind of muscular resistance (stiffness) to movement. In particular, spastic means a resistance that increases the more rapidly a muscle is extended; tendon reflexes are also hyperactive and Babinski's sign (abnormal reflexes of the toes) must be present. Babinski's sign reveals the death of neurons in the corticospinal tracts, which signals the occurrence of upper motor neuron death. The presence of fasciculations reveals lower motor neuron death.

Progressive spinal muscular atrophy (SMA) will show only lower motor neuron signs—namely, muscular weakness, fasciculations, and atrophy. Babinski's sign or spasticity is not found. The early symptoms may include increased clumsiness in using the fingers for fine movements (including writing or using kitchen utensils), stiffness of the fingers and hands, and cramping of the upper and lower limbs. Once the brain-stem nerves become involved, difficulty in speaking and swallowing occur. Of all persons afflicted with one of the motor neuron diseases, 7 to 15 percent will have lower motor neuron signs only and are presumed to have the progressive spinal muscular atrophy form.

Progressive bulbar palsy literally means progressive brain-stem paralysis. This form of motor neuron disease accounts for 20 to 25 percent of all cases. The tongue is usually the first place to show muscular wasting and fasciculations. As the nerves controlling the tongue die, the tongue shrivels and shrinks so that speaking, chewing, and moving solids or liquids to the back of the mouth for swallowing become difficult or impossible.

Children can be afflicted with spinal muscular atrophy. This disease is believed by many experts to be completely unique from the adult form. The childhood form seems to be more associated with environmental and genetic factors. (This concept is greatly debated, however, since the actual cause of any of the motor neuron diseases is unknown.)

Three forms of childhood SMA have been identified: type 1, or acute infantile SMA (also known as Werdnig-Hoffman disease); type 2, or intermediate SMA; and type 3, or juvenile SMA (also known as Kugelberg-Welander disease).

Of children afflicted with SMA, 25 percent have type 1. This form of the disease is an autosomal recessive genetic disorder which occurs in 1 of 15,000 to 25,000 births. In an experienced mother, there may be awareness of minimal fetal movement in the last trimester of pregnancy; the fetus tends to stay still as a result of muscular weakness. Upon birth, the newborn may be a "floppy" baby of great weakness and may immediately have trouble with nursing and breathing. In other cases, it may take three to six months before symptoms begin. Because of the eventual weakening of the muscles of respiration, the child becomes prone to respiratory infections that cannot be cleared because of a lost cough reflex. Death usually occurs at two to three years of age.

When a child fails to stand or walk between six to twelve months of age, the physician considers the possibility that the child has type 2 SMA. An abnormal curvature of the spine to the forward and sideways position (kyphoscoliosis) is often seen, but rarely is there any problem with feeding or breathing. It is generally the case that very fine tremors of the child's hands can be noticed, and sometimes contractures of the hips and knees can occur. There is no delay in terms of mental health or intellect for these children.

Type 3 SMA is most often seen in the adolescent, but this disease can be observed in some children as early as five years of age. The predominant feature is weakness of the hip muscles. Since these children have been walking for some time, a change in their walking gait to a waddle can be seen over the course of years. Most people with type 3 SMA must use wheelchairs in their mid-thirties, but some may lose their ability to walk earlier. Type 3 SMA has been shown to be an autosomal recessive disorder in many cases, but there are also reported cases of sporadic occurrences within families that have previously been unaffected. Clearly, there are unanswered questions about this disease.

It should be noted that controversy abounds on the assigned classifications of motor neuron diseases. This controversy arises from the fact that the origins of the diseases are not known. Since cause has not been established for any form of motor neuron disease, physicians must use clusters of symptoms to sort the differences in disease manifestation. This sorting is used to plan the best possible treatment programs for the circumstances; nevertheless, these distinctions may seem arbitrary once more is known about the causes of motor neuron death.

### TREATMENT AND THERAPY

Perhaps one of the most frustrating attributes of motor neuron diseases is that neither prevention nor effective treatment and cures are available. For a person living with motor neuron disease, physicians and health care professionals must work as a team to manage the symptoms of the diseases and offer palliative care.

In general, patients are encouraged to use and exercise their muscles cautiously in order to avoid disuse atrophy, but activity to the point of fatigue is forbidden since it is believed to aggravate the progression of muscular wasting. In addition, exposure to cold may worsen muscular contractures. Physical therapy facilitates a delay in the total loss of willed body movement by allowing the use of braces, walkers, and wheelchairs as modes of locomotion. Adults are encouraged to continue nonexertive work for as long as possible; it aids both the body and the mind to maintain independence and a sense of wholeness, well-being, and dignity.

As muscular control of the voice wanes, sketch pads, word boards, and computers can aid the ill person in communicating with loved ones, doctors, nurses, and colleagues. In addition, respiratory therapy aids in maintaining healthy breathing in spite of ever-weakening respiratory muscles. Prophylactic immunizations for influenza and pneumococci are given, especially to those who are wheelchair-dependent or bedridden. Forced deep breathing and coughing are needed at least once every four hours to bring up any congestion that may otherwise lead to grave consequences. Almost all persons with motor neuron diseases die from respiratory insufficiency. For this reason, it is imperative that the patient and physician discuss respiratory care early after diagnosis to determine whether the patient wants to be placed on mechanical ventilators in the later stages of the disease. Other issues such as tube feedings should be discussed while the patient is still able to voice an opinion and express any concerns about the dying process associated with the disease.

### PERSPECTIVE AND PROSPECTS

Life can be socially difficult for people with motor neuron diseases. Others tend to assume that persons who must use wheelchairs and are unable to control mouth movements (so that speech and swallowing are lost and drooling may occur) are not intelligent, thinking, or aware. This is a sad misperception.

Many persons suffering from a motor neuron disease rise above its physical challenges to conquer in spirit that which the body cannot. For example, former United States senator Jacob Javits labored hard to improve the awareness of and funding for ALS in spite of being on a ventilator and completely immobile because of his battle with the disease. Another example of how well the intellect is preserved in this physically tragic disease can be seen in the life and work of the world-renowned astrophysicist Stephen Hawking.

Until there is an established cause or causes for these diseases effective treatments or cures are likely to remain hidden. The research continues in hopes of pinning down the ever-elusive motor neuron diseases. —*Mary C. Fields*

*See also* Aphasia and dysphasia; Paralysis.

### FOR FURTHER INFORMATION:

Bannister, Roger. *Brain and Bannister's Clinical Neurology.* 7th ed. Oxford, England: Oxford University Press, 1992. Although much of this text is advanced, chapter 27 ("Motor Neuron Disease") is more descriptive than technical. The black-and-white photographs provide memorable images of the destruction that these diseases cause.

Calne, Donald B. *Neurodegenerative Diseases.* Philadelphia: W. B. Saunders, 1994. An excellent book with a section devoted to amyotrophic lateral sclerosis and related motor neuron diseases.

Ferguson, Kitty. *Stephen Hawking: Quest for a Theory of Everything.* New York: Bantam Books, 1992. Ferguson describes Dr. Hawking's brilliant and complex theories in simple language, as well as how he and those around him cope with ALS.

Parsons, Malcolm. *Color Atlas of Clinical Neurology.* 2d ed. St. Louis: Mosby Year Book, 1993. Impeccably assembled, this atlas shows the most distinguishing clinical features associated with motor neuron diseases, such as muscular wasting of the hands and tongue.

Ringel, Steven P. *Neuromuscular Disorders: A Guide for Patient and Family.* New York: Raven Press, 1987. Written by a physician whose brother, also a medical doctor, died of a neuromuscular disease. Offers a thorough, yet nontechnical, account of the struggles and challenges facing persons with motor neuron diseases.

# MULTIPLE SCLEROSIS

**SYSTEMS AFFECTED:** Muscular, nervous
**SPECIALISTS:** Internists, neurologists, pediatricians
**DEFINITION:** An incurable, debilitating disease of the nervous system.

### CAUSES AND SYMPTOMS

Multiple sclerosis, which is usually abbreviated as MS, results from an inflammation of the fatty material, myelin, which insulates the nerves. This inflammation occurs at multiple locations in the brain and spinal cord, leading first to demyelination (the removal of the myelin) and then to scarring (sclerosis). MS commences as a series of attacks on the myelin, which has a limited ability to repair itself. Eventually, the myelin breaks down completely, the scarring process occurs, and the affected nerves lose their ability to conduct impulses.

MS does not affect the same nerves in all people; therefore, it is difficult to predict how severe the disease will be in a particular patient. Some experience only mild discomfort with no permanent disabilities; others may become severely paralyzed and require full-time care. Even in those who experience the most debilitating forms of MS, however, life expectancy is not shortened by more than a few years, although quality of life may be dramatically compromised at a relatively early age. The disease is most common in working-age adults, between the ages of twenty and

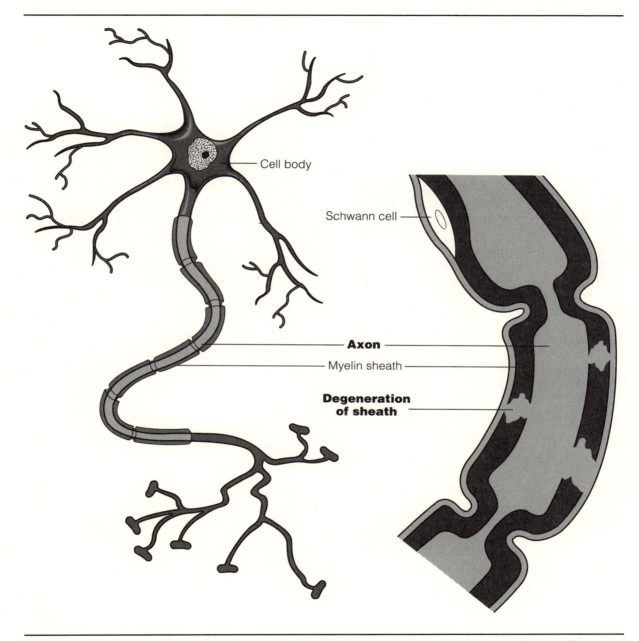

Cell body

Schwann cell

**Axon**

Myelin sheath

**Degeneration
of sheath**

*Multiple sclerosis is caused by degeneration of the myelin sheath (right) that insulates the axons of nerve cells; a nerve cell is shown on the left.*

forty, and is more prevalent in women than in men. There is also an increased incidence in people of western European ancestry living in temperate zones.

There are two main types of MS: exacerbating-remitting disease and the less common chronic progressive disease. In the former, attacks of MS are followed by periods of relative recovery, although over time the general trend is

one of deterioration. In the chronic progressive form of the disease, the patient becomes increasingly ill, with no periods of temporary recovery. It is not uncommon for the fluctuating form of the disease to develop into the chronic form.

The symptoms of MS are diverse, because any part of the brain or spinal cord may be affected. Commonly, symptoms include fatigue, loss of muscle strength, increased muscle stiffness, a tingling sensation in the extremities, loss of bladder control, double vision, and a general loss of sensation in the limbs (resulting from scarring of the sensory nerves). Because these symptoms accompany many other disorders as well, MS may be overlooked at first, especially because the first attack may be too mild to be remarkable. The next attack may not take place for another three to four years, at which point they become more and more frequent. This attack-remission cycle is characteristic of the disease. Another indication of MS is a worsening of the symptoms when the patient's body temperature increases, as with a hot bath, exercise, or time out in the sun; high temperatures further slow the conduction of impulses in the nerve fibers. For this reason, cold baths have proven therapeutic in relieving the discomfort of MS.

The causes of MS are unknown. Possibilities include a virus, genetic factors, or an immune system disturbance.

Although a specific MS virus has not yet been found, there is another virus called human T-cell lymphotropic virus type I (HTLV-I) that causes demyelination of the spinal cord, leading to an illness similar to MS. Some researchers therefore reason that other viruses might exist which cause the type demyelination and sclerosis found in MS.

The ...ence of the disease in families of MS patients is highe. han in families with no incidences of MS. This finding suggests a genetic aspect to the disease. In identical twins, if one member of the pair has MS, the other has a 25 to 50 percent chance of developing the disease. Because identical twins share the same genes, one or several of these genes might play a role in the development of the disease.

Significant evidence exists for classifying MS as an autoimmune disease, that is, a disease in which the body's infection-fighting mechanism mistakes the body's own tissues for foreign invaders. Scientists have noted an increase in immune system cells in the central nervous system (brain and spinal cord) prior to the onset of MS symptoms. It is possible that these cells, for some unknown reason, mistake the myelin surrounding the nerves for foreign tissue and begin to attack it.

It has been suggested that all three factors—viral, genetic, and autoimmune—may play a role in the development of MS: A virus may mimic the body's own proteins so well that the immune system cannot discriminate between the two and attacks its own tissues as well as the virus. A certain gene or genes may make an individual susceptible to such viral deception.

### TREATMENT AND THERAPY

There is no cure for multiple sclerosis, and neither can the progression of the disease be stopped. Approximately 50 percent of all patients develop significant disability about ten years after onset. The treatment of MS has three objectives: to reduce inflammation of the nerves, to sup-

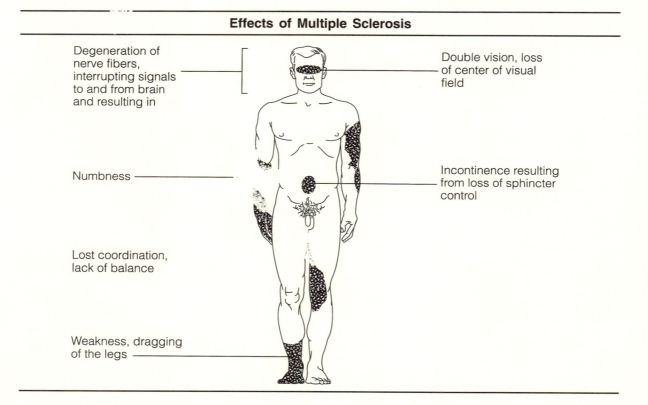

**Effects of Multiple Sclerosis**

Degeneration of nerve fibers, interrupting signals to and from brain and resulting in

Double vision, loss of center of visual field

Numbness

Incontinence resulting from loss of sphincter control

Lost coordination, lack of balance

Weakness, dragging of the legs

press the presumed autoimmune attack, and to relieve the symptoms.

Inflammation can be combated to some extent with drugs. In the case of exacerbating-remitting MS, synthetic steroids can be administered, or a hormone called adreno-corticotropic hormone (ACTH) can be given to stimulate the body to produce its own steroid, cortisol. Chronic progressive MS is more resistant to treatment. Strong immunosuppressive drugs are sometimes given, but their side effects can be so severe that many physicians have questioned whether their benefits outweigh their disadvantages. One of these agents is cyclophosphamide, which is highly toxic and gives some relief to only about a third of MS patients.

Symptoms may be relieved with drugs that treat painful muscle spasms and stiffness, fatigue, and loss of bladder control. As a last resort to relieve facial pain, which may interfere with chewing or speaking, specific facial nerves can be severed, although this will result in numbness over part of the face. Exercise for MS sufferers is important, for both physical and emotional reasons, but only if done in cold water, which rapidly dissipates the heat that tends to worsen the patient's neurological symptoms.

—*Robert Klose*

**See also** Paralysis.

**FOR FURTHER INFORMATION:**

Larson, David E., ed. "Multiple Sclerosis." In *Mayo Clinic Family Health Book*. New York: William Morrow, 1990.

National Institutes of Health (U.S.). Clinical Center. *Multiple Sclerosis*. No. 90-3015. Bethesda, Md.: U.S. Department of Health and Human Services, Public Health Service, National Institutes of Health, Warren Grant Magnuson Clinical Center, 1990.

Schroeder, Steven A., et al., eds. *Current Medical Diagnosis and Treatment*. 30th ed. Norwalk, Conn.: Appleton and Lange, 1991.

Tapley, Donald T., et al., eds. *The Columbia University College of Physicians and Surgeons Complete Home Medical Guide*. Rev. ed. New York: Crown, 1989.

# MUMPS

**SYSTEMS AFFECTED:** Gastrointestinal, reproductive (male), immune

**SPECIALISTS:** Family physicians, pediatricians, public health specialists

**DEFINITION:** A contagious childhood disease caused by a virus, mumps is diagnosed by the characteristic swelling of the salivary (parotid) glands in front of and below the ears. Direct contact and airborne droplets are responsible for spreading the infection, sometimes causing epidemics. During childhood, infection with mumps is usually not serious. In addition to the swelling, the symptoms include fever, fatigue, neck pain, and headache, and the risk of complications exists. In males, epididymorchitis may occur, in which there is swelling and tenderness in

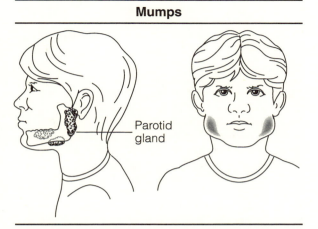

**Mumps**

*Mumps cause a characteristic swelling of the parotid (salivary) glands.*

the testicles, lower abdominal pain, vomiting, nausea, and chills; these symptoms are usually more severe in men or adolescents who contract mumps, and in rare cases, sterility may result. Most infections are not serious, however, and one episode confers lifelong immunity. A vaccine for mumps is available.

**See also** Childhood infectious diseases.

# MUSCLE SPRAINS, SPASMS, AND DISORDERS

**SYSTEM AFFECTED:** Muscular

**SPECIALISTS:** Family physicians, physiatrists, physical therapists, sports medicine physicians

**DEFINITION:** Injuries, defects, or disorders of the muscles of the body.

## CAUSES AND SYMPTOMS

There are three kinds of muscle tissue in the human body: smooth muscle, cardiac muscle, and striated muscle. Smooth muscle tissue is found around the intestines, blood vessels, bronchioles in the lung, and in other areas. These muscles are controlled by the autonomic nervous system, which means that their movement is not subject to voluntary action. They have many functions: They maintain the airway in the lungs, regulate the tone of blood vessels, and move foods and other substances through the digestive tract. Cardiac muscle is found only in the heart. Striated muscles are those that move body parts. They are also called voluntary muscles because they must receive a conscious command from the brain in order to work. They supply the force for physical activity, and they also prevent movement and stabilize body parts.

Muscles are subject to many disorders: Muscle sprains, strains, and spasms are common events in everyone's life and, for the most part, they are harmless, if painful, results of overexercise, accidents, falls, bumps, or countless other events. Yet these symptoms can also signal serious myopathies, or disorders within muscle tissue.

Myopathies constitute a wide range of diseases. They are classified as inflammatory myopathies or metabolic myopathies. Inflammatory myopathies include infections by bacteria, viruses, or other microorganisms, as well as other diseases that are possibly autoimmune in origin (that is, resulting from and directed against the body's own tissues). In metabolic myopathies, there is some failure or disturbance in the body's ability to maintain a proper metabolic balance or electrolyte distribution. These conditions include glycogen storage diseases, in which there are errors in glucose processing; disorders of fatty acid metabolism, in which there are derangements in fatty acid oxidation; mitochondrial myopathies, in which there are biochemical and other abnormalities in the mitochondria of muscle cells; endocrine myopathies, in which an endocrine disorder underlies muscular symptoms; and the periodic paralyses, which can be the result of inherited or acquired illnesses. This is only a partial list of the myopathies, the symptoms of which include weakness and pain.

Muscular dystrophies are a group of inherited disorders in which muscle tissue fails to receive nourishment. The result is progressive muscular weakness and the degeneration and destruction of muscle fibers. The symptoms include weakness, loss of coordination, impaired gait, and impaired muscle extensibility. Over the years, muscle mass decreases and the arms, legs, and spine become deformed.

Neuromuscular disorders include a wide variety of conditions in which muscle function is impaired by faulty transmission of nerve impulses to muscle tissue. These conditions may be inherited; they may be attributable to toxins, such as in food poisoning (for example, botulism) or by pesticide poisoning; or they may be side effects of certain drugs. The most commonly seen neuromuscular disorder is myasthenia gravis.

The muscular disorders most often seen are those that result from overexertion, exercise, athletics, accidents, and trauma. As a matter of fact, injuries sustained during sports and games have become so significant that sports medicine has become a recognized medical subspecialty. Besides the muscles, the parts of the body involved in these disorders include tendons (tough, stringy tissue that attaches muscles to bones), ligaments (tissue that attaches bone to bone), synovia (membranes enclosing a joint or other bony structure), and cartilage (soft, resilient tissue between bones). A sprain is an injury in which ligaments are stretched or torn. In a strain, muscles or tendons are stretched or torn. A contusion is a bruise that occurs when the body is subjected to trauma; the skin is not broken, but the capillaries underneath are, causing discoloration. A spasm is a short, abnormal contraction in a muscle or group of muscles. A cramp is a prolonged, painful contraction of one or more muscles.

Sprains can be caused by twisting the joint violently or by forcing it beyond its range of movement. The ligaments that connect the bones of the joint stretch or tear. Sprains occur most often in the knees, ankles, and arches of the feet. There is pain and swelling, and at least some immobilization of the joint.

A strain is also called a pulled muscle. When too great a demand is placed on a muscle, it and the surrounding tendons can stretch and/or tear. The main symptom is pain; swelling and muscle spasm may also occur.

Muscle spasms and cramps are common. Sometimes they occur spontaneously, such as the calf muscle cramps that occur at night. Sometimes they are attributable to muscle strain (the charley horse that tightens thigh muscles in runners and other athletes). Muscles that are used often will go into spasm, such as those in the thumb and fingers of writers (writers' cramp), as can muscles that have remained in one position for too long. Muscle spasm and cramps can also occur as a direct consequence of dehydration; they are common in athletes who perspire excessively during hot weather.

Some injuries to muscles and joints occur so regularly that they are named for the activities associated with them. A good example is tennis elbow, a condition that results from repeated, vigorous movement of the arm, such as swinging a tennis racket, using a paintbrush, or pitching a baseball. Runners' knee can afflict joggers and other athletes. It is usually caused by sprains in the knee ligaments; there is pain and there may be partial or total immobilization of the knee. Achilles tendinitis, as the name suggests, is inflammation of the Achilles tendon in the heel. It is usually the result of excessive physical activity that causes small tears in the tendon. Pain and immobility are symptoms. Tendinitis can occur in other joints as well; elbows and shoulders are common sites. Tenosynovitis is inflammation of the synovial membrane that sheaves the tendons in the hand. It may be caused by bacterial infection or may be attributable to overexertion.

Tumors and cancerous growths in muscle tissue are rare. If a lump appears in muscle, it is usually a lipoma, a fatty deposit that is benign. One tumor, called rhabdomyosarcoma, however, is malignant and can be fatal.

## TREATMENT AND THERAPY

The myopathies are a wide group of diseases, and treatment varies considerably among them. The muscular dystrophies also vary in their treatment methods. Physical therapy is recommended to prevent contractures, the permanent, disfiguring muscular contractions that are a feature of the disease. Orthopedic appliances and surgery are also used. Because these diseases are genetic, it is sometimes recommended that people with a familial history of muscular dystrophy be tested for certain genetic markers that would suggest the possibility of disease in their children.

Myasthenia gravis is treated with drugs that increase the amount of neurotransmitters available where nerves and muscles come together. The drugs help improve the transmission of information from the brain to the muscle tissue. In some cases, a procedure called plasmapheresis is used to eliminate blood-borne substances that may contribute to the disease. Surgical removal of the thymus gland is helpful in alleviating symptoms in some patients.

In treating the many muscle disorders that are caused by athletic activity and excessive wear and tear on the muscle, the R-I-C-E formula is recommended. The acronym stands for rest-ice-compression-elevation: The patient must rest and not use or exercise the limb or muscle involved; an ice pack is applied to the injury; compression is supplied by wrapping a moist bandage snugly over the ice, reducing the flow of fluids to the injured area; and the injured limb is elevated. If there is a fracture involved, the limb must be properly splinted or otherwise immobilized before elevation. The ice pack is held in place for twenty minutes and removed, but the bandage is held in place. Ice therapy can be resumed every twenty minutes.

Heat is also part of the therapy for strains and sprains, but it is not applied until after the initial swelling has gone down, usually after forty-eight to seventy-two hours. Heat raises the metabolic rate in the affected tissue. This brings more blood to the area, carrying nutrients that are needed for tissue repair. Moist heat is preferred, and it can be supplied by an electrical heating pad, a chemical gel in a plastic bag, or as hot baths and whirlpools. In using pads and chemical gels, there should be a layer of toweling or other material between the heat source and the body. Temperature for a whirlpool or hot bath should be about 106 degrees Fahrenheit. Only the injured part should be immersed, if possible. As in the ice treatments, heat should be applied for twenty minutes and can be repeated after twenty minutes of rest.

Analgesics are given for pain. Over-the-counter preparations such as aspirin, acetaminophen, or ibuprofen are used most often. Sometimes, when pain is severe, more potent medications are required. Steroids are sometimes prescribed to reduce inflammation, and nonsteroidal anti-inflammatory drugs (NSAIDs) can alleviate both pain and inflammation. If a strained muscle or tendon is seriously torn or otherwise damaged, surgery may be required. Similarly, if a sprain involves torn or detached ligaments, they may have to be surgically repaired.

Muscle spasms and cramps may require both manipulation and the application of heat or cold. The affected limb is gently extended to stretch the contracted muscle. Massage and immersion in a hot bath are useful, as are cold packs.

Tennis elbow, runners' knee, and tendinitis respond to R-I-C-E therapy. Ice is applied to the injured site, and the limb is elevated and allowed to rest. When tenosynovitis is caused by bacterial infection, prompt antibiotic therapy may be necessary to avoid permanent damage. When it is attributable to overexertion, analgesics may help relieve pain and inflammation. Rarely, a corticosteroid is used when other drugs fail.

Often, the injured site requires physical therapy for the full range of motion to be restored. The physical therapist analyzes the patient's capability and develops a regimen to restore strength and mobility to the affected muscles and joints. Physical therapy may involve massage, hot baths, whirlpools, weight training, and/or isometric exercise. Orthotic devices may be required to help the injured area heal.

An important aspect of sports medicine and the treatment of sports-related muscle disorders is prevention. Many painful, debilitating, and immobilizing episodes can be avoided by proper training and conditioning, intelligent exercise practice, and restriction of exertion. Before undertaking any sport or strenuous physical activity, the individual is advised to warm up by gentle stretching, jogging, jumping, and other mild muscular activities. Arms can be rotated in front of the body, over the head, and in circles perpendicular to the ground. Knees can be lifted and pulled up to the chest. Shoulders should be gently rotated to relax upper-back muscles. Neck muscles are toned by gently and slowly moving the head from side to side and in circles. Back muscles are loosened by bending forward and continuing around in slow circles.

If a joint has been injured, it is important to protect it from further damage. Physicians and physical therapists often recommend that athletes tape, brace, or wrap susceptible joints, such as knees, ankles, elbows, or wrists. Sometimes a simple commercial elastic bandage, available in various configurations specific to parts of the body, is all that is required. Neck braces and back braces are used to support these structures.

Benign muscle tumors require no treatment, or may be surgically removed. Malignant tumors may require surgery, radiation, and chemotherapy.

### PERSPECTIVE AND PROSPECTS

With the increased interest in physical exercise in the United States has come increasing awareness of the dangers of muscular damage that can arise from improper exercise, as well as of the cardiovascular risks that lie in wait for weekend athletes. Warm-up procedures are universally recommended. Individual exercisers, those in gym classes, professional athletes, and schoolchildren, are routinely taken through procedures to stretch and loosen muscles before they start strenuous activity.

Greater attention is being paid to the special needs of young athletes, such as gymnasts. Over the years, new athletic toys and devices are constantly being developed for the young: Skateboards, roller skates, and bicycles expose children to a wide range of bumps, falls, bruises, strains, and sprains. Protective equipment and devices have been designed especially for them: Helmets, padding, and special uniforms give children more security against accidents. Similarly, adults should take the time and trouble to outfit themselves correctly for the sports and athletics in which they engage: Joggers should tape, wrap, and brace their joints; and cyclists should wear helmets.

Nevertheless, the incidence of sport- and athletic-related muscular damage is relatively high, pointing to the necessity for increased attention to prevention. The growth of sports medicine as a medical specialty helps considerably in this endeavor. Physicians and nurses in this area are trained to deal with the various problems that arise, and they are often expert commentators on the best means to prevent problems. —*C. Richard Falcon*

*See also* Arthritis; Burns and scalds; Bursitis; Dystrophy; Fracture and dislocation; Hypertrophy; Motor neuron diseases; Multiple sclerosis; Muscular dystrophy; Obesity; Paralysis; Tendon disorders; Wounds.

**FOR FURTHER INFORMATION:**

Abraham, Edward A. *Freedom from Back Pain*. Emmaus, Pa.: Rodale Press, 1986. Damage to the muscles of the back, particularly the lower back, is a common affliction. Abraham gives the lay reader a concise description of the causes of back pain and clear instructions on how to deal with it.

Dragoo, Jason J. *Handbook of Sports Medicine*. Tempe, Ariz.: Renaissance, 1993. Dragoo covers the wide range of sport- and athletics-related disorders with clarity and precision. The text is intended for the lay reader, and the illustrations are simple and clear.

Larson, David E., ed. *Mayo Clinic Family Health Book*. New York: William Morrow, 1990. Chapter 32 discusses both muscles and bones, underscoring the intimate relationship between disorders in the two systems. The text and illustrations are complete and easy to understand.

Ryan, Allan J., and Fred L. Allman, eds. *Sports Medicine*. 2d ed. San Diego: Academic Press, 1989. Directed to the professional, but the text can be understood by the lay reader. Particularly useful in outlining the contemporary status of sports medicine and how it relates to the training and care of the athlete.

# MUSCULAR DYSTROPHY

**SYSTEMS AFFECTED:** Muscular, skeletal
**SPECIALISTS:** Pediatricians, physiatrists, physical therapists
**DEFINITION:** A group of related diseases that attack different muscle groups which are progressive, genetically determined, and have no known cure.

**KEY TERMS:**

*disease:* an interruption, cessation, or disorder of a body function or system, usually identifiable by a group of signs and symptoms and characterized by consistent anatomical alterations

*distal:* situated away from the center of the body; the farthest part from the midline of the body

*DNA (deoxyribonucleic acid):* a type of protein found in the nucleus of a cell comprising chromosomes that contain the genetic instructions of an organism

*dystrophy:* an improper form of a tissue or group of cells (literally, "bad nourishment")

*enzyme:* a protein secreted by a cell that acts as a catalyst to induce chemical changes in other substances, remaining apparently unchanged itself in the process

*genetic:* imparted at conception and incorporated into every cell of an organism

*fiber:* a slender thread or filament; the elongated, threadlike cells that collectively constitute a muscle

*muscle:* a bundle of contractile cells that is responsible for the movement of organs and body parts

*muscle group:* a collection of muscles that work together to accomplish a particular movement

## CAUSES AND SYMPTOMS

Muscles, attached to bones through tendons, are responsible for movement in the human body. In muscular dystrophy, muscles become progressively weak. As individual muscle fibers become so weak that they die, they are replaced by connective tissue, which is fibrous and fatty rather than muscular. These replacement fibers are commonly found in skin and scar tissue and are not capable of movement, and the muscles become progressively weak. There are several different recognized types of muscular dystrophy. These have in common degeneration of muscle fibers and replacement with connective tissue. They are distinguished from one another on the basis of the muscle group or groups involved and the age at which individuals are affected.

The most common type is Duchenne muscular dystrophy. In this disease, the muscles involved are in the upper thigh and pelvis. The disease strikes in early childhood, usually between the ages of four and seven. It is known to be genetic and occurs only in boys. Two-thirds of affected individuals are born to mothers who are known to carry a defective gene; one-third are simply new cases whose mothers are genetically normal. Individuals afflicted with Duchenne muscular dystrophy suffer from weakness in their hips and upper thighs. Initially, they may experience difficulty in sitting up or standing. The disease progresses to involve muscle groups in the shoulder and trunk. Patients lose the ability to walk during their early teens. As the disease progresses, portions of the brain become affected, and intelligence is reduced. Muscle fibers in the heart are also affected, and most individuals die by the age of twenty.

Normally, muscle cells make a small amount of a protein called dystrophin, which helps to maintain the integrity of muscle fiber membranes. The gene for the Duchenne variety of muscular dystrophy inhibits the production of dystrophin. As a result, the muscle fiber membrane breaks down and leaks, allowing fluid from outside of the cell to enter the muscle cell. In turn, the contents of affected cells are

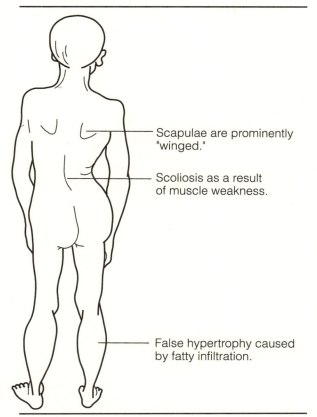

Scapulae are prominently "winged."

Scoliosis as a result of muscle weakness.

False hypertrophy caused by fatty infiltration.

*Duchenne muscular dystrophy, the most common type, is characterized by prominently "winged" scapulae, scoliosis, false hypertrophy of the calves, and other less visible effects; children are the victims, usually not surviving beyond age twenty.*

broken down by other chemicals called proteases that are normally stored in the muscle cell. The dead pieces of muscle fiber are removed by scavenging cells called macrophages. The result of this process is a virtually empty and greatly weakened muscle cell.

A second type is Becker's muscular dystrophy, which is similar to the Duchenne form of the disease. Approximately 3 in 200,000 people are affected, and it too is found only among males. The major clinical difference is the age of onset. Becker's muscular dystrophy typically first appears in the early teenage years. The muscles involved are similar to those of Duchenne muscular dystrophy, but the course of the disease is slower. Most individuals require the use of a wheelchair in their early thirties and eventually die in their forties.

Myotonic dystrophy is a form of muscular dystrophy that strikes approximately 5 out of 100,000 people in a population. Myotonia is the inability of a muscle group to relax after contracting. Individuals with myotonic dystrophy ex-

perience this difficulty in their hands and feet. On average, the disease first appears at the age of nineteen. The condition is benign, in that it does not shorten an affected person's life span. Rather, it causes inconveniences to the victim. Affected persons also experience a variety of other problems, including baldness at the front of the head and malfunction of the ovaries and testes. The muscles of the stomach and intestines can become involved, leading to a slowing down of intestinal functions and diarrhea.

Another type is limb-girdle muscular dystrophy. The muscles of both upper and lower limbs—the shoulders and the pelvis—are involved. The onset of this dystrophy form is variable, from childhood to middle age. While the disorder is not usually fatal, it does progress, and victims experience severe disability about twenty years after the disease first appears. While this variant is also genetically transmitted, men and women are about equally affected.

One type of muscular dystrophy found almost exclusively among individuals of Scandinavian descent is called distal dystrophy. It first appears relatively early in adult life, between the thirties and fifties. The muscles of the forearm and hand become progressively weak and decrease in size. Eventually, the muscles of the lower leg and foot also become involved. This form of muscular dystrophy is not usually fatal.

Oculopharyngeal muscular dystrophy is a particularly serious form that involves the muscles of the eyes and throat. In this disease, victims are affected in their forties and fifties. There is progressive loss of control of the muscles that move the eyes and loss of the ability to swallow. Death usually results from starvation or from pneumonia acquired when the affected individual accidentally inhales food or drink.

A type of muscular dystrophy for which the location of the genetic abnormality is known is facioscapulohumeral muscular dystrophy; the defect is confined to the tip of the fourth chromosome. This disease initially involves the muscles of the face and later spreads to the muscles of the posterior or back of the shoulder. Eventually, muscles in the upper thigh are involved. The affected person loses the ability to make facial expressions and assumes a permanent pout as a result of loss of muscle function. As the condition advances, the shoulder blades protrude when the arms are raised. Weakness and difficulty walking are eventually experienced. As with other forms of muscular dystrophy, there is some variability in the degree to which individuals are affected. Occasionally, a variety of deafness occurs involving the nerves that connect the inner ear and the brain. Less commonly, victims become blind.

There are other variants of muscular dystrophy that have been recognized and described. These forms of the disease, however, are rare. The main problem facing physicians is differentiating accurately the variety of muscular dystrophy seen in a particular patient so as to arrive at a correct diagnosis.

## TREATMENT AND THERAPY

The diagnosis of muscular dystrophy is initially made through observation. Typically, parents notice changes in their affected children and bring these concerns to the attention of a physician. The physician takes a careful family history and then examines a suspected victim to make a tentative or working diagnosis. Frequently, knowledge of other family members with the condition and observations are sufficient to establish a firm diagnosis. Occasionally, a physician may elect to order physiological or genetic tests to confirm the tentative diagnosis. As Duchenne muscular dystrophy is the most common form of muscular dystrophy, it provides a convenient example of this process.

A diagnosis of Duchenne or any other form of muscular dystrophy is rarely made before the age of three. This form of the disease almost always occurs in boys. (Variants, rather than true Duchenne type of muscular dystrophy, are seen in girls, but this situation is extremely rare.) The reason for this finding is that the genetic defect occurs on the X chromosome that is found only in males. Approximately two-thirds of all victims inherit the defective chromosome from their mothers, who are asymptomatic carriers; thus, the condition is recessive and said to be X-linked. The disease occurs in the remaining one-third of victims as a result of a fresh mutation, in which there is no family history of the disease and the parents are not carriers.

Victims usually begin to sit, walk, and run at an older age than normally would be expected. Parents describe walking as waddling rather than the usual upright posture. Victims have difficulty climbing stairs. They also have apparently enlarged calf muscles, a finding called muscular hypertrophy. While the muscles are initially strong, they lose their strength when connective and fatty tissues replace muscle fibers. The weakness of muscles in the pelvis is responsible for difficulties in sitting and the unusual way of walking. Normal children are able to go directly from a sitting position to standing erect. Victims of Duchenne muscular dystrophy first roll onto their stomachs, then kneel and raise themselves up by pushing their hands against their shins, knees, and thighs; they literally climb up themselves in order to stand. These children also have a pronounced curvature of their lower backs, an attempt by the body to compensate for the weakness in the muscles of the hips and pelvis.

There is frequently some weakness in the muscles of the shoulder. This finding can be demonstrated by a physician, but it is not usually seen by parents and is not an early problem for the victim. A physician tests for this weakness by lifting the child under the armpits. Normal children will be able to support themselves using the muscles of the shoulder. Individuals with Duchenne muscular dystrophy are unable to hold themselves up and will slip through the physician's hands. Eventually, these children will be unable to lift their arms over their heads. Most victims of Du-

chenne muscular dystrophy are unable to walk by their teen years. The majority die before their twentieth birthday, although about one-quarter live for a few more years. Most victims also have an abnormality in the muscles of the heart that leads to decreased efficiency of the heart and decreased ability to be physically active; in some cases, it also causes sudden death. Most victims of Duchenne muscular dystrophy suffer mental impairment. As their muscles deteriorate, their measured intelligence quotient (IQ) drops approximately twenty points below the level that it was at the onset of the disease. Serious mental handicaps are experienced by about one-quarter of victims.

Other forms of muscular dystrophy are similar to Duchenne muscular dystrophy. Their clinical courses are also similar, as are the methods of diagnosis. The critical differences are the muscles involved and the age of onset.

Laboratory procedures used to confirm the diagnosis of muscular dystrophy include microscopic analysis of muscle tissue, measurement of enzymes found in the blood, and measurement of the speed and efficiency of nerve conduction, a process called electromyography. Some cases have been diagnosed at birth by measuring a particular enzyme called creatinine phosphokinase. It is possible to diagnose some types of muscular dystrophy before birth with chorionic villus sampling or amniocentesis.

There is no specific treatment for any of the muscular dystrophies. Physical therapy is frequently ordered and used to prevent the remaining unaffected muscles from losing their tone and mass. In some stages of the disease, braces, appliances, and orthopedic surgery may be used. These measures do not reverse the underlying pathology, but they may improve the quality of life for a victim. The cardiac difficulties associated with myotonic dystrophy may require treatment with a pacemaker. For victims of myotonic dystrophy, some relief is obtained by using drugs; the most commonly used pharmaceuticals are phenytoin and quinine. The inability to relax muscles once they are contracted does not usually present a major problem for sufferers of myotonic dystrophy.

More useful and successful is prevention, which involves screening individuals in families or kinship groups who are potential carriers. Carriers are persons who have some genetic material for a disease or condition but lack sufficient genes to cause an apparent case of a disease or condition; in short, they appear normal. When an individual who is a carrier conceives a child, however, there is an increased risk of the offspring having the disease. Genetic counseling should be provided after screening, so that individuals who have the gene for a disease can make more informed decisions about having children.

Chemical tests are available for use in diagnosing some forms of muscular dystrophy. Carriers of the gene for Duchenne muscular dystrophy can be detected by staining a muscle sample for dystrophin; a cell that is positive for

Duchenne muscular dystrophy will have no stained dystrophin molecules. The dystrophin stain test is also used to diagnose Becker's muscular dystrophy, but the results are not quite as consistent or reliable. Approximately two-thirds of carriers and fetuses at risk for both forms of muscular dystrophy can be identified by analyzing DNA. Among individuals at risk for myotonic dystrophy, nine out of ten who carry the gene can be identified with DNA analysis before they experience actual symptoms of the disease.

### PERSPECTIVE AND PROSPECTS

Muscular dystrophy has been recognized as a medical entity for several centuries. Initially, it was considered to be a degenerative disease only of adults, and it was not until the nineteenth century that the disease was addressed in children with Guillaume-Benjamin-Amand Duchenne's description of progressive weakness of the hips and upper thighs. An accurate classification of the various forms of muscular dystrophy depended on accurate observation and on the collection of sets of cases. Correct diagnosis had to wait for the development of accurate laboratory methods for staining muscle fibers. The interpretation of laboratory findings depended on the development of biochemical knowledge. Thus, much of the integration of knowledge concerning muscular dystrophy is relatively recent.

Genes play an important role in the understanding of muscular dystrophy. All forms of muscular dystrophy are hereditary, although different chromosomes are involved in different forms of the disease. The development of techniques for routine testing and diagnosis has also occurred relatively recently. Specific chromosomes for all forms of muscular dystrophy have not yet been developed. Considering initial successes of the Human Genome Project, an effort to identify all human genes, it seems likely that more precise genetic information related to muscular dystrophy will emerge.

There still are no cures for muscular dystrophies, and many forms are relentlessly fatal. Cures for many communicable diseases caused by bacteria or viruses have been discovered, and advances have been made in the treatment of cancer and other degenerative diseases by identifying chemicals that cause the conditions or by persuading people to change their lifestyles. Muscular dystrophy, however, is a group of purely genetic conditions. Many of the particular chromosomes involved are known, but no techniques are available to cure the disease once it is identified. Muscular dystrophy continues to cause human suffering and to cost victims, their families, and society large sums of money. The disease is publicized on an annual basis via efforts to raise money for research and treatment, but there is little publicity on an ongoing basis. For these reasons, muscular dystrophy remains an important medical problem in contemporary society. —*L. Fleming Fallon, Jr.*

*See also* Dystrophy; Genetic diseases; Hypertrophy; Muscle sprains, spasms, and disorders; Scoliosis.

### FOR FURTHER INFORMATION:

Behrman, Richard E., ed. *Nelson Textbook of Pediatrics.* 14th ed. Philadelphia: W. B. Saunders, 1992. The forms of muscular dystrophy found in children are discussed in a logical and complete format. Pictures clearly depict the difficulties in movement experienced by victims of Duchenne muscular dystrophy. The authors are experts in their fields; this work is known internationally as an excellent resource on pediatric medicine.

Berkow, Robert, ed. *The Merck Manual of Diagnosis and Therapy.* 16th ed. Rahway, N.J.: Merck Sharp & Dohme Research Labs, 1992. The more common forms of muscular dystrophy are discussed in clear, relatively nontechnical language. The entries are brief and succinct. This work is useful for an overview of muscular dystrophy; the more unusual and rarer forms of muscular dystrophy are not included.

Blacklow, Robert S., ed. *MacBryde's Signs and Symptoms.* 6th ed. Philadelphia: J. B. Lippincott, 1983. Provides a useful discussion of the diagnosis of muscular dystrophy that has significant depth. A succinct summary of signs and symptoms is provided in tabular form, allowing the reader to distinguish between muscular dystrophy and other related diseases involving muscles.

Cotran, Ramzi S., Vinay Kumar, and Stanley L. Robbins. *Robbins Pathologic Basis of Disease.* 4th ed. Philadelphia: W. B. Saunders, 1989. A complete discussion about the pathology of several forms of muscular dystrophy. Technical language is employed, but the book is well written. Photographs of microscopic sections of muscle are included, as well as descriptions of the clinical course of muscular dystrophy.

Engel, Andrew G., and Betty Q. Banker, eds. *Myology.* New York: McGraw-Hill, 1986. This work describes the study of muscles and contains an excellent, comprehensive description of the different variants of muscular dystrophy. The terminology is precise and technical, and the scope of the work is wide. Also includes discussions of other muscle diseases related to muscular dystrophy.

Schroeder, Steven A., et al. *Current Medical Diagnosis and Treatment 1989.* 28th ed. Norwalk, Conn.: Appleton and Lange, 1989. In a brief and concise format, the diagnosis and management of muscular dystrophy is discussed. The section authors are recognized experts in their fields. Treatment protocols are included. As this book is comprehensive, only an overview of muscular dystrophy is included.

Wyngaarden, James B., Lloyd H. Smith, and J. Claude Bennett, eds. *Cecil Textbook of Medicine.* 19th ed. Philadelphia: W. B. Saunders, 1992. The descriptions of muscular dystrophy are clear and detailed. The language used in the book is precise. Using multiple authors, each section is written by an internationally recognized expert.

**MYOCARDIAL INFARCTION.** *See* **HEART ATTACK.**

## MYOPIA

**SYSTEM AFFECTED:** Visual

**SPECIALISTS:** Ophthalmologists

**DEFINITION:** Myopia, commonly known as nearsightedness or shortsightedness, is a condition in which only light rays that are a certain close distance to the eye are focused on the retina. Vision impairment usually starts in childhood or adolescence as the eye grows; if it becomes too long or the cornea is overly curved, then myopia results. Nearsightedness can be easily corrected with glasses or contact lenses, but the prescription may change many times, especially during childhood. Some people choose to have corrective surgery known as radial keratotomy, in which cuts are made with a scalpel or laser in order to flatten the cornea; however, many physicians consider the procedure to be flawed or experimental. *See also* Visual disorders.

---

**Myopia**

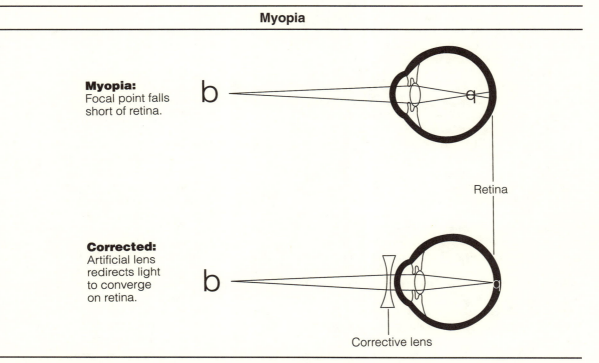

**Myopia:**
Focal point falls short of retina.

**Corrected:**
Artificial lens redirects light to converge on retina.

Retina

Corrective lens

---

*Myopia is commonly termed "nearsightedness" because most light rays entering the eye will not resolve, or focus, on the retina unless they are coming from a very near distance; corrective lenses are required.*

# NARCOLEPSY

**SYSTEM AFFECTED:** Brain

**SPECIALISTS:** Sleep specialists

**DEFINITION:** A disorder characterized by brief, numerous, and overwhelming attacks of sleepiness throughout the day, an apparently inherited disorder of the nervous system.

**KEY TERMS:**

*cataplexy:* brief periods of partial or total loss of skeletal muscle tone, usually triggered by emotional stimuli, which can cause the person to collapse

*electroencephalogram (EEG):* a recording of brain-wave activity using electrodes attached to the scalp

*excessive daytime sleepiness:* a strong tendency to fall asleep, accompanied by reduced energy and lack of alertness during the entire day

*hypnogogic hallucination:* a bizarre, sometimes frightening, dreamlike occurrence just as one is falling asleep or just after waking

*maintenance of wakefulness test:* a polysomnographic technique to measure a person's ability to remain awake during repeated trials throughout the day

*multiple sleep latency test:* a polysomnographic technique to measure how quickly one falls asleep during repeated trials throughout the day

*polysomnography:* the continuous recording of brain waves, eye movements, skeletal muscle movements, and other body functions to determine bodily changes during the stages of sleep

*REM sleep:* a period of intense brain activity, often associated with dreams; named for the rapid eye movements that typically occur during this time

*sleep paralysis:* an inability to move voluntarily, occurring just at the beginning of sleep or upon awakening

## CAUSES AND SYMPTOMS

Narcolepsy (*narco* meaning "numbness" and *lepsy* meaning "seizure") consists primarily of attacks of irresistible sleepiness in the daytime. The sleepiness is extreme; it has been described as the feeling that most people would experience if they tried to add columns of numbers in the middle of the night after forty-eight hours without sleep.

The narcoleptic's day is broken up by a series of brief and repetitive sleep attacks, perhaps even two hundred attacks in a single day. These transient, overpowering attacks of sleepiness may last from a few seconds to thirty minutes, with an average spell lasting two minutes. It is excruciatingly difficult, and frequently impossible, to ignore the urge to sleep, no matter how inconvenient or inappropriate. Narcoleptics typically fall asleep suddenly, on the job, in conversation, standing up, and even while eating, driving, or making love.

These sleep attacks result from an abrupt failure in resisting sleep, as opposed to a sudden surge in sleepiness, because narcoleptics are actually sleepy all day. The misconception that their daytime sleepiness is caused by insufficient nighttime sleep prompts undiagnosed patients to spend inordinately long hours in bed. Narcoleptics will be sleepy during the day regardless of how much sleep they get at night.

One of the most prominent and troubling features of narcolepsy is cataplexy, a sudden loss of muscle tone which causes the person to collapse. Cataplexy occurs during the daytime while the person is awake. It may involve all the muscles at once or only a select few, so the severity may range from total collapse to the ground to partial collapse of a limb or the jaw. The cataplectic sometimes remains conscious, able to think, hear, and see, although vision may be blurred. At other times, there is a brief loss of consciousness, associated with an experience of dreaming. Although most attacks of cataplexy last less than a minute, occasionally they go on for as long as twenty minutes. Cataplexy is often triggered by enjoyable feelings, laughter, or excitement during which the person suddenly crumples into a heap. For other patients, a strong negative emotion, such as fear or anger, precipitates an attack.

Many narcoleptics notice the symptom of excessive daytime sleepiness for as much as a year before the onset of cataplexy. After many years of experiencing cataplexy, some patients find that less emotional stimulus is required to induce the muscle collapse and that increasingly more muscles are involved. Others find that this symptom diminishes, possibly because they have become adept at anticipating and avoiding the situations that trigger attacks. It has been noted that other hypersomnias—that is, other diseases of excessive sleepiness—do not include cataplexy; only narcoleptics suffer from this embarrassing and troubling symptom of muscle collapse.

Many narcoleptics also experience hypnogogic hallucinations, dreams that intrude into the waking state. In normal sleep, dreaming generally occurs approximately ninety minutes after falling asleep; narcoleptics begin their sleeping episodes with vivid dreams. These hallucinations are extremely realistic and often violent. The patient sees someone else in the room or hears someone calling his or her name, for the hallucinations are nearly always visual and are usually auditory. The vivid sights, sounds, and feelings characteristic of hypnogogic hallucinations are thought to occur while the person is awake, both during the day and just at the edges of nighttime sleep. Since narcoleptics typically fall asleep dozens if not hundreds of times a day, they can experience these disturbing hallucinations with great frequency. Somewhat more than 50 percent of daytime sleep attacks include hallucinations, while only about 7 percent are usually marked by cataplexy.

Approximately 40 to 60 percent of narcoleptics suffer another frightening symptom: sleep paralysis. This condition occurs at the beginning or end of sleep and renders immobile virtually every voluntary muscle, except those around the eyes. During sleep paralysis, the mind is awake and one is aware of the external surroundings, but the muscles refuse to move. The paralysis usually lasts only a few seconds, but it may continue for as long as twenty minutes. Sleep researchers find that almost everyone has a few-second-long episode of sleep paralysis sometime during his or her lifetime. When the paralysis continues for more than a few seconds, however, it is usually a sign of narcolepsy. Although either sleep paralysis or hypnogogic hallucinations alone are distressing enough, they often happen simultaneously.

Because of their frequent, irresistible sleep attacks, narcoleptics often wobble back and forth between sleep and wakefulness in a state that has been likened to sleepwalking and is termed automatic behavior. When in this state, the person seems to behave normally but later does not remember extended periods of time. For example, narcoleptics might find themselves in a different building or several exits farther down a highway than they last remembered. Obviously, automatic behavior is very anxiety-producing; it is very troubling to narcoleptics to be unable to remember what they have done in the minutes or hours that have just passed.

In addition to these memory difficulties, some narcoleptics experience constant eye fatigue, difficulty focusing, and double vision. They also have a higher incidence of the heart abnormality called mitral valve prolapse, which affects blood flow to the left ventricle. The reason for this association is not clear.

Although narcolepsy is an illness of excessive daytime sleepiness, the nighttime sleep of those afflicted is far from normal as well. It is often troubled by restlessness and frequent awakenings, which are brief or may last for hours. Patients also experience many nightmares about murder and persecution. Many narcoleptics talk, cry out, or thrash about periodically during the night.

One narcoleptic in ten has the added complication of suffering from sleep apnea. This sleep disorder consists of recurrent interruptions in breathing during sleep. This further disturbance of nighttime sleep aggravates the narcoleptic's tendency to excessive daytime sleepiness.

Narcolepsy was once thought to be extremely rare. By 1989, however, the United States Department of Health estimated that 250,000 Americans suffer from this disease, which is more than the number afflicted by multiple sclerosis. The American Medical Association considers 250,000 to be a very conservative estimate and believes the number to be between 400,000 and 600,000.

Males and females are equally affected by narcolepsy. Although the disorder has been diagnosed in a five-year-old, its symptoms most frequently appear for the first time during adolescence. In about 75 percent of cases, the attacks begin between the ages of fifteen and twenty-five; only 5 percent of cases begin before the age of ten. Onset is rare after the age of forty; if narcolepsy seems to appear in an older person, it has probably existed undiagnosed for years. Sleep researchers believe that the extra need for sleep characteristic of adolescence may make this stage of development particularly vulnerable for the onset of narcolepsy. Thus, this disorder may typically begin in adolescence because it is somehow triggered by the brain changes associated with sexual maturation.

Between two and five persons in one thousand in the general population of the United States have scattered episodes of excessive daytime sleepiness but are not considered narcoleptics. It is not until a person has one to several attacks each day that narcolepsy is suspected.

### TREATMENT AND THERAPY

Narcolepsy is now known to be a disease of the nervous system. Although incurable, it can be successfully treated with various medications once it has been diagnosed. The diagnosis of narcolepsy, however, is often slow to occur. The average interval between the first appearance of symptoms and diagnosis is often as long as thirteen years. Because early symptoms are usually mild, narcoleptics typically spend years wondering whether they are sick or whether they merely lack initiative. They are often called lazy because they repeatedly nap during the day and are lethargic even when awake. Diagnosis is made more difficult by the wide range of severity of symptoms. For example, excessive daytime sleepiness may trouble a person for ten or twenty years before cataplexy appears. Patients may even occasionally experience a temporary or partial remission in their condition. Narcoleptics often fight off their sleep attacks by ingesting large amounts of caffeine and never realize that they have an actual disease until years later.

If narcolepsy is suspected, a polysomnographic study is done at a sleep disorders center to confirm the diagnosis. The most reliable confirmation of narcolepsy can be obtained by what is called the multiple sleep latency test (MSLT). The MSLT is easy, convenient, inexpensive, and very informative. The person is given four or five opportunities to lie down and fall asleep during the daytime. Normal individuals take fifteen to thirty minutes to fall asleep. In the MSLT, falling asleep in less than five minutes is considered abnormal. Those afflicted with narcolepsy always fall asleep in less than five minutes and often within a minute. The maintenance of wakefulness test (MOWT) is also used in the confirmation of narcolepsy. In the MOWT, the person is kept all day in a comfortable reclining position. Polysomnography is used to measure the patient's ability to stay awake and how many times he or she falls asleep.

Along with the MSLT and the MOWT, a thorough physical examination is needed to discover if the person has some other disorder that can mimic narcolepsy; an underactive thyroid gland, diabetes, chronic low blood sugar, anemia, and a malfunctioning liver can each cause excessive daytime sleepiness. Similarly, drug use, poor nutrition, emotional frustration, dissatisfaction, or poor motivation can also result in the type of sleepiness that a narcoleptic experiences.

When the diagnosis of narcolepsy is confirmed, treatment usually consists of stimulant medications such as dextroamphetamine, pemoline, or methylphenidate (Ritalin) during the daytime. These stimulant drugs can increase alertness and cut down the number of sleep attacks from perhaps several per day to several per month. Unfortunately, patients can quickly develop tolerance to these medications.

Even on low doses, some patients become irritable, aggressive, or nervous, or they may develop obesity and sexual problems. It is very important, therefore, to monitor a narcoleptic carefully, determining the lowest effective dose and the best times of day to take it. It may be months before the positive effects of drug therapy are fully experienced. The MSLT will often be given on a day that one takes the medication and on another when it is not taken, in order to evaluate the success of a given treatment.

Because specific drug and dosage schedules may have to be altered frequently, patients may repeatedly have to face drug withdrawal symptoms such as intensified sleepiness and disturbing dreams. To prevent adverse reactions, narcoleptics must often avoid certain foods and common medications. Their use of stimulant drugs may even be viewed as morally wrong, in these days of widespread drug abuse, by neighbors or coworkers who do not comprehend that narcolepsy is a disabling disease.

If cataplexy is present, medications other than amphetamines or Ritalin are required and useful. The class of drugs called tricyclic antidepressants, including protriptyline and imipramine, or the class of drugs called monoamine oxidase inhibitors may alleviate cataplexy. These medicines can often reduce attacks—for example, from three a day to three a month. In addition, effective treatment for cataplexy usually also relieves sleep paralysis and hypnogogic hallucinations.

Since the development of tolerance is common and these drugs can aggravate the symptom of sleepiness, determining the best timing and dose is critical. Another side effect of cataplexy drugs is impaired sexual function in males. Some men even discontinue these medications periodically for a day or two in order to sustain sexual relations. In addition, none of the drugs used for any symptoms of narcolepsy are safe to take during pregnancy.

In some cases, narcoleptics can be treated without medication if they carefully space naps during the day to relieve excessive sleepiness. Patients keep nap diaries to rate their alertness at regular intervals during the day. They then schedule short, strategically timed naps during those daytime periods when their sleep attacks are most likely to occur.

Naps are particularly valuable in treating children with narcolepsy because the consequences of a lifetime of medication on their development or on the course of their illness

is unknown. Some children who show hyperactive behavior actually have narcolepsy; they are working frantically to overcome their persistent sleepiness and to keep themselves awake. Children with narcolepsy may also justifiably fear falling asleep, day or night, because of hallucinations and sleep paralysis.

It is evident that supportive counseling must be a strong component of treatment, whatever the patient's age. Sensitive medical monitoring can offer narcoleptics a measure of satisfactory daily living, but the use of stimulants to improve alertness may also make them more aware of their limitations and, therefore, more frustrated. Depression is not the cause of narcolepsy but may result primarily from the disruption in their lives and the feeling that they are denied the right to a "normal" life. Their constant sleepiness engenders feelings of inferiority and inadequacy. Narcoleptics usually refrain from mentioning their hallucinations and try to hide their automatic behavior for fear of being labeled insane. Loss of work, broken marriages, and social isolation are often witnesses to the crippling effects of narcolepsy.

Of all the people with narcolepsy seen at major sleep disorders centers, more than one-half have been completely disabled with respect to regular employment by the age of forty. With part-time, homebound, or self-employment, however, most narcoleptics can gain self-respect and help support themselves through work that is safe and tailored to their needs. They must be given tasks that can be divided into parts performed in relatively short time periods.

Drug and nap therapy can do little for narcoleptics without education of their families, friends, acquaintances, employers, and coworkers about the reality of this neurological disease. Most people find it hard to accept the notion that sleepiness cannot be controlled and insist that narcoleptics could be more alert if they tried harder. Narcoleptics are often stigmatized as slackers or incompetents, or assumed to be drug abusers or closet drinkers. It is most important that patients and all the people in their lives comprehend that excessive daytime sleepiness is not the patients' "fault."

Further help for narcoleptics seems to lie in animal studies, which may fill in many important pieces of the narcolepsy puzzle. The effects of the disease on behavior, the way in which it is inherited, and the benefits and risks of specific drugs continue to be evaluated in narcoleptic dogs.

### PERSPECTIVE AND PROSPECTS

Once viewed as "all in the mind," narcolepsy is now recognized as a neurological disorder. Its origin is unknown, but research has already discovered evidence of possible causes. An understanding of narcolepsy both depended on and advanced the understanding of normal sleep and of other sleep disorders. Scientists define sleep as a reduction in awareness of and interaction with the environment, lowered movement and muscle activity, and partial or complete suspension of voluntary behavior and consciousness.

Although narcolepsy was named and described in 1880, it could not be genuinely studied until the 1930's, when the electroencephalograph (EEG) was developed to record brain activity during the various stages of sleep. By the 1940's, this advancement led to a description of the narcoleptic tetrad, the four usual symptoms of narcolepsy: excessive daytime sleepiness, cataplexy, sleep paralysis, and hypnogogic hallucinations.

In the 1950's, narcolepsy still only rated a paragraph in one neurology textbook, which mistakenly called it a rare variety of epilepsy. A major discovery occurred in 1960: Narcoleptics bypass the normal stages of light and deep sleep and fall directly into rapid eye movement (REM) sleep. Thus, sudden-onset REM period (or SOREMP) became the major distinguishing feature of this brain disorder.

It was soon noted that relatives of narcoleptics are sixty times more likely to have the disease than members of the general population. Clearly, there is a hereditary factor involved, and geneticists have joined the hunt for narcolepsy's cause. The hereditary aspects of the disease are particularly important to counselors because parents with narcolepsy may feel guilty if their child develops it. (Indeed, some patients abandon plans to have children.) Geneticists have found a gene which may be responsible for narcolepsy. Since the gene produces an antigen called DR2 on patients' white blood cells, which is not found in non-narcoleptics, immunologists have also begun to search for the origins of narcolepsy.

The disease is thought to arise from a biochemical imbalance in the brain which disturbs the mechanism that activates the on/off cycle of sleep. Biochemists are studying the possible relationship of various brain chemicals called neurotransmitters to narcolepsy. A defect in the way in which the body produces or uses dopamine, acetylcholine, or some other neurotransmitter is suspected to precipitate narcolepsy, which never spontaneously disappears once it is developed.

Two interesting discoveries may help in the diagnosis of narcolepsy even before the classical clinical symptoms develop. There is some evidence that REM sleep is entered with abnormal rapidity years before the disorder develops. The drug physostigmine salicylate has no effect on normal dogs but elicits cataplexy in puppies with narcolepsy. Both these discoveries may be useful in screening the children of narcoleptics.

Because narcolepsy involves the fundamental processes of sleep, the combined efforts of neuroscientists, geneticists, biochemists, immunologists, and other scientists to unravel its mysteries will continue to yield important information about the basic mechanism of sleep—that state in which humans spend almost one-third of their lives.

—*Grace D. Matzen*

**See also** Hallucinations; Paralysis; Sleep disorders; Sleeping sickness.

**FOR FURTHER INFORMATION:**

Anch, A. Michael, Carl P. Browman, Merrill M. Mitler, and James K. Walsh. *Sleep: A Scientific Perspective*. Englewood Cliffs, N.J.: Prentice-Hall, 1988. A more technical volume than usually recommended to the general reader, this book can provide more detailed information to those who desire it. Contains a useful glossary, an extensive list of references, and an index of scientists involved in sleep research.

Dement, William C., *The Sleepwatchers*. Stanford, Calif.: Stanford Alumni Association, 1992. A lively and often amusing book by the chair of the National Commission on Sleep Disorders Research. Traces the story of such research since the 1950's, when Dement first studied narcolepsy. Solid science that reads like a novel.

Dotto, Lydia. *Losing Sleep*. New York: William Morrow, 1990. The intent of the author is to provide lay readers with basic scientific information to understand the impact of sleep problems on daily life. Dotto has a highly interesting style of writing. Includes a bibliography.

Dryer, Bernard, and Ellen S. Kaplan. *Inside Insomnia*. New York: Villard Books, 1986. Provides the general reader with basic information about sleep, including a brief but accurate discussion of narcolepsy. A fifty-page reader's guide lists sleep centers and laboratories, as well as often-used and often-abused sleep medications. An annotated glossary is provided.

Hartmann, Ernest. *The Sleep Book*. Glenview, Ill.: Scott, Foresman, 1987. An easily understood discussion by a well-known pioneer in normal sleep and sleep disorders research. Contains a forty-page appendix of sleep disorders classification, centers, and specialists.

Hauri, Peter, and Shirley Linde. *No More Sleepless Nights*. New York: John Wiley & Sons, 1990. Contains only a brief description of narcolepsy, but there is an easy-to-understand chapter on basic sleep facts. Ends with a unique chapter explaining the need for and work of sleep disorders centers.

Lamberg, Lynne. *The American Medical Association Guide to Better Sleep*. Rev. ed. New York: Random House, 1984. Includes an excellent and extensive explanation of narcolepsy. A well-written, highly readable, and scientifically thorough discussion of all aspects of sleep. Contains a glossary.

Sweeney, Donald R. *Overcoming Insomnia*. New York: G. P. Putnam's Sons, 1989. Although the major focus of this book is insomnia, its discussion of narcolepsy is quite adequate. Contains a bibliography and a useful list of the drugs used to treat sleep disorders.

# NASOPHARYNGEAL DISORDERS

**SYSTEM AFFECTED:** Respiratory

**SPECIALISTS:** Allergists, family physicians, occupational medicine physicians, otolaryngologists

## Anatomy of the Nasopharyngeal Region

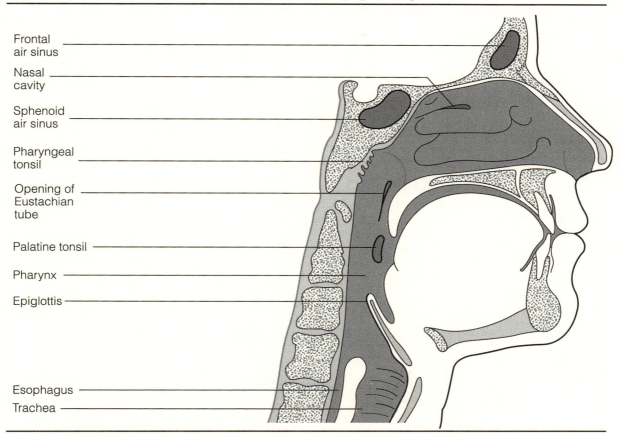

Frontal air sinus
Nasal cavity
Sphenoid air sinus
Pharyngeal tonsil
Opening of Eustachian tube
Palatine tonsil
Pharynx
Epiglottis
Esophagus
Trachea

**DEFINITION:** Disorders of the nose, nasal passages (sinuses), and pharynx (mouth, throat, and esophagus).

**KEY TERMS:**

*acute disease:* a short and sharp disease process

*chronic disease:* a lingering illness

*esophagus:* the tube that leads from the pharynx to the stomach

*larynx:* the organ that produces the voice, which lies between the pharynx and the trachea; commonly called the voice box

*nasopharyngeal:* referring to the nose and pharynx (the upper part of the throat that leads from the mouth to the esophagus)

*trachea:* a tube that leads from the throat to the lungs; commonly called the windpipe

### CAUSES AND SYMPTOMS

Nasopharyngeal disorders include all the diseases that can be present in the nasal cavity and the pharynx. These include the common cold, pharyngitis (sore throat), laryngitis (inflammation of the larynx), epiglottitis (inflammation of the lid over the larynx), tonsillitis (inflammation of the

lymph nodes at the rear of the mouth), sinusitis (inflammation of the sinus cavities that surround the nose), otitis media (earache that is often associated with nasopharyngeal infection), nosebleed, nasal obstruction, halitosis (bad breath), and various other disorders.

The common cold is one of the most prevalent diseases that afflict humankind. Pharyngitis, or sore throat, often accompanies the common cold, or it may appear by itself. Acute infections can be caused by viruses or bacteria, often by certain streptococcus strains—hence the common term for the disorder, strep throat. Acute pharyngitis can also be caused by chemicals or radiation. As a chronic disorder, pharyngitis can be caused by lingering infection in other organs such as the lungs and sinuses, or it can be attributable to constant irritation from smoking, drinking alcohol, or breathing polluted air. The usual symptoms of pharyngitis include sore throat, difficulty in swallowing, and fever. The infected area appears red and swollen. Ordinarily, pharyngitis is not serious. If certain strains of streptococcus are the cause, however, then the infection may progress to rheumatic fever. This disease appears to be the result of an immune system reaction to some streptococcus bacteria. It can have painful effects in many parts of the body, such as in joints, and can do permanent damage to parts of the heart. In rare cases, rheumatic fever can be fatal.

Acute laryngitis is usually caused by a viral infection, but bacteria, outside irritants, or misuse of the voice are other causes. Ordinarily, the vocal cords produce sounds by vibrating in response to the air passing over them. When inflamed or irritated, they swell, causing distortion in the sounds produced. The voice becomes hoarse and raspy and may even diminish to a soft whisper. This distortion of sound is the main symptom of laryngitis, but there may also be a sore throat and congestion that causes constant coughing. The condition generally resolves itself and requires no treatment. Chronic laryngitis has the same symptoms but does not go away spontaneously. It may be caused by an infectious agent, but more likely is attributable to some irritant activity, such as constantly misusing the voice, smoking, drinking alcohol, or breathing contaminated air.

The epiglottis is a waferlike tissue covered by a mucous membrane that sits on top of the larynx. It can become infected by such microorganisms as the bacteria *Haemophilus influenzae* type b in a condition called epiglottitis. Although the symptoms of epiglottitis can resemble pharyngitis, the infection can quickly progress to a very serious, life-threatening disorder. Epiglottitis usually afflicts children from two to four years of age, but adults can also be affected. The infection can begin rapidly, causing the epiglottis to swell and obstruct the airway to the lungs, creating a major medical emergency. Within twelve hours of the onset of symptoms, 50 percent of patients require hospitalization and intubation (insertion of a breathing tube into the trachea). The symptoms are high fever, severe sore throat, difficulty in breathing, difficulty in swallowing, and general malaise. As the airway becomes more and more occluded, the patient begins to gasp for air. The lack of oxygen may cause cyanosis (blue color in the lips, fingers, and skin), exhaustion, and shock.

Another disease associated with the larynx is croup, or laryngotracheobronchitis. As the medical name indicates, croup involves the larynx, the trachea, and the bronchi (the large branches of the lung). It is usually caused by a virus, but some cases are attributable to bacterial infection. Children from three to five years of age are the usual victims. This disease causes the airways to narrow because of inflammation of the inner mucosal surfaces. Inflammation causes coughing, but the narrowed airway causes the cough to be sharp and brassy, like the barking of a seal. Croup is usually relatively benign, but sometimes it progresses to a severe disease requiring hospitalization.

Various other disorders can afflict the larynx, such as damage to the vocal cords because of infection by bacteria, fungi, or other microorganisms. The vocal cords can also be damaged by misusing the voice, smoking, or breathing contaminated air. Polyps (masses of tissue growing on the surface), nodes (little knots of tissue), or "singers' nodules" may develop. Sores called contact ulcers may form on the vocal cords.

Tonsillitis is an inflammation of two large lymph nodes located at the back of the throat, the tonsils. It may also involve the adenoids, lymph nodes located at the top of the throat. The function of these lymph nodes is to remove harmful pathogens (disease-causing organisms) from the nasopharyngeal cavity. At times, the load of microorganisms that they absorb becomes more than they can handle and they become infected. The tonsils and adenoids may then become enlarged. A sore throat develops, along with a headache, fever, and chills. Glands of the neck and throat feel sore and may become enlarged. Young adults can also suffer from quinsy, or peritonsillar abscess. In this condition, one of the tonsils becomes infected and pus forms between the tonsil and the soft tissue surrounding it. Quinsy is characterized by pain in the throat and/or the soft palate, pain on swallowing, fever, and a tendency to lean the head toward the affected side.

The nasal sinuses are four pairs of cavities in the bone around the nose. There are two maxillary sinuses, so called because they are found in the maxilla, or upper jaw. Slightly above and behind them are the ethmoid sinuses, and behind them are the sphenoid sinuses. Sitting over the nose in the lower part of the forehead are the two frontal sinuses. All these sinuses are lined with a mucous membrane and have small openings that lead into the nasal passages. Air moves in and out of the sinuses and allows mucus to drain into the nose. In acute sinusitis, infection builds up in the mucous membrane of any or all of the sinuses. The membrane lining the sinus swells and shuts the opening into the nasal passages. At the same time, membranes of the nose swell and become congested. Mucus and pus build up inside the sinuses, causing pain and pressure. Most often, sinusitis accompanies the common cold: The mucous membrane that lines the nose extends into the sinuses, so the infection of a cold can readily spread into the sinuses. The various viruses responsible for the common cold may be involved, as well as a wide group of bacteria. Chronic sinusitis can be caused by repeated infections that have allowed scar tissue to build up, closing the sinus openings and impeding mucus drainage, or may be the result of allergies.

Tissues in the nasopharyngeal cavity may be affected by conditions occurring in other parts of the body. For example, vocal cord paralysis may be caused by vascular accidents, certain cancers, tissue trauma, and other events.

Some infections in the nasopharyngeal cavity can spread to the ear through the Eustachian tubes that connect the two areas. Chief among the diseases of the ear that can be associated with nasopharyngeal disorders are the various forms of acute otitis media, an earache occurring in the central part of the ear. There are four basic types of otitis media. With the first type, serous otitis media, there is usually no infection, but fluid accumulates inside the middle ear because of the blockage of the Eustachian tube or the overproduction of fluid; the condition is usually mild, with some pain and temporary loss of hearing. The second type is otitis media with effusion; with this condition comes both infection and accumulation of fluid. The third form is acute purulent otitis media, the most serious type. Pus builds up inside the middle ear, and its pressure may rupture the eardrum, allowing discharge of blood and pus. The fourth type is secretory otitis media, which usually occurs after several bouts of otitis media. Cells within the middle ear start producing a fluid that is thicker than normal and produced in greater amounts.

Chronic otitis media is bacterial in origin. It is characterized by a perforation of the eardrum and chronic pus discharge. The eardrum is a flat, pliable disk of tissue that vibrates to conduct sounds from the outside to the inner-ear structures. The perforation that occurs in chronic otitis media can be one of two types: a relatively benign perforation occurring in the central part of the eardrum or a potentially dangerous perforation occurring near the edges of the eardrum. The latter perforation can be associated with loss of hearing, increased discharge of pus and other fluids, facial paralysis, and the spread of infection to other tissues. When the perforation of chronic otitis media is near the edges of the eardrum, something called a cholesteatoma develops. This accumulation of matter grows in the inner ear and can be destructive to bone and other tissue.

The same organisms that cause otitis media can be responsible for a condition called mastoiditis. The mastoid process is a bone structure lined with a mucous membrane. Infection from otitis media can spread to this area and in severe cases can destroy the bone. Mastoiditis used to be a leading cause of death in children.

Nosebleeds are common and most often result from a blow to the nose, but they can also be caused by colds, sinusitis, and breathing dry air. The septum (the cartilaginous tissue that separates the nostrils) and the surrounding intranasal mucous membrane contain many tiny blood vessels that are easily ruptured. If an individual receives a blow to the nose, these vessels can break and bleed. They can also rupture because of irritation from a cold or other condition. Breathing very dry air sometimes causes the nasal mucous membrane to crust over, and bleeding can follow. Nosebleeds are not usually serious, but sometimes they are indicative of an underlying condition, such as hypertension (high blood pressure), a tumor, or another disease.

Nasal obstruction is common during colds and allergy attacks, but it can also be caused by a deviated septum, a malformation in the cartilage between the nostrils that can be congenital or caused by a blow to the nose. Also, nasal obstruction can be attributable to nasal polyps, nasal tumors, or swollen adenoids. A common source of nasal ob-

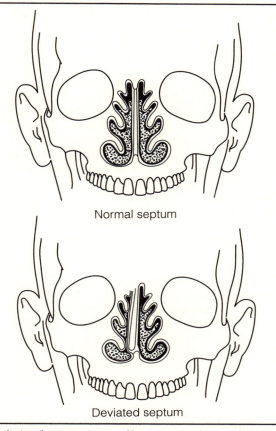

Normal septum

Deviated septum

*A deviated septum is a malformation in the cartilage between the nostrils, either present at birth or caused by a blow to the nose.*

struction is overuse of nasal decongestants. These agents relieve nasal congestion by reducing intranasal inflammation and swelling. If used too often or too long, however, they can cause the very problem that they were intended to cure: Intranasal blood vessels dilate, the area swells, secretions increase, and the nose becomes blocked. This is known as rebound congestion, or in medical terminology, rhinitis medicamentosa (nasal inflammation that is caused by a medication).

Halitosis, or bad breath, can be considered a nasopharyngeal disorder in the sense that it can originate in the mouth. It can be caused by diseases of the teeth and/or gums, but the most common causes are smoking or eating aromatic foods such as onions and garlic. Bad breath may also be a sign of disease conditions in other parts of the body, such as certain lung disorders or cancer of the esophagus. Hepatic failure, a liver dysfunction, may be accompanied by a fishy odor on the breath. Azotemia, the retention of nitrogen in the blood, may give rise to an ammonia-like odor. A sweet, fruity odor on the breath of diabetic patients may accompany ketoacidosis, a condition that occurs when there are high levels of glucose in the blood. Sometimes, young children stick foreign objects or other materials into their noses; it has been reported that these materials can fester, causing severe halitosis. Bad breath is rarely apparent to the individual who has it, however offensive it may be to others. A good way to check one's breath is to lick the back of one's hand and smell the spot; malodor, if it exists, will usually be apparent.

## TREATMENT AND THERAPY

Nasopharyngeal disorders are most often mild illnesses that can be treated at home. For example, acute pharyngitis or sore throat is easily managed most of the time. The patient is advised to rest, gargle with warm salt water several times a day, and soothe the pain with lozenges or anesthetic gargles. If the infection is caused by a virus, it usually will clear without further treatment. If the physician suspects, however, that the infection is bacterial in origin, throat smears may be taken so that the organism can be identified. If bacteria are discovered, antibiotic therapy will be undertaken to eradicate the pathogens. This is particularly important if the infection is caused by certain strains of streptococcus bacteria. In this case, it is vital to destroy the organism in order to avoid the development of rheumatic fever.

In acute laryngitis caused by viral infection, the patient is advised to rest the voice, inhale steam, and drink warm liquids. If bacteria are the cause of the laryngitis, antibiotic therapy is undertaken. In treating chronic laryngitis, the physician must discover the cause and remove it. If allergy is the cause, antihistamine therapy could help. If the cause is bacterial, antibiotic therapy is used. If smoking or drinking alcohol is the problem, the patient should be counseled to stop. The simple palliative measures used for acute laryngitis—resting the voice, drinking warm liquids, and breathing steam—are also useful for chronic laryngitis.

Symptoms of epiglottitis are often similar to those of sore throat. If there is any evidence of difficulty in breathing, however, the patient should be seen by a physician quickly because an emergency situation may be developing. If epiglottitis is obstructing the airway, the patient should be treated in an intensive care setting. It is important to make an airway for the patient, and it may be necessary to insert a tube into the trachea to allow the patient to breathe.

Before the age of antibiotics, tonsillitis was often treated surgically, with both tonsils and adenoids removed. This procedure is now rare because the infection usually responds to antibiotic therapy. Similarly, in peritonsillar abscess or quinsy, antibiotics usually clear the condition satisfactorily. In some cases, accumulations of pus may be removed surgically. If the abscesses return, it may be advisable to remove the tonsils.

As a rule, the child with croup is treated at home. Because the disease is usually caused by viruses, antibiotics are not used unless bacteria are known to be involved. Steam is often used to help liquefy mucus deposits on the interior walls of the trachea, the larynx, and the bronchi. The patient is given warm liquids to drink and is closely watched so that any signs that the condition is getting worse will be detected. The following symptoms should alert the caregiver to the possibility that an emergency situation is developing and that medical help is needed quickly: drooling, difficulty in swallowing, difficulty in breathing, inability to bend the neck forward, blue or dark color in the lips, high-pitched sounds when inhaling, rapid heartbeat, and loss of consciousness. These symptoms could mean the patient is in danger.

The main goals of therapy for sinusitis are to control infection, relieve the blockage of the sinus openings to permit drainage, and relieve pain. When sinusitis is known to be of bacterial origin, an appropriate antibiotic will be used to eradicate the organism. Often, however, sinusitis is attributable to viral infection, and other procedures are used to treat it. Inhaling steam is useful for reducing swelling and promoting drainage, as are decongestant sprays and oral decongestants. Analgesics can be given for pain. In certain circumstances, the sinuses are drained surgically.

Acute otitis media is most often diagnosed with the aid of an otoscope, an instrument that the doctor uses to look at the eardrum and surrounding tissues. The eardrum will be a dull red color, bulging, and perhaps perforated. While a viral infection may precede otitis media, the causative microorganisms for this and related ear infections, such as mastoiditis, are usually bacteria. Antibiotics are used both to treat the infections and to prevent the spread of disease to other areas. The drugs are usually taken orally, although antibiotic ear drops are often given as well. Penicillin and its derivatives are used, as are erythromycin and sulfisoxazole. Antibiotic therapy for acute otitis media is usually continued for ten days to two weeks. Sometimes, pus and other fluids and solid matter build up in the inner ear. It may be necessary to pierce the eardrum in order to remove these deposits. To help relieve blockage of the Eustachian tubes, a topical vasoconstrictor may be used in the nose to reduce the swelling of blood vessels. Antihistamines could be helpful to patients with allergies, but otherwise they are not indicated.

For chronic otitis media, it is necessary to clean both the outer ear canal and the middle ear thoroughly. A mild acetic acid solution with a corticosteroid is used for a week to ten days. Meanwhile, aggressive oral antibiotic therapy is undertaken to eradicate the pathogen. The perforated eardrum associated with chronic otitis media can usually be repaired surgically with little or no loss of function, and the cholesteatoma must be surgically removed.

Simple nosebleed can be treated by pinching the nose with the fingers and breathing through the mouth for five or ten minutes, to allow the blood to clot. Also, a plug of absorbent paper or cloth can be inserted into the bleeding nostril. A nosebleed that does not stop easily should be seen by a physician.

Nasal obstruction resulting from colds or allergies is treated by appropriate medications, decongestants for colds, and antihistamines for allergies. A deviated septum may require surgery. The only therapy for rhinitis medicamentosa, or rebound congestion caused by overuse of nasal decongestants, is to stop the medication and endure the congestion for as long as it takes the condition to clear. Sometimes, it is necessary to consult a physician.

For simple halitosis caused by smoking or food, breath fresheners (with or without "odor-fighting" chemicals) are often used, even though they usually simply replace a "bad" odor with a "good" one. Some people firmly believe that chewing parsley or other leaves rich in chlorophyll will counteract the smell of garlic. When halitosis is attributable to tooth or gum disease, it will persist until the condition is cured. Halitosis may be of diagnostic value in certain situations where a characteristic odor could alert the physician to the possibility of a disease condition.

### PERSPECTIVE AND PROSPECTS

Diseases and infections of the nasal cavity and throat have always been common among human populations, as have therapies to deal with them. Until the advent of antibiotics, some of these disorders were quite serious, especially in young children, but modern medications and surgeries, where appropriate, have greatly lessened the danger. Many over-the-counter drugs are now used to combat sore throats, sinus congestion, and other nasopharyngeal symptoms of the common cold, although colds themselves remain incurable because of the hundreds or thousands of different microorganisms that may be responsible. Despite the numerous medications that can be taken, however, more serious infections or diseases, such as chronic tonsillitis or laryngitis, require a doctor's care, with more potent, prescription drugs and surgery if needed. The treatments available to physicians and patients for the symptoms of nasopharyngeal disorders are many, but the search continues for better drugs and perhaps preventive measures such as vaccinations to address the causes of these conditions.

—*C. Richard Falcon*

*See also* Choking; Common cold; Ear infections and disorders; Halitosis; Laryngitis; Pharyngitis; Rhinitis; Sinusitis; Sore throat; Strep throat; Tonsillitis; Voice and vocal cord disorders.

### FOR FURTHER INFORMATION:

Larson, David E., ed. *Mayo Clinic Family Health Book.* New York: William Morrow, 1990. A thorough and up-to-date medical text for the lay reader. The section on nasopharyngeal diseases—part 4, chapter 25, "The Ears, Nose, and Throat"—is quite complete and offers excellent anatomic illustrations.

Scott, Andrew. *Pirates of the Cell.* Oxford, England: Basil Blackwell, 1985. Useful for understanding the virus families that are often responsible for nasopharyngeal disorders.

Smith, Lendon H. *The Encyclopedia of Baby and Child Care.* Rev. ed. Englewood Cliffs, N.J.: Prentice Hall, 1980. Nasopharyngeal diseases strike babies and children most often. This reference work lists all the familiar disorders with Smith's descriptions of their symptoms and his recommendations for treatment.

Wagman, Richard J., ed. *The Complete Illustrated Book of Better Health.* Chicago: J. G. Ferguson, 1986. Contains good advice on how to care for common disease conditions, such as nasopharyngeal disorders.

_____. *The New Complete Medical and Health Encyclopedia.* 4 vols. Chicago: J. G. Ferguson, 1993. The chapters on upper respiratory diseases in this work are thorough and clear, with good illustrations.

## NAUSEA AND VOMITING

**SYSTEMS AFFECTED:** Gastrointestinal, brain

**SPECIALISTS:** Gastroenterologists, neurologists, otolaryngologists

**DEFINITION:** Nausea is the unpleasant subjective sensation, accompanied by epigastric and duodenal discomfort, which often culminates in vomiting, the regurgitation of the contents of the stomach.

**KEY TERMS:**

*affect:* the emotional reactions associated with experience

*antiemetics:* drugs that prevent or relieve the symptoms of nausea and/or vomiting

*chemoreceptor trigger zone:* a sensory nerve ending in the brain which is stimulated by and reacts to certain chemical stimulation localized outside the central nervous system

*emesis:* the act of vomiting

*psychogenic:* of mental origin

*psychotropics:* drugs that affect psychic function, behavior, or experience

### CAUSES AND SYMPTOMS

Nausea is defined as a subjectively unpleasant sensation associated with awareness of the urge to vomit. It is usually felt in the back of the throat and epigastrium and is accompanied by the loss of gastric tone, duodenal contractions, and reflux of the intestinal contents into the stomach. Retching is defined as labored, spasmodic, rhythmic contractions of the respiratory muscles (including the diaphragm, chest wall, and abdominal wall muscles) without the expulsion of gastric contents. Vomiting, or emesis, is the forceful expulsion of gastric contents from the mouth and is brought about by the powerful sustained contraction of the abdominal muscles, the descent of the diaphragm, and the opening of the gastric cardia (the cardiac orifice of the stomach).

Nausea and vomiting are important defense mechanisms against the ingestion of toxins. The act of emesis involves a sequence of events that can be divided into three phases: preejection, ejection, and postejection. The preejection phase includes the symptoms of nausea, along with salivation, swallowing, pallor, and tachycardia (an abnormally fast heartbeat). The ejection phase comprises retching and vomiting. Retching is characterized by rhythmic, synchronous, inspiratory movements of the diaphragm, abdominal, and external intercostal muscles, while the mouth and the glottis are kept closed. As the antral (cavity) portion of the stomach contracts, the proximal (nearest the center) portion relaxes and the gastric contents oscillate between the stomach and the esophagus. During retching, the hiatal portion of the diaphragm does not relax, and intraabdominal pressure increases are associated with a decrease in intrathoracic pressure.

In contrast, relaxation of the hiatal portion of the diaphragm (near the esophagus) permits a transfer of intraabdominal pressure to the thorax during the act of vomiting. Contraction of the muscles of the anterior abdominal wall, relaxation of the esophageal sphincter, an increase in intrathoracic and intragastric pressure, reverse peristalsis (movement of the contents of the alimentary canal), and an open glottis and mouth result in the expulsion of gastric contents. The postejection phase consists of autonomic and visceral responses that return the body to a quiescent phase, with or without residual nausea.

The complex act of vomiting, involving coordination of the respiratory, gastrointestinal, and abdominal musculature, is controlled by what researchers label the emetic center. This center in the brain stem has access to the motor pathways responsible for the visceral and somatic output involved in vomiting, and stimuli from several areas within the central nervous system can affect this center. These include afferent (inward-directed) nerves from the pharynx and gastrointestinal tract, as well as afferents from the higher cortical centers (including the visual center) and the chemoreceptor trigger zone (CTZ) in the area postrema (a highly vascularized area of the brain stem). The CTZ can be activated by chemical stimuli received through the blood or the cerebrospinal fluid. Direct electrical stimulation of the CTZ, however, does not result in emesis.

Clinical assessment of nausea and vomiting usually focus on the occurrence of vomiting, that is, the frequency and number of episodes. Nausea, however, is a subjective phenomenon unobservable by another. Few data collection instruments that measure separately the patient's experience of nausea and vomiting and his or her symptom distress have been reported in the literature. In fact, the Rhodes Index of Nausea and Vomiting (INV) Form 2 is the only available tool that measures the individual components of nausea, vomiting, and retching. This index measures the patient's perception of the duration, frequency, and distress from nausea; the frequency, amount, and distress from vomiting; and the frequency, amount, and distress from retching

(dry heaves). The INV score provides a measurement of the total symptom experience of the patient.

While the causes of nausea and vomiting are numerous—they include gastrointestinal diseases, infections, intracranial disease, toxins, radiation sickness, psychological trauma, migraines, and circulatory syncope—three of the most common causes are motion sickness (air, sea, land, or space), pregnancy, and anesthesia administered during operative procedures.

The sequence of symptoms and signs that constitute motion sickness is fairly characteristic. Premonitory symptoms often include yawning or sighing, lethargy, somnolence, and a loss of enthusiasm and concern for the task at hand. Increasing malaise is directed toward the epigastrium, a sensation best described as "stomach awareness," which progresses to nausea. Diversion of the blood flow from the skin toward the muscles results in pallor. A feeling of warmth and a desire for cool air is often accompanied by sweating. Frontal headache and a sensation of disorientation, dizziness, or light-headedness may also occur. As symptoms progress, vomiting occurs early in the sequence of symptoms for some; in others, malaise is severe and prolonged and vomiting is delayed. After vomiting, there is often a temporary improvement in well-being; however, with continued provocative motion, symptoms build again and vomiting recurs. The symptoms may last for minutes, hours, or even days.

The most coherent explanation for the development of motion sickness is provided by sensory conflict theory. Motion sickness is generally thought to occur as the result of a "sensory conflict" between information arising from the semicircular canals and organs of the vestibular system, visual, and other sensory input and the input that is expected on the basis of past experience or exposure history. It is argued that conflicts between current sensory inputs are by themselves insufficient to produce motion sickness since adaptation occurs even though the conflicting inputs continue to be present. Visual input alone, however, can produce symptoms of motion sickness, such as watching motion pictures shot from a moving vehicle or looking out of the side window (as opposed to the front window) of a moving vehicle.

Nausea and/or vomiting in the early morning during pregnancy, so-called morning sickness, is so common that it is accepted as a symptom of normal pregnancy. Occurring soon after waking, it is often retching rather than actual vomiting and usually does not disturb the woman's health or her pregnancy. The symptoms nearly always cease before the fourteenth week of pregnancy. In a much smaller proportion of cases, approximately 1 in 1,000 births, the vomiting becomes more serious and persistent, occurring throughout the day and even during the night. The term "hyperemesis gravidarum" is given to this serious form of vomiting. Theories on the etiology of morning sickness have tended to be grouped under four main areas: endocrine (caused by estrogen and progesterone levels), psychosomatic (a conscious or unconscious wish not to become pregnant), allergic (a histamine reaction), and metabolic (a lack of potassium).

Nausea and vomiting occur frequently as unpleasant side effects of the administration of anesthesia in many clinical procedures. Most postoperative vomiting is mild, and only in a few cases will the problem persist so as to cause electrolyte disturbances and dehydration. The factors affecting postoperative nausea and vomiting may be divided into two categories: by the type of patient and surgery, and by the anesthetic and preoperative and postoperative medication uses. Patients with a history of motion sickness have a predisposition to postoperative vomiting. Nearly 43 percent of patients who vomited following previous surgery vomited again, whereas slightly more than 14 percent of those who did not vomit previously had an emetic episode at their next operation. Patients undergoing their first anesthetic procedure had an incidence of vomiting of approximately 30 percent.

No direct association between vomiting and age has been found. That vomiting may be hormonally related, however, is suggested by the higher incidence of nausea and vomiting in the latter half of the menstrual cycle. Other factors that may affect nausea and vomiting associated with anesthesia include patient weight (female obese patients being particularly more vulnerable), amount of hydration, metabolic status, and psychological state.

With regard to the type of surgery performed, the highest incidence of nausea and vomiting appears to be associated with abdominal surgery, as well as ear, nose, and throat surgery, with middle-ear surgery being the major category. The length of surgery, and therefore the duration of anesthesia, also has a direct effect on nausea and vomiting. Short (thirty-minute to sixty-minute) operations using cyclopropane had an emetic incidence of 17.5 percent, while operations lasting one and a half to three and a half hours had an incidence of 46.4 percent.

Most of the causes of vomiting associated with general anesthesia are expected to be eliminated with regional or spinal anesthesia. The type of anesthesia used also has an effect on nausea and vomiting. Research indicates that cyclopropane, ether, and nitrous oxide are potent emetics.

### TREATMENT AND THERAPY

Since the generation of sensory conflict underlies all motion environments that give rise to motion sickness, practical measures that reduce conflict are likely to reduce motion sickness incidence. Motion sickness can be minimized if the subject has the widest possible view of an earth-stable visual reference. Passengers aboard ships are less likely to be seasick if they remain on deck at midship, where vertical motion is minimized, and view the horizon. In a car or bus, individuals should be in a position to see the road directly ahead, since the movement of this visual scene will correlate with the changes in the direction of the vehicle. While head movements in a rotating environment are known to precipitate motion sickness, there is no clear experimental evidence that they elicit nausea in mild linear oscillation. Thus, some nonpharmacologic remedies for motion sickness are restricting head movements, lying in a supine position, or closing the eyes. In addition, the use of acupressure wrist bands have proven effective in combating motion sickness.

Pharmacologically, the drug hyoscine hydrobromide (also called hyoscine or scopolamine) emerged as a valuable prophylactic drug following extensive research during World War II into the problems of motion sickness in troops transported in aircraft, ships, and landing craft. It remains one of the most effective drugs for short-duration exposures to provocative motion. Doses in excess of 0.6 milligram, however, are very likely to lead to drowsiness, and there is much experimental evidence that hyoscine impairs short-term memory. Hyoscine can be absorbed transdermally, and in order to extend the duration of action, a controlled-release patch was developed to deliver 1.2 milligrams on application and 0.01 milligram hourly thereafter. There is substantial evidence of its sustained effectiveness, but, perhaps as a result of variable absorption rates, there is an increased risk of blurred vision after more than twenty-four hours of use.

Amphetamines, ephedrine, and a number of antihistamines (such as dimenhydrinate) have been found to be clinically useful in motion sickness. Following oral administration, these drugs are generally slower than hyoscine in reaching their peak efficacy, but they have a longer duration of action.

For most susceptible subjects, whose exposure to motion sickness-inducing stimuli is infrequent, prophylactic drugs offer the only useful treatment. When exposure to provocative stimuli is more frequent, as for example in professional aircraft pilots, spontaneous adaption occurs during training and an initially high incidence of motion sickness decreases with time.

In medical conditions in which the cause is relatively unknown, it is usual to find a wide variety of suggested therapies, and nausea and vomiting during pregnancy and hyperemesis gravidarum (the serious, persistent form of vomiting in pregnancy) are no exception. Prior to 1968, treatments numbered approximately thirty. In subsequent years, however, suggested therapy has been mainly drugs of the antiemetic variety. Yet since the thalidomide tragedy (in which severe deformities occurred in the children of women who took this drug), there has been a reluctance to use drugs of any kind during early pregnancy. Probably the only value of drug therapy is at the stage of morning sickness, when antiemetics or mild sedatives may counter the feeling of nausea and prevent women from experiencing excessive vomiting and entering the vicious cycle of dehydration, starvation, and electrolyte imbalance. Once the patient has reached the stage of hyperemesis gravidarum, much more basic therapy is required, and the regimen calls for correction of dehydration, carbohydrate deficiency, and ionic deficiencies. This program is best managed by intravenous therapy, with or without the addition of vitamin supplements and sedative agents.

Nonpharmacologic self-care actions for morning sickness fall into the three broad categories of manipulating diet, adjusting behavior, and seeking emotional support. Some of the most effective self-care actions are getting rest, eating several small meals rather than three large ones, avoiding bad smells, avoiding greasy or fried foods, avoiding cooking, and receiving extra attention and support.

In terms of postoperative nausea and vomiting caused by anesthesia, it has been found that routine antiemetic prophylaxis of patients undergoing elective surgical procedures is not indicated, since fewer than 30 percent of patients experience postoperative nausea and vomiting. Of those who develop these symptoms, many have transient nausea or only one or two bouts of emesis and do not require antiemetic therapy. In addition, commonly used antiemetic drugs can produce significant side effects, such as sedation. Nevertheless, antiemetic prophylaxis may be justified in those patients who are at greater risk for developing postoperative nausea and/or vomiting. Such therapy is often given to patients with a history of motion sickness or to those undergoing gynecologic procedures, inner-ear procedures, oral surgery (in which the jaws are occluded by wires, causing a high risk of breathing in vomitus), and operations on the ear or eye and plastic surgery operations (in order to avoid disruption of delicate surgical work).

Many different antiemetic drugs are available for the treatment of postoperative nausea and vomiting. Researchers have found it difficult to interpret the results of antiemetic drug studies because the severity of postoperative vomiting and the response to therapeutic agents can be influenced by many variables in addition to the antiemetic drug being studied. Even with the use of the same drugs in a homogenous population undergoing the same procedure, the severity of emesis varies from individual to individual.

Because antiemetic drugs have differing sites of action, better results can be obtained by using a multidrug approach. If a combination of drugs with a similar site of action is used, however, the incidence of side effects may be increased. There are few data regarding combination antiemetic prophylaxis or therapy for postoperative nausea and emesis. Drug combinations have been avoided in postsurgical patients because of concerns about additive central nervous system toxicity. An exception is the combination of low-dose droperidol and metoclopramide, which appears to be more effective than droperidol alone for outpatient gynecologic procedures.

Although a full stomach is best avoided before any operative procedure, with situations such as emergencies, in which danger from vomiting is acute, a rapid sequence of administering anesthesia (induction) and clearing the air passage (intubation) remains the method of choice to avoid nausea and vomiting in patients with a full stomach. After the procedure, it is recommended that the patient minimize movement in order to avoid nausea and vomiting. Also, it has been found that avoiding eating solid food for at least eight hours after a surgical procedure is helpful in preventing postoperative nausea and vomiting.

## PERSPECTIVE AND PROSPECTS

Though it has existed for as long as there have been human beings, the symptom of nausea has never received much attention in health care practice or research. In fact, until the early 1970's the sensation of nausea was frequently dismissed as merely a passing phenomenon. The rationale for this dismissal was most likely the understanding that nausea is self-limiting (it always passes with time), is never life-threatening in itself, is probably psychogenic in nature (at least to some degree), and being subjective, is very difficult to measure. In addition, in the past the most predictable nausea was pregnancy-related, which may also explain the lack of attention given to it.

Until the late 1980's, there was still little research being conducted on the nausea associated with pregnancy, although it is a common symptom. The historical lack of interest in nausea and vomiting during pregnancy may be traced to the fact that, since the symptoms generally persist only through the first trimester, health care professionals have viewed the problem as relatively insignificant. As more pregnant women work outside the home in demanding positions, however, these women have exhibited less tolerance for illness. Demands upon the health care industry and upon personal physicians for more research and effective treatment have become more widespread.

While it is surprising that nausea has received scant attention in the history of clinical research, it is even more astonishing that vomiting, an observable behavior, has received so little attention as well. Although vomiting is a primitive neurologic process that has remained almost unchanged in the evolution of animals, the mechanisms that regulate the behavior remain virtually unknown.

One reason for the paucity of information on the subject of nausea in particular stems from the lack of a reliable animal model. This fact has hampered research aimed at establishing the etiological basis for nausea and its relationship to vomiting. While some species of lower animals, for example rats, cannot vomit, it is not known whether rats experience the phenomenon of nausea. Thus no effective means of measuring nausea in lower animals has been devised.

Since the early 1970's, there has been a noticeable increase in research on nausea as a drug side effect because it was so frequently seen in cancer chemotherapy clinical trials sponsored by the National Cancer Institute and the American Cancer Society. As more powerful chemotherapy agents and aggressive combinations were clinically investigated, patients began to experience severe, potentially life-threatening nausea and vomiting. Yet it was still the symptom of vomiting that began to receive attention; nausea was either coupled with the investigation of vomiting, with the two treated as a unit, or it was ignored. Nevertheless, efforts continued to improve antiemetic drugs until nausea began to be seen as a separate but related symptom.

Aside from the pharmacological investigations of new drugs and drug combinations in the treatment of nausea and vomiting, an interesting branch of scientific investigation has begun the process of exploring alternative ways of managing these symptoms. Behavioral interventions, such as progressive muscle relaxation, biofeedback, imagery, or music therapy have been used to alleviate postchemotherapy anxiety. These methods may also be used to treat other patients suffering from the symptoms of nausea and vomiting, such as pregnant women.

Another noninvasive, nonpharmacologic measure that has been considered in the relief of nausea and vomiting is transcutaneous electrical nerve stimulation (TENS). Several research studies indicate that TENS may be useful in alleviating chemotherapy-related nausea and vomiting, including delayed nausea and vomiting. Side effects from using TENS units are negligible, and with further study they may prove to be an acceptable, helpful relief measure.
—*Genevieve Slomski*

*See also* Food poisoning; Iatrogenic disorders; Influenza; Motion sickness; Pregnancy and gestation; specific diseases.

**FOR FURTHER INFORMATION:**

Davis, C. J., G. V. Lake-Bakaar, and D. G. Grahame-Smith, eds. *Nausea and Vomiting: Mechanisms and Treatment.* New York: Springer-Verlag, 1986. A multidisciplinary approach to the topics of nausea and vomiting is presented in this collection of essays. Section 1 discusses anatomy, physiology, and pharmacology; section 2 discusses mechanisms of treatment and new approaches to therapy. Contains numerous charts, graphs, and illustrations.

Funk, Sandra G., ed. *Key Aspects of Comfort.* New York: Springer, 1989. This work, which discusses the management of pain, fatigue, and nausea, functions both as an introduction to these topics and as a sourcebook for treatment. The various authors argue that just as both psychosocial and biological factors play a role in the etiology of these phenomena, so must the interventions reflect both behavioral and biological dimensions. Includes charts, tables, illustrations, and a list of references following each of the book's three sections.

Kucharczyk, John, et al. *Nausea and Vomiting.* Boca Raton, Fla.: CRC Press, 1991. A comprehensive work on recent research and clinical advances in the areas of nausea and vomiting. After an introductory chapter on pioneers in emesis research, discusses the mechanisms of emesis, including respiratory muscle control, digestive tract, and neural mechanisms; the clinical characteristics and consequences of vomiting; and antiemetic therapies. In addition to summarizing already existing data, the authors put forth new concepts in the management and treatment of nausea and vomiting. Extensive references are provided.

Laszlo, John, ed. *Antiemetics and Cancer Chemotherapy.* Baltimore: Williams & Wilkins, 1983. This work focuses on pharmacologic prophylaxis and treatment of the symptoms of nausea and vomiting experienced by patients undergoing cancer chemotherapy. Age, gender, and medical history are some of the factors considered in choosing a drug or combination of drugs to alleviate the symptoms of nausea and vomiting.

Levine, Seymour, and Holger Ursin, eds. *Coping and Health.* New York: Plenum Press, 1980. This work for the general reader on psychosocial mechanisms for coping with serious illness offers an insightful discussion of nausea and vomiting in the context of cancer chemotherapy. Contains a useful bibliography.

## NECK INJURIES AND DISORDERS. *See* HEAD AND NECK DISORDERS.

## NECROSES. *See* FROSTBITE; GANGRENE.

## NEPHRITIS

**SYSTEM AFFECTED:** Kidneys

**SPECIALISTS:** Internists, nephrologists

**DEFINITION:** Nephritis refers to an inflammation of the kidneys. Pyelonephritis is caused by a bacterial infection and may be acute or chronic; it is generally the result of bladder infection that has spread to the kidneys or from the reflux of urine to the kidneys because of a congenital defect. Nephritis can also be caused by glomerulonephritis, an inflammation of the glomeruli (the functioning units of the kidneys) that may result from an improper response of the immune system to bacteria. Metabolic disorders, such as kidney stones and gout, may also be responsible for kidney infection. Renal failure can result from many of these conditions.

*See also* Glomerulonephritis; Gout; Kidney disorders; Renal failure; Stones.

## NEURALGIA, NEURITIS, AND NEUROPATHY

**SYSTEM AFFECTED:** Nervous

**SPECIALISTS:** Neurologists

**DEFINITION:** Pathological conditions affecting the peripheral nerves of the body and interfering with the proper functioning of those nerves.

**KEY TERMS:**

*autonomic neuropathy:* a disorder involving the nerves that work independently of conscious control, and including those nerves that go to small blood vessels, sweat glands, the urinary bladder, the gastrointestinal tract, and the genital organs

*axon:* the portion of a neuron that carries electrical impulses away from the nerve cell body

*mononeuropathy:* a neuropathy involving only one peripheral nerve

*nerve:* a bundle of sensory and motor neurons held together by layers of connective tissue

*neuralgia:* pain associated with a nerve, often caused by inflammation or injury

*neuritis:* inflammation of a nerve

*neuron:* a nerve cell that is capable of conducting electrical impulses; several different types of neurons exist, including motor neurons, sensory neurons, and interneurons

*neuropathy:* a disorder that causes a functional disturbance of a peripheral nerve, brought about by any cause

*peripheral nervous system:* the portion of the nervous system found outside the brain and spinal cord

*polyneuropathy:* a disease that involves a disturbance in the function of several peripheral nerves

### CAUSES AND SYMPTOMS

Peripheral nerves, those nerves found outside the brain and spinal cord, function to carry information between the central nervous system and the other portions of the body. These peripheral nerves consist of a bundle of nerve cells, also called neurons, which are wrapped in a protective sheath of connective tissue. A nerve consisting of neurons that only carry impulses toward the central nervous system is termed a sensory nerve. Nerves that contain only neurons that carry information from the central nervous system to the periphery of the body are called motor nerves, because they usually carry information telling a particular body part to move. Most nerves, however, consist of both sensory and motor neurons and are thus called mixed nerves.

The nerves of the peripheral nervous system can be divided into two different categories, cranial nerves and spinal nerves. Cranial nerves come directly out of the brain and supply information to and about the head and neck. There are twelve pairs of cranial nerves. Spinal nerves come directly out of the spinal cord and provide information to and from the arms, legs, chest, gut, and all other parts of the body not supplied by cranial nerves. In humans, there are usually thirty-one pairs of spinal nerves. Both cranial and spinal nerves can be affected by neuropathies.

Neurons (nerve cells) are highly specialized structures designed to convey information from one part of the body to another. This information is passed along in the form of electrical impulses. Neurons consist of three main parts: a cell body, which contains the nucleus and is the control center of the entire neuron; dendrites, which are slender, fingerlike extensions that convey electrical impulses toward the cell body; and an axon, which is a slender extension that carries electrical impulses away from the cell body.

Most of the dendrites and axons of peripheral nerves are covered with a white, fatty substance called myelin. Myelin acts to protect and insulate axons and dendrites. By insulating the axons and dendrites, myelin actually speeds up the rate at which an electrical impulse can be carried along these two structures. Damage to the myelin sheath surrounding axons and dendrites can greatly impair the function of a nerve.

Often, when a nerve becomes pinched, damaged, or inflamed, the result is excessive electrical stimulation of the nerve, which will be registered as pain. The pain associated with the damaged nerve is referred to as neuralgia. One of

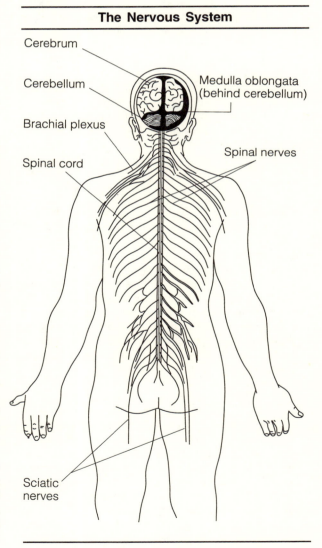

**The Nervous System**

Cerebrum

Cerebellum

Medulla oblongata
(behind cerebellum)

Brachial plexus

Spinal nerves

Spinal cord

Sciatic
nerves

the most common forms of neuralgia occurs upon the striking of the "funny bone." This area around the elbow is the spot where the ulnar nerve is easily accessible. The ulnar nerve runs from just under the shoulder to the little finger, and when the ulnar nerve is struck near the elbow it is compressed or pinched, leading to pain or a tingling sensation from the elbow down to the little finger.

Compression of nerves for prolonged periods can also lead to neuralgia. The most common example of compression neuralgia is carpal tunnel syndrome. In this syndrome, the median nerve becomes compressed at the wrist, usually as a result of an inflammation of the tendon sheaths of the tendons located on either side of the median nerve. The swelling of these tendon sheaths causes the compression of the median nerve, which may initially lead to neuralgia. As this condition progresses, it can lead to a loss of feeling along the palm side of the thumb and the index and middle fingers. This condition is most common in people who use their fingers for rigorous work over prolonged periods of time, such as operators of computer terminals.

Sciatica is another common form of neuralgia, in which pain is associated with the sciatic nerve. The sciatic nerve is the longest nerve in the human body, running from the pelvis down the back of the thigh to the lower leg and then down to the soles of the feet. The symptoms of sciatica include sharp pains along the sciatic nerve. The pain may involve the buttocks, hip, back, posterior thigh, leg, ankle, and foot. Sciatica can result from many different causes, but the most common cause is from a ruptured intervertebral disk which puts pressure on, or causes a pinching of, the sciatic nerve.

Neuritis is defined as the inflammation of a nerve or of the connective tissue that surrounds the nerve. Many diseases can lead to the inflammation of peripheral nerves. Perhaps the most common disease leading to neuritis is shingles. Shingles are caused by the occurrence of herpes zoster, a virus that attacks the dorsal root ganglion, a place near the spinal cord that houses the cell bodies of neurons. A rash, swelling, and pain progress from the dorsal root ganglion along one or more spinal nerves. The rash along the course of the spinal nerves usually disappears within two or three days, but the pain along this path can persist for months.

Leprosy is another disease that leads to the inflammation of nerves. Leprosy is a bacterial disease caused by *Mycobacterium leprae*. These bacteria invade the cells that make up the myelin sheath that surrounds the nerve. The result is a noticeable swelling of the nerves affected, primarily those that are close to the skin. Many times, this swelling will lead to neuralgia and, if left untreated, to muscle wasting.

"Neuropathy" is a general term used to describe a decrease in the function of peripheral nerves which may be caused by many factors. The first signs of a neuropathy are usually a tingling, prickling, or burning sensation in some part of the body. This is followed by a sensory loss; the inability to perceive touch, heat, cold, or pressure; and a weakness in the muscles in the area affected. This weakness may eventually lead to a loss of muscle termed muscular atrophy. Neuropathies may affect sensory neurons, motor neurons, or both and can occur in both spinal and cranial nerves. A neuropathy may develop over a few days or many years. Neuropathies can be caused by a number of factors, including toxic exposure to solvents, pesticides, or heavy metals; viral illness; certain medications; metabolic disturbances such as diabetes mellitus; excessive use of alcohol; vitamin deficiency; loss of blood to the nerve; or cold exposure.

Neuropathies can be categorized based on the number of nerves that they affect, whether it is the myelin sheath surrounding the axon that is affected or the axon itself is destroyed, and the amount of time before symptoms of the neuropathy occur and progress. Thus, neuropathies are usually broken down into four different types: polyneuropathy, in which more than one nerve is affected; mononeuropathy, in which only one nerve is affected; axonal neuropathy, in which the axon is affected and degenerates; and demyelinating neuropathy, in which the myelin sheath surrounding the nerve is destroyed. Each of the four categories can be further subdivided based on the time frame in which the symptoms occur. Those neuropathies that appear over days are termed acute, those that appear over weeks are termed subacute, and those neuropathies whose symptoms slowly appear over months or years are termed chronic.

Another type of neuropathy is autonomic neuropathy, a condition which affects the nerves of the autonomic nervous system. These are the peripheral nerves that go to the sweat glands, small blood vessels, gastrointestinal tract, urinary bladder, and genital organs. These nerves are referred to as autonomic since they automatically provide information between these organs and the central nervous system without the individual's conscious effort. The symptoms associated with this form of neuropathy include loss of control over urination, difficulty swallowing food, occasional stomach upset, diarrhea, impotence, and excessive sweating.

The most common cause of neuropathies in the Western world is diabetes mellitus, while leprosy is the more common cause of neuropathies elsewhere. It is estimated that at least 70 percent of all diabetics have some degree of peripheral neuropathy. In most of these cases, the neuropathy is very slight and causes the patient no noticeable symptoms. In about 10 percent of those diabetics with a neuropathy, however, the symptoms will be serious.

### TREATMENT AND THERAPY

Often, the first notable feature of a neuropathy that prompts a patient to seek medical attention is a tingling, prickling, or burning sensation in a particular area of the body. The occurrence of these sensations without any external stimuli is termed paresthesias. Since diabetes is the most common cause of neuropathy in the Western world, the sensations experienced by a diabetic patient can serve as an example of the symptoms that are associated with common neuropathies. These patients may first notice the above-mentioned symptoms in the balls of the feet or tips of the toes. As the neuropathy progresses, patients may lose feeling in their feet and experience a weakness in the muscles of the feet leading to a difficulty in flexing the toes upward. This makes walking difficult, and many patients remark that they feel as if they are walking on stumps. This condition may lead to difficulties in maintaining balance. The neuropathy will begin to affect the legs above the ankles and then travel up the legs, eventually leading to atrophy of the leg muscles.

As the neuropathy worsens, it is critical that patients seek help because they can no longer feel pain. This situation is dangerous, as the patient may no longer sense the pain that can be caused by injuries from sharp objects or even a pebble in the shoe. If unnoticed, these injuries lead to ulcers that can easily become infected.

The first step in treating a neuropathy is to diagnose the type of neuropathy affecting the patient. A patient's medical history is taken to identify any recent viral or bacterial illness, any exposure to toxic substances such as pesticides or heavy metals, the patient's habits concerning alcohol use, or any other illness or injury that might have brought about a possible neuropathy. Next, a physical exam will be performed to determine if the patient's sensations regarding touch, pain, pressure, or temperature have been affected, as well as the ability of the patient to react to these stimuli. The physician may also feel the affected area to determine if the nerve or nerves are inflamed and enlarged.

If the patient's history and the physical examination point toward a neuropathy, further testing using electrodiagnostic tests will be performed. These tests measure the speed at which an electrical impulse travels down a nerve, which is called the nerve conduction velocity. Motor nerve conduction velocity is measured by stimulating the nerve with electrodes placed on the skin above the nerve. Stimulation of the nerve is typically done at two different sites. Using the arm as an example, one electrode would be placed on the inside of the arm at the elbow. The time that it takes for the impulse to reach a recording electrode on the thumb would be measured. A second site at the wrist would be tested to determine the time that it takes for the electrical impulse to reach the recording electrode on the thumb. The time that it took for the impulse to travel from the wrist to thumb would be subtracted from the amount of time that it took for the impulse to go from the inside of the arm at the elbow to the thumb. The resulting value would then be divided by the distance between the site at the wrist and the site at the elbow, giving a nerve conduction velocity value measured in meters per second.

The typical nerve conduction velocity for the motor and sensory peripheral nerves of adults is approximately 40 to 80 meters per second. If a neuropathy is the result of demyelination, the affected nerve will have a much slower nerve conduction velocity. If the neuropathy is a result of axonal damage, then the nerve conduction velocity is usually not altered from normal. Thus, electrodiagnostic testing helps to determine if the neuropathy is a demyelination neuropathy or an axonal neuropathy. Such a determination is important because they are caused by different diseases and are thus treated differently. Electrodiagnostic tests can also provide useful information regarding the site of the neuropathy and whether the neuropathy is affecting sensory neurons, motor neurons, or both.

The last diagnostic test to be performed, if other methods are inconclusive, is a biopsy of the affected nerve. This procedure involves the surgical removal of a portion of the afflicted nerve. The small sample of nerve will be placed under a microscope and examined for specific changes in the nerve. The nerve sample may also be subjected to various biochemical studies to determine if metabolic disturbances have occurred. Nerve biopsies are rarely performed, however, and are usually not recommended.

Once the type of neuropathy afflicting the patient has been determined, treatment can begin. Unlike axons in the central nervous system, axons in the peripheral nervous system are capable of regenerating under certain conditions. If the neuropathy is the result of exposure to toxic substances such as pesticides or heavy metals, removal of the patient from the exposure to such substances is the simple cure. If the neuropathy is the result of viral or bacterial infections, the treatment and recovery from these infections will also usually correct the neuropathy. The same principle applies to neuropathies caused by metabolic diseases and vitamin deficiencies: Corrections of these problems will lead to the correction of the neuropathy.

Should the neuropathy be of the mononeuropathy type and caused by trauma, anti-inflammatory drugs such as corticosteroids may be used or surgery may be performed to repair the nerve. If the mononeuropathy is caused by compression, as in carpal tunnel syndrome, surgery may also be needed to increase the space around the nerve and thus relieve the compression. Surgery is also used to remove tumors on the nerve that might be causing a neuropathy.

The time required to recover from a neuropathy is dependent on the severity and type of neuropathy. Recovery from demyelination is typically quicker than recovery from axonal neuropathies. If only the myelin surrounding the axon is damaged, and not the axon itself, the axon can quickly replace the damaged myelin. Demyelinating neuropathies usually require three to four weeks for recovery. In contrast, recovery from axonal neuropathies may take from two months to more than a year, depending on the severity of the neuropathy.

## PERSPECTIVE AND PROSPECTS

Perhaps the earliest documentation of peripheral neuropathies occurred during biblical times, when the term "leprosy" was coined. It is likely, however, that this term was employed rather loosely, as it was used to describe not only the disease leprosy but also a number of skin diseases not involving neuropathies, such as psoriasis.

The actual diagnosis of neuropathies and their subsequent categorization did not occur until the advent of electrical diagnostic testing. The earliest use of electricity to study nerve function occurred in 1876 when German neurologist Wilhelm Erb noted that the electrical stimulation of a damaged peripheral nerve below the site of injury resulted in muscular contraction. In contrast, electrical stimulation at a site above the injured nerve brought about no activity in the muscle. Erb concluded that the injury blocked the flow of electrical impulses down the nerve.

The actual use of electrical diagnostic testing did not take place until the late 1940's when electrodes and an oscilloscope, an instrument that measures electrical activity, were used to measure the rate at which an electrical impulse could travel down a nerve. This discovery allowed the testing of nerve function and would become useful in the discrimination between axonal and demyelinating neuropathies. During this period, the invention of the electron microscope and the discovery of better nerve-staining techniques enhanced the ability of scientists to study the physiological and anatomical changes that occur in nerves with the onset of neuropathies.

Neuropathies received considerable attention in 1976 when approximately five hundred cases of the neuropathy called Guillain-Barré syndrome occurred in the United States following a national vaccination program for swine flu. The reason that the swine flu vaccine caused this neuropathy has never been discovered, but this syndrome often occurs after an upper-respiratory tract or gastrointestinal infection.

Those suffering from neuropathies that result from exposure to toxic substances, viral or bacterial infections, or metabolic diseases have a good prognosis of recovery if the underlying cause of the neuropathy is treated. The prognosis of recovery is not as good for those who suffer neuropathies as a result of hereditary diseases. Advances made in genetic research and continued research in gene therapy may someday greatly increase the prognosis of recovery for those suffering from hereditary neuropathies.
—*David K. Saunders*

***See also*** Brain disorders; Cerebral palsy; Cluster headaches; Diabetes mellitus; Encephalitis; Epilepsy; Guillain-Barré syndrome (GBS); Hallucinations; Headaches; Hemiplegia; Lead poisoning; Leprosy; Meningitis; Migraine headaches; Motor neuron diseases; Multiple sclerosis; Numbness and tingling; Pain, types of; Palsy; Paralysis; Paraplegia; Parkinsonism; Quadriplegia; Sciatica; Seizures; Shingles; Tics.

## FOR FURTHER INFORMATION:

Kandel, Eric R., James H. Schwartz, and Thomas M. Jessell. *Principles of Neural Science*. 3d ed. New York: Elsevier, 1991. Although this book is used in many college graduate courses, the discussion involving peripheral neuropathies should be understandable to the general reader. Provides examples of neuropathies, their syndromes, causes, diagnosis, and history.

Margolis, Simeon, and Hamilton Mosses III, eds. *The Johns Hopkins Medical Handbook: The One Hundred Major Medical Disorders of People over the Age of Fifty*. New York: Rebus, 1992. This book deals primarily with neuropathies associated with diabetes mellitus, discussing the symptoms and dangers of neuropathies in diabetic patients. Written for the general reader without a medical background.

Marieb, Elaine N. *Essentials of Human Anatomy and Physiology*. 3d ed. Redwood City, Calif.: Benjamin/Cummings, 1991. An excellent book to begin the study of the peripheral nervous system. This text is easy-to-understand, as it uses little technical jargon and explains the jargon that it does use. Provides good descriptions and drawings of most parts of the peripheral nervous system.

National Institute of Neurological and Communicative Disorders and Stroke. Office of Scientific and Health Reports. *The Diabetic Neuropathies*. Bethesda, Md.: Department of Health, Education, and Welfare; Public Health Service; National Institutes of Health; National Institute of Neurological and Communicative Disorders and Stroke; Office of Scientific and Health Reports, 1978. A guide to the different types of diabetic neuropathies and their syndromes. Does an excellent job of describing the different types of diabetic neuropathies in easy-to-understand, nontechnical language. Provides an excellent introduction to neuropathies in general and their effects on peripheral nerves.

Stedman, Thomas Lathrop. *Stedman's Medical Dictionary*. Edited by William R. Hensyl. 25th ed. Baltimore: Williams & Wilkins, 1990. This dictionary not only defines medical and medically related terms but also provides an overview of many of the different types of neuropathies and diseases that result in, or cause, neuropathies.

# NEUROSIS

**SYSTEM AFFECTED:** Psychic-emotional

**SPECIALISTS:** Psychiatrists, psychologists

**DEFINITION:** A chronic mental disorder characterized by distressing and unacceptable anxiety.

## CAUSES AND SYMPTOMS

A neurosis is experienced at a level of severity that is less than psychotic but significant enough to impair a person's functioning. The term "neurosis" includes nine psychological states: hysteria, obsessions and compulsions, phobias, some depressions, some traumatic reactions, addictions, psychosomatic disorders, some sexual disorders, and anxiety. A person tends to continue suffering from one of the recurrent and continuing reactions noted above, if not treated for the neurosis.

Hysteria features somatic symptoms resembling those of a physical disease without actual physical illness (for example, a headache without organic cause). Phobias are abnormal fears that arise because an inner fear is displaced onto an object or situation outside the individual (for example, impotence to deal with fear of intimacy). Obsessions (recurrent thoughts) and compulsions (repetitively performed behaviors) bear little relation to the person's needs and are experienced by the person as foreign or intrusive (for example, repeated hand washing). Depression is a mood of sadness, unhappiness, hopelessness, loss of interest, difficulty concentrating, and lack of a sense of self-worth. Addictions are the use of substances or self-defeating behaviors to fulfill one's need for love instead of loving self or another person (for example, addiction to gambling). Psychosomatic disorders are organic illnesses caused by psychological distress (for example, peptic ulcer). Sexual disorders are the avoidance of developing adult sexual competency by immature sexual behavior (for example, exhibitionism). Traumatic reactions in the past delay or impair normal development in the present (for example, childhood sexual abuse leads to difficulty with intimacy as an adult). Anxiety is experienced as a generalized anxious affect which is pervasive and without a known cause (for example, a person chronically worrying that "something bad will happen").

## Treatment and Therapy

All the forms of neuroses listed above need treatment to be resolved. All have the potential to become borderline or overtly psychotic disorders under stress. Treatment involves entering psychotherapy to understand better and therefore manage neurotic symptoms. It often can require the use of psychoactive medications for the treatment of anxieties, depressions, obsessions, and addictions. Treatment can be received from family physicians and general internists at the first level of intervention. Patients refer to psychiatrists, psychologists, social workers, and substance counselors for more advanced interventions.

## Perspective and Prospects

Sigmund Freud (1856-1939), Alfred Adler (1870-1937), Carl Jung (1875-1961), and Karen Horney (1885-1952) all made major contributions toward understanding neuroses. All four were Austrian-born physicians who helped invent modern psychology, eventually leaving Austria to work in either Great Britain or America.

Freud founded psychoanalysis with his work on the causes and treatment of neurotic and psychopathic states. The methods that he developed form the root of all "talking therapies." Freud proposed that psychological conflicts pro-

duce neuroses according to the following pattern. Inner conflicts are produced by fears or guilt around one's emerging sexual drives. The conflicts, if not resolved on a conscious level, are repressed on the unconscious level, where they drive a person to act according to one or more of the various neurotic symptoms.

Adler was one of the four original members of Freud's psychoanalytic school. With his emphasis on the person as a whole being and on the importance of willpower, he created an individual psychology for the twentieth century. Adler said that neurotic persons form a rigid way of thinking about themselves and others. They then project that rigid thought process onto the world. They proceed to operate as though the world accepted their rigid thinking as real. This tendency is at the basis of the neurotic thought processes of sadism, hatred, intolerance, envy, and irresponsibility.

Jung was the only member of Freud's inner circle who was formally trained as a psychiatrist. He founded analytic psychology, which studies mental behavior as complexes of behavior, emotion, thought, and imagery. He opened up psychology to religious and mystical experiences. Jung wrote that neuroses are a dissociation of the personality caused by splitting. A person has a conscious set of values or beliefs which conflict with an opposite set of feelings. The person, rather than resolving the problem, maintains the rational-emotive split as one or more of the forms of neuroses.

Horney developed a psychoanalytic theory of humans who evolve within their culture, family, and environment. She was sensitive to the negative effects of a male-dominated psychology, attempting to explain women's experiences. Horney believed that neuroses are disturbances in the relationship of self-to-self and self-to-other. If one's development in childhood is disturbed from its normal pattern, the adult will use one of three neurotic coping styles: compliance, aggressiveness, or detachment.

These four psychologists agreed that neuroses are a childhood developmental defect which impairs the adult's rational-emotional integration, appearing as one or more of the indirect symptoms of anxiety. —*Gerald T. Terlep*

***See also*** Anxiety; Depression; Hypochondriasis; Manic-depressive disorder; Midlife crisis; Obsessive-compulsive disorder; Panic attacks; Paranoia; Phobias; Postpartum depression; Psychiatric disorders; Psychosis; Psychosomatic disorders; Schizophrenia; Stress.

## For Further Information:

Cleve, Jay. *Out of the Blues.* Minneapolis: CompCare, 1989. Presents methods of coping with neurotic depression, stemming from Alfred Adler's belief that neurosis comes from overly rigid thinking.

Rapoport, Judith. *The Boy Who Couldn't Stop Washing.* New York: Penguin Group, 1989. A classic description of the neurosis of obsessive-compulsive behaviors. Based upon Sigmund Freud's understanding of neurosis as an illness.

Roth, Geneen. *When Food Is Love*. New York: Plume, 1991. Reviews the neurotic abuse of foods as an addiction. Roth's work reflects Carl Jung's understanding of the importance of love and spirit for each person.

Sheehy, Gail. *Passages*. New York: E. P. Dutton, 1976. Presents an explanation of how and why neuroses are developmental. Sheehy's classic work is a follow-up to Karen Horney's theories of neurosis.

## NUMBNESS AND TINGLING

**SYSTEMS AFFECTED:** Muscular, nervous, skin

**SPECIALISTS:** Neurologists, physiatrists

**DEFINITION:** Abnormalities of sensation that are attributable to nerve damage or disorders.

*Symptoms.* Patients commonly report various sensory aberrations that are often described as "pins and needles," tingling, prickling, burning of varying severity, or sensations resembling electric shock. The accepted term for these symptoms is "paresthesias" or "dysesthesias." When severe enough to be painful, they can be referred to as painful paresthesias.

The other major sensory symptom is a reduction or loss of feeling in an area of skin. Most patients use the relatively unambiguous term "numbness"; however, the more formal medical term is "hypesthesia." Paresthesias and hypesthesias are usually restricted to a part rather than all of the cutaneous territory of a damaged root or nerve.

The distribution of nonparesthetic pain is seldom as anatomically specific as the paresthesias themselves. Patients with carpal tunnel syndrome, for example, often have arm and shoulder pain that suggests compression of a cervical root rather than of the distal median nerve (a combined motor and sensory nerve). The paresthesias, by contrast, are usually localized to the tips of the fingers innervated by the median nerve. Similarly, in patients with cervical or lumbosacral radiculopathies (any diseased condition of the roots of spinal nerves), the distribution of pain in the upper or lower limbs often correlates poorly with the root involved. The paresthesias, however, are felt usually either along the entire area or, more commonly, in the distal part of the skin area innervated by the damaged root (the dermatome).

*Examination.* In attempting to localize the site of a lesion, the physician innervates major muscles from the spinal nerve roots (myotomes) through the plexuses, the individual peripheral nerves and their branches, and also the cutaneous areas supplied by each of these components of the peripheral nervous system. Traditionally, the site of the lesion can be deduced from which muscles and nerves are involved and from where the various branches of the peripheral nerves arise.

In motor examination, the muscles and tendon reflexes are examined first because weakness and reflex changes are often easier to elicit than are sensory signs. The muscles are first examined for atrophy, since muscles become atrophic when denervated, the focal atrophy can sometimes identify accurately a nerve lesion. The lack of atrophy in a weak muscle either indicates an upper motor neuron lesion or raises the suspicion of spurious weakness. A systematic examination of individual muscles is then performed.

In sensory examination, the patient describes the area of sensory abnormality, which often tells as much as a formal examination. Testing light touch with the examiner's finger is frequently all that is required for confirmation. If this reveals no abnormality, retesting with a pin may disclose an area of sensory deficit. Pinpricks in normal and abnormal areas are compared.

It is important to examine the entire course of an affected nerve for bone, joint, or other abnormalities that may be causing the nerve damage. Local tenderness of the nerve and/or a positive Tinel's sign (paresthesias produced in the area of the nerve when the nerve is tapped or palpated) may also help to identify the site. Many normal persons experience mild tingling when nerves such as the ulnar at the elbow or the median at the wrist are tapped lightly, so this finding is significant only when the nerve is very sensitive to light percussion. Conversely, a badly damaged nerve may be totally insensitive to percussion or palpation.

Nerve conduction studies and the electromyographic examination of muscles evaluate the function of large-diameter, rapidly conducting motor and sensory nerve fibers. These two complimentary techniques are valuable tools in the accurate assessment of focal peripheral neuropathies, helping in the localization of the nerve lesion and the assessment of its severity.

*Diagnosis.* Peripheral nerves causing sensory symptoms may be damaged anywhere along their course from the spinal cord to the muscles and skin that they innervate. The site of a focal neuropathy (the focus of neurologic disease) may therefore be in the nerve roots, the spinal nerves, the ventral or dorsal rami (branches), the plexuses (network of nerves), the major nerve trunks, or their individual branches. The character, site, mode of onset, spread, and temporal profile of sensory symptoms must be established and precipitating or relieving factors identified. These features—and the presence of any associated symptoms—help identify the origin of sensory disturbances, as do the physical signs. Sensory symptoms or signs may conform to the territory of individual peripheral nerves or nerve roots. Involvement of one side of the body, or of one limb in its entirety, suggests a central lesion. Distal involvement of all four extremities suggests polyneuropathy (several neurologic disorders), a cervical cord or brain-stem lesion, or, when symptoms are transient, a metabolic disturbance such as hyperventilation syndrome. Short-lived sensory complaints may be indicative of sensory seizures or cerebral ischemic phenomena (local and temporal deficiency of blood supply caused by obstruction of the circulation to a part) as well as metabolic disturbances. In patients with cord lesions, there may be a transverse sensory level. Dissociated sensory loss is characterized by the loss of some sensory modalities and the preservation of others. Such findings may be encountered in patients with either peripheral or central disease and must therefore be interpreted in the clinical context in which they are found.

The absence of sensory signs in patients with sensory symptoms does not mean that symptoms have a nonorganic basis. Symptoms are often troublesome before signs of sensory dysfunction have had time to develop.

—*Genevieve Slomski*

*See also* Neuralgia, neuritis, and neuropathy; Pain, types of; Spinal disorders.

**FOR FURTHER INFORMATION:**

Chou, Shelley N., and Edward Seljeskoy, eds. *Spinal Deformities and Neurological Dysfunction*. New York: Raven Press, 1978.

Mathers, Lawrence H. *The Peripheral Nervous System: Structure, Function, and Clinical Correlations*. Menlo Park, Calif.: Addison-Wesley, 1985.

Rothman, Richard H., and Frederick Simeone. *The Spine*. 3d ed. Philadelphia: W. B. Saunders, 1992.

Wienir, Michael A., ed. *Spinal Segmental Pain and Sensory Disturbance*. Philadelphia: Hanley and Belfus, 1988.

**NUTRITIONAL DISORDERS.** *See* **MALNUTRITION; VITAMIN AND MINERAL DEFICIENCIES.**

# HEALTH
# AND
# ILLNESS

# ALPHABETICAL LIST OF CONTENTS

# ENTRIES BY MEDICAL SPECIALIZATION

AEROSPACE PHYSICIANS
Altitude sickness
Motion sickness

ALL
Disease
Iatrogenic disorders

ALLERGISTS
Allergies
Asthma
Bites and stings
Eczema
Itching
Nasopharyngeal disorders
Pulmonary diseases
Rhinitis
Viral infections

ANESTHESIOLOGISTS
Hyperthermia and hypothermia

AUDIOLOGISTS
Aging
Ear infections and disorders
Hearing loss
Ménière's disease
Speech disorders

BURN SPECIALISTS
Burns and scalds
Electrical shock
Inflammation
Radiation sickness
Wounds

CARDIOLOGISTS
Aging
Aneurysms
Angina
Anxiety
Arrhythmias
Atherosclerotic disease
Cholesterol
Congenital heart disease
Dizziness and fainting
Endocarditis
Heart attack
Heart disease
Heart failure
Hypertension
Ischemia

Mitral insufficiency
Palpitations
Rheumatic fever
Thrombosis and thrombus
Varicosis
Venous insufficiency

CHILD PSYCHIATRISTS
Autism
Dyslexia
Speech disorders

COLORECTAL SURGEONS
Abdominal disorders
Colon cancer
Cysts and ganglions
Diverticulitis and diverticulosis
Hemorrhoids
Intestinal disorders
Malignancy and metastasis

DENTISTS
Caries, dental
Dental diseases
Endodontic disease
Gingivitis
Halitosis
Head and neck disorders
Periodontitis
Toothache

DERMATOLOGISTS
Abscesses
Acne
Albinism
Athlete's foot
Carcinoma
Chickenpox
Cysts and ganglions
Dermatitis
Eczema
Fungal infections
Hair loss and baldness
Itching
Keratoses
Lice, mites, and ticks
Lupus erythematosus
Malignancy and metastasis
Pimples
Poisonous plants
Psoriasis
Puberty and adolescence

Rashes
Rosacea
Scabies
Skin cancer
Skin disorders
Warts

DIETITIANS, REGISTERED
Anorexia nervosa
Beriberi
Cholesterol
Malnutrition
Obesity
Vitamin and mineral deficiencies
Weight loss and gain

EMBRYOLOGISTS
Birth defects
Brain disorders
Cerebral palsy
Down syndrome

EMERGENCY PHYSICIANS
Abdominal disorders
Aging
Altitude sickness
Aneurysms
Appendicitis
Asphyxiation
Bites and stings
Bleeding
Botulism
Burns and scalds
Choking
Coma
Concussion
Diphtheria
Dizziness and fainting
Domestic violence
Electrical shock
Fracture and dislocation
Frostbite
Head and neck disorders
Heart attack
Heat exhaustion and heat stroke
Hyperthermia and hypothermia
Intoxication
Meningitis
Peritonitis
Plague
Pneumonia
Poisoning

Rheumatic fever
Rubella
Rubeola
Scabies
Scarlet fever
Sciatica
Sexuality
Shingles
Shock
Sibling rivalry
Sinusitis
Sore throat
Strep throat
Stress
Tetanus
Tonsillitis
Ulcers
Viral infections
Vitamin and mineral deficiencies
Wounds

GASTROENTEROLOGISTS
Abdominal disorders
Appendicitis
Bulimia
Cholecystitis
Cholera
Colitis
Colon cancer
Constipation
Crohn's disease
Cysts and ganglions
Diarrhea and dysentery
Diverticulitis and diverticulosis
Food poisoning
Gallbladder diseases
Gastrointestinal disorders
Heartburn
Hemorrhoids
Indigestion
Intestinal disorders
Liver cancer
Liver disorders
Nausea and vomiting
Obstruction
Pancreatitis
Poisonous plants
Roundworm
Salmonella
Shigellosis
Stomach, intestinal, and pancreatic
  cancers
Tapeworm
Trichinosis

Ulcers
Weight loss and gain
Worms

GENETICISTS
Aging
Albinism
Alzheimer's disease
Birth defects
Breast cancer
Breast disorders
Color blindness
Down syndrome
Dwarfism
Genetic diseases
Hemophilia
Immunodeficiency disorders
Mental retardation
Phenylketonuria
Porphyria
Sexuality

GERIATRIC SPECIALISTS
Aging
Alzheimer's disease
Amnesia and memory loss
Bed-wetting
Blindness
Bone disorders
Brain disorders
Death and dying
Dementia
Domestic violence
Fatigue
Hearing loss
Incontinence
Osteoporosis
Parkinsonism
Visual disorders

GYNECOLOGISTS
Amenorrhea
Anorexia nervosa
Breast cancer
Breast disorders
Breast-feeding
Cervical, ovarian, and uterine
  cancers
Childbirth
Chlamydia
Conception
Cystitis
Cysts and ganglions
Dysmenorrhea

Endometriosis
Female genital disorders
Gonorrhea
Herpes
Incontinence
Infertility in females
Mastitis
Menopause
Menorrhagia
Menstruation
Ovarian cysts
Pelvic inflammatory disease (PID)
Peritonitis
Postpartum depression
Pregnancy and gestation
Premenstrual syndrome (PMS)
Sexual dysfunction
Sexuality
Sexually transmitted diseases
Syphilis
Urethritis
Urinary disorders
Warts

HEMATOLOGISTS
Anemia
Bleeding
Chronic fatigue syndrome
Hemophilia
Hodgkin's disease
Hyperlipidemia
Infection
Jaundice
Leukemia
Lymphadenopathy and lymphoma
Malaria
Septicemia
Sickle-cell anemia
Thalassemia
Thrombosis and thrombus
Toxemia

IMMUNOLOGISTS
Acquired immunodeficiency
  syndrome (AIDS)
Allergies
Asthma
Autoimmune disorders
Bacterial infections
Bites and stings
Candidiasis
Childhood infectious diseases
Chronic fatigue syndrome
Fungal infections

Phlebitis
Pneumonia
Psoriasis
Puberty and adolescence
Rashes
Renal failure
Reye's syndrome
Rheumatic fever
Rheumatoid arthritis
Rubella
Rubeola
Scabies
Scarlet fever
Schistosomiasis
Sciatica
Scurvy
Septicemia
Sexuality
Sexually transmitted diseases
Shingles
Shock
Sickle-cell anemia
Sinusitis
Sore throat
Staphylococcal infections
Stones
Strep throat
Streptococcal infections
Stress
Strokes and TIAs
Tetanus
Thrombosis and thrombus
Tonsillitis
Toxemia
Tumors
Ulcers
Viral infections
Vitamin and mineral deficiencies
Wounds

MAXILLOFACIAL SURGEONS
Head and neck disorders

MICROBIOLOGISTS
Abscesses
Bacterial infections
Protozoan diseases
Smallpox
Tuberculosis

NEONATOLOGISTS
Childbirth
Childbirth, complications of
Chlamydia

Congenital heart disease
Fetal alcohol syndrome
Hydrocephalus
Jaundice
Premature birth

NEPHROLOGISTS
Cysts and ganglions
Edema
Glomerulonephritis
Hypertension
Kidney disorders
Lupus erythematosus
Nephritis
Renal failure
Stones

NEUROLOGISTS
Aging
Altitude sickness
Alzheimer's disease
Amnesia and memory loss
Aphasia and dysphasia
Apnea
Ataxia
Bell's palsy
Botulism
Brain disorders
Cerebral palsy
Claudication
Cluster headaches
Concussion
Death and dying
Dementia
Dizziness and fainting
Dyslexia
Dystrophy
Ear infections and disorders
Electrical shock
Encephalitis
Epilepsy
Guillain-Barré syndrome (GBS)
Hallucinations
Head and neck disorders
Headaches
Hearing loss
Hemiplegia
Ischemia
Lead poisoning
Learning disabilities
Ménière's disease
Meningitis
Migraine headaches
Motor neuron diseases

Multiple sclerosis
Nausea and vomiting
Neuralgia, neuritis, and neuropathy
Numbness and tingling
Pain, types of
Palsy
Paralysis
Paraplegia
Parkinsonism
Phenylketonuria
Poliomyelitis
Porphyria
Quadriplegia
Rabies
Reye's syndrome
Sciatica
Seizures
Snakebites
Spina bifida
Spinal disorders
Strokes and TIAs
Stuttering
Tetanus
Thrombosis and thrombus
Tics
Trembling and shaking
Tumors
Unconsciousness
Visual disorders

NEUROSURGEONS
Brain disorders
Cysts and ganglions
Epilepsy
Gigantism
Head and neck disorders
Spinal disorders
Tics

OBSTETRICIANS
Birth defects
Breast-feeding
Cervical, ovarian, and uterine
  cancers
Childbirth
Childbirth, complications of
Conception
Down syndrome
Eclampsia
Ectopic pregnancy
Female genital disorders
Fetal alcohol syndrome
Genetic diseases
Gonorrhea

Growth
Incontinence
Menstruation
Miscarriage
Postpartum depression
Pregnancy and gestation
Premature birth
Rubella
Sexuality
Spina bifida
Stillbirth
Toxoplasmosis

OCCUPATIONAL MEDICINE
  PHYSICIANS
Altitude sickness
Asphyxiation
Environmental diseases
Hearing loss
Interstitial pulmonary fibrosis (IPF)
Lead poisoning
Lung cancer
Nasopharyngeal disorders
Pulmonary diseases
Radiation sickness
Skin disorders
Tendon disorders

ONCOLOGISTS
Aging
Bone cancer
Bone disorders
Breast cancer
Cancer
Carcinoma
Cervical, ovarian, and uterine
  cancers
Colon cancer
Female genital disorders
Hodgkin's disease
Liver cancer
Lung cancer
Lymphadenopathy and lymphoma
Male genital disorders
Malignancy and metastasis
Prostate cancer
Pulmonary diseases
Radiation sickness
Sarcoma
Skin cancer
Stomach, intestinal, and pancreatic
  cancers
Stress
Tumors

OPHTHALMOLOGISTS
Albinism
Astigmatism
Blindness
Cataracts
Color blindness
Conjunctivitis
Dystrophy
Glaucoma
Macular degeneration
Myopia
Visual disorders

ORTHOPEDISTS AND
  ORTHOPEDIC SURGEONS
Arthritis
Bone cancer
Bone disorders
Cancer
Cerebral palsy
Dwarfism
Foot disorders
Fracture and dislocation
Osteoporosis
Paget's disease
Scoliosis
Slipped disk
Tendon disorders

OTOLARYNGOLOGISTS
Common cold
Ear infections and disorders
Halitosis
Head and neck disorders
Hearing loss
Laryngitis
Ménière's disease
Motion sickness
Nasopharyngeal disorders
Nausea and vomiting
Pharyngitis
Rhinitis
Sinusitis
Sore throat
Strep throat
Tonsillitis
Voice and vocal cord disorders

PATHOLOGISTS
Breast cancer
Inflammation
Malignancy and metastasis

PEDIATRICIANS
Acne
Bed-wetting
Birth defects
Childhood infectious diseases
Cholera
Cleft palate
Cystic fibrosis
Domestic violence
Down syndrome
Fever
Genetic diseases
Growth
Hydrocephalus
Kwashiorkor
Learning disabilities
Measles, red
Menstruation
Multiple sclerosis
Mumps
Muscular dystrophy
Pertussis
Phenylketonuria
Poliomyelitis
Premature birth
Puberty and adolescence
Reye's syndrome
Rheumatic fever
Rickets
Roseola
Rubella
Rubeola
Scarlet fever
Seizures
Sexuality
Sibling rivalry
Sore throat
Stammering
Streptococcal infections
Sudden infant death syndrome
  (SIDS)

PERINATOLOGISTS
Birth defects
Breast-feeding
Childbirth
Fetal alcohol syndrome
Premature birth

PHYSIATRISTS
Muscle sprains, spasms, and
  disorders
Muscular dystrophy
Numbness and tingling

Legionnaires' disease
Leishmaniasis
Leprosy
Lice, mites, and ticks
Lyme disease
Malaria
Malnutrition
Measles, red
Meningitis
Mumps
Parasitic diseases
Pertussis
Plague
Poliomyelitis
Protozoan diseases
Rabies
Radiation sickness
Roundworm
Rubella
Rubeola
Salmonella
Schistosomiasis
Sexually transmitted diseases
Shigellosis
Sleeping sickness
Smallpox
Syphilis
Tetanus
Toxoplasmosis
Trichinosis
Tuberculosis
Typhoid fever and typhus
Worms
Zoonoses

PULMONOLOGISTS
Asthma
Bronchitis
Coughing
Cystic fibrosis
Emphysema
Fungal infections
Interstitial pulmonary fibrosis (IPF)
Lung cancer
Pleurisy
Pneumonia
Pulmonary diseases
Tuberculosis
Tumors

RADIATION ONCOLOGISTS
Cancer
Liver cancer
Lung cancer

Prostate cancer
Radiation sickness
Sarcoma

RADIOLOGISTS
Cancer
Radiation sickness

RHEUMATOLOGISTS
Arthritis
Autoimmune disorders
Bone disorders
Bursitis
Gout
Inflammation
Lyme disease
Osteoarthritis
Rheumatic fever
Rheumatoid arthritis
Spondylitis

SLEEP SPECIALISTS
Apnea
Narcolepsy
Sleep disorders

SPEECH PATHOLOGISTS
Aphasia and dysphasia
Autism
Cerebral palsy
Dyslexia
Speech disorders
Stammering
Stuttering

SPEECH THERAPISTS
Cleft palate
Voice and vocal cord disorders

SPORTS MEDICINE PHYSICIANS
Athlete's foot
Head and neck disorders
Heat exhaustion and heat stroke
Muscle sprains, spasms, and
  disorders
Tendon disorders

SURGEONS, GENERAL
Aging
Appendicitis
Burns and scalds
Cancer
Cholecystitis
Cirrhosis

Colon cancer
Crohn's disease
Diverticulitis and diverticulosis
Ectopic pregnancy
Female genital disorders
Frostbite
Gallbladder diseases
Gangrene
Hernia
Hyperthermia and hypothermia
Intestinal disorders
Malignancy and metastasis
Obstruction
Peritonitis
Phlebitis
Stomach, intestinal, and pancreatic
  cancers
Stones
Tumors
Varicosis
Wounds

THORACIC SURGEONS
Aneurysms
Hyperthermia and hypothermia

TOXICOLOGISTS
Bites and stings
Botulism
Eczema
Environmental diseases
Food poisoning
Hepatitis
Intoxication
Itching
Lead poisoning
Leukemia
Poisoning
Poisonous plants
Rashes
Snakebites
Staphylococcal infections
Streptococcal infections
Toxemia
Toxoplasmosis

TROPICAL MEDICINE
  PHYSICIANS
Arthropod-borne diseases
Cholera
Diarrhea and dysentery
Elephantiasis
Itching
Leishmaniasis

# ENTRIES BY SYSTEM AFFECTED

Strokes and TIAs
Thrombosis and thrombus
Varicosis
Venous insufficiency

CONNECTIVE TISSUE
Lupus erythematosus
Sarcoma
Slipped disk
Tendon disorders

ENDOCRINE
Addison's disease
Diabetes mellitus
Dwarfism
Eating disorders
Endocrine disorders
Gigantism
Goiter
Hair loss and baldness
Hyperparathyroidism and
    hypoparathyroidism
Hypoglycemia
Obesity
Postpartum depression
Thyroid disorders
Weight loss and gain

GALLBLADDER
Cholecystitis
Gallbladder diseases
Stones

GASTROINTESTINAL
Abdominal disorders
Appendicitis
Arthropod-borne diseases
Bacterial infections
Botulism
Bulimia
Candidiasis
Childhood infectious diseases
Cholera
Colitis
Colon cancer
Constipation
Crohn's disease
Diabetes mellitus
Diarrhea and dysentery
Diverticulitis and diverticulosis
Eating disorders
Food poisoning
Gallbladder diseases
Gastrointestinal disorders

Halitosis
Heartburn
Hemorrhoids
Hernia
Incontinence
Indigestion
Intestinal disorders
Kwashiorkor
Motion sickness
Mumps
Nausea and vomiting
Obesity
Obstruction
Pancreatitis
Poisoning
Poisonous plants
Premenstrual syndrome (PMS)
Protozoan diseases
Radiation sickness
Roundworm
Salmonella
Shigellosis
Stomach, intestinal, and pancreatic
    cancers
Tapeworm
Trichinosis
Typhoid fever and typhus
Ulcers
Weight loss and gain
Worms

GUMS
Dental diseases
Endodontic disease
Gingivitis
Periodontitis
Toothache

HEART
Angina
Anxiety
Arrhythmias
Atherosclerotic disease
Beriberi
Bites and stings
Congenital heart disease
Depression
Diphtheria
Down syndrome
Electrical shock
Embolism
Endocarditis
Heart attack
Heart disease

Heart failure
Hypertension
Lyme disease
Mitral insufficiency
Paget's disease
Palpitations
Reye's syndrome
Rheumatic fever
Shock
Strokes and TIAs
Thrombosis and thrombus
Toxoplasmosis

IMMUNE
Acquired immunodeficiency
    syndrome (AIDS)
Allergies
Arthritis
Autoimmune disorders
Bacterial infections
Bites and stings
Candidiasis
Chronic fatigue syndrome
Fungal infections
Human immunodeficiency virus
    (HIV)
Immunodeficiency disorders
Measles, red
Mumps
Poisonous plants
Rubella
Rubeola
Scarlet fever
Smallpox
Stress

JOINTS
Arthritis
Bursitis
Chlamydia
Fracture and dislocation
Gout
Lyme disease
Osteoarthritis
Rheumatoid arthritis
Spondylitis

KIDNEYS
Diphtheria
Glomerulonephritis
Hypertension
Kidney disorders
Lead poisoning
Malaria